TEXTBOOK OF PEDIATRIC RHEUMATOLOGY

SECOND EDITION

TEXTBOOK OF PEDIATRIC RHEUMATOLOGY

SECOND EDITION

James T. Cassidy, M.D.
Professor, Department of Child Health
Chief, Division of Pediatric Rheumatology
University of Missouri—Columbia School of Medicine
Columbia, Missouri

Ross E. Petty, M.D., Ph.D.
Professor, Department of Paediatrics
Head, Division of Paediatric Rheumatology
University of British Columbia Faculty of Medicine
Vancouver, British Columbia, Canada

Churchill Livingstone
New York, Edinburgh, London, Melbourne

Library of Congress Cataloging-in-Publication Data

Cassidy, James T.
    Textbook of pediatric rheumatology. — 2nd ed. / James
T. Cassidy, Ross E. Petty.
        p.   cm.
    Includes bibliographical references.
    ISBN 0-443-08640-0
    1. Rheumatism in children.   I. Petty, Ross E.   II. Title.
    [DNLM: 1. Arthritis—in infancy & childhood.
    2. Collagen Diseases—in infancy & childhood.
    3. Rheumatism—in infancy & childhood.   WE 544 C345t]
RJ482.R48C37   1990
618.92'723—dc20
DNLM/DLC
for Library of Congress   89-22236
                                                              CIP

Second edition © Churchill Livingstone Inc.   1990
First edition © Churchill Livingstone Inc.   1982

Distributed in the United Kingdom by Churchill Livingstone,
Robert Stevenson House, 1–3 Baxter's Place, Leith Walk, Edinburgh
EH1 3AF, and by associated companies, branches, and
representatives throughout the world.

Accurate indications, adverse reactions, and dosage schedules for
drugs are provided in this book, but it is possible that they may
change. The reader is urged to review the package information data
of the manufacturers of the medications mentioned.

The Publishers have made every effort to trace the copyright holders
for borrowed material. If they have inadvertently overlooked any,
they will be pleased to make the necessary arrangements at the first
opportunity.

Acquisitions Editor: *Kim Loretucci*
Copy Editor: *Kamely Dahir*
Production Designer: *Marci Jordan*
Production Supervisor: *Sharon Tuder*

Printed in the United States of America

First published in 1990

To
Nan and Beryl

Preface

It has been seven years since the publication of the first edition of the *Textbook of Pediatric Rheumatology*. The passing of time has changed the face of the specialty of pediatric rheumatology and deepened our understanding of many of the rheumatic disorders of childhood to the extent that a second edition of the book is in order. This edition of the *Textbook of Pediatric Rheumatology* has undergone extensive reorganization and complete revision under the joint authorship of two of the original contributors.

The aim of this book is to provide a comprehensive but focused source of information and reference for physicians involved in the care of children with rheumatic diseases. This edition has, we hope, benefitted from the constructive criticism of the first edition given to us by our colleagues and students. As a result, organizational changes are extensive, and an attempt to unify style and emphasis has been made. We believe that this has eliminated unnecessary duplication and minimized unintentional omissions. We have made every attempt to provide a comprehensive and balanced view of the specialty with extensive references to the current literature. We recognize that chapters 2 and 3 do not intend to deal comprehensively with all aspects of basic science related to understanding and treating rheumatic diseases of childhood. Instead, they are intended to provide a framework with particular emphasis on those aspects of anatomy, physiology, and pharmacology that are of specific significance in children.

Preparation of this edition of the *Textbook of Pediatric Rheumatology* would not have been possible without the ground-breaking work of the other contributors to the first edition— Drs. Donita B. Sullivan, Carol G. Ragsdale, and Lyubica Dabich, all of the University of Michigan Medical School. We also acknowledge the encouragement and support of our colleagues, in particular, Dr. Peter Malleson, Division of Rheumatology, Department of Paediatrics, University of British Columbia Faculty of Medicine, Vancouver, and Dr. Russell Hopp, Department of Pediatrics, Creighton University School of Medicine, Omaha, who were frequently the sounding boards for first (and sixth) drafts. Finally, the book would not have been possible without the patience and understanding of our families and colleagues to whom we are indebted during our preoccupation with this work.

James T. Cassidy, M.D.
Ross E. Petty, M.D., Ph.D.

Contents

1

An Introduction to the Study of the Rheumatic Diseases of Children

The rheumatic diseases are a group of diverse afflictions that have as their common denominator inflammation of the connective tissues. The cardinal features of inflammation are redness, swelling, heat, pain, and loss of function. It is the presence of these objective signs of inflammation involving a joint that we refer to as *arthritis*, one of the most frequent manifestations of these diseases, to be distinguished from *arthralgia*, which is simply pain in a joint without objective findings on physical examination.

HISTORY

The term *rheumatism* is used today to refer to inflammatory or degenerative diseases affecting joints, bones, muscles, or bursae. It is derived from the Greek word *rheumatismos*, which signified suffering from a flux of evil catarrh into the joints. *Rheumatic* as an adjective was first used in the English language about 1563 to refer to rheumatic fever, took on a broader meaning by 1727, and was distinguished from *rheumatoid* around 1859. The term *arthritis* is derived from the Greek word *arthron*. It came into English use about 1544 and at first referred only to gout.

Guillaume Baillou (1558–1616) was the first to use the term *rheumatism* to mean acute arthritis, as distinguished from gout. Hippocrates in the fourth century BC may have recognized rheumatoid arthritis as a disease. It was identified as a distinct entity by Alfred E. Garrod (1819–1909),[1] but even he may have confused the nodal arthritis of Heberden as part of the syndrome. Chronic arthritis has been diagnosed in the spine of ancient humans (Java and Lansing) and is documented in Egyptian mummies dating to 8000 BC before the Old Kingdom and the recorded dynasties.

The first English language reference to rheumatism in children is contained in the 1560 text *The Regiment of Life Whereunto Is Added a Treatise of the Pestilence, with the Booke of Chyldren* by Thomas Phaire. In this work he refers to "the stiffness of the lymmes'" resulting from exposing a child to cold.[2,3] Cornil in 1864 described a woman who had developed chronic arthritis as a child.[4] At the age of 12 years, she had had the onset of polyarthritis, which pursued a chronic relapsing course and terminated in her death in uremic coma at the age of 28 years. Autopsy revealed myocardial degeneration, nephrotic syndrome, bony ankylosis of some joints, and synovial proliferation with marked destruction of cartilage in others. It may be that this girl had amyloidosis complicating chronic polyarticular juvenile rheumatoid arthritis. Diamant-Berger published a detailed account of 38 arthritic children whom he had seen personally or whose cases had been documented in the literature.[5] He observed the heterogeneity of onset of the disease, its predominance in girls, and the occurrence of cervical spine and temporomandibular joint disease as well as ocular involvement. He also noted the generally good prognosis relative to that of adults with chronic arthritis.

Six years after the publication of Diamant-Berger's findings, George Frederic Still, in a paper read to the Royal Medical and Chirurgical Society in London in 1896, described 22 cases of acute and chronic arthritis in children, almost all of whom were observed at the Hospital for Sick Children, Great Ormond Street, London.[6] This treatise carefully documented the clinical characteristics of these children and pointed out the differing modes of onset. Still (1868–1941) was the first English physician to confine his practice to diseases of children and was also the first professor of paediatrics at King's College Hospital Medical School, London. Unfortunately, after his classic study published in 1897, he rarely returned to the field of pediatric rheumatology; this is remarkable, considering his scholarly work in the context of the time—108 papers and 5 books, including his *History of Paediatrics* and *Common Diseases in Children.*

As a clinical discipline, the study of rheumatic diseases in children was established in earnest only in the last 50 years. The roots of contemporary pediatric rheumatology are found in adult rheumatology and in the post–World War II establishment of the Rheumatism Research Unit at Taplow in England. As rheumatic fever declined in the midtwentieth century, chronic rheumatic diseases of childhood became the focus of this institution, and a small group of physician-scientists, including Professor E. G. L. Bywaters and later B. M. Ansell, laid the foundation for the development of the specialty of pediatric rheumatology. In North America a focus on pediatric rheumatology began to develop in the early 1950s and has accelerated to the present time. Reminiscences of three of the pioneers of pediatric rheumatology in the United States, J. Sidney Stillman, Virgil Hanson, and Joseph E. Levinson, are recorded for the interested reader.[7–9]

CLASSIFICATION OF THE PEDIATRIC RHEUMATIC DISEASES

Without a clear definition of the extent, etiology, and pathogenesis of the rheumatic diseases of childhood, it is difficult to provide a meaningful classification. A few of these diseases, such as infectious arthritis, can be classified on the basis of etiology; most cannot. They can be grouped into taxonomic divisions on the basis of their clinical manifestations or postulated pathogenesis. This approach is unsatisfactory at best but is a necessary interim step in order to place diseases into logical diagnostic, therapeutic, and prognostic categories.

A committee of the American Rheumatism Association has classified the more than 80 rheumatic diseases. In Table 1-1 we have modified this listing to reflect pediatric interest and some of the newly described diseases. This list is not complete. It is not unchangeable. As our basic understanding grows, it will be modified.

CLASSIFICATION CRITERIA

Diagnosis of a disease whose etiology is unknown is based principally upon clinical manifestations. The criteria vary with each disease but include elements from the history and physical, laboratory, radiologic, or pathologic examinations. In a few cases, only the course or outcome of the disease reveals the correct diagnosis. In order to ensure reasonable uniformity, clinicians (and, more recently, committees) have used a number of different approaches to selecting key diagnostic features for these classifications. In most instances, choices are empiric and are accepted by other expert clinicians if the criteria agree with their clinical experience. In a few selected cases, studies have been performed in cooperating clinics to substantiate by statistical analysis the validity of each item in the schema. The purpose of these criteria is to ensure that studies of a specified disease are composed of similar cases in all clinics; they are not intended for diagnosis of the disease in individual children. The latter process remains a matter of experienced, mature clinical judgment.

The only such criteria that were developed specif-

Table 1-1 Diagnostic Classification of Juvenile Arthritis and Pediatric Rheumatic Diseases

Connective-tissue diseases
  Juvenile rheumatoid arthritis
  Systemic lupus erythematosus
  Scleroderma
  Dermatomyositis
  Necrotizing vasculitis
    Polyarteritis (includes Kawasaki disease)
    Hypersensitivity vasculitis (includes Henoch-Schön-
      lein purpura and serum sickness
    Wegener granulomatosis
    Giant cell arteritis
    Behçet's disease
    Miscellaneous
      Mixed connective-tissue disease and overlap syn-
        dromes
      Eosinophilic fasciitis
      Sjögren's syndrome

Seronegative spondyloarthropathies
  Juvenile ankylosing spondylitis
  Inflammatory bowel disease
    Regional enteritis
    Ulcerative colitis
  Psoriatic spondyloarthritis
  Reiter's syndrome

Degenerative joint disease

Arthritis, tenosynovitis, and bursitis associated with infec-
  tious agents
  Direct
    Bacterial arthritis
      Gram-positive cocci (staphylococcus and others)
      Gram-negative cocci (gonococcus and others)
      Gram-positive rods
      Mycobacteria
    Viral arthritis (rubella, mumps, Epstein-Barr virus)
    Fungal arthritis
    Lyme arthritis
    Unknown, suspected (Whipple's disease, toxic syn-
      ovitis of the hip)
  Indirect (reactive arthritis)
    Bacterial (includes acute rheumatic fever, intestinal by-
      pass, postdysenteric *Shigella, Yersinia*)
    Viral (hepatitis B)

Rheumatic diseases associated with immunodeficiency
  Selective IgA deficiency
  Agammaglobulinemia and hypogammaglobulinemia
  Complement component deficiencies

Metabolic and endocrine diseases associated with rheumatic
  states
  Crystal-induced arthritis (gout, pseudogout, chondro-
    calcinosis)
  Biochemical abnormalities
    Amyloidosis (includes familial Mediterranean fever)
    Vitamin C deficiency (scurvy)
    Specific enzyme deficiency states (including Fabry's
      disease, Farber's disease, alkaptonuria, Lesch-
      Nyhan syndrome)
    Hyperlipidemias (types II, IV)
    Mucopolysaccharidoses
    Hemoglobinopathies (sickle cell anemia, thalassemia)
    Hemophilia
    Connective-tissue disorders (Ehlers-Danlos syn-
      drome, Marfan's syndrome, pseudoxanthoma elas-
      ticum, and others)
  Endocrine diseases
    Diabetes mellitus
    Acromegaly
    Hyperparathyroidism
    Thyroid disease (hyperthyroidism, hypothyroidism)
  Other hereditary or congenital disorders
    Arthrogryposis multiplex congenita
    Hypermobility syndromes
    Myositis ossificans progressiva

Neoplasms
  Malignant
    Primary (e.g., synovioma, synoviosarcoma)
    Metastatic (osteosarcoma)
  Benign
    Osteoid osteoma
  Diffuse
    Leukemia and lymphoma
    Neuroblastoma
    Histiocytosis

Neuropathic disorders
  Charcot's joints
  Compression neuropathies
  Reflex sympathetic dystrophy

Continued

Table 1-1 Diagnostic Classification of Juvenile Arthritis and Pediatric Rheumatic Diseases *(Continued)*

Bone and cartilage disorders associated with articular manifestations
  Osteoporosis
    Generalized
    Localized (regional)
  Osteomalacia
  Hypertrophic osteoarthropathy
  Avascular necrosis (includes Legg-Calvé-Perthes disease)
  Osteochondritis dissecans
  Congenital dysplasia of the hip
  Slipped capital femoral epiphysis
  Costochondritis (includes Tietze's syndrome)
  Osteolysis and chondrolysis

Nonarticular rheumatism
  Myofascial pain syndromes
    Generalized (fibromyalgia)
    Regional
  Low back pain and intervertebral disc disorders
  Tendinitis (tenosynovitis) or bursitis

Ganglion cysts
Fasciitis
Chronic ligament and muscle strain
Vasomotor disorders
  Erythromelalgia
  Raynaud's phenomenon

Miscellaneous disorders
  Trauma (the result of direct trauma)
  Plant-thorn synovitis
  Pancreatic disease
  Sarcoidosis
  Villonodular synovitis
  Internal derangement of joints (includes chondromalacia patellae, loose bodies)

Arthromyalgia
  Growing pains
  Psychogenic rheumatism

ically for the classification of rheumatic diseases in childhood are the revised, modified Jones criteria for the identification of acute rheumatic fever[10] and the criteria for the classification of juvenile rheumatoid arthritis (JRA) of the American Rheumatism Association.[11,12] Other diagnostic criteria (e.g., those for systemic lupus erythematosus [SLE] and juvenile ankylosing spondylitis [JAS]), were developed in relation to studies of adults, although they are frequently applied to the study of such diseases in childhood.

To an increasing but still limited extent, laboratory evaluations (histocompatibility antigens, antinuclear antibody specificities, enzyme deficiencies, etc.) provide information that is useful for classification of disease. This is particularly true for identifying subtypes of a disease. Thus pauciarticular arthritis associated with the presence of human leukocyte antigen B27 (HLA-B27) may represent a different subset of patients than similar disease in children lacking HLA-B27. Certain antinuclear antibodies (anti-nDNA, anti-Ro) are associated with specific complications in patients with SLE. These clinical subtypes emphasize the indistinct boundaries within and among the connective-tissue diseases and the variable nature of their presentation and course.

Subtypes are also useful in providing the physician with a guide to an expected course and prognosis of a disease. The recognition of distinct subtypes of onset of JRA (polyarticular, pauciarticular, or systemic) has led to the suggestion that each represents a unique and separate disease. This hypothesis may or may not be substantiated by future research.

Classification criteria must be evaluated from two aspects: sensitivity and specificity. *Sensitivity* of a clinical characteristic or laboratory test is an expression of the frequency with which the characteristic correctly identifies an individual with the disease in question. *Specificity* is an expression of the ability of the criterion to identify correctly those individuals who do *not* have the disease in question. These relationships are shown in Table 1-2.

Classification of rheumatic diseases by either clinical or laboratory criteria is also complicated by the fact that some rheumatic syndromes appear to be "overlaps" between two or more distinct disease entities. Mixed connective-tissue disease, described by Sharp et al,[13] is the best known example of this problem. Furthermore, the fact that diseases evolve over time, both clinically and serologically, necessitates a constant reevaluation of the diagnostic category. A further example of this phenomenon is demonstrated by the apparent transition from JRA to SLE in a small number of children.[14] In such cases, is it correct to believe that these children always had SLE, that they

Table 1-2 Relationships of Sensitivity and Specificity

Test Result	True Diagnosis		
	Disease Present	Disease Absent	
Positive	a	b	$a + b$
Negative	c	d	$c + d$
	$a + c$	$b + d$	

$$\text{Sensitivity} = \frac{a}{a + c}$$

$$\text{Specificity} = \frac{d}{b + d}$$

$$\text{Predictive value of a positive test} = \frac{a}{a + b}$$

$$\text{Predictive value of a negative test} = \frac{d}{c + d}$$

had two distinct diseases in sequence, or that the same disease has expressed different manifestations at different points in time? These questions are largely unanswerable at the present time but indicate some of the complexities and pitfalls of classifications.

UNIQUE FACTORS THAT MODIFY THE PRESENTATION AND COURSE OF RHEUMATIC DISEASES IN CHILDREN

One of the fundamental questions that has pervaded research in pediatric rheumatology is the extent to which rheumatic diseases in childhood are the same as, or different from, similar diseases in adults. It is important to attempt to differentiate semantic from biologic similarities. Simply because two diseases bear the same name (e.g., rheumatoid arthritis [RA] and JRA), should not necessarily imply that they are the same diseases biologically. Application of such names was usually made in ignorance of contemporary epidemiology, genetics, or biology and may lead to a narrow vision of the true nature of a disease, and its relationship to other disorders. A complete distinction between RA and JRA based upon age of onset alone is arbitrary and unlikely to represent accurately the biologic "truth." There is no age at

which the manifestations of these diseases abruptly change from one to another, and yet, if one examines JRA and its subtypes there are clear age-related changes. There is little doubt that some rheumatic diseases occur only in young children (e.g., pauciarticular JRA with uveitis), and others appear almost exclusively in adults (e.g., gout). More commonly, however, diseases with similar names and similar biologic characteristics occur in both pediatric and adult populations (e.g., SLE, scleroderma, and ankylosing spondylitis). Age-related differences in the frequency of many of the manifestations of these diseases are well recognized and may be influenced by a number of factors.

Table 1-3 lists some of the prominent differences between children and adults that may modify the clinical expression of a rheumatic disease on an age-related basis. Figure 1-1 presents classic observations of general and systemic growth in children from birth to young adulthood.[15] In particular, development of the lymphoid system until the pubertal years and its gradual involution thereafter represent an important age-related change central to considerations of the rheumatic diseases.

The degree of skeletal immaturity is one of the most important but most poorly understood differences between children and adults with rheumatic diseases. It seems probable that physical and biochemical differences between young cartilage and bone and old cartilage and bone profoundly influence the effect of an inflammatory process involving those structures. Because physes are not fused in the child with arthritis, they lead to local growth abnormalities, such as leg length inequality and mandibular asymmetry, that are not seen in adults. Short stature is a frequent result of chronic inflammatory arthritis in the child but is obviously not a problem in the skeletally mature adult. The anatomy of the blood supply to the physis and epiphysis in the infant is reflected in the

Table 1-3 Connective-Tissue Diseases in Children: Modifying Factors

Potential for growth and development
Gonadal immaturity
Proliferating lymphoid system
Less complex antigenic exposure
Early expression of immunogenetic predisposition

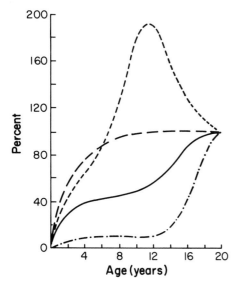

Fig. 1-1 Idealized growth curves drawn to a uniform scale by computing values at each successive age in terms of their average sequential increments. Lymphoid --- (thymus, lymph nodes, intestinal lymphoid tissue). Neural —— (brain, dura, spinal cord, eyes, head dimensions). General body —— (whole body [with exception of head and neck] skeleton, musculature, lungs, gastrointestinal tract, kidneys, spleen, blood volume). Genital ·—· (testes, prostate, ovaries, uterus). (Modified from Harris,[15] with permission.)

predisposition to septic arthritis as a complication of osteomyelitis in that age group.

The influence of gonadal immaturity in causing differences between the expression of rheumatic diseases in children and adults is unclear. The generalization that most rheumatic diseases are more common in females than in males is true at any age, although there are important exceptions. In SLE, the female to male ratio increases with advancing age. In early childhood, girls and boys are affected with equal frequency; in adulthood, women are affected eight to nine times more than men. That this observation may reflect the role of sex hormones in the pathogenesis of SLE is supported by studies of adult males with Klinefelter's syndrome (who have two X chromosomes and one Y chromosome and who have a high incidence of SLE)[16] and by studies of lupuslike disease in mice.[17] In contrast, the sex ratios in children and adults with ankylosing spondylitis do not appear to be different.

Many genetically determined diseases have their expression in childhood. This is particularly true for the inherited dysplasias of bone and cartilage and biochemical disorders such as the mucopolysaccharidoses and hemophilia. The influence of disease predispositions associated with or linked to histocompatibility antigens is less clear, however. The strongest HLA association is that of HLA-B27 with ankylosing spondylitis, a disease that begins in childhood in only about 10 percent of cases.[18] That this genetic predisposition does not more frequently result in childhood onset of disease may reflect yet another factor that differentiates the child from the adult: the extent of environmental antigenic exposure and the ability of the immune system to respond to that experience.

One argument in support of the significance of antigenic experience and immune reactivity might be exemplified by pauciarticular onset JRA. This disease has a strikingly narrow age-at-onset distribution, with onset of disease in the vast majority of children between the ages of 1 and 4 years.[19] Another characteristic age restriction is seen in Kawasaki disease, which occurs most frequently in the 1- to 3-year age group.[20] It is tempting to speculate that these diseases might reflect the age of initial exposure to an environmental pathogen such as a virus or bacterium, together with the absence of specific protective immunity.

EPIDEMIOLOGIC ASPECTS OF RHEUMATIC DISEASES IN CHILDREN

Data on the frequency of the rheumatic diseases in children, even the more common ones, are incomplete. Epidemiologic studies have focused either on the complaint of *arthritis* in a population of children or on the frequency of *JRA* per se.

Population studies of rheumatic diseases distinguish between two measurements. *Incidence* is the rate of occurrence of a disease in a population based upon a time scale (horizontal frequency). It is the number of patients who have onset of disease within a period of 1 year per 100,000 of the population at risk. *Prevalence* is the proportion of a population that is affected with a disease at a given time (vertical frequency). It is the number of cases of the disease per 100,000 of the population at risk.

Table 1-4 Incidence of the Connective-Tissue Diseases

Rheumatic Disease in Adults	Annual Rate/ 10^5	Sex Ratio F:M	Race Ratio W:B	Peak Age at Risk (Years)	Childhood Onset of Similar Disease (%)
Ankylosing spondylitis	130–1,000	1:3	W > B	Young adult	10
Rheumatoid arthritis	40	3:1	Equal	Increases with age (20–50)	5
Systemic lupus erythematosus	6	8:1	1:4	15–45	18
Dermatomyositis/ polymyositis	0.8	2:1	1:3	45–65	20
Scleroderma	0.4	3:1	Equal	Increases with age (30–50)	3
Polyarteritis	0.2	1:3	Equal	Midadult	Rare[a]

[a] Except for Kawasaki disease.

For the most part, reasonable estimates of either incidence or prevalence of most of the rheumatic diseases in children are unavailable or are often based upon their relative frequency in comparison to that of adults with similar diseases. The frequency of some of the more important systemic rheumatic diseases in adults is illustrated in Table 1-4.[21] Ankylosing spondylitis is probably the most common form of arthritis in the population. Rheumatoid arthritis is the most frequent inflammatory peripheral joint disease. Various estimates based upon relatively strict diagnostic criteria have placed its incidence at 0.04 to 1 percent of the U.S. population.

A 1976 survey by the National Center for Health Statistics on the prevalence of chronic skin and musculoskeletal conditions in the United States provided an estimate of chronic arthritis and rheumatic complaints in children of 2.2 cases per 1,000 (Tables 1-5 and 1-6).[22] In a similar study, the Canada Health Survey of 1978–1979 indicated that the number of children with rheumatic complaints less than 15 years of age was 1.3 percent.[23] In both of these surveys, the presence of a rheumatic complaint was determined by questionnaires or interviews and was not confirmed by a formal history and physical examination. Inevitably, therefore, some or many of the individuals reporting a rheumatic complaint had no defined rheumatic disease, and the data should be interpreted to indicate the frequency of occurrence of any complaint referable to the musculoskeletal system.

A prospective study of the incidence of arthritis in children in Finland has been recently reported and provides an overview of the extent of the problem (Table 1-7).[24] Included in this 1-year survey were all children under 16 years of age who had swelling or limitation of motion of a joint, walked with a limp,

Table 1-5 Relative Prevalences of Chronic Childhood Diseases

Epilepsy	2.9/1,000
Arthritis	2.2/1,000
Cerebral palsy	1.3/1,000
Diabetes	1.0/1,000

(From National Center for Health Statistics.[22])

Table 1-6 Prevalence of Chronic Conditions among Children (< 17 Years of Age) 1979–81

Condition	Prevalence per 100,000
Diseases of the respiratory system	1079
Mental and nervous system disorders	454
Diseases of the eye and ear	288
Endocrine, nutritional, metabolic, and blood disorders	163
Diseases of the circulatory system	151
Certain congenital anomalies and causes of perinatal morbidity	150
Diseases of the musculoskeletal system and connective tissue	132
Disease of the skin and subcutaneous tissue	114

(From National Health Interview Survey. J Chronic Dis 39:63, 1986, with permission.)

Table 1-7 Incidence of Arthritis in Children in a Finnish Community

Diagnostic Group	n	Percentage of Total	Incidence[a]
Transient synovitis of the hip	77	47.8	51.9 (41.4–64.9)
Acute transient arthritis	38	23.6	25.8 (18.1–35.6)
Juvenile rheumatoid arthritis	27	16.8	18.2 (10.8–28.7)
Septic arthritis	10	6.2	6.7 (3.2–12.3)
Reactive arthritis	8	5.0	5.4 (2.3–10.6)

[a] Per 100,000 children < 16 years of age (95% confidence limits). (Adapted from Kunnamo et al,[24] with permission.)

or had hip pain, as determined by a primary care physician, pediatrician, or orthopedic surgeon. All patients were subsequently evaluated by a single group of pediatric rheumatologists. Overall, the incidence of arthritis was estimated at 109/100,000. Transient synovitis of the hip and other self-limited disorders (Henoch-Schönlein purpura, serum sickness, etc.) were most common. Chronic arthritis, mostly JRA, had an incidence of 18.9/100,0000. Septic arthritis and reactive arthritis were much less frequent. Children with connective-tissue diseases such as SLE were not detected in this survey.

A number of studies have investigated the prevalence and incidence of chronic arthritis. Data collected on children in the state of Michigan in 1973 noted a minimal incidence rate for JRA of 9.2 new cases per 100,000 children at risk per year (Fig. 1-2).[19] This study included only those patients referred to the University of Michigan Pediatric Rheumatology Clinic and therefore represented the more serious, chronic cases. Estimates of the total number of children with JRA in the state were 100 to 200 percent higher than the cited frequency would indicate.

More recent data from Rochester, Minnesota indicated an incidence for JRA of 13.9 cases per 100,000 per year.[25] The prevalence of JRA in the Rochester survey was 113.4 cases per 100,000 children with 95

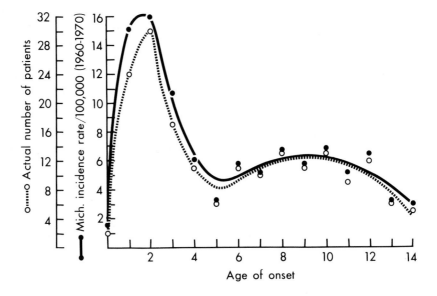

Fig. 1-2 Incidence of juvenile rheumatoid arthritis (JRA) in Michigan children. Illustrated is the incidence-rate curve for age of onset for children living in Michigan compared with the number of children with JRA for each age of onset. These curves represent minimal estimates and cannot be projected to the actual frequency of this disease within the state. From 1960 to 1970 the mean incidence rate for JRA, determined from these data, was 9.2 children per 100,000 at risk per year. The incidence rate curves for boys and girls were similar. The fact that this incidence rate projection and the expected age of onset curve were similar indicated that children included in our study probably did not represent a group biased for age of onset. (From Sullivan et al.,[19] with permission.)

percent confidence limits of 69.1 to 196.3.[9] Both the Ann Arbor and the Rochester studies based a diagnosis of JRA on classification criteria of the American Rheumatism Association (ARA) (see Table 5-1).[11]

A Swedish study used the European League Against Rheumatism (EULAR) criteria for the diagnosis of juvenile chronic arthritis (JCA) in an outpatient clinic population.[26] JCA includes children with JRA (based on the ARA criteria) and those with seronegative spondyloarthropathies, so these data are not strictly comparable to those derived from studies based on the ARA criteria. These investigators estimated an incidence of JCA of 12/100,000 and a prevalence of 56/100,000.

Another approach to the problem is to compare the relative frequencies with which various connective-tissue diseases are encountered in established pediatric rheumatology clinics. Table 1-8 includes data from the University of Michigan, the University of Southern California, and the University of British Columbia. Possible and probable diagnostic categories were not included. At each clinic the relative incidence of each of these rheumatic diseases has remained essentially constant during the period of observation. However, these data do not totally take into consideration the increasing importance of Kawasaki disease, the emergence of new entities such as Lyme arthritis, and the other various forms of juvenile arthritis and soft tissue rheumatism that are seen in a diagnostic clinic and represent an important aspect of the clinical workload of a pediatric rheumatologist. The major connective-tissue diseases and JRA make up only approximately one-third to one-half of the children who are seen on referral each year. Therefore any estimate of the total frequency of these conditions must be adjusted accordingly.

Finally, for the population of children 15 years of age or less in the United States in 1986, the frequency of all forms of juvenile arthritis on the basis of the Ann Arbor and the Rochester studies, including JRA, the other major connective-tissue diseases, and the various other rheumatic diagnoses, is calculated in Table 1-9. On the basis of this estimate, it seems accurate to state that the total number of children in the United States with a rheumatic disease is approximately 160,000 to 190,000 children.[27] In Canada the numbers would be between 16,000 and 19,000. Prevalence in other countries depends on the proportion of the population in the childhood age range and can be calculated from recent vital statistics.

These pediatric-specific estimates do not include patients who have continuation of chronic unremitting disease or residual disability into the late teenage or adult years and do not reflect the long-term impact of these diseases (e.g., problems such as inability to care for oneself, psychosocial aspects of chronic disease and peer deprivation, and blindness from chronic uveitis). It is clear that a problem for national health planning agencies is that there are no totally reliable epidemiologic data for these important diseases of

Table 1-8 Frequency of the Major Pediatric Connective-Tissue Diseases (%)

	University of Michigan[a]	University of Southern California[b]	University of British Columbia[c]
Juvenile rheumatoid arthritis	75	83	65
Systemic lupus erythematosus	10	8.5	6
Dermatomyositis	6	4	2
Spondyloarthritis	5	—	15[d]
Scleroderma	3	3.5	2
Vasculitis	1	1	10[e]

[a] 1961–1979, 618 children.
[b] 1952–1977, 1,450 children.
[c] 1979–1987, 466 children.
[d] Reflects in part the high frequency of these diseases in the North American Indian population.
[e] Increase includes the diagnosis of Kawasaki disease.

Table 1-9 Estimates of the Prevalence of the Various Forms of Juvenile Arthritis for the United States[a]

Forms of Juvenile Arthritis	Source of Data	
	Ann Arbor, Michigan	Olmsted Co, Minnesota
Juvenile rheumatoid arthritis	77,000	63,000
Major connective tissue diseases	19,000	16,000
Other rheumatic diseases	96,000	79,000
Total	190,000	160,000

[a] Calculations are based on a US population in 1986 of 55,745,000 children ≤ 15 years of age.
(From Cassidy and Nelson,[27] with permission.)

childhood. Furthermore, we are unlikely to obtain such data in the foreseeable future since these disorders represent relatively uncommon diseases in a community. An epidemiologic survey designed to determine their frequency is therefore destined to be inefficient statistically, time-consuming, and costly.

APPROACH TO THE STUDY OF THE RHEUMATIC DISEASES OF CHILDHOOD

Much of the information that forms the basis of our understanding of pediatric rheumatic diseases has been derived from clinical observation and analysis of reported series of patients. It should be remembered, however, that there are a number of largely uncontrolled variables, such as referral bias, time of initial observation, and duration of follow-up, that influence the conclusions of such studies.

Figure 1-3 shows two sets of theoretic clinical observations. Figure 1-3A represents a child with a rheumatic disease seen immediately after onset. Diagnostic evaluation and appropriate period of follow-up ensure correct diagnosis. The child is followed throughout the course of the disease until outcome, whether total remission or death. Evaluation of a reasonably circumscribed disease based upon a large number of children observed in this manner would represent an ideal sequential study. That this paragon is seldom achieved is obvious to all who participate

in clinical studies. First, it usually takes too long to do such a study, since the diseases in which we are interested have courses measured in years. Second, a child usually remains in a study for a limited period of time because of a variety of unpredictable factors, including family mobility.

Figure 1-3B summarizes the construct of the usual published series. Children have entered and left the study at varying times. This report must, therefore, reach its conclusions by cohort analysis. Since all children do not have uniform manifestations or disease duration, averages, weighted means, and standard deviations are used to define characteristics of the group at a specified period.

Evaluation of outcome can be greatly altered if consideration is not given to the number of children leaving a study before reaching the specified endpoint. One statistical method of accounting for this problem is survivorship analysis.[28] By this technique estimates of outcome are partially adjusted toward a negative result, for example, death, by accounting for losses from the original patient group that are otherwise unexplained (i.e., lost to follow-up).

Estimates of prognosis based on our knowledge of a disease are important factors in influencing decisions on choice of therapy and management. Outcome may be specified in a number of ways. The care and specificity with which we select outcomes to be evaluated are crucial to study design.

One of the unknown qualities in studies of rheumatic diseases is the bias of referral. Studies of these

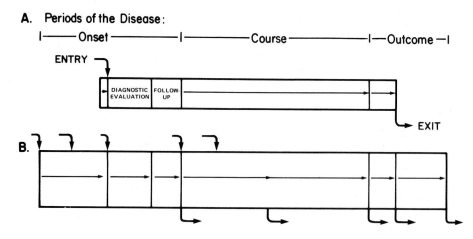

Fig. 1-3 Evaluation of children with rheumatic disease for onset, course, and outcome. (**A**) Ideal study design. Child enters at onset and exits at remission. (**B**) Actual clinical study consisting of many children who have entered at uncontrolled times and exited at equally unpredicted intervals.

relatively rare diseases are usually not possible except in large clinics or medical centers. We suspect that an incorrect impression of the seriousness of some rheumatic diseases has been created although in actuality the milder cases are seldom referred and studied. Community-based epidemiologic studies are often, however, an unsatisfactory method of determining the clinical spectrum of a rare disease.

APPROACH TO THE TREATMENT OF RHEUMATIC DISEASES OF CHILDHOOD

Care of the chronically ill child is best provided by family-centered, community-based, coordinated care.[29] Team care is directed at facilitating the enormous challenge of the management of these children. The therapeutic team required for optimal treatment of a child with a rheumatic disease includes a pediatric rheumatologist, nurse, physical therapist, occupational therapist, and social worker. In addition, consultation with ophthalmologists and specialists in oral medicine, orthopedics, physiatry, nephrology, dermatology, and other disciplines is frequently necessary. Support for the patient and family may come from psychologists, psychiatrists, and other community resources. Family-centered organizations such as the American Juvenile Arthritis Organization provide an opportunity for peer interaction. Education of patients, parents, health professionals, educators, and community organizations constitutes an important additional requirement in order to optimize the care of children with rheumatic diseases, minimize the global effects of the disease, and foster the normal psychological and physical growth and development of our patients.

SUMMARY

The scope of pediatric rheumatology is broad and embraces all branches of medicine. Although one of the newer specialities, pediatric rheumatology can now begin to be established on a sound scientific basis with developments in our knowledge of immunology, immunogenetics, and biochemical and physiologic control mechanisms of the inflammatory response, together with the establishment of a "critical mass" of clinicians and scientists with related expertise.

REFERENCES

1. Garrod AE: A Treatise on Rheumatism and Rheumatoid Arthritis. Charles Griffin, London, 1890, pp. 251, 265
2. Phaire T: The Regiment of Life Whereunto Is Added a Treatise of the Pestilence, with the Booke of Children, Newly Corrected and Enlarged. London, Edw Whitchurch, 1560 (probably printed circa 1553)
3. Bywaters EGL: The history of pediatric rheumatology. Arthritis Rheum 20:145, 1977
4. Cornil MV: Mémoire sur des coincidences pathologiques du rhumatisme articulaire chronique. C R Soc Biol (Paris), Series 4, 3:3, 1864
5. Diamant-Berger M-S: Du Rhumatisme Noueux (Polyarthrite Déformante) Chez Les Enfants. Paris, Lecrosnier et Babe, 1891 (reprinted by Editions Louis Parente, Paris in 1988)
6. Still GF: On a form of chronic joint disease in children. Med-Chirurg Trans 80:47, 1897 (reprinted in Am J Dis Child 132:195, 1978)
7. Stillman JS: The history of pediatric rheumatology in the United States. Rheum Dis Clin North Am 13:143, 1987
8. Levinson JE: Reflections of a pediatric rheumatologist. Rheum Dis Clin North Am 13:149, 1987
9. Hanson V: Pediatric rheumatology: a personal perspective. Rheum Dis Clin North Am 13:155, 1987
10. Stollerman GH, Markowitz M, Taranta A et al: Jones criteria (revised) for guidance in the diagnosis of rheumatic fever. Circulation 32:664, 1965
11. Brewer EJ, Bass J, Baum J et al: Current proposed revision of JRA criteria. Arthritis Rheum 20:195, 1977
12. Cassidy JT, Levinson JE, Bass JC et al: A study of classification criteria for a diagnosis of juvenile rheumatoid arthritis. Arthritis Rheum 29:274, 1986
13. Sharp GG, Irvin WS, Tan EM et al: Mixed connective tissue disease—an apparently distinct rheumatic syndrome associated with a specific antibody to an extractable nuclear antigen (ENA). Am J Med 52:148, 1972
14. Ragsdale CG, Petty RE, Cassidy JT et al: The clinical progression of apparent juvenile rheumatoid arthritis to systemic lupus erythematosus. J Rheumatol 7:50, 1980
15. Harris JA: The Measurement of Man. University of Minnesota Press, Minneapolis, 1930
16. Ortiz-New C, LeRoy EC: The coincidence of Klinefelter's syndrome and systemic lupus erythematosus. Arthritis Rheum 12:241, 1969

17. Roubinian JR, Talal N, Greenspan JS et al: Sex hormone modulation of autoimmunity in NZB/NZW mice. Arthritis Rheum 22:1162, 1979

18. Bennett PH, Wood PHN: Population Studies of the Rheumatic Diseases. Excerpta Medica Foundation, New York, 1968, p. 456

19. Sullivan DB, Cassidy JT, Petty RE: Pathogenic implications of age of onset in juvenile rheumatoid arthritis. Arthritis Rheum 18:251, 1975

20. Morens DM, O'Brien RJ: Kawasaki disease in the United States. J Infect Dis 137:91, 1978

21. Lawrence RC, Shulman LE (eds): Epidemiology of the Rheumatic Diseases: Proceedings of the Fourth International Congress. Gower Medical Publications, New York, 1984

22. National Center for Health Statistics: Prevalence of Chronic Skin and Musculoskeletal Conditions. United States Health Interview Study, 1976, Series 10, No 124, DHSW (PHA) Pub No 79-1552

23. Lee P, Helewa A, Smythe HA et al: Epidemiology of musculoskeletal disorders (complaints) and related disability in Canada. J Rheumatol 12:1169, 1985

24. Kunnamo I, Kallio P, Pelkonen P: Incidence of arthritis in urban Finnish children. Arthritis Rheum 29:1232, 1986

25. Towner SR, Michet CJ, Jr, O'Fallon WM et al: The epidemiology of juvenile arthritis in Rochester, Minnesota. Arthritis Rheum 26:1208, 1983

26. Gäre BA, Fasth A, Andersson J et al: Incidence and prevalence of juvenile chronic arthritis: a population survey. Ann Rheum Dis 46:;277, 1987

27. Cassidy JT, Nelson AM: The frequency of juvenile arthritis. J Rheumatol 15:535, 1988

28. Merrell M, Shulman LE: Determination of prognosis in chronic disease, illustrated by systemic lupus erythematosus. J Chronic Dis 1:12, 1955

29. Surgeon General's Report: Children with Special Health Care Needs. United States Department of Health and Human Services, Public Health Service, Washington DC, 1987

2

Etiology and Pathogenesis of Rheumatic Diseases: Basic Concepts

STRUCTURE AND PHYSIOLOGY

Rheumatic diseases frequently affect many different organ systems. Inflammation of the structures of the musculoskeletal system, particularly joints, connective tissues, and muscles, is common to all rheumatic diseases, however. This brief discussion focuses on selected aspects of the anatomy, histology, and biochemistry of those tissues that are of particular importance to the study of rheumatic diseases of childhood.

Joints

CLASSIFICATION OF JOINTS

Joints may be classified as fibrous, cartilaginous, or synovial (Table 2-1). Fibrous joints are those in which little or no motion occurs and in which the bones are separated by fibrous connective tissue. Cartilaginous joints are those in which little or no motion occurs but in which the bones are separated by cartilage. Synovial joints are those in which considerable motion occurs and a joint space between the bones that is lined with a synovial membrane is present. It is the synovial joint that is the site of inflammation in most of the chronic arthritides of childhood such as juvenile rheumatoid arthritis (JRA) and the seronegative arthropathies. In the latter group, however, cartilaginous joints such as those at the symphysis pubis and the manubrium sterni may also be affected.

DEVELOPMENT OF JOINTS

Diarthrodial joints (joints in which motion occurs) develop in the fetus by cavitation of the cartilage core of the limb bud. The "cavity" is occupied by joint fluid. Further development of the diarthrodial joint is apparently dependent on fetal movement that induces formation of cartilage and synovial membrane, and without which the "cavity" regresses and becomes filled with fibrous tissue.[1] The synovial lining begins to form subsequent to cavitation, and the development of other structures, such as bursae, intra-articular fat, tendons, muscle, and capsule, quickly ensues. The whole process takes place from the fourth to seventh weeks of gestation, except for the temporomandibular joint, which develops much later.[2]

Table 2-1 Classification of Joints

Type	Motion	Characteristics	Examples	Disease Target
Fibrous	No	Bones separated by fibrous connective tissue	Sutures of skull	None
Cartilaginous	No	Bones separated by cartilage	Symphysis pubis	Ankylosing spondylitis
Synovial	Yes	Bones separated by joint space lined with synovial membrane	Joints of extremities	Juvenile rheumatoid arthritis

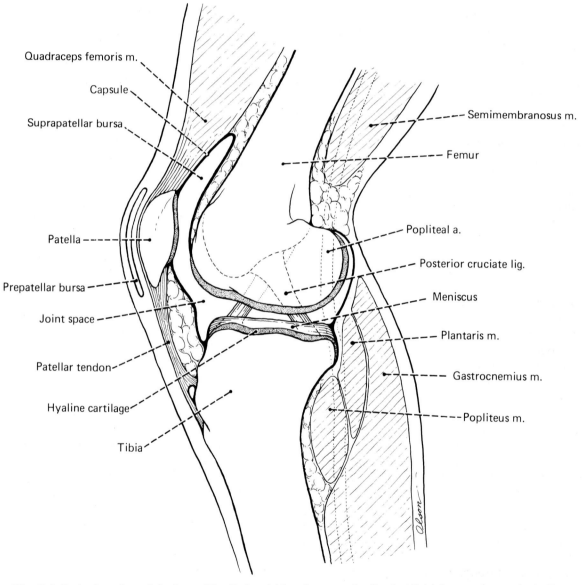

Fig. 2-1 Sagittal section of the knee. The distinguishing features of a diarthrodial joint are shown, including bone, hyaline cartilage, synovial space, fibrocartilage, capsule, bursae, ligaments, tendons, muscles, vascular and nervous supply. The rheumatic diseases affect all of these structures individually or in concert.

THE ANATOMY OF SYNOVIAL JOINTS

The anatomy of a typical synovial joint is illustrated in Figure 2-1. The bones of such joints are almost always covered by hyaline cartilage. The synovial membrane attaches at the cartilage-bone junction so that the entire joint "space" is covered by either hyaline cartilage or synovium. The temporomandibular joint is unusual in that the articular surfaces are covered by fibrocartilage rather than by hyaline cartilage. In some synovial joints, intra-articular fibrocartilage structures are present. Thus the knee joint contains two menisci, which separate the peripheral hyaline articular surfaces of the tibia and femur; the triangular fibrocartilage of the wrist joins the distal radioulnar surfaces; and a disc (or meniscus) separates the temporomandibular joint into two spaces. Other intra-articular structures include the anterior and posterior cruciate ligaments of the knee, the interosseous ligaments of the talocalcaneal joint, and the ligament of the head of the femur. These structures are actually extrasynovial, although they cross through the joint space.

ARTICULAR CARTILAGE

Hyaline cartilage facilitates relatively frictionless motion and absorbs the compressive forces generated by weight bearing. The cartilage is firmly fixed to subchondral bone, and its margins blend with the periosteum of the metaphysis of the bone and with the synovial membrane. In children hyaline cartilage is white or slightly blue, is somewhat compressible, and becomes progressively less cellular throughout the period of growth.[3] It is composed of chondrocytes within an acellular matrix consisting of collagen fibers that contribute tensile strength and of ground substance comprising water and proteoglycan that contributes resistance to compression. The articular cartilage is organized into four zones (Fig. 2-2).[4] Zones 1, 2, and 3 represent a continuum from the most superficial zone (zone 1), in which the chondrocyte long axis and collagen fibers are tangential to the surface; through zone 2, where the chondrocytes become rounder and the collagen fibers are oblique; to zone 3, where the chondrocytes tend to be arranged in columns perpendicular to the surface.

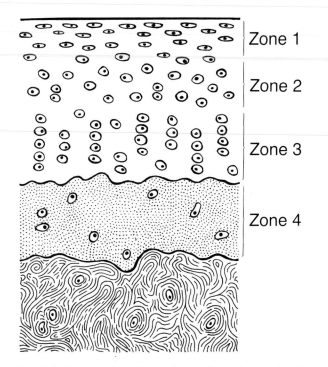

Fig. 2-2 Organization of articular cartilage. In zone 1, adjacent to the joint space, the chondrocytes are flattened. In zone 2, the chondrocytes are more rounded, and in zone 3 they are arranged in perpendicular columns. The tide mark separates zone 3 from zone 4, which is impregnated with calcium salts. Bone is beneath zone 4.

The tide mark, a blue line of staining by hematoxylin and eosin, represents the level at which calcification of the matrix occurs and separates zone 3 from zone 4.

Chondrocytes are responsible for the synthesis of the two major constituents of the matrix, collagen and proteoglycan, as well as enzymes that have the ability to degrade matrix components (collagenase, neutral proteinases, and cathepsins) and are capable of phagocytosis.[5] This dual function places the chondrocytes in the role of regulating cartilage synthesis and degradation. Whether or not they have any reparative function mediated by cell division is less clear.[6] In the child, end-capillaries proliferate in zone 4, leading eventually to replacement of this zone by bone. It is likely that nourishment of the chondrocytes occurs in this manner, although in the adult, nourishment through the exchange of synovial fluid constituents with cartilage matrix may play the predominant role.

SYNOVIUM

Synovial Membrane

The synovial membrane is a vascular connective-tissue structure that lines the capsule of all diarthrodial joints and has important intra-articular regulatory functions. The synovium consists of specialized fibroblasts, one to three cells in depth, overlying a loose meshwork of type I collagen fibers containing blood vessels, lymphatics, fat pads, unmyelinated nerves, and isolated cells such as mast cells. There is no basement membrane separating the joint space from the subsynovial tissues. The synovial membrane is discontinuous, and within the joint space there are so-called bare areas, which are areas of bone between the edge of the cartilage and the attachment of the synovial membrane to the periosteum of the metaphysis. These bare areas are vulnerable to damage (erosion) by inflamed synovium. Folds or villi of

the synovium provide for unrestricted motion of the joint and for augmented absorptive area. The synoviocytes are of two types, a subdivision that may reflect different functional states rather than different origins. Synovial A cells, the most common synoviocytes, are capable of phagocytosis and pinocytosis, have numerous microfilopodia and a prominent Golgi complex, and may synthesize hyaluronic acid. B cells are more fibroblastlike, have a prominent rough endoplasmic reticulum, and synthesize fibronectin, laminin, and types I and III collagen, as well as enzymes (collagenase, neutral proteinases) and catabolin (Fig. 2-3).

Synovial Fluid

Synovial fluid, present in very small quantities in normal synovial joints, has two functions: lubrication

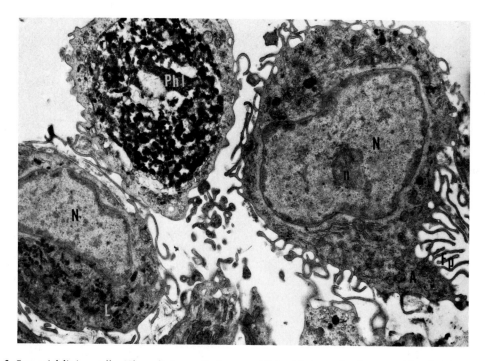

Fig. 2-3 Synovial lining cells. These lining cells from a child with juvenile rheumatoid arthritis (JRA) show marked phagocytic activity. One lining cell contains a partially degraded cell, probably a neutrophil with lysosomal granules. Another lining cell shows many filopodia (Fp). These cells, which often contain many lysosomal granules and well-developed Golgi complex, have been called *A (phagocytic) cells*. They contrast to *B (synthetic) cells* (not shown), which contain well-developed rough endoplasmic reticulum lamellae. Cells intermediate between these two principal types of the synovial lining layer have been called *C (intermediate) cells*. Another phagocytic cell (lower left) contains many lysosomes (L). Nucleus (N), phagolysosome (Phl), nucleolus (n). Lead citrate and uranyl acetate, ×7,260. (Courtesy of Dr. C.R. Wynne-Roberts.)

and nutrition. It is a combination of a filtrate of plasma, reaching the joint space from the subsynovial capillaries, and hyaluronic acid secreted by the synoviocytes. It is the hyaluronic acid that confers the high viscosity and, with water, the lubricating properties of synovial fluid. The concentrations of small molecules (electrolytes, glucose) are similar to those in plasma, but larger molecules are present in low concentrations relative to plasma unless an inflammatory state alters vasopermeability. Notably absent from synovial fluid are components of the coagulation pathway (fibrinogen, prothrombin, factors V and VII, tissue thromboplastin, and antithrombin),[7] thus rendering normal synovial fluid resistant to clotting. There appears to be free exchange of small molecules between synovial fluid of the joint space and water bound to collagen and proteoglycan of cartilage. Characteristics of normal synovial fluid are listed in Table 2-2.[8-17]

Synovial Structures

Synovium lines bursae and tendon sheaths as well as joints. Bursae facilitate frictionless movement between surfaces, such as subcutaneous tissue and bone, or between two tendons. Bursae located near synovial joints frequently communicate with the joint space. This is particularly evident at the shoulder, where the subscapular bursa or recess communicates with the glenohumeral joint, and around the knee, where the suprapatellar pouch, the posterior femoral recess, and occasionally other bursae communicate with the knee joint. Tendon sheaths lined with synovial cells are prominent around tendons as they pass under the extensor retinaculum at the wrist and the ankle. Although closely associated with joints, tendon sheaths do not communicate with the joint space.

VASCULAR SYSTEM

The arterial supply to the diaphysis and metaphysis of long bones arises from a nutrient artery that penetrates the diaphysis and subdivides in the medulla,

Table 2-2 Normal Synovial Fluid

Characteristics	Mean or Representative Value[a]	Reference
Volume	0.13–3.5 ml (adult knee)	8
pH	7.3–7.4	9
Relative viscosity	235	8
Cl, HCO₃	Slightly higher than serum	8
Na, K, Ca, Mg	Slightly lower than serum	8
Glucose	Serum value ±10%	10
Total protein	1.7–2.1 g/dl	11
Albumin	1.2 g/dl	12
Alpha1	0.17 g/dl	
Alpha2	0.15 g/dl	
Beta	0.23 g/dl	
Gamma	0.38 g/dl	
IgG	13% serum value	13
IgM	5% serum value	
IgE	22% serum value	14
Alpha2 macroglobulin	3% serum value	13
Transferrin	24% serum value	
Ceruloplasmin	16% serum value	
CH₅₀	30–50% plasma value	15
Hyaluronic acid	300 mg/dl	16
Cholesterol	7.1 mg/dl	17
Phospholipid	13.8 mg/dl	

[a] These values represent different adult synovial fluid studies. Similar data are not available for children.

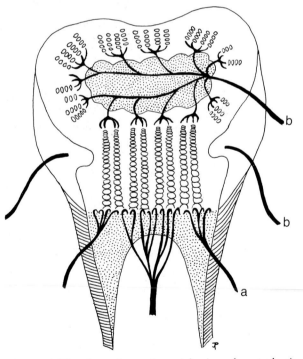

Fig. 2-4 Blood supply to the epiphysis and metaphysis. End-arteries at the epiphyseal plate arising from the medullary arteries, *a*. Juxta-articular arteries, *b*, supply epiphysis and synovium.

terminating in end-arteries at the epiphyseal plate in the child. The epiphyseal blood supply arises from juxta-articular arteries that also supply the synovium via a complex network of arterial and arteriovenous anastomoses and capillary beds, called the *circulus articuli vasculosus* by William Harvey.[18] Not until growth has ceased and the epiphyseal plate has ossified is there arterial communication between the metaphyseal and epiphyseal-synovial circulations, a phenomenon of importance in explaining the predisposition of the immature diaphysis to infection and aseptic necrosis following trauma[18] (Fig. 2-4).

Connective Tissues

COLLAGEN

Collagens are glycoproteins with high proline and hydroxyproline content and are the most abundant structural proteins in connective tissues. There are at least 10 types of collagen[19] (Table 2-3) of which only types II and V are found in articular cartilage. Type

Table 2-3 Types of Collagen

Type	Composition	Tissue Distribution
I	$[\alpha_1(I)]_2\alpha_2$	Skin, bone, tendon, ligament, fascia, dentin, cornea, lung, liver, muscle, annulus fibrosis synovium
II	$[\alpha_1(II)]_3$	Cartilage, vitreous, nucleus pulposus, notochord
III	$[\alpha_1(III)]_3$	Muscle, aorta, tendon, skin, liver, lung, intestine
IV	$[\alpha_1(IV)]_3$	Basement membrane, anterior lens capsule
V	$[\alpha_1(V)]_2[\alpha_2(V)]$	Placenta, skin, bone, tendon, synovium, cornea, aorta, lung, liver, muscle
VI	$[\alpha_1(VI)][\alpha_2(VI)]$ $[\alpha_3(VI)]$	Aortic intima, placenta, skin, kidney, muscle
VII	$[\alpha_1(VII)]_3$	Amnion
VIII	$[\alpha_1(VIII)]_3$	Endothelial cells, Descemet's membrane
IX	$[\alpha_1(IX)][\alpha_2(IX)]$ $[\alpha_3(IX)]$	Cartilage
X	$[\alpha_1(X)]_3$	Cartilage

(Adapted from Murray,[19] with permission.)

II collagen, the principal constituent, is a trimer of three identical alpha-helical chains. Type V collagen, a trimer consisting of two alpha chains and one $alpha_2$ chain (or in some tissues, one $alpha_1$, one $alpha_2$, and one $alpha_3$ chain), is found in small quantities around chondrocytes. Collagen types VI through X are present in very minute quantities. Collagen synthesis

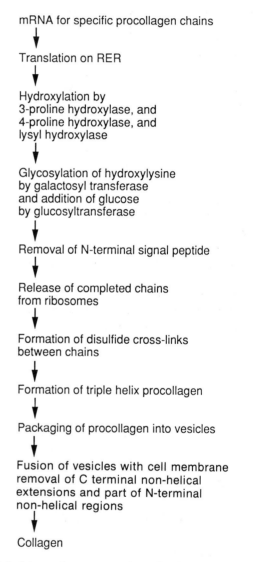

mRNA for specific procollagen chains

↓

Translation on RER

↓

Hydroxylation by
3-proline hydroxylase, and
4-proline hydroxylase, and
lysyl hydroxylase

↓

Glycosylation of hydroxylysine
by galactosyl transferase
and addition of glucose
by glucosyltransferase

↓

Removal of N-terminal signal peptide

↓

Release of completed chains
from ribosomes

↓

Formation of disulfide cross-links
between chains

↓

Formation of triple helix procollagen

↓

Packaging of procollagen into vesicles

↓

Fusion of vesicles with cell membrane
removal of C terminal non-helical
extensions and part of N-terminal
non-helical regions

↓

Collagen

Fig. 2-5 Schematic representation of collagen biosynthesis. Triple helical procollagen is secreted from the fibroblast. Specific procollagenases produce collagen by removing the ends of these molecules. The collagen molecules (except for type IV collagen) then form fibrils that undergo cross linking to form collagen fibers. (Adapted from Nimni,[127] with permission.)

appears to be minimal in the mature animal. The degree of stable cross linking of collagen fibers increases with increasing age up to the fourth decade.[20] This results in increased resistance to pepsin degradation and may contribute to increased rigidity and decreased tensile strength of old cartilage.

Collagen is an unusual protein in that it undergoes extensive changes in primary and tertiary structure after it is secreted from the fibroblast into the extracellular space as the triple helix procollagen. Specific peptidases cleave off the amino and carboxyl extention peptides, yielding collagen molecules that in some collagen types form fibrils and cross links between fibrils via lysyl and hydroxylysyl residues. Glycosylation also occurs at this posttranslational stage (Fig. 2-5).

PROTEOGLYCANS

Proteoglycans are macromolecules consisting of a protein core to which are attached 50 to 100 unbranched sulfated carbohydrates called *glycosaminoglycans*. The proteoglycans are attached via a link protein to a nonsulfated glycosaminoglycan, hyaluronic acid, to form large proteoglycan aggregates with molecular weights of several million. This structure is shown schematically in Figure 2-6, and the constituents are listed in Table 2-4. With increasing age, the size of the proteoglycan aggregates increases, the pro-

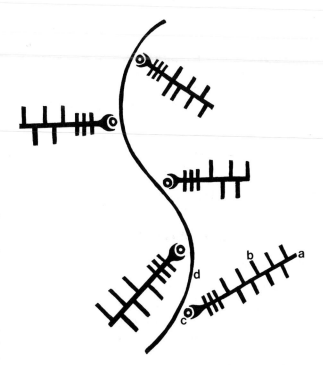

Fig. 2-6 The structure of proteoglycan. The proteoglycan monomer consists of a core protein, *a*, to which are attached glycosaminoglycan molecules, *b*. The proteoglycan is attached via a link protein, *c*, to a hyaluronic acid backbone, *d*, to form a proteoglycan aggregate.

Table 2-4 Glycosaminoglycans: Composition and Distribution

GAG	Amino Sugar[a]	Hexuronic Acid or Monosaccharide	Distribution
Hyaluronic acid	NAGlu	D-Glucuronic acid	Most connective tissues
Chondroitin-4-SO₄	NAGal	D-Glucuronic acid	Cartilage, skin, bone
Chondroitin-6-SO₄	NAGal	D-Glucuronic acid	Cartilage, skin, aorta Nucleus pulposus, umbilical cord
Dermatan sulfate	NAGal	D-Glucuronic acid L-Iduronic acid	Heart valves, vessels Skin, tendon, ligament
Heparan sulfate	NAGlu	D-Glucuronic acid L-Iduronic acid	Cell membranes All connective tissue
Heparin	NAGlu	D-Glucuronic acid L-Iduronic acid	An anticoagulant Mast cells, liver capsule
Keratan sulfate	NAGlu	D-Galactose	Cornea, skeletal tissues

[a] Abbreviations: NAGlu: *N*-acetyl-D-glucosamine; NAGal: *N*-acetyl-D-galactosamine.

tein and keratan sulfate content increases, and the chondroitin sulfate content decreases.[21,22]

OTHER CONNECTIVE-TISSUE CONSTITUENTS

In addition to collagens there are a number of specialized tissues derived from embryonic mesoderm that contribute to connective-tissue structures.

Elastin occurs in association with collagen in many tissues, especially in the walls of blood vessels and in certain ligaments. Fibers of elastin lack the tensile strength of collagens but have the ability to stretch and return to their original length. Elastin is produced by fibroblasts and smooth muscle cells.[23]

Fibronectin is a dimeric glycoprotein with a molecular weight of 450,000 produced by many different cell types, including macrophages, dedifferentiated chondrocytes, and fibroblasts, and acts as an attachment protein in the extracellular matrix. It has the ability to bind to collagens, proteoglycans, fibrinogen, and actin as well as to cell surfaces and to bacteria. It is present in the plasma and as an insoluble matrix throughout loose connective tissues, especially between basement membranes and cells.[24]

Laminin is, together with type IV collagen, a major constituent of the basement membrane. *Reticulin* may be an embryonic form of type III collagen. It is present as a fine branching network of fibers widespread in spleen, liver, bone marrow, and lymph nodes.

Connective tissues have diversified to provide the supporting structures of the body (bone, periosteum, cartilage), to permit the action of muscles on the supporting structure (tendons, ligaments, fasciae), to support internal organs (dermis, capsules, serosal membranes, basement membranes), and to provide support for blood vessels, lymphatics and the bronchopulmonary tree.

CONNECTIVE-TISSUE STRUCTURES

Tendons

Tendons are specialized connective-tissue structures that attach muscle to bone. They contain, in addition to water, type I collagen and small amounts of elastin and type III collagen, the latter forming the epitenon and endotenon. The type III collagen fibers themselves are densely packed in a parallel manner in a proteoglycan matrix containing elongated fibroblasts.

Ligaments and Fasciae

Ligaments and fasciae join bone to bone and, like tendons, are composed of type I collagen. So-called elastic ligaments, such as the ligamenta flava and li-

gamenta nucha, predominantly contain elastin, however.

Entheses

An enthesis is the site of attachment of tendon, ligament, fascia, or capsule to bone. Unlike the tendon or ligament, the enthesis is an active metabolic site, particularly in the child. It includes the peritenon, which is continuous with the periosteum; the collagen fibers of the tendon or ligament that insert into the bone (Sharpey's fibers); the adjoining cartilage; and bone not covered by periosteum.[25]

The Growing Skeleton

Bones change in size, shape, and microstructure throughout the period of growth. Bones of the appendicular and axial skeleton develop initially by ossification of preexisting cartilage that has developed from mesenchymal condensations in the embryo (endochondral ossification). In contrast, bones of the face, skull, and, initially, the mandible and clavicle develop by ossification of the fibrocellular tissue (membranous ossification). All axial and appendicular bones also have secondary membranous ossification: the diaphyseal cortex is continuously modified by periosteal bone deposition.

BONE ANATOMY

Long bones consist of four parts. The diaphysis consists of the long tubular midportion of bone that ends in the metaphyses, the flared portions of bone that are separated from the epiphyses by the growth plates or physes. At birth the diaphysis is relatively short. It grows in length by endochondral ossification. Cartilage cells proliferate toward the ends of bone; those closest to the middle of the bone ossify. Periosteal deposition of new bone increases the diameter of the diaphysis. The newborn diaphysis consists of laminar bone that lacks the Haversian canal system characteristic of mature bone, and as the child ages, increased intercellular matrix, decreased porosity, and increased hardness of the bone occur. All epiphyses, except that of the distal femur, are completely cartilaginous at birth. The cartilage is gradually replaced by bone, until in the mature individual only the articular cartilage remains unossified. The physis is a cellular zone in which mitoses are frequent and new cells are being formed. Factors influencing growth at the physis include thyroxine, growth hormone, and testosterone. Thyroxine and growth hormone act synergistically to induce cell division. Testosterone stimulates the physis to undergo rapid cell division with resultant physeal widening during the growth spurt (the anabolic effect) but eventually slows growth (androgenic effect). Estrogens suppress the growth rate by increasing calcification of the matrix, a prerequisite to epiphyseal closure. There do not appear to be receptors for these steroids on physeal cells, although there are receptors for somatomedin, insulin, and prolactin. It is probably through these molecules and their receptors that the steroid effects are mediated.[26] Hydrocortisone affects physeal physiology indirectly, by suppressing growth hormone release.[27-29]

The relative contributions of individual epiphyses to limb length are summarized in Table 2-5. Growth in the bones of the appendicular skeleton ceases coincident with completion of the ossification of the iliac apophyses, although increase in the height of the vertebral bodies may continue to contribute to overall height until the third decade.[30]

Skeletal age can be determined by radiographic identification of the onset of secondary ossification in the long bones and by physeal closure. In general, ossification centers appear earlier and physes fuse earlier in girls than in boys.

Table 2-5 Relative Contributions of Individual Physes to Length of the Bone and of the Limb

Growth Area		Contribution to Total Growth (%)	
		of Bone	of Limb
Humerus	Proximal	80	40
	Distal	20	10
Radius/ulna	Proximal	20	10
	Distal	80	40
Femur	Proximal	30	15
	Distal	70	40
Tibia/fibula	Proximal	55	27
	Distal	45	18

(Data from Ogden.[30])

Muscle

A skeletal muscle is surrounded by the connective tissue epimysium that in turn surrounds a number of fascicles that are covered by connective tissue perimysium. Each fascicle contains many individual muscle fibers that are the basic structural units of skeletal muscle (Fig. 2-7). Muscle fibers are elongated mul-

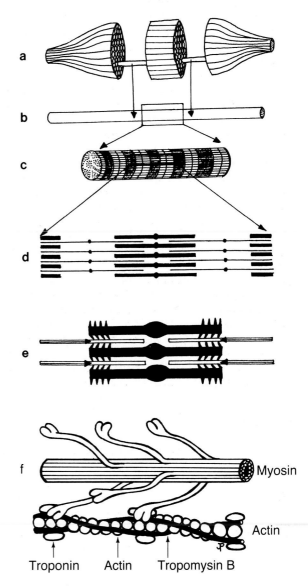

Fig. 2-7 Schematic representation of the anatomy of skeletal muscle. *a*, fascicle; *b*, fiber; *c*, myofibrils; *d*, actin and myosin; *e* and *f*, enlargement of actin and myosin filaments showing the actin filaments coiled around each other and associated with tropomysin B lying in the groove.

tinucleated cells surrounded by connective-tissue endomysium (reticulin, collagen) that is richly supplied with capillaries. Within each fiber are a large number of myofibrils consisting of highly organized interdigitated myofilaments of actin and myosin. Each myofilament has approximately 180 myosin molecules with a molecular weight of 500,000, a long tail, and a double head. The myofilament is composed of the myosin tails; the myosin heads project in a spiral arrangement. Lying parallel to the myosin molecules are actin filaments (F-actin) composed of globular subunits of G-actin with a molecular weight of 42,000. Two actin filaments are coiled around each other as a helix, with a second protein, tropomyosin B, lying in the groove. A regulatory protein, troponin, is located at intervals along this structure. This complex structure is demonstrable by light or electron microscopy as striations. The relationship of the contractile molecules to the striated appearance is shown schematically in Figure 2-7.[31] Creatine kinase is bound at regular intervals to the myosin filaments.[32]

There are two types of muscle fibers, which differ in their structure and biochemistry (Table 2-6).[33] Most muscles contain both types: type I (slow) fibers are narrower, have poorly defined myofibrils, are irregular in size, have thick Z bands, and are rich in mitochondria and oxidative enzymes but poor in phosphorylases. Type II (fast) fibers have fewer mitochondria and are poor in oxidative enzymes, but rich in phosphorylases and glycogen. These two muscle fiber types are demonstrable histochemically (Fig.

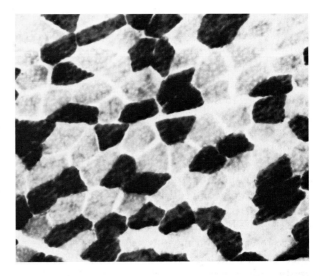

Fig. 2-8 Frozen section of normal skeletal muscle stained with ATP-ase, pH 9.2. Type I fibers are pale and type II fibers are dark. Magnification 800×. (Photomicrograph courtesy of Dr. M. Norman).

2-8). Muscles differ in the proportions of each fiber type that they contain; diaphragm contains predominantly "slow" fibers and small muscles contain predominantly "fast" fibers.

INFLAMMATION

HISTORICAL REVIEW

Whenever tissue is injured there occurs at the site of injury a series of host defense reactions to limit the spread of the injurious agent and to repair damaged tissue, i.e., the acute inflammatory response.[34–36] The cardinal signs of inflammation were defined by Celsus as "rubor et tumor cum calore et dolore," and Virchow added "et functio laesa"—redness and swelling with heat, pain, and loss of function.[37]

The in vivo studies of Cohnheim using frog mesentery or tongue marked the first important analysis of the phenomenon of inflammation.[38] Under the microscope, he examined mesentery that had become irritated by exposure to air and noted a sequence of events beginning with arteriolar dilatation, increased rate of blood flow, margination of white blood cells in venules, and diapedesis of leukocytes through the venule wall into the extravascular space. He noted also that plasma escaped from the vessel wall because

Table 2-6 Comparison of Muscle Fiber Types

	Type 1	Type 2
Size	Smaller	Larger
Color	Red	White
Myoglobin content	High	Low
Oxidative enzymes (NADH)	High	Low
Myophosphofructokinase	High	Low
Myofibrillar ATP-ase	Low	High
Myophosphorylase	Low	High
Lipid	High	Low
Glycogen	Low	High
Metabolic characteristics	Oxidative (aerobic)	Glycolytic (anaerobic)
Function	Sustained	Brief

(Adapted from Heffner,[33] with permission.)

of increased vascular permeability. In 1891, Elie Metchnikoff published *Lectures on the Comparative Pathology of Inflammation,* delivered at the Pasteur Institute, the culmination of 25 years of intense study. He regarded all the other phenomena of inflammation as secondary to the phagocytic reaction in ridding the body of the "infectious" agents. The phagocytic theory had to wait another 10 years, however, for full exposition in his second book, *Immunity in Infective Diseases,*[46] which distilled into one monumental work the biologic thought that had begun with the experiments of Pasteur and colleagues in 1879 on fowl cholera. Metchnikoff's theory of immunity, although one-sided, was nevertheless an important stimulus to future research. During this period of time, the science of immunology was born. The two fields of study, inflammation and immunology, although not synonymous, have become increasingly intertwined. Understanding the inflammatory response, and why it becomes self-perpetuating in the connective tissue diseases instead of limited as in wound healing, is a basic research area in rheumatology.

Phases of Inflammation

The inflammatory response can be reduced to three component phases: (1) vascular, (2) exudative, and (3) proliferative, which are followed by regeneration and repair, the formation of a scar. In addition to the three phases of the local inflammatory response, systemic reactions are usual and are characterized by fever and an acute phase response of the serum proteins. The febrile reaction is in part related to the release of endogenous pyrogens and is a predominant constitutional reaction in most acute rheumatic diseases.

THE VASCULAR PHASE OF INFLAMMATION

As a consequence of tissue injury, there is a release of chemical mediators such as histamine that produce dilatation of the venules of the terminal vascular bed. Arteriolar dilatation follows reflexly, occasionally preceded by a brief phase of constriction. These acute vascular changes persist for hours. The slowing of blood flow through the injured site initiates exudation of plasma into the perivascular tissues. Phagocytes enter the interstitium by passing between the endothelial cells and through ultrastructural discontinuities in the basement membrane at sites populated by primitive cells called *pericytes.* Accelerated transudation of the extracellular constituents of plasma follows this hyperemic stage and is perpetuated by other chemical mediators such as kinins. The accumulation of fibrinogen at the inflammatory site triggers coagulation. The terminal lymphatics, in response to vascular stasis and increased tissue hydrostatic pressure, transport a markedly increased amount of protein-rich lymph away from the site of the injury. Antigenic materials arising from the injury reach the regional lymph nodes first through these channels and initiate or provoke chronicity of the immune response. Local transudation of immunoglobulin E (IgE) may play a major role in the initial phases of increased vascular permeability. Later, host defenses are dependent on IgG for completion of these initial immunologic events.

THE CELLULAR OR EXUDATIVE PHASE OF INFLAMMATION

Accumulation of leukocytes at the inflammatory site, the morphologic hallmark of the second stage of inflammation, involves several mechanisms, among which release of chemotactic substances plays a central role. Lysosomal hydrolytic enzymes are released at the inflammatory site by the phagocytic cells during ingestion and, later, with cell death. Other proinflammatory mediators also accumulate at the injured site during this phase of exudation. Although polymorphonuclear granulocytes are not essential to the total sequence of the cellular events associated with wound healing, their absence can have obvious deleterious consequences if the noxious stimulus is infectious. Macrophages, derived principally from circulating monocytes, predominate in the later stages of the cellular response and augment phagocyte activity, including the eventual engulfment of other leukocytes, the cleaning-up process of local injury. They participate in processing antigen and are attracted to the inflammatory site by specific chemotactic substances and restricted there by the action of specific lymphokines. The plasma cell is a recognizable component only in chronic inflammatory lesions. The eosinophil is a minor constituent of these reactions except in special circumstances in which allergic phenomena have a recognized role or in certain types of inflammation involving parasites.

THE PROLIFERATIVE PHASE OF INFLAMMATION

Provided the inflammatory stimulus has been controlled by exudation and phagocytosis, repair of damaged tissue is initiated with increasing fibroblastic and angioblastic activity. The fibroblast is derived from the perivascular connective tissue and is stimulated by derivatives of the cellular inflammatory response. The regenerative phase reaches maturity with formation of a scar.

Simultaneous with the emergence of fibroblastic activity, angioblasts derived from endothelial cells form new capillary channels through the thrombosed terminal vascular bed and initiate normal blood flow into the injured region. Vascular continuity is reestablished, and the new capillary network provides the nutrients and environment that will lead to the completion of the reparative process.

Chronic Inflammation

Chronic inflammation may be of two types. The first type follows an acute inflammatory response that fails to resolve completely, and inflammation is prolonged for several months. The second type of chronic inflammation is that which is chronic ab initio, that is, from the beginning. This type of chronic inflammation characterizes rheumatic and other diseases.[39] The histologic characteristics of chronic inflammation are those shown in Table 2-7.[40] Chronic granulomatous inflammation is characterized by a predominant mononuclear phagocytic cell infiltrate and the presence of multinucleated foreign body giant cells derived from cytoplasmic fusion of macrophages.[41] These cells frequently predominate in chronic inflammation when the initiating stimulus is not satisfactorily terminated or repair is delayed by local or systemic factors.[42] Granulation tissue, typi-

fied by the rheumatoid pannus, consists of various constitutents (fibroblasts, angioblasts, giant cells, and newly formed connective tissue) and is a result of chronic inflammation. Continuing stimulation by the persistence of foreign material (or altered host proteins) is too simple and incomplete an explanation for the chronicity of the inflammatory diseases in humans. The chronic inflammatory response and autoimmunity come together in self-perpetuation of a destructive response that evolved in vertebrates as a protective and reparative function of phagocytes and immunologic mechanisms.

Mediators of the Inflammatory Response

THE COMPLEMENT SYSTEM

The complement system consists of two converging pathways of sequential enzymatic activation of specific plasma proteins resulting in a wide range of biologic functions, including cell activation, opsonization, and cell lysis. The pathways are outlined in Figure 2-9, and the characteristics of the individual components of both pathways are shown in Table 2-8. A central characteristic of the complement system is that it is an amplification mechanism: a membrane-bound enzyme molecule can activate many precursor

Table 2-7 Characteristics of Chronic Inflammation

1. The process is characterized more by the infiltration of cells than by the accumulation of fluid.

2. There is coexistent destruction and repair.

3. The cellular infiltrate consists of polymorphonuclear and mononuclear cells and their derivatives.

(Adapted from Hurley,[40] with permission.)

Table 2-8 Characteristics of Components of Complement System

Component	MW ($\times 10^3$)	Serum Level (μg/ml)
C1q	400	70
C1r	83	34
C1s	83	31
C2	117	25
C3	195	1,200
C4	206	600
C5	180	85
C6	128	60
C7	120	55
C8	150	55
C9	79	60
Factor B	95	225
Factor D	25	1
Factor H	150	500
Factor I	90	34
Factor P	190	25

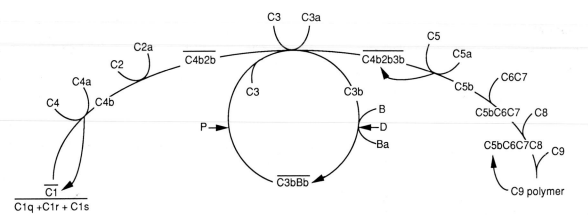

Fig. 2-9 The complement activation pathways. See text for a description of the sequence of activation and the functions of the intermediates.

enzyme molecules by limited proteolysis. Each of these activated enzyme molecules subsequently activates the next precursor, and so on. Accompanying this activation system is an equally important system of inhibitors. Except for C1, which is synthesized by the epithelium of the gastrointestinal and genitourinary tracts, complement components are synthesized by hepatic parenchymal cells.

In the activation of the classical complement pathway, the initial event is the binding of complement protein C1q to the second domain of two molecules of IgG1, IgG2, IgG3, or the fourth domain of one molecule of IgM. C1q then binds to C1r, which activates C1s, forming a trimolecular complex, which remains attached to the membrane or activating immune complex. C1s cleaves plasma C4 into C4a and C4b, which attaches to the cell membrane. C2 interacts with membrane-bound C4b and is then cleaved by C1s to yield C4b2b (C3 convertase) and the small C2a fragment. C1 esterase inhibitor binds to C1s and C1r and, in so doing, limits the action of C1s, especially in the fluid phase.

The third complement component, C3, marks the point where the classical and alternative pathways merge. C4b2b splits C3 into C3a (anaphylatoxin) and C3b. C3b either attaches to membrane-bound C4b2b to form a trimolecular complex C4b2b3b or attaches directly to cells that have receptors for this molecule (neutrophils, eosinophils, monocytes, Kupffer cells, alveolar macrophages, erythrocytes, and B lymphocytes), thus promoting phagocytosis through immune adherence.

The C4b2b3b complex splits C5 into C5a (anaphylatoxin) and C5b, which is the initial component of the C5–9 membrane attack complex. Membrane-bound C5b binds C6 and C7, forming C5b67. Addition of C8 initiates lysis of the cell membrane. The C5b678 complex facilitates the polymerization of C9 into a tubule (collectively termed the membrane attack complex), which traverses the membrane lipid bilayer to allow free passage of extracellular water and sodium into the cell with resultant cell lysis.

The anaphylatoxins C3a and C5a are important mediators of histamine release from mast cells and contraction of smooth muscle. In addition, C5a is chemotatic for neutrophils, activates the oxidative burst, and induces leukotriene production, all factors of significance in inflammation. C3a and C5a are inactivated by carboxypeptidase B by removal of the terminal arginine group to yield the des-arg form of the molecule.

The alternative pathway, as its name implies, provides an alternate mechanism for activation of C3. Although IgA can apparently initiate this pathway, C3 may be activated without the participation of antibody, by proteinases such as trypsin, plasmin, thrombin, and elastase, all of which are generated in inflammatory responses, or by polysaccharide components of bacterial cell wall (similar to zymosan, or inulin). Protein B then attaches to membrane-bound C3b to form C3bB. Factor B in this complex is enzymatically cleaved by factor D to form a membrane-bound C3 convertase (C3bBb) and a small fragment, Ba. Properdin (factor P) stabilizes C3bBb, thus contributing to the effectiveness of the activation of C3 by C3Bb in the feedback loop. This system is limited by factor H, which competes with factor B for the binding site on C3b. C3b is further inactivated in a series of steps by C3b inactivator (factor I) and by proteolytic enzymes yielding a membrane-bound C3d fragment and an inactive fluid phase component, C3c. The biologic activities resulting from the activation of the complement system are summarized in Table 2-9. See the references for current reviews of the complement pathways and their role in inflammation.[43,44]

INTERACTIONS WITH THE COAGULATION AND KININ-GENERATING PATHWAYS

In inflammation, there are important interrelationships between the complement system and the coagulation, kinin-generating, and fibrinolytic systems (Fig. 2-10). For example, C3b is generated by the action of plasmin or thrombin on C3. Hageman factor (factor XII) is activated by exposure to crystals, collagen, protein-polysaccharide complexes, and immune complexes to generate enzymatic functions in a variety of proinflammatory pathways, including the conversion of prekallikrein to kallikrein, which is chemotactic for polymorphs and degrades kininogen to form bradykinin, which in turn contributes to the increase of vascular permeability and production of pain.

DERIVATIVES OF ARACHIDONIC ACID

A crucial link in the explanation of the anti-inflammatory activity of the nonsteroidal anti-inflammatory drugs, especially that of aspirin, was forged by

Table 2-9 Biologic Activities Resulting from Complement Activation

Component	Biologic Activity
C1q	Aggregation of immune complexes
C4b	Virus neutralization
C2a	Kininlike activity
C3a	Anaphylatoxin
C3b	Opsonization, immune adherence (via receptors on B lymphocytes, granulocytes, and macrophages)
C5a	Anaphylatoxin, chemotactin
C8, C9	Cytolysis

the discovery of the prostaglandins and their roles in the acute inflammatory response.[45-47] Subsequently, the other metabolites of arachidonic acid metabolism, hydroperoxyeicosatetraenoic acids (HPETEs) and hydroxyeicosatetraenoic acids (HETEs), have been included in this family of inflammatory mediators (Fig. 2-11). The initial step in the generation of these mediators is the release by the action of phospholipase A_2 of arachidonic acid from cell membrane phospholipid of cells participating in the immunologic reaction to the inflammatory stimulus.

The prostaglandins are a family of labile 20-carbon dienes that result from the action of molecular oxygen on arachidonic acid in the presence of cyclooxygenase. The unstable endoperoxide prostaglandin G_2 (PGG_2) is reduced by hydroperoxidase to a second unstable endoperoxide, PGH_2, which breaks down nonenzymatically to form PGE_2 and PGD_2 or is acted upon by PGI_2 synthase to produce PGI_2 (prostacyclin) or by thromboxane synthase to produce thromboxane A_2.

HPETEs are generated by the action of lipoxygenases on arachidonic acid.[47] The products of the action of 5-lipoxygenase, the leukotrienes, are of particular importance in inflammation. The unstable intermediate leukotriene A_4 (LTA_4) is hydrolyzed to LTB4 or acted upon by glutathione to form LTC_4. LTC_4 is subsequently metabolized to LTD_4, LTE_4, and LTF_4.

Actions of the prostaglandins are often centered in tissues containing smooth muscle, such as the vasculature and gastrointestinal and genitourinary tracts, and are mediated by an increase in intracellular cyclic adenosine monophosphate (cAMP). The fever that is characteristic of inflammatory reactions results from the action of interleukin 1 (IL1) from macrophages on the thermoregulatory center in the preoptic area of the anterior hypothalamus. The hypothalamic effect is mediated by PGE_2 and $PGF_{2\alpha}$.

Pain, one of the cardinal symptoms of inflammation, is generated by a number of chemical mediators, including the prostaglandins PGE_1, PGE_2, and PGI_2 and the leukotrienes LTB_4, LTC_4, and LTD_4, which appear to sensitize pain receptors to the action of other mediators such as histamine and bradykinin. Vasodilatation is increased by PGE_2 and PGI_2 and by LTC_4 and LTD_4. PGE_2 and PGI_2 also act synergistically with other mediators (histamine, bradykinin, C5a) to increase vasopermeability and cause edema. The leukotriene LTB_4 has a number of important effects on

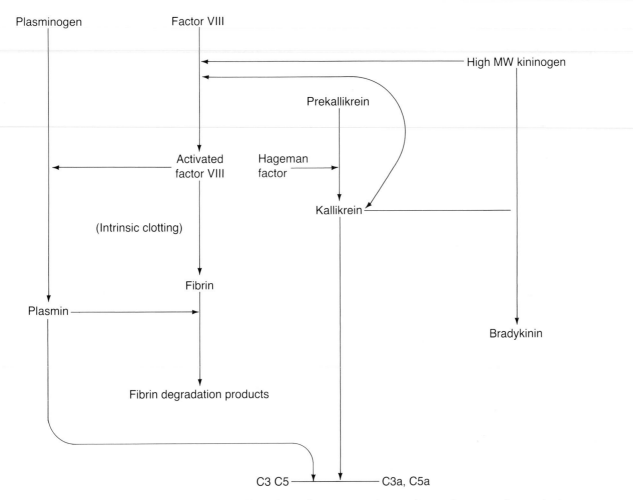

Fig. 2-10 Interactions among coagulation, fibrinolytic, kinin-generating, and complement pathways in inflammation.

polymorphs and macrophages. It enhances polymorph chemotaxis,[48] lysosomal enzyme release,[49] and other functions.[50]

In addition to these proinflammatory functions, however, prostaglandins appear to have anti-inflammatory properties in some circumstances. In general, PGE_1 and PGE_2 suppress antibody-dependent cell-mediated cytotoxicity (ADCC) by K cells and decrease migration inhibition factor (MIF) production and lymphocyte response to mitogens.[51]

Reactive Oxygen Species

The biosynthesis of the prostaglandins may also be accompanied by the generation of highly reactive species of oxygen that participate in tissue injury (superoxide, peroxide, hydroxyl, and singlet oxygen).[52,53] The role of activated oxygen in tissue inflammation remains unproved; the hydroxyl ion may be the most injurious. Superoxide is reduced to hydrogen peroxide and oxygen by the action of the superoxide dismutases. Peroxide, an injurious intermediate, is disposed of by catalases and peroxidases. These same oxygen intermediates are generated during phagocytosis and subserve the function of bacterial killing in the phagolysosome. Boys with chronic granulomatous disease lack the ability to generate this type of bactericidal action, a phenomenon mimicked by the effect of corticosteroids on normal phagocytes.[54] Certain NSAIDs as well as acute phase reactants (e.g., ceruloplasmin) may serve as scavengers of oxygen radicals at the inflammatory sites.[55]

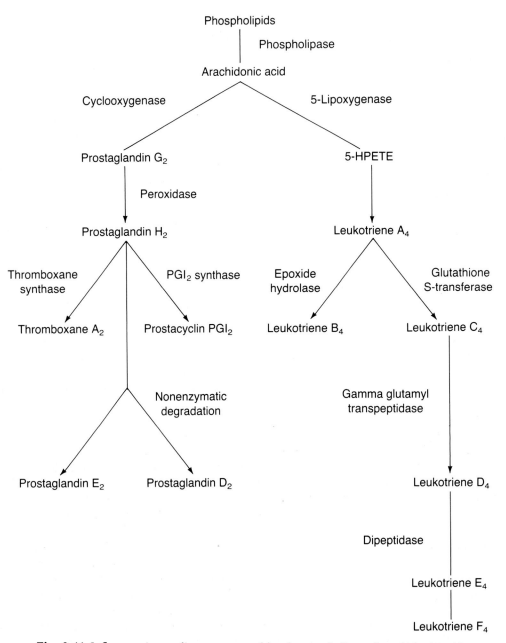

Fig. 2-11 Inflammatory mediators generated by the metabolism of arachidonic acid.

ACUTE PHASE PROTEINS

The term *acute phase* was first used by Abernathy and Avery[56] to describe changes in the serum of patients with acute bacterial infection. The acute phase reactants are those plasma proteins that undergo changes in concentration as a result of an inflammatory stimulus (Table 2-10).[57] Most acute phase proteins are synthesized in the hepatocytes in response to the effect of interleukin 1 (IL 1) or interleukin 6 (IL 6).

In humans, the most important acute phase proteins are C-reactive protein (CRP) and serum amyloid A (SAA), which increase several hundredfold within

Table 2-10 Acute Phase Proteins

Proteins increased in inflammation
    C-reactive protein
    Serum amyloid A protein
    Fibrinogen
    Haptoglobin
    Alpha1 antichymotrypsin
    Alpha1 proteinase inhibitor
    Ceruloplasmin
    C3
    C1 inactivator

Proteins decreased in inflammation
    Albumin
    Transferrin
    Alpha2 HS glycoprotein
    Alpha1 lipoprotein
    Prealbumin

(Adapted from Koj,[57] with permission.)

hours of a stimulus. The acute phase proteins are used as laboratory indicators of the presence and extent of inflammation. The most commonly used quantitator of inflammation, the erythrocyte sedimentation rate (ESR), reflects changes in several of these reactants, particularly increased fibrinogen and immunoglobulins, and decreased albumin, all of which contribute to rouleaux formation. CRP is a pentamer with a molecular weight of 105 kD. It is present in very low concentrations in normal serum (<0.2 mg/dl) but increases rapidly to levels in the 10- to 25-mg/dl range in acute inflammation. CRP binds to phosphocholines, galactans, and polycations with resultant complement activation.[58] Some functions of other acute phase proteins are shown in Table 2-11.

CELLULAR ELEMENTS OF THE INFLAMMATORY RESPONSE

Although any tissue injury results in an inflammatory response, the mechanisms of injury believed to be of paramount importance in the etiology and pathogenesis of rheumatic diseases are immunologic. These mechanisms are the result of a response of the immune system to an exogenous or endogenous antigen. The cells involved are derived from a hematopoietic stem cell by one of two major pathways: one by way of the common lymphoid cell progenitor gives rise to lymphocytes; the other by way of the common myeloid cell progenitor gives rise to phagocytic cells, including polymorphonuclear leukocytes and macrophages (Fig. 2-12).

Lymphocytes

The cells of the immune system are organized into the lymphoid tissues that are widespread throughout the body. Cooper and co-workers originally proposed the two-component concept of lymphoid differentiation.[59] The common lymphoid cell progenitor differentiates under the influence of the thymus into T lymphocytes or in the fetal liver, spleen, or adult bone marrow into B lymphocytes and thereafter into mature plasma cells. The enormous complexity of the characteristics and functions of the cells of the T- and B-lymphocyte types is documented in Table 2-12.

T Lymphocytes

T lymphocytes are influenced by the thymus that is derived from the third and fourth pharyngeal pouch endoderm and branchial cleft ectoderm. T cells consist of at least four types characterized by different functions and different surface markers demonstrable by the use of monoclonal antibodies (Table 2-13).

The interactions of T cells, B cells, and antigen presenting cells are mediated by soluble products of T lymphocytes or macrophages or by direct cell-to-cell contact. The soluble products of lymphocytes, called lymphokines, and of monocytes and macrophages, called monokines, are listed in Tables 2-14 and 2-15. Most of these factors are characterized by

Table 2-11 Functions of the Acute Phase Proteins

Acute Phase Protein	Functions
Haptoglobin, alpha1-antichymotrypsin	Inhibition of proteinases
Fibrinogen, C-reactive protein, C1 inactivator	Coagulation and fibrinolysis
C-reactive protein, serum amyloid A protein, C3, fibrinogen	Phagocytosis
Proteinase inhibitors, haptoglobin, ceruloplasmin	Anti-inflammatory
Haptoglobin, transferrin, albumin, ceruloplasmin	Binding of biologically active compounds

Table 2-12 Characteristics of T and B Lymphocytes

Characteristic	T Cell	B Cell
Anatomic		
Origin	Bone marrow	Bone marrow
Maturation	Thymus	Bone marrow, spleen, liver
Lifespan	Months to years	Days to weeks
Recirculating pool	Majority	Minority
Distribution		
Lymph node	Paracortical Perifollicular	Subcapsular Medullary cords Germinal centers
Spleen	Periarteriolar sheaths	Peripheral white and red pulp
Peyer's patches	Perifollicular	Follicular
Peripheral blood	60–80%	20–30%
Thoracic duct	90%	10%
Membrane receptors		
Immunoglobulin	−	+
Fc gamma	+	+
Fc mu	+	−
Fc epsilon	+	−
HLA class I	+	+
HLA class II	+	+
Complement receptor 1	−	+
Complement receptor 2	−	+
T 1	−	+
EBV-R	−	+
ME-R	−	+
Sheep RBC receptor	+	−
Mitogen responses		
Phytohemagglutinin	+	±
Concanavalin A	+	±
Pokeweed	±	+
Lipopolysaccharide	±	+
MLR	+	−
AMLR	+	−

their effect on in vitro systems, and only a few have been isolated and completely characterized biochemically.[60–62]

Macrophages, derived from the common myeloid progenitor, have a central role in the immune response, since they function both as antigen presenting cells in inducing the lymphocytes to mount an immune response and as effector cells in responding to the signals of the activated T lymphocytes.

Helper and cytotoxic T cells respond to antigen only when it is presented by an antigen presenting cell such as the macrophage or dendritic cell together with products of the major histocompatibility locus. Cytotoxic T cells respond to class I MHC antigens (HLA-A, HLA-B, HLA-C), which are present on all nucleated cells, whereas most other T lymphocytes respond to antigen when presented in conjunction with class II MHC antigens (HLA-DR), which are more restricted in their distribution, being present on antigen presenting cells (macrophages, dendritic cells, and some B lymphocytes), although their expression on other cells participating in the immune

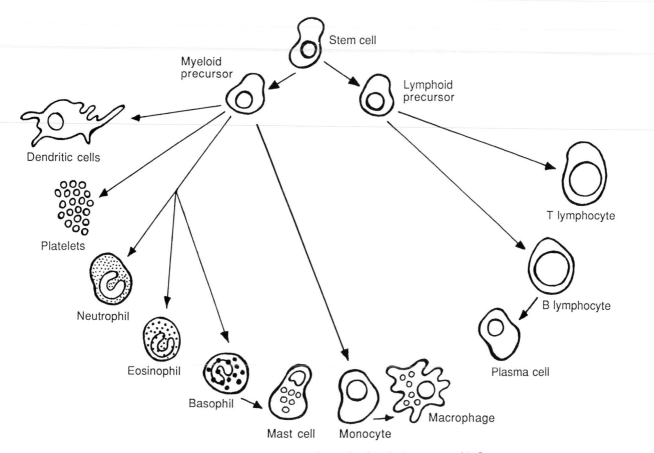

Fig. 2-12 A schematic representation of the lineage of cells involved in the immune and inflammatory responses.

response can be induced under appropriate circumstances.

The interaction between antigen presenting cell and T lymphocyte results in release of IL 1 by the antigen presenting cell. IL1 activates the T cell to release IL 2, which causes the T cell to proliferate in response to antigenic stimulation.[60]

B Lymphocytes

B lymphocytes synthesize and secrete antibody in response to signals from T lymphocytes and macrophages. The isotype (heavy chain class) of the antibody determines its role in the immunoinflammatory response. Characteristics of the antibody classes and subclasses are listed in Table 2-16.

In chickens, the central lymphoid tissue for B lymphocytes is located in a hindgut organ, the bursa of Fabricius. The bursa-equivalent organ in humans may be Peyer's patches within the gastrointestinal tract. B cells are located in the cortex of the lymph nodes, where they form follicles. B lymphocytes can be recognized in the peripheral blood by detection of surface immunoglobulin markers that react with anti-

Table 2-13 T-Lymphocyte Subsets

Subset	Function	Surface Markers
T suppressor	Down-regulates B-cell response to T-dependent antigens	T 3, 8, 11
T helper	Up-regulates B-cell response to T-dependent antigens	T 1, 3, 4, 11
T cytotoxic	Kills target cells	T 3, 8, 11
T dth	Mediates delayed hypersensitivity reactions	T 1, 3, 4, 11

Table 2-14 Interleukins

Interleukin	Source	Target	Function
Interleukin 1 (LAF)	Macrophage, epithelial, endothelial cells	T and B cells	Stimulates thymocytes, fibroblasts, osteoclasts; promotes production of some acute phase proteins; is a pyrogen and induces slow wave sleep
Interleukin 2 (TCGF)	T helper	T cells	Promotes cell division of lymphokine activated T killer cells
Interleukin 3 (multi CSF)	T helper	Stem cells	Promotes growth and maturation of PMNs, eosinophils, basophils, RBCs, and megakaryocytes
Interleukin 4 (BCGF)	T helper (2)	Stem cells	Promotes proliferation of B cells, expression of Ia on B cells and macrophages, and proliferation of T helper (2) cells
Interleukin 5 (BCGF II) (TCRF)	T helper (2)	B cells, eosinophils	Growth factor for B cells and eosinophils
Interleukin 6 (IFN beta$_2$)	Monocytes and fibroblasts	B cells, some T cells	Stimulates B-cell maturation and antibody production; regulates acute phase responses; pyrogenic

immunoglobulin antisera. After surface Ig binds with a specific antigen, a B cell matures into a plasma cell that secretes antibody with the antigenic specificity of the surface Ig. The basic immunoglobulin structure consists of two heavy chains that determine the isotype (IgG1, IgG2, IgG3, IgG4, IgA1, IgA2, IgM, IgD, IgE) and two light chains (either kappa or lambda). The heavy chains are joined to each other by one or more disulfide bridges. The light chains are joined to the N-terminal regions of the heavy

Table 2-15 Other Soluble Mediators of Cell Growth and Activity

Monokines	Source	Target	Function
Tumor necrosis factor alpha	Macrophage	Fibroblasts, chondrocytes	Stimulates collagenase and PGE$_2$ production, cytotoxic
Tumor necrosis factor beta (lymphotoxin)	T lymphocytes	Some tumors	Cytotoxic
Migration inhibition factor (MIF)	T lymphocytes	Macrophage	Increases cAMP and reduces cell migration
Plasminogen activator	Macrophage	T cell	Promotes cell division, lyses fibrinogen, activates complement
Macrophage activating factor (MAF)	T lymphocytes	Macrophage	Activates macrophages (same as interferon gamma)
Leukocyte migration inhibition factor (LMIF)	T lymphocytes	Polymorphs	Prevents migration of PMNs from site
Macrophage chemotactic factor	T lymphocytes	Macrophage	Recruits macrophages to inflammatory site
Transfer factor	T lymphocytes	Lymphocyte	Confers antigenic specificity
Interferon gamma	T lymphocytes	Macrophage	Activates macrophages

Table 2-16 Immunoglobulins

	IgG1	IgG2	IgG3	IgG4	IgA1	IgA2	IgM	IgD	IgE
Normal adult serum level (mg/ml)	9	3	1	0.5	3	0.5	1.5	0.03	0.00005
Sedimentation coefficient	7S	7S	7S	7S	7S	7S	19S	7S	8S
Molecular weight ($\times 10^3$)	146	146	170	146	160	160	970	184	188
Carbohydrate (%)	3	3	3	3	8	8	12	10	12
Intravascular (%)	45	45	45	45	40	40	75	75	50
Total circulating pool (mg/kg)	325	115	35	20	80	15	37	1	0.02
Half-life (days)	23	23	9	25	6		5	3	3
Synthetic rate (mg/kg/day)	30				25		7	0.5	0.2
Biologic function									
Crosses placenta	+	±	+	+	−	−	−	−	−
Complement fixation	+ +	+	+ + +	−	−	−	+ + +	−	−
Cell binding									
Mononuclears	+	−	+	−	−	−	−	−	−
Neutrophils	+	−	+	+	+	+	−	−	−
Lymphocytes	+	+	+	+	±	±	±	−	±
Mast cells	−	−	−	−	−	−	−	−	+ + +
Platelets	+	+	+	+	−	−	−	−	−

chains by additional disulfide bridges, except for IgA2, in which the light chains are noncovalently bound to the heavy chains.

The structure of the immunoglobulin molecule is related to its function (Fig. 2-13). Antigen binding is the function of the N-terminal variable region of the molecule, the antigen-binding fragment (Fab). The constant portions of the heavy chains are divided into three domains centered around disulfide bridges. The first domain, N-terminal to the hinge region, binds the C4b fragment of complement. The second domain binds C1q and, together with the third domain, contains the site that binds to the crystallizable fragment (Fc) receptor on neutrophils, to K cells, and to staphylococcal protein A. The third domain has the site for binding to the Fc receptor on macrophages and monocytes.

Two other molecules are important in immunoglobulin structure. The joining (J) chains (molecular weight 15,000), which are synthesized by the plasma cell, covalently bind the C-terminal octapeptide of one heavy chain to its counterpart on a heavy chain of a second immunoglobulin molecule. Heavy chains of the mu and alpha classes form pentamers or dimers

in this way. A second molecule, secretory component (molecular weight 70,000), which is synthesized by the mucosal epithelial cells, attaches to a heavy chain of each of two IgA molecules. Secretory component facilitates transportation of IgA into the secretions and protects it from proteolytic degradation.

Genetic polymorphism is characteristic of immunoglobulin molecules. The genes for individual immunoglobulin isotypes for heavy and light chains are present in all individuals. Allotypes are not present in all members of the population but represent the products of alternative genes at a given genetic locus, resulting in differences in the amino acid sequences of heavy chains. Such differences (e.g., gamma [Gm] allotypes) are recognized as foreign by the immune system of other members of the species having a different allotype. Idiotypic variation is the representation of the polymorphism of the antigen-binding site in the hypervariable region of the light and heavy chains. The total diversity generated by differences in isotype, allotype, and idiotype is enormous and reflects the complexity of the genetic machinery devoted to the synthesis and control of these important molecules.

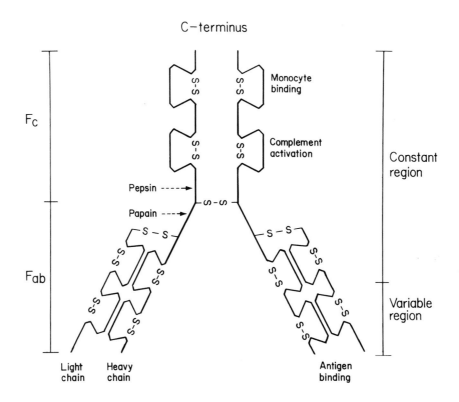

C-terminus

N-terminus

Fig. 2-13 Basic immunoglobulin structure. Linear and tertiary configurations of a typical immunoglobulin G molecule are suggested in this diagram based upon enzymatic analysis, amino acid composition, and electron microscopy. The variable regions of the light and heavy chains are shown by the brackets. Critical S-S bonds are indicated at the junction of the variable and constant regions of these chains and in the hinge area at the junction of the Fc and Fab portions of the molecule. The loops of the heavy and light chains are stabilized by interchain and intrachain hydrogen bonding. The Fab and Fc regions are defined by analysis with papain and pepsin. Reaction of an immunoglobulin molecule with pepsin destroys the larger part of the Fc portion, leaving an $F(ab')_2$ divalent molecule. The Fd region of the heavy chains is represented by the portion of these chains enclosed within the Fab fragment.

PHAGOCYTIC CELLS IN INFLAMMATION

Polymorphonuclear Leukocytes

Neutrophils Activation of the complement pathway at the inflammatory site yields C5a, one of the most active chemotactic peptides, which diffuses to adjoining blood vessels, thus initiating the following sequence of events: pavementing of the neutrophil against the endothelial cell, diapedesis between endothelial cells, and accumulation of cells at the site of inflammation. Although C5a is the most potent chemotactic agent, many other products of complement activation (C567, C3bBb), protein degradation

(fragments of collagen or fibrin), mast cell (histamine) or lymphocyte (lymphokine) activation, and breakdown of cell membrane lipid (leukotrienes) are chemotactic for neutrophils.[74] The second phase of neutrophil involvement in the inflammatory process is phagocytosis, which is initiated by interaction of receptors on the phagocytic cell with ligands on the immune complex or cellular debris. This process is facilitated by opsonization, which may be of two types. Nonspecific opsonization is accomplished by way of the C3b molecule in the immune complex or attached to the target cell and the receptor for C3b on the polymorph. This interaction facilitates contact

Table 2-17 Lysosomal Granules, Their Contents and Functions

Type of Lysosome	Enzyme	Function
Azurophil granules	Myeloperoxidase	Generates toxic oxidants from H_2O_2.
	β-glucuronidase	Cleaves glucuronic acid from oligosaccharides
	Lysozyme	Cleaves glucosidic link in bacterial cell walls
	Phospholipase	Degrades membrane phospholipids
	Ribonuclease	Degrades ribonucleic acid
	Elastase	Degrades cartilage proteoglycan, types I–IV collagen, elastin, fibronectin, clotting factors, complement components, IgG, IgM
	Cathepsin G	Degrades cartilage proteoglycan and types II and IV collagen, fibrinogen, clotting factors, complement components, IgG
Specific granules	Lactoferrin	Binds plasma iron taken up by RES of liver and stored as ferritin; promotes adhesion of neutrophils to endothelium
	Lysozyme	Degrades bacterial cell walls
	Latent collagenase	Collagenolytic, especially for type I collagen

(From Ohlsson K: Granulocyte proteases and their inhibitors in inflammation: basic concerns and clinical implications. In Venge P, Lindbom A (eds): Inflammation. Almqvist and Wiksell International, Stockholm, Sweden, 1985, p. 379, with permission.)

between the particle and the phagocytic cell. Specific opsonization involves specific antibody in the immune complex or attached to the target cell and the receptor for the Fc end of the immunoglobulin molecule on the polymorph. The IgG-Fc receptor interaction not only facilitates contact between particle and phagocytic cell but promotes ingestion of the particle.[63] Following receptor ligand binding, the polymorph engulfs the attached particle into a phagosome. Lysosomes, which contain proteolytic enzymes, fuse with the phagosome to form a phagolysosome in which the ingested material is degraded by enzymatic and other chemical actions. There are two types of lysosomes: azurophilic granules and specific granules. The enzyme contents of these granules and their specific actions are outlined in Table 2-17. In the process of phagocytosis, the contents of the phagolysosome are released into the tissues, where the degradative enzymes are tissue destructive. Collagenase, neutral proteases, and elastase activate certain components of the complement system such as C1 and C5, thereby releasing chemotactic and anaphylatoxic activities.

Eosinophils The eosinophils have a prominent role in certain inflammatory disorders. They have surface membrane receptors for the Fc of IgG and IgE and for C3b and C3d.[64] They migrate to sites of inflammation in response to eosinophil chemotactic factor of anaphylaxis (ECF-A). Eosinophils are triggered to

degranulate by fusion of the granular membranes with the cytoplasmic membrane. In this way the enzymatic contents of the granules are released into the extracellular milieu, where they function to degrade nonphagocytosable tissue constituents or foreign material such as parasites (Table 2-18).[66,67,68] Eosinophils are also capable of phagocytosing mast cell granules containing histamine and other proteases.[65]

Basophils and Mast Cells Basophils are the least common cell type in the peripheral blood but have great importance in the mediation of immediate (IgE-mediated) hypersensitivity. The mast cell is believed

Table 2-18 Inflammatory Mediators from Eosinophils

Mediator	Effect
Histaminase	Inactivates histamine
Aryl sulfatase	Neutralizes slow-reacting substance of anaphylaxis (S-RSA)
Phospholipase D	Neutralizes platelet activating factor (PAF)
Prostaglandins E_1 and E_2	Inhibit leukocyte histamine release[66]
Major basic protein	Neutralizes heparin[67]
Eosinophil peroxidase	Degrades leukotrienes[68]

to be the tissue counterpart of the basophil. They are both characterized by a high affinity membrane receptor for IgE and by the presence of abundant intracytoplasmic granules containing proteoglycans to which histamine, acid hydrolases, and neutral proteases are bound (Table 2-19). Degranulation is initiated by the binding of antigen to the IgE molecule on the mast cell membrane or by the action of anti-IgE. In addition to the preformed constituents of basophils listed in Table 2-19, mast cells (and to a lesser extent, basophils) secrete metabolites of the arachidonic acid pathway (leukotrienes and prostaglandins) and platelet activating factor (PAF).

Mononuclear Phagocytes

The macrophage and other accessory cells are emerging as an infinitely more central and complex system that was initially envisioned. The understanding of these cells is undergoing rapid expansion, and the reader is referred to recent reviews of this subject.[69,70] The circulating mononuclear phagocyte is the monocyte; those in tissues are Kupffer cells (liver), alveolar macrophages (lung), microglia (central nervous system), osteoclasts (bone), fixed macrophages (bone marrow, lymph node), type A syn-

oviocytes (synovium), and other undifferentiated tissue macrophages in serous cavities, nodes, spleen, and perivascular connective tissue. Although some controversy persists, it is generally believed that tissue macrophages are derived from blood monocytes that have become resident in tissue and developed characteristics peculiar to their microenvironment. Tissue macrophages can give rise to epithelioid cells or multinucleated giant cells characteristic of chronic inflammatory lesions. The macrophage membrane is the site of a multiplicity of receptors reflecting the complexity of functions ascribed to this cell (Table 2-20).

Monocytes are attracted to sites of inflammation by chemotactic agents such as C5a and by factors arising from kinin and coagulation system activation. They are facilitated in their egress from the capillaries and postcapillary venules by the vasodilating effects of histamine released from mast cells, basophils, and platelets.

The synthetic capability of macrophages places them in a central position in any inflammatory state. Complement components (C1, C2, C3, C4, C5; factors B, D, H, I; and properdin) and coagulation pathway components (factors V, VII, IX, X; prothrom-

Table 2-19 Inflammatory Constituents of Basophils

Mediator	Effect
Histamine	Increases vascular permeability
Eosinophilic chemotactic factor of anaphylaxis	Chemotactic for eosinophils
Neutrophil chemotactic factor	Chemotactic for neutrophils
Acid hydrolases β-glucuronidase β-galactosidase β-hexosaminidase Aryl sulfatase	Hydrolysis of carbohydrates
Neutral proteases (tryptase)	Generates anaphylatoxins from C3
Platelet activating factor	Causes platelet aggregation, hypotension, and potentiation of leukotriene generation

Table 2-20 Molecules with Receptors on Macrophages

Immunoglobulin
  Fc IgG$_1$, IgG$_3$, IgE

Complement
  C3b, C3d, C3bi
  C4b
  C5a

Other regulatory proteins
  Lactoferrin
  Fibrin
  Fibronectin
  Interferons
  Migration inhibition factor
  Migration activation factor

Other
  Some lipoproteins
  Lipopolysaccharide endotoxin
  Some glycoproteins
  Histamine
  Insulin

bin; thromboplastin) are synthesized by tissue macrophages (principally in the liver) but also in the inflammatory site. Macrophages also synthesize interleukin 1 (IL-1), which stimulates T-cell proliferation by initiating interleukin 2 (IL-2) production by T cells stimulated with antigen or lectin. IL-1 also increases body temperature, induces synthesis of acute phase proteins, stimulates cartilage resorption by connective-tissue cells, and causes proliferation of fibroblasts leading to fibrosis in some circumstances.[60] Nonimmune interferons (alpha, beta), synthesized by macrophages, cause increased phagocytosis by macrophages. Arachidonic acid from macrophage membrane phospholipid is metabolized to prostaglandins or leukotrienes that have important pro- and anti-inflammatory effects, as described previously.

One of the key roles of these accessory cells is that of antigen presentation. In order for an antigen to induce an immune response, it must be "presented" to lymphocytes by an antigen presenting cell that bears class II histocompatibility antigens on the surface, such as a dendritic cell (for a primary response) or a macrophage, dendritic cell or B lymphocyte (for a secondary response). In most instances the macrophage processes the antigen after phagocytosis in such a way that when it is presented on the cell surface together with a class II molecule, it is immunogenic.

IMMUNOLOGIC MECHANISMS OF TISSUE DAMAGE

Autoimmunity is a term that is the modern equivalent of Erlich's "horror autotoxicus." It describes a situation in which the immune system causes tissue damage as a consequence of failure to differentiate self from nonself. Such failure of self-recognition could result from an intrinsic failure of the immune system to recognize a normal self-component, from alteration of the self-antigen by its combination with drug or infectious agent, or from exposure of a neoantigen by degradation of self-antigens as a result of inflammatory processes. An autoimmune disease may also result from immunologic cross-reactivity between an extrinsic antigen and a self-antigen.

It is convenient to divide immunologic effector mechanisms into four types based upon the classification of Coombs and Gell.[71]

Type I: Anaphylactic Reaction

In the anaphylactic type of hypersensitivity reaction, mast cells in tissue (basophils in blood) bind IgE molecules via their Fc receptors. When specific antigen binds to the IgE molecules, cross linking them, the mast cell is induced to undergo degranulation with release of vasoactive substances contained in the granules (histamine and slow-reacting substance of anaphylaxis) into the immediate environment of the cell (Fig. 2-14). These pharmacologically active mediators are responsible for the principal clinical manifestations of allergic rhinitis, asthma, urticaria, and anaphylaxis. The immediate wheal-flare skin reaction is the prototype of a type I response. IgE may subserve another component of the humoral system by localizing the antibody response. By reacting with antigen in tissue sites, IgE produces increased capillary permeability that allows an influx of serum antibodies into the target organ to participate further in the immunologic defense of the host. Mast cell degranulation can also be brought about by the anaphylatoxins C3a and C5a; by drugs such as codeine, morphine, and calcium ionophores; and by T-cell products (histamine releasing factors). Activation of the mast cell leads to the synthesis of prostaglandin A_2, thromboxane A_2, and leukotrienes, from catabolism of arachidonic acid from the cell membrane.

Type II: Cytotoxic Reaction

Serum antibody, primarily IgG, interacts with antigen that either is part of a cell surface or has become attached to a cell (Fig. 2-15). Cell lysis results through activation of the complement system or by the cytotoxic action of K cells. K cells (cells that have Fc receptors and participate in cell lysis) are joined to the target cell antigen by an immunoglobulin bridge. The proximity of K cell and target permits the lysosomal enzymes released by the K cell to lyse the target cell membrane, independent of the cytolytic complement components. In the case of drugs, two mechanisms have been recognized: antibody reacting against a drug-cell surface protein complex (e.g., penicillin) and antibody reacting against a surface membrane that has been altered by a drug (e.g., alpha methyldopa). Disorders characterized by type II reactions include autoimmune hemolytic anemia, thrombocytopenia and leukopenia, inactivation of certain hor-

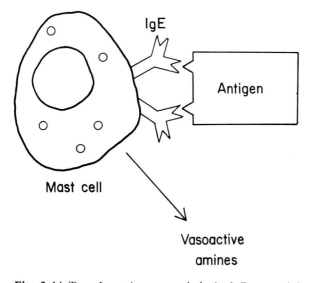

Fig. 2-14 Type I reaction or anaphylaxis. IgE or reaginic antibodies are bound to target cells in tissues that in most instances are mast cells. Upon reaction with specific antigen, release of vasoactive substances (bradykinin, histamine, SRS-A) occurs, leading to the classic allergic reactions.

mones, blood clotting factors and enzymes, and Goodpasture's syndrome.

Type III: Immune Complex Reaction

The formation of immune complexes is a physiologic event. The elimination of complexes by phagocytic cells ordinarily prevents the development of tissue damage involving immune complexes, although some complexes, under certain circumstances, can induce widespread tissue damage—immune complex disease.

Immune complexes may contain antibody of any class bound noncovalently (and hence, reversibly) to an antigen. Immune complex disease involves either extrinsic or self-antigens. Replicating organisms such as bacteria or viruses may cause a persisting infection with constant release of antigen. Infective endocarditis is an example of this type of immune complex disease. When the inciting antigen is a self-antigen, or an antigen that cross-reacts with a self-antigen, an autoimmune immune complex disease may result.

Not all immune complexes are pathogenic. The circumstances that lead to immune complex disease

include increased vascular permeability, appropriate immune complex size and composition, and activation of complement. Increased vascular permeability is mediated by vasoactive amines (especially histamine) released from basophils and mast cells (and in some species, platelets), after activation by mechanisms described previously. Immune complexes that are potentially pathogenic are those that are formed under conditions of slight antigen excess, contain at least two IgG molecules, and activate complement.

The location of immune complex deposition is influenced by immune complex size, specific characteristics of the antigen, and hemodynamic factors. Immune complex size is influenced by both the size of the antigen and the number of immunoglobulin molecules in the immune complex lattice. The latter depends on the number of antigenic determinants on the antigen and the affinity of the antigen-antibody interaction. Complexes of relatively small size (i.e.,

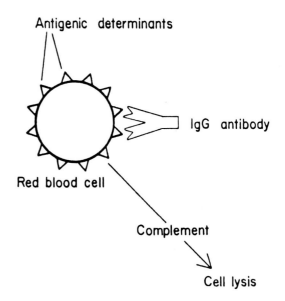

Fig. 2-15 Type II reaction or immune cytolysis. Specific antibodies, usually IgG, react with antigens and form antigen-antibody complexes. These are normally removed from the circulation by the mononuclear phagocytic system. However, if the antigen is located on a cell surface or is bound to a cell, cell lysis occurs through activation of complement. If the antigen is an essential enzyme, blood clotting factor, or hormone, this reaction will lead to inactivation of that substance.

two IgG molecules plus antigen) are more likely to pass through basement membrane of the vasculature and deposit in tissue. Such immune complexes are represented by the subepithelial deposits of glomerulonephritis. Larger immune complexes do not pass through the basement membrane and hence deposit in a subendothelial location (the subendothelial deposits of glomerulonephritis) (Fig. 2-16). In some circumstances charge characteristics of the antigen may predispose immune complexes to deposit in certain locations. Thus DNA in immune complexes carries

a strong negative charge and may therefore attach via this nonimmune mechanism to positively charged basement membrane, preventing its passage through the basement membrane irrespective of complex size.[72] Antigen charge may also provide a mechanism for in situ formation of immune complexes: free DNA may bind to basement membrane and form the focus for attachment of free IgG anti-DNA antibodies or of other immune complexes that contain free antigen-binding sites. Hemodynamic characteristics influence immune complex localization. Areas of tur-

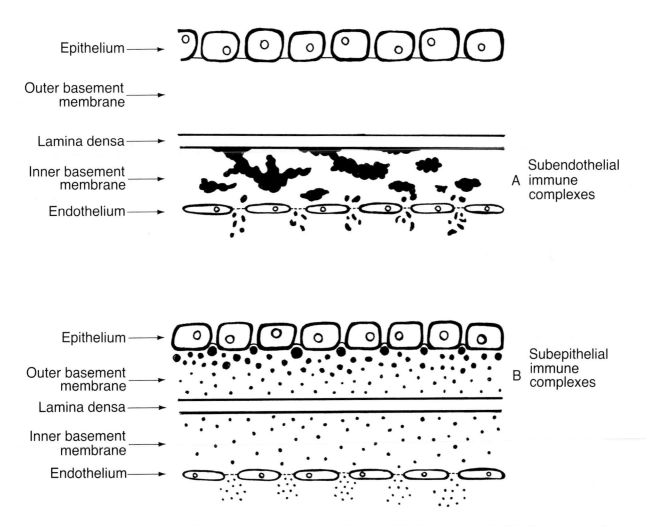

Fig. 2-16 The deposition of immune complexes in the subendothelial **(A)** and subepithelial **(B)** locations of a blood vessel.

Table 3-25 Pharmacologic Actions of the Immunosuppressive Agents

	Prednisone	Cyclophosphamide	Azathioprine	Methotrexate
Anti-inflammatory effects				
Inflammatory response	+ + +	±	+	+
Wound healing	+	−	−	−
Granulocyte function	+	±	±	±
Immunosuppressive effects				
Macrophages	+	±	±	±
B lymphocytes	+	+ +	±	±
Immunoglobulin concentration	+ +	+ +	+	+
T lymphocytes	+ +	+	±	±
Delayed hypersensitivity	+ +	−	±	±
Lymphocyte transformation	+	±	+	+
Homograft rejection	+ +	+	+ +	+

is replicating. Both cyclophosphamide and azathioprine are maximally effective in inhibiting immunologic responses when their administration coincides with the period of proliferation of the specific immunologically competent cells.

Azathioprine

Cytotoxic agents were developed for treatment of neoplastic diseases. Their primary mode of action is to prevent replication of rapidly dividing cells. Azathioprine is converted in vivo to 6-mercaptopurine, which is an analogue of hypoxanthine.[333] The metabolic ribonucleotides lead to feedback inhibition of phosphoribosyl pyrophosphate conversion in purine nucleotide synthesis, inhibition of the inosinic acid to xanthylic acid pathway (purine nucleoside phosphorylase), and incorporation of nucleotide triphosphates into cellular DNA.

Azathioprine suppresses cell-mediated immune function and inhibits monocyte activity.[334–336] These immunosuppressive effects are related primarily to inhibition of cell growth during the S phase of division. A measurable decrease in antibody synthesis occurs with long-term administration, and occasionally a decrease in serum antibody concentration is observed.

The drug is administered orally with approximately 50 percent absorption. The plasma half-life is approximately 75 min. The kidneys are the major route of excretion. Oral and GI ulcerations are important manifestations of toxicity. Nausea may be prominent in some patients. A major form of dose-related toxicity is depression of the bone marrow with leukopenia and less commonly thrombocytopenia and anemia. An idiosyncratic arrest of granulocyte maturation that occurs shortly after initiation of therapy has been described. Other side effects include hepatitis with abnormal liver function tests, fever, and rash. Oncogenic effects are predominantly related to a statistical increase in the occurrence of lymphoma, including disease of the CNS. Other tumors include those of the skin and cervix.

Experience with azathioprine in the rheumatic diseases of childhood is limited.[337,338] Although the usual dose in cancer chemotherapy is 3 mg/kg/day, children with rheumatic diseases (JRA, SLE) appear to be sensitive to the marrow suppressing effects of the drug and should be initially treated at a lower level (for example, 1 mg/kg/day).

Cyclophosphamide

The alkylating agents such as cyclophosphamide and chlorambucil are examples of non-cell-cycle-dependent drugs and substitute alkyl radicals into DNA, RNA, and proteins.[339] These agents act potentially on all cells including those that are mitotically inactive (G_0 interphase) at the time of administration, for example, memory T cells.[340–342]

Cyclophosphamide has prominent anti-inflammatory actions by its effect upon mononuclear cells and cellular immunity. Alkylating agents are capable of depleting the pool of immunologically competent small lymphocytes and lead to B- and T-cell lymphopenia. In humans, depression of IgG and IgM synthesis occurs, and there is a measurable decrease of serum antibody concentration after chronic administration.[340,341]

Cyclophosphamide is metabolized in the liver to the active product by the P-450 mixed-function oxidase system of the smooth endoplasmic reticulum. Excretion is primarily urinary; therefore, the dose must be reduced in patients with renal impairment. The half-life of cyclophosphamide is approximately 7 h.

The alkylating agents are very potent drugs for the treatment of severe rheumatic disease in children and have prominent toxic effects.[343–346] Alopecia following cyclophosphamide appears to be related to dose and duration of treatment and is usually reversible. In our experience it has not been a significant problem. Sterility has been reported and is an important consideration in treatment of children.[347,348] Granulocytopenia is dose-dependent, and thrombocytopenia is less common than with chlorambucil. (As with azathioprine, the initial oral dose in children with rheumatic diseases should be low, approximately 1 mg/kg/day). Pulmonary fibrosis has been reported in a small number of patients on daily cyclophosphamide therapy. The alkylating agents have been associated with an increased risk of leukemia and lymphomas, which has been estimated at 0.1 to 1.0 percent in patients with rheumatic diseases on oral therapy.[349]

Cyclophosphamide and its metabolic products are direct irritants to the mucosa of the bladder and may cause hemorrhagic cystitis, fibrosis, or carcinoma.[350] Adequate hydration should be maintained in the child receiving daily cyclophosphamide. This is particularly true during the summer months. The child should always urinate before going to bed so that the metabolic by-products of this drug are not allowed to have prolonged contact with the mucosa of the bladder. Because cystitis is a significant threat, some physicians prefer the use of chlorambucil as an alkylating agent or use cyclophosphamide as IV-pulse therapy and avoid oral administration (Chs. 7 and 9). IV-pulse therapy places the child at less risk for toxicities including hemorrhagic cystitis and confines those risks to a short period of time each month instead of every day. Hydration during pulse therapy should be with isotonic saline in order to prevent inappropriate antidiuretic hormone (ADH) secretion.[351] Some patients develop nausea and vomiting even after IV-pulse therapy.

The total granulocyte count is used to determine the maximum IV pulse that can be administered.[323] The dose should be adjusted to maintain the total count at $\geq 1,500/mm^3$ ($\geq 1.5 \times 10^9/L$). The nadir of granulocytopenia with IV therapy occurs between the first and second week. There is no direct association between the degree of granulocytopenia and the clinical effectiveness of the drug. Once determined, the monthly dose that a patient will tolerate generally remains the same over an extended period. Corticosteroids are synergistic with cyclophosphamide and probably aid in protecting the bone marrow from the cytopenic effects of the drug.

Methotrexate

Methotrexate was introduced into the therapy of hematologic malignancies in 1948, and subsequently in RA,[352] as an effective and relatively safe cytostatic agent. It is a potent inhibitor of dihydrofolate reductase and interferes thereby with the metabolic transfer of single carbon units in methylation reactions, especially those involved in synthesis of thymidylate and purine deoxynucleotides, essential components of DNA. Methotrexate may act as an anti-inflammatory agent in RA by inhibiting the proliferation of synovial cells.

Sixty percent of the orally administered drug is absorbed with a direct relationship between dose and plasma concentration. The plasma half-life is approximately 2 h.[354] Approximately 50 percent of the drug is protein-bound and can be displaced by salicylates and sulfa drugs,[354] and 80 percent is excreted unchanged in the urine within 8 to 48 h. The dose must be lowered in patients with renal insufficiency.

The advantages of methotrexate in JRA or JDM are its apparent efficacy at doses well below those known to produce predictable toxicity and its demonstrated safety from the standpoint of long-term oncogenesis.[355] Toxicity includes bone marrow suppression,[356,357] GI ulcerations, diarrhea and hemorrhagic enteritis, alopecia, dermatitis, and hepatic cirrhosis.[358] Folinic acid is a specific anecdote, especially for aplastic crises. Neurotoxicity and nephrotoxicity do not appear to be problems at antirheumatic dose levels. Acute renal toxicity occurs only at very high blood levels, e.g., 10^{-4} molar.

Progressive cirrhosis of the liver is not an expected toxic effect in patients on weekly therapy as long as certain risks—alcoholism, malnutrition, viral hepatitis, diabetes mellitus, and obesity[359]—are meticulously excluded. The development of hepatic disease appears to be related to these predisposing factors, frequency of administration, weekly dose, and duration of therapy in adults.[358,359] Hepatic fibrosis seems to be essentially prevented by low-dose, once-a-week regimens.

Methotrexate has been used extensively in adult RA after trials that documented the efficacy of low-dose weekly oral pulse therapy.[360–364] Approximately 1 percent of adults with RA can develop, early or late, acute pulmonary insufficiency and interstitial pneumonitis with effusions as an idiosyncratic reaction to methotrexate therapy.[365]

In JRA, current studies have employed doses of 5 or 10 mg/M²/wk given orally.[366,367] A double-blind randomized placebo-controlled trial has recently been completed in children with JRA by the Pediatric Rheumatology Collaborative Study Group.[367a] The study included two methotrexate groups, 5 mg/M²/wk and 10 mg/M²/wk, and a placebo group. To be eligible for enrollment, patients had to have failed NSAID therapy and to have clinically active, poorly controlled disease. Up to two concurrent NSAIDs were allowed, as was prednisone at a dose $\leq$ 10 mg/day. Sixty-six patients were randomized and 63 were evaluated for efficacy. Only 31 percent of the placebo patients were judged to be improved after 6 months of therapy, whereas 78 percent of the children in the 5 mg/M²/wk group and 79 percent in the 10 mg/M²/wk group were. The change from baseline in the sum of severity score averaged -2.8 for the placebo group, -17 for the 5 mg/M²/wk methotrexate group (NS), and -75 for the 10 mg/M²/wk methotrexate group ($P = 0.027$). Dropouts due to adverse reactions included 1 child for proteinuria in the 5 mg/M² group, and 2 in the 10 mg/M² group: 1 for hematuria and 1 for an increase in the concentrations of the liver enzymes.

In other diseases such as JDM, oral weekly pulse therapy has been administered in doses that have ranged from 0.3 to 0.6 mg/kg/wk. The bioavailability of orally administered methotrexate, although questioned in children compared to adults, probably does not pertain to doses of this level. Methotrexate can be given in a variety of protocols. Generally the oral weekly pulse dose is currently preferred and IV pulse or IM administration is used only when oral therapy is not tolerated because of nausea or is not possible. The drug should be given on an empty stomach with clear liquids early in the morning at least 60 min before breakfast.

An extensive protocol for monitoring methotrexate toxicity has been developed by the Pediatric Rheumatology Collaborative Study Group. Baseline studies include complete blood count (CBC), urinalysis, blood urea nitrogen (BUN), creatinine, total serum bilirubin, AST, ALT, alkaline phosphatase, and albumin. Additional studies that are performed periodically are a creatinine clearance, ophthalmologic examination, pulmonary function tests, and chest radiograph. Monitoring during the course of the treatment should consist of a CBC, urinalysis, and enzyme studies every 2 weeks for the first 3 months and then every month thereafter.

It is important to realize that measurement of liver enzyme levels guards against the infrequent occurrence of acute hepatic toxicity and not the progressive development of cirrhosis. Additional monitoring to prevent toxicity in one study employed assays of methotrexate drug levels; the serum concentration of methotrexate was measured in order to ensure that there had been complete clearance of the drug from the vascular compartment in 1 day.[368] Levels were determined 1 h after the morning oral dose and 24 h later. Acceptable concentrations at 1 h were approximately 6×10^{-7} molar (range 0.22 to 12×10^{-7} molar) and undetectable levels at 24 h, preferably $< 2.2 \times 10^{-8}$ molar but no greater than 1×10^{-7} molar.

There are many drug interactions that may occur with methotrexate; one of the more important in children is with salicylates and other NSAIDs.[369] Salicylates are known to block the renal tubular excretion of methotrexate and displace methotrexate from plasma proteins. Both of these factors increase the bioavailability of methotrexate and therefore its potential toxicity. Salicylates should either not be used when methotrexate is given or used cautiously with strict adherence to monitoring plasma levels. The child's parents should be made aware of the many over-the-counter products that contain salicylates. NSAIDs may not produce this same effect, or at least not so pronounced a one as ASA.[370]

IMMUNOREGULATORY DRUGS

New classes of agents for the treatment of autoimmune disease are being developed. Among these are enzyme inhibitors that exert their effects at key steps in the purine pathway (adenosine deaminase, purine nucleoside phosphorylase, S-adenosyl homocysteine hydrolase, etc.), have specific immunologic actions (anti-T-cell serum, transfer factor, thymosin, etc.), degrade toxic oxygen radicals (superoxide dismutase), or produce ameliorating effects through mechanisms not completely understood (certain antihelminthic drugs, interleukins, etc.). Among the latter agents, levamisole, an immunostimulant, has been used in children with SLE and JRA in small trials.[371,372] Initial reports in JRA were not encouraging, and there have been a number of deaths. Pharmacologic modifications may produce analogues of more therapeutic promise.

Antilymphocyte sera in general use are heterogeneous agents or, if sufficiently purified, may be directed specifically against the T-cell population. They are maximally effective as immunosuppressive agents if administered before antigenic challenge. They are frequently used in transplant surgery, but efficacy in the pediatric autoimmune diseases has not been evaluated to any extent. Adverse reactions include hypersensitivity reactions, serum sickness, hepatitis, and potential oncogenic effects.

Cyclosporin A

Cyclospirin A is a cyclic compound that consists of 11 amino acids and is resistant to proteolytic digestion in the GI tract. In interferes primarily with interleukin 2 (Il-2) production and cell-mediated immune responses.[373–376] It has been used to prevent rejection of renal allografts and to treat inflammatory diseases such as RA and uveitis.[377] Major toxicities include nephropathy,[378,379] hypertension, and hepatotoxicity.[380] Hypertrichosis and gingival hyperplasia have been observed. Renal toxicity is related to high doses of the drug and may result in hypertension from interstitial fibrosis or tubular atrophy, even in adults treated with relatively low doses (3 to 5 mg/kg/day orally). Concomitant use of NSAIDs may exacerbate this toxic effect of the drug. The risk of lymphoma has been reported at approximately 0.5 percent. Reports of trials in JRA[381] and other rheumatic diseases in children are beginning to appear.

REFERENCES

1. Lindsley CB: Pharmacotherapy of juvenile rheumatoid arthritis. Pediatr Clin North Am 28:161, 1981
2. Laxer RM, Shore AD, Silverman ED: Drug therapy in juvenile rheumatoid arthritis. In Kean WF (ed): Sulfasalazine in Rheumatic Disease. Proceedings of the International Rheumatology Conference. Medicöpea, Quebec, 1987, p. 45
3. Huskisson EC (ed): Anti-Rheumatic Drugs. Praeger Scientific, New York, 1983
4. American Hospital Formulary Service: Drug Information 88. American Society of Hospital Pharmacy, Bethesda, Md, 1988, p. 978
5. Lamont-Havers RW, Wagner BM (eds): Proceedings of the Conference on Effects of Chronic Salicylate Administration. U.S. Government Printing Office, Washington D.C., 1966, p. 199
6. Furst DE: Salicylates in pediatric rheumatology. In Moore TD (ed): Arthritis in Childhood. Report of the Eightieth Ross Conference in Pediatric Research. Ross Laboratories, Columbus, Ohio, 1981, p. 104
7. Hollister JR: Aspirin in juvenile rheumatoid arthritis (editorial). Am J Dis Child 139:866, 1985
8. Dromgoole SH, Furst DE, Paulus HE: Rational approaches to the use of salicylates in the treatment of rheumatoid arthritis. Semin Arthritis Rheum 11:257, 1981
9. Lasagna L, McMahon FG (eds): New perspectives on aspirin therapy. Proceedings of a symposium. Am J Med 18, suppl., 1983
10. Oates JA, FitzGerald GA, Branch RA et al: Clinical implications of prostaglandin and thromboxane A_2 formation. N Engl J Med 319:689, 761, 1988
11. Burch JW, Stanford N, Majerus PW: Inhibition of platelet prostaglandin synthetase by oral aspirin. J Clin Invest 61:314, 1978
12. Preston FE, Whipps S, Jackson CA et al: Inhibition of prostacyclin and platelet thromboxane A_2 after low-dose aspirin. N Engl J Med 304:76, 1981
13. Pedersen AK, FitzGerald GA: Dose-related kinetics of aspirin. Presystemic acetylation of platelet cyclooxygenase. N Engl J Med 311:1206, 1984
14. Levy G: Clinical pharmacokinetics of aspirin. Pediatrics, suppl., 62:867, 1978
15. Done AK, Yaffe SJ, Clayton JM: Aspirin dosage for infants and children. J Pediatr 95:617, 1979
16. Mandelli M, Tognoni G: Monitoring plasma concentration of salicylate. Clin Pharmacokinet 5:424, 1980
17. Kvien TK, Olsson B, Høyeraal HM: Acetylsalicylic acid and juvenile rheumatoid arthritis. Effect of dosage interval on the serum salicylic acid level. Acta Paediatr Scand 74:755, 1985
18. Pachman LM, Olufs R, Procknal JA et al: Pharmacokinetic monitoring of salicylate therapy in children with juvenile rheumatoid arthritis. Arthritis Rheum 22:826, 1979
19. Bergman GE, Phillippidis P, Naiman JL: Severe gas-

trointestinal hemorrhage and anemia after therapeutic doses of aspirin in normal children. J Pediatr 88:501, 1976

20. Fromm D: Salicylate and gastric mucosal damage. Pediatrics, suppl., 62:938, 1978
21. Lanza FL, Royer GL, Jr, Nelson RS: Endoscopic evaluation of the effects of aspirin, buffered aspirin, and enteric-coated aspirin on gastric and duodenal mucosa. N Engl J Med 303:136, 1980
22. Manso C., Taranta A, Nydick I: Effect of aspirin administration on serum glutamic oxaloacetic and glutamic pyruvic transaminases in children. Proc Soc Exp Biol Med 93:83, 1956
23. Kornreich H, Maloug NN, Hanson V: Acute hepatic dysfunction in juvenile rheumatoid arthritis. J Pediatr 79:27, 1971
24. Rich RR, Johnson JS: Salicylate hepatotoxicity in patients with juvenile rheumatoid arthritis. Arthritis Rheum 16:1, 1973
25. Seaman WE, Ishak KG, Plotz PH: Aspirin-induced hepatotoxicity in patients with systemic lupus erythematosus. Ann Intern Med 80:1, 1974
26. Zucker P, Daum F, Cohen MI: Aspirin hepatitis. Am J Dis Child 129:1433, 1975
27. Schaller JG: Chronic salicylate administration in juvenile rheumatoid arthritis: aspirin "hepatitis" and its clinical significance. Pediatrics, suppl., 62:916, 1978
28. Ulshen MH, Grabd RJ, Crain JD et al: Hepatotoxicity with encephalopathy associated with aspirin therapy in rheumatoid arthritis. J Pediatr 93:1034, 1978
29. Rachelefsky GS, Kar NC, Coulson A et al: Serum enzyme abnormalities in juvenile rheumatoid arthritis. Pediatrics 58:730, 1976
30. Athreya BH, Moser G, Cecil HS et al: Aspirin-induced hepatotoxicity in juvenile rheumatoid arthritis. A prospective study. Arthritis Rheum 18:347, 1975
31. Miller JJ, III, Weissman DB: Correlations between transaminase concentrations and serum salicylate concentration in juvenile rheumatoid arthritis. Arthritis Rheum 19:115, 1976
32. Bernstein BH, Singsen BH, King KK et al: Aspirin-induced hepatotoxicity and its effect on juvenile rheumatoid arthritis. Am J Dis Child 131:659, 1977
33. Hadchouel M, Prieur A-M, Griscelli C: Acute hemorrhagic, hepatic and neurologic manifestations in juvenile rheumatoid arthritis: possible relationship to drugs or infection. J Pediatr 106:561, 1985
34. Silverman ED, Miller JJ, Bernstein B et al: Consumption coagulopathy associated with systemic juvenile rheumatoid arthritis. J Pediatr 103:872, 1983
35. Starko KM, Ray CG, Dominguez LB et al: Reye's syndrome and salicylate use. Pediatrics 66:859, 1980
36. Diagnosis and treatment of Reye's syndrome. Consensus Conference. JAMA 246:2441, 1981
37. Remington PL, Shabino CL, McGee H et al: Reye syndrome and juvenile rheumatoid arthritis in Michigan. Am J Dis Child 139:870, 1985
38. Kauffman RE, Roberts RJ: Asprin use and Reye syndrome (commentary). Pediatrics 79:1049, 1987
38. Arrowsmith JB, Kennedy DL, Kuritsky JN et al: National patterns of aspirin use and Reye syndrome reporting, United States, 1980–1985. Pediatrics 79:858, 1987
40. Rennebohm RM, Heubi JE, Daugherty CC et al: Reye's syndrome in children receiving salicylate therapy for connective tissue disease. J Pediatr 107:877, 1985
41. Hurwitz ES, Barrett MJ, Bregman D et al: Public Health Service study of Reye's syndrome and medications. JAMA 257:1905, 1987
42. Committee on Infectious Diseases: Aspirin and Reye syndrome. Pediatrics 69:810, 1982
43. Lawson AAH, MacLean N: Renal disease and drug therapy in rheumatoid arthritis. Ann Rheum Dis 25:441, 1966
44. Clive DM, Stoff JS: Renal syndromes associated with nonsteroidal anti-inflammatory drugs. N Engl J Med 310:563, 1984
45. Kimberly RP, Plotz PH: Aspirin-induced depression of renal function. N Engl J Med 296:418, 1977
46. Plotz PH: Analgesic nephropathy. Arch Intern Med 143:1676, 1983
47. Nanra RS, Stuart-Taylor J, DeLeon AH et al: Analgesic nephropathy: etiology, clinical syndrome and clinicopathologic correlations in Australia. Kidney Int 13:79, 1978
48. Wortmann DW, Kelsch RC, Kuhns L et al: Renal papillary necrosis in juvenile rheumatoid arthritis. J Pediatr 97:37, 1980
49. Allen RC, Petty RE, Lirenman DS et al: Renal papillary necrosis in children with chronic arthritis. J Pediatr 140:16, 1986
50. Spuehler O, Zollinger HU: Die chronisch-interstitielle nephritis. Z Klin Med 151:1, 1953
51. Murray T, Goldberg M: Chronic interstitial nephritis: etiologic factors. Ann Intern Med 83:453, 1975
52. Mihatsch MJ, Hofer HO, Gudap F et al: Capillary sclerosis of the urinary tract and analgesic nephropathy. Clin Nephrol 20:285, 1983
53. Kimberly RP, Bowden RE, Keiser HR et al: Reduction of renal function by newer nonsteroidal anti-inflammatory drugs. Am J Med 64:804, 1978
54. Shelley JG: Pharmacological mechanisms of analgesic nephropathy. Kidney Int 13:15, 1978
55. Muther RS, Bennett W: Effects of aspirin on GFR in normal humans. Ann Intern Med 92:386, 1980
56. Muther RS, Potter DM, Bennett WM: Aspirin-induced depression of glomerular filtration rate in nor-

mal humans: role of sodium balance. Ann Intern Med 94:317, 1981

57. Lifschitz MD: Renal effects of nonsteroidal anti-inflammatory agents. J Lab Clin Med 102:313, 1983

58. Garella S, Matarese RA: Renal effects of prostaglandins and clinical adverse effects of nonsteroidal antiinflammatory agents. Medicine 63:165, 1984

59. Dubach UC, Rosner B, Pfister E: Epidemiologic study of abuse of analgesics containing phenacetin. Renal morbidity and mortality (1968–1979). N Engl J Med 308:357, 1983

60. Murray TG, Stolley PD, Anthony JC: Epidemiologic study of regular analgestic use and end-stage renal disease. Arch Intern Med 143:1687, 1983

61. Slepian IK, Mathews KP, McLean JA: Aspirin-sensitive asthma. Chest 87:386, 1985

62. Rachelefsky GS, Coulson A, Siegel SC et al: Aspirin intolerance in chronic childhood asthma: detected by oral challenge. Pediatrics 56:443, 1975

63. Fischer TJ, Guilfoile TD, Kesarwala HH et al: Adverse pulmonary responses to aspirin and acetaminophen in chronic childhood asthma. Pediatrics 71:313, 1983

64. Brandt KG, Palmoski MJ: Effects of salicylates and other nonsteroidal anti-inflammatory drugs on articular cartilage. Amer J Med 77:suppl. 1A, 65, 1984

65. Mäkelä A-L, Yrjänä T, Mattila M: Dosage of salicylates for children with juvenile rheumatoid arthritis. Acta Paediatr Scand 68:423, 1979

66. Poe TE, Mutchie KD, Saunders GH et al: Total and free salicylate concentrations in juvenile rheumatoid arthritis. J Rheumatol 7:717, 1980

67. Bardara M, Cislaghi GU, Mandelli M et al: Value of monitoring plasma salicylate levels in treating juvenile rheumatoid arthritis. Arch Dis Child 53:381, 1978

68. Brewer EJ: Nonsteroidal anti-inflammatory agents. Arthritis Rheum 20:513, 1977

69. Simon LS, Mills JA: Nonsteroidal antiinflammatory drugs. N Engl J Med 302:1179, 1237, 1980

70. Schlegel SI, Paulus HE: Nonsteroidal antiinflammatory drugs—use in rheumatic disease, side effects and interactions. Bull Rheum Dis 36:1, 1986

71. Bombardier C, Chalmers A, Jamali F et al: Proceedings of workshops. The monitoring of clinical and pharmacological effects of antiinflammatory drugs in populations. J Rheumatol 15:suppl. 17, 1988

72. Baum C, Kennedy DL, Forbes MB: Utilization of nonsteroidal antiinflammatory drugs. Arthritis Rheum 28:686, 1985

73. Brewer EJ, Jr, Arroyo I: Use of nonsteroidal antiinflammatory drugs in children. Pediatr Ann 15:575, 1986

74. Pediatric Rheumatology Collaborative Study Group (PRCSG): Methodology and studies of children with juvenile rheumatoid arthritis. J Rheumatol 9:107, 1982

75. Bass JC, Athreya BH, Brewer EJ et al: A once-daily antiinflammatory drug, oxaprozin, in the treatment of juvenile rheumatoid arthritis. The Pediatric Rheumatology Collaborative Study Group (letter). J Rheumatol 12:384, 1985

76. Lempiäinen M, Mäkelä A-L: Determination of proquazone and its m-hydroxy metabolite by high-performance liquid chromatography. Clinical application: pharmacokinetics of proquazone in children with juvenile rheumatoid arthritis. J Chromatogr 31:105, 1985

77. Bass J, Athreya B, Brandstrup N et al: Flurbiprofen in the treatment of juvenile rheumatoid arthritis. J Rheumatol 13:1081, 1986

78. Paulus HE: Pharmacological considerations. In Roth, SH (ed): Handbook of Drug Therapy in Rheumatology. PSG Publishing, Littleton, Mass, 1985, p. 39

79. Barron KS, Person DA, Brewer EJ: The toxicity of nonsteroidal antiinflammatory drugs in juvenile rheumatoid arthritis. J Rheumatol 9:149, 1982

80. O'Brien WM, Bagby GF: Rare adverse reactions to nonsteroial antiinflammatory drugs. J Rheumatol 12:13, 1985

81. Lovell DJ, Giannini EH, Brewer EJ, Jr: Time course of response to nonsteroidal antiinflammatory drugs in juvenile rheumatoid arthritis. Arthritis Rheum 27:1433, 1984

82. Lanza FL: Endoscopic studies of gastric and duodenal injury after the use of ibuprofen, aspirin, and other nonsteroidal antiinflammatory agents. Am J Med 76:19, 1984

83. Miller TA, Jacobson ED: Gastrointestinal cytoprotection by prostaglandins. Gut 20:75, 1979

84. Dunn MJ, Patrono C (eds): Renal Effects of Nonsteroidal Antiinflammatory Drugs. Proceedings of a Symposium. Am J Med 81:2B, 1986

85. Husserl FE, Lange RK, Kantrow CM: Renal papillary necrosis and pyelonephritis accompanying fenoprofen therapy. JAMA 242:1896, 1979

86. Ray PE, Rigolizzo D, Wara DR et al: Naproxen nephrotoxicity in a 2-year-old child. Am J Dis Child 142:524, 1988

87. Mitchell H, Muirden KD, Kincaid-Smith P: Indomethacin-induced renal papillary necrosis in juvenile chronic arthritis (letter). Lancet 2:558, 1982

88. Sedor JR, Davidson EW, Dunn MJ: Renal effects of nonsteroidal antiinflammatory drugs in healthy subjects. Am J Med 81:suppl. 81B, 58, 1986

89. Blockshear JL, Napier HS, Davidman M et al: Renal complications of nonsteroidal antiinflammatory drugs: identification and monitoring of those at risk. Semin Arthritis Rheum 14:163, 1985

90. Price T, Venning H, Ansell BM: Ibuprofen in juvenile chronic arthritis. Clin Exp Rheumatol 3:59, 1985

91. Samuelson CO, Williams HJ: Ibuprofen-associated aseptic meningitis in systemic lupus erythematosus. West J Med 131:57, 1979

92. Mamus SW, Burton JD, Groat JD et al: Ibuprofen-associated pure white-cell aplasia. N Engl J Med 314:624, 1986

93. Guidry JB, Ogburn CI, Jr, Griffin FM, Jr: Fatal autoimmune hemolytic anemia associated with ibuprofen. JAMA 242:68, 1979

94. Lee CY, Finkler A: Acute intoxication due to ibuprofen overdose. Arch Pathol Lab Med 110:747, 1986

95. Court H, Volans GH: Poisoning after overdose with nonsteroidal antiinflammatory drugs. Adver Drug 3:1, 1984

96. Moran H, Hanna DB, Ansell BM et al: Naproxen in juvenile chronic polyarthritis. Ann Rheum Dis 38:152, 1979

97. Cashman TM, Starns RJ, Johnson J et al: Comparative effects of naproxen and aspirin on fever in children. J Pediatr 95:626, 1979

98. Mäkelä A-L: Naproxen in the treatment of juvenile rheumatoid arthritis. Scand J Rheumatol 6:193, 1977

99. Ansell BM, Hanna B, Moran H et al: Naproxen in juvenile chronic polyarthritis. Eur J Rheumatol Inflam 2:79, 1979

100. Nicholls A, Hazelman B, Todd RM et al: Long-term evaluation of naproxen suspension in juvenile chronic arthritis. Curr Med Res Opin 8:204, 1982

101. Kvein TK, Høyeraal HM, Sandstad B: Naproxen and acetylsalicylic acid in the treatment of pauciarticular and polyarticular juvenile rheumatoid arthritis. Scand J Rheumatol 13:342, 1984

102. Lo TCN, Martin MA: Autoimmune haemolytic anaemia associated with naproxen suppositories (unreviewed report). Br Med J 292:1430, 1986

103. Mayou S, Black MM: Pseudoprophyria due to naproxen (letter). Br J Dermatol 114:519, 1986

104. Fredell EW, Strand LJ: Naproxen overdose (letter). JAMA 238:938, 1977

105. Orudis (ketoprofen). Product monograph. Wyeth Laboratories, Philadelphia, 1986

106. Lempiäinen M, Mäkelä A-L: Determination of ketoprofen by high-performance liquid chromatography from serum and urine: clinical application in children with juvenile rheumatoid arthritis. Int J Clin Pharmacol Res 7:265, 1987

107. Brewer EJ, Jr: A comparative evaluation of indomethacin, acetaminophen and placebo as antipyretic agents in children. Arthritis Rheum 11:645, 1968

108. Sherry DD, Patterson MWH, Petty RE: The use of indomethacin in the treatment of pericarditis in childhood. J Pediatr 100:995, 1982

109. Roth SH, Englund DW: Indomethacin in the treatment of juvenile rheumatoid arthritis (abstract). Arthritis Rheum 10:307, 1967

110. Jacobs JC: Sudden death in arthritic children receiving large doses of indomethacin. JAMA 199:932, 1967

111. Merck, Sharp & Dohme Research Laboratories: Use of indomethacin in children. Report to the FDA, 1976

112. Weiss B, Hair WN: Selective cyclic nucleotidephosphodiesterase inhibitors as potential therapeutic agents. Annu Rev Pharmacol Toxicol 17:441, 1977

113. Mielke K, Otto P, Platz CM (eds): Current Concepts of Antiinflammatory Drugs. Biomedical Information, New York, 1980

114. Kantor TG: Ibuprofen. Ann Intern Med 91:877, 1979

115. Huskisson EC, Franchimont P (eds): Clinoril in the Treatment of Rheumatic Disorders: A New Nonsteroidal Antiinflammatory/Analgesic Agent. Proceedings of a Symposium, VIII European Rheumatology Congress, Helsinki, 1975. Raven Press, New York, 1976

116. Bhettay E: Double-blind study of sulindac and aspirin in juvenile chronic arthritis. S Afr Med J 70:724, 1986

117. Brater DC, Anerson S, Baird B et al: Sulindac does not spare the kidney. Clin Pharmacol Ther 35:229, 1984

118. Ciabattoni G, Cinotti GA, Pierucci A et al: Effects of sulindac and ibuprofen in patients with chronic glomerular disease. Evidence for the dependence of renal function on prostacyclin. N Engl J Med 310:279, 1984

119. Ehrlich GE: Tolmetin sodium: meeting the clinical challenge. Clin Rheum Dis 5:481, 1979

120. Levinson JE, Baum J, Brewer E, Jr et al: Comparison of tolmetin sodium and aspirin in the treatment of juvenile rheumatoid arthritis. J Pediatr 91:799, 1977

121. Gewanter HL, Baum J: The use of tolmetin sodium in systemic onset juvenile rheumatoid arthritis. Arthritis Rheum 24:1316, 1981

122. Feinfield DA, Olesnicky L, Perani C et al: Nephrotic syndrome associated with use of the nonsteroidal antiinflammatory drugs. Case report and review of the literature. Nephron 37:174, 1984

123. Squires JE, Mintz PD, Clark S: Tolmetin-induced hemolysis. Transfusion 25:410, 1985

124. Brewer EJ, Giannini EH, Baum J et al: Sodium meclofenamate (Meclomen[R]) in the treatment of juvenile rheumatoid arthritis. A segment I study. J Rheumatol 9:129, 1984

125. Todd PA, Sorkin EM: Diclofenac sodium. A reappraisal of its pharmacodynamic and pharmacokinetic properties, and therapeutic efficacy. Drugs 35:244, 1988

126. Sanger L: Long-term treatment of juvenile chronic arthritis (juvenile rheumatoid arthritis) and systemic

juvenile chronic arthritis (Still's syndrome) with diclofenac. Aktuel Rheumatol 3:5, 1978

127. Chiappo GF, Mignone F, Oggero R et al: Diclofenac sodium in the treatment of juvenile rheumatoid arthritis. Minerva Pediatr 30:1773, 1978

128. Haapasaari J, Wuolijoki E, Ylijoki H: Treatment of juvenile rheumatoid arthritis with diclofenac sodium. Scand J Rheumatol 12:325, 1983

129. DeVere-Tyndall AG, Ansell BM: Piroxicam in juvenile chronic arthritis: a pilot study. Symposium Proceedings, Malaga. Excerpta Medica, New York 1980, p. 45

130. DeLaTorre IG, Cetina JA: Piroxicam in the treatment of juvenile rheumatoid arthritis. Curr Ther Res 38:309, 1985

131. Williams PL, Ansell BM, Bell A et al: Multicentre study of piroxicam versus naproxen in juvenile chronic arthritis, with special reference to problem areas in clinical trials of nonsteroidal antiinflammatory drugs in childhood. Br J Rheumatol 25:67, 1986

132. Garcia-Morteo O, Maldonado-Cocco JA, Cuttica R et al: Piroxicam in juvenile rheumatoid arthritis. Eur J Rheumatol Inflamm 9:49, 1987

133. Bunch TW, O'Duffy JD: Disease modifying drugs for progressive rheumatoid arthritis. Mayo Clin Proc 55:161, 1980

134. Iannuzzi L, Dawson N, Zein N et al: Does drug therapy slow radiographic deterioration in rheumatoid arthritis? N Engl J Med 309:1023, 1983

135. Proceedings of a symposium: a reassessment of plaquenil in the treatment of rheumatoid arthritis. Am J Med 18, suppl., 1983

136. Maksymowych W, Russell AS: Antimalarials in rheumatology: efficacy and safety. Semin Arthritis Rheum 16:206, 1987

137. Hughes GRV, Rynes RI (eds): Antimalarials in rheumatic disease: opportunity for an expanding role? Br J Clin Pract 41:suppl. 52, 1987

138. Salmeron G, Lipsky PE: Immunosuppressive potential of antimalarials. Am J Med 75:19, 1983

139. Matsuzawa Y, Hostetler KY: Inhibition of lysosomal phospholipase A and phospholipase C by chloroquine and 4,4'-bis-(diethylaminoethyoxy) α,β-diethyldiphenylethane. J Biol Chem 255:5190, 1980

140. Miyachi Y, Yoshioka A, Imamura S et al: Antioxidant action of antimalarials. Ann Rheum Dis 45:244, 1986

141. Greaves MW, McDonald-Gibson W: Effect of nonsteroidal antiinflammatory drugs and antipyretic drugs on prostaglandin biosynthesis by human skin. J Invest Dermatol 61:127, 1973

142. Stillman JS: Antimalarials in the treatment of juvenile rheumatoid arthritis. In Moore TD (ed): Arthritis in Childhood. Report of the Eightieth Ross Conference in Pediatric Research. Ross Laboratories, Columbus, Ohio, 1981, p. 125

143. Laaksonen A-L, Koskiahde V, Juva K: Dosage of antimalarial drugs for children with juvenile rheumatoid arthritis and systemic lupus erythematosus. A clinical study with determination of serum concentrations of chloroquine and hydroxychloroquine. Scand J Rheumatol 3:103, 1974

144. Brewer EJ, Giannini EH, Kuzmina H et al: Penicillamine and hydroxychloroquine in the treatment of severe juvenile rheumatoid arthritis. Results of the U.S.A.–U.S.S.R. double-blind placebo-controlled trial. N Engl J Med 314:1269, 1986

145. Dubois E: Antimalarials in the management of discoid and systemic lupus erythematosus. Semin Arthritis Rheum 8:33, 1978

146. Markowitz HA, McGinley JM: Chloroquine poisoning in a child. JAMA 189:950, 1964

147. Henkind P, Rothfield NF: Ocular abnormalities in patients treated with synthetic antimalarial drugs. N Engl J Med 269:433, 1963

148. Rynes RI, Krohel G, Falbo A et al: Ophthalmologic safety of long-term hydroxychloroquine treatment. Arthritis Rheum 22:832, 1979

149. Rynes RI: Side effects of antimalarial therapy. Br J Clin Pract 41:suppl. 52, 42, 1987

150. Sassaman FW, Cassidy JT, Alpern M et al: Electroretinography in patients with connective tissue diseases treated with hydroxychloroquine. Am J Ophthalmol 70:515, 1970

151. Forestier J: L'aurotherapie dans les rheumatismes chroniques. Bull Soc Méd Hop Paris 53:323, 1929

152. Forestier J: Rheumatoid arthritis and its treatment with gold salts. J Lab Clin Med 20:827, 1935

153. Lewis AJ, Walz DT: Immunopharmacology of gold. In Ellis JP, West GB (eds): Progress in Medicinal Chemistry. Vol. 19. Elsevier Biomedical, New York, 1982, p. 1

154. Lipsky PE, Ugai K, Ziff M: Alterations in human monocyte structure and function induced by incubation with gold sodium thiomalate. J Rheumatol 6:suppl. 5, 130, 1979

155. Martini A, De Amici M, Visconti L et al: Immunological evaluation in children with juvenile chronic arthritis treated with auranofin. Int J Clin Pharmacol Res 5:149, 1985

156. Fantini F, Cottafava F, Martini A et al: Changes of immunological parameters during auranofin treatment in children affected with juvenile chronic arthritis. Int J Clin Pharmacol Res 6:61, 1986

157. Sadler PJ: The comparative evaluation of the physical and chemical properties of gold compounds. J Rheumatol 9:suppl. 8, 71, 1982

158. Gottlieb NL: Comparative pharmacokinetics of parenteral and oral gold compounds. J Rheumatol 9:suppl. 8, 99, 1982

159. Blocka K, Furst D, Landau E et al: Single dose pharmacokinetics of auranofin in rheumatoid arthritis. J Rheumatol 9:suppl. 8, 110, 1982

160. Giannini EH, Person DA, Brewer EJ et al: Blood and serum concentration of gold after a single dose of auranofin in children with juvenile rheumatoid arthritis. J Rheumatol 10:496, 1983

161. Mäkelä A-L, Peltola OL, Mäkelä P: Gold serum levels in children with juvenile rheumatoid arthritis. Scand J Rheumatol 7:161, 1978

162. Giannini EH, Brewer EJ, Person DA: Blood gold concentrations in children with juvenile rheumatoid arthritis undergoing long-term oral gold therapy. Ann Rheum Dis 43:228, 1984

163. Nuki G, Gumpel JM (eds): Myocrisin. 50 Years Experience. Proceedings of an International Symposium. Medi-Ciné Communications International, London, 1985

164. Sairanen E, Laaksonen A-L: The results of gold therapy in juvenile rheumatoid arthritis. Ann Paediatr Fenn 10:274, 1963

165. Hicks RM, Hanson V, Kornreich HK: The use of gold in the treatment of juvenile rheumatoid arthritis. Arthritis Rheum 13:323, 1970

166. Kvien TK, Høyeraal HM, Sandstad B: Slow acting antirheumatic drugs in patients with juvenile rheumatoid arthritis—evaluated in a randomized, parallel 50-week clinical trial. J Rheumatol 12:533, 1985

167. Kvien TK, Høyeraal HM, Sandstad B: Gold sodium thiomalate and D-penicillamine. A controlled, comparative study in patients with pauciarticular and polyarticular juvenile rheumatoid arthritis. Scand J Rheumatol 14:346, 1985

168. Manners PJ, Ansell BM: Slow-acting antirheumatic drug use in systemic onset juvenile chronic arthritis. Pediatrics 77:99, 1986

169. Grondin C, Malleson P, Petty RE: Slow-acting antirheumatic drugs in chronic arthritis of childhood. Semin Arthritis Rheum 18:38, 1988

170. Brewer EJ, Jr, Giannini EH, Barkley E: Gold therapy in the management of juvenile rheumatoid arthritis. Arthritis Rheum 23:404, 1980

171. Thompson DM, Pegelow CH, Singsen BH et al: Neutropenia associated with chrysotherapy for juvenile rheumatoid arthritis. J Pediatr 93:871, 1978

172. Coblyn JS, Weinblatt M, Holdsworth D et al: Gold-induced thrombocytopenia. A clinical and immunogenetic study of twenty-three patients. Ann Intern Med 95:178, 1981

173. Gold therapy in RA: A multicentre controlled trial conducted by the research sub-committee of the Empire Rheumatism Council. Bull Rheum Dis 11:235, 1960

174. Research Subcommittee of the Empire Rheumatism Council: Gold therapy in rheumatoid arthritis: final report of a multicentre controlled trial. Ann Rheum Dis 20:315, 1961

175. Cooperating Clinics Committee of the American Rheumatism Association: A controlled trial of gold salt therapy in rheumatoid arthritis. Arthritis Rheum 16:353, 1973

176. Kvien TK, Larheim TA, Høyeraal HM et al: Radiographic temporomandibular joint abnormalities in patients with juvenile chronic arthritis during a controlled study of sodium aurothiomalate and D-penicillamine. Br J Rheumatol 25:59, 1986

177. Sairanen E, Laaksonen A-L: The toxicity of gold therapy in children suffering from rheumatoid arthritis. Ann Paediatr Fenn 8:105, 1962

178. Kean WF, Anastassiades TP: Long-term chrysotherapy: incidence of toxicity and efficacy during sequential time periods. Arthritis Rheum 22:495, 1979

179. Debendetti C, Tretbar H, Corrigan JJ: Gold therapy in juvenile rheumatoid arthritis. Ariz Med 33:373, 1976

180. Levinson JF, Balz GP, Bondi S: Gold therapy. Arthritis Rheum 20:531, 1977

181. Levinson JE: Gold salts in the rheumatic diseases. In Moore TD (ed): Arthritis in Childhood. Report of the Eightieth Ross Conference in Pediatric Research. Ross Laboratories, Columbus, Ohio, 1981, p. 120

182. Malleson PN, Grondin C, Petty RE et al: Outcome of gold therapy in juvenile rheumatoid arthritis. Arthritis Rheum 30:528, 1987

183. Wooley PH, Griffin J, Panayi GS: HLA-DR antigens and toxic reaction to sodium aurothiomalate and D-penicillamine in patients with rheumatoid arthritis. N Engl J Med 303:300, 1980

184. Fan AG, Gordon DA, Sarkozi J et al: Neurologic complications associated with gold therapy for rheumatoid arthritis. J Rheumatol 11:700, 1984

185. Aron S, Davis P, Percy J: Neutropenia occurring during the course of chrysotherapy. A review of 25 cases. J Rheumatol 12:897, 1985

186. Pik A, Cohen N, Yona E et al: Should acute gold overdose be invariably treated? J Rheumatol 12:1174, 1985

187. Gambari P, Ostuni P, Lazzarin P et al: Neurotoxicity following a very high dose of oral gold (auranofin) (letter). Arthritis Rheum 27:1316, 1984

188. Garland JS, Sheth KJ, Wortman DW: Poor clearance of gold using peritoneal dialysis for the treatment of gold toxicity (letter). Arthritis Rheum 29:450, 1986

189. Jacobs JC, Gorin LJ, Hanissian AS et al: Consumption

coagulopathy after gold therapy for JRA. J Pediatr 105:674, 1984

190. Favreau M, Tannenbaum H, Lough J: Hepatic toxicity associated with gold therapy. Ann Intern Med 87:717, 1977

191. Howrie DL, Gartner JC, Jr: Gold-induced hepatotoxicity: case report and review of the literature. J Rheumatol 9:727, 1982

192. Ghishan FK, LaBrecque DR, Younoszai K: Intrahepatic cholestasis after gold therapy in juvenile rheumatoid arthritis. J Pediatr 93:1042, 1978

193. Harats N, Shalit M, Ehrenfeld M et al: Gold-induced granulomatous hepatitis. Isr J Med Sci 21:753, 1985

194. Olsen JL, Lovell DJ, Levinson JE: Hypogammaglobulinemia associated with gold therapy in a patient with juvenile rheumatoid arthritis. J Rheumatol 13:224, 1986

195. Tarp U, Graudal H: A follow-up study of children exposed to gold compounds in utero. Arthritis Rheum 28:235, 1986

196. Winterbauer RH, Wilske KR, Wheelis RF: Diffuse pulmonary injury associated with gold treatment. N Engl J Med 294:919, 1976

197. Gould PW, McCormack PL, Palmer DG: Pulmonary damage associated with sodium aurothiomalate therapy. J Rheumatol 4:252, 1977

198. Husserl FE, Shuler SE: Gold nephropathy in juvenile rheumatoid arthritis. Am J Dis Child 133:50, 1979

199. Merle LJ, Reidenberg MM, Camacho MT et al: Renal injury in patients with rheumatoid arthritis treated with gold. Clin Pharmacol Ther 28:216, 1980

200. Paulus HE: Government affairs: FDA Arthritis Advisory Committee meeting: auranofin. Arthritis Rheum 28:450, 1985

201. Brewer EJ, Jr, Giannini EH, Person DA: Early experiences with auranofin in juvenile rheumatoid arthritis. Am J Med 75:152, 1983

202. Giannini EH, Brewer EJ, Person DA: Auranofin in the treatment of juvenile rheumatoid arthritis. J Pediatr 102:138, 1983

203. Giannini EH, Brewer EJ, Person DA et al: Long-term auranofin therapy in patients with juvenile rheumatoid arthritis. J Rheumatol 13:768, 1986

204. Garcia-Morteo O, Sugrez-Almazo ME, Maldonado-Cocco JA et al: Auranofin in juvenile rheumatoid arthritis: an open label, non-controlled study. Clin Rheumatol 3:223, 1984

205. Kvien TL, Høyeraal HM, Sandstad B et al: Auranofin therapy in juvenile rheumatoid arthritis: a 48-week phase II study. Scand J Rheumatol 63:79, 1986

206. Marcolongo R, Mathieu A, Pala R et al: The efficacy and safety of auranofin in the treatment of juvenile rheumatoid arthritis. A long-term open study. Arthritis Rheum 31:979, 1988

207. Brewer EJ, Giannini EH: Oral gold (auranofin) in juvenile rheumatoid arthritis—results of the double-blind, placebo controlled trial (abstract). Arthritis Rheum 30:S31, 1987

208. Howard-Lock HE, Lock CJL, Mewa A et al: D-penicillamine: chemistry and clinical use in rheumatic disease. Semin Arthritis Rheum 15:261, 1986

209. Jaffe IA: D-penicillamine. Bull Rheum Dis 28:948, 1978

210. Multicenter Trial Group: Controlled trial of D-penicillamine in severe rheumatoid arthritis. Lancet 1:275, 1980

211. Theyboom RHB, Jaffe IA: Metal antagonists. Side Effects Drugs Annu 11:211, 1987

212. Lipsky PE: Immunosuppression by D-penicillamine in vitro. Inhibition of human T lymphocyte proliferation by copper- or ceruloplasmin-dependent generation of hydrogen peroxide and protection by monocytes. J Clin Invest 73:53, 1984

213. Sheikh IA, Kaplan AP: Assessment of kinases in rheumatic diseases and the effects of therapeutic agents. Arthritis Rheum 30:138, 1987

214. Bresnihan GP, Ansell BM: Effect of penicillamine treatment on immune complexes in two cases of seropositive juvenile rheumatoid arthritis. Ann Rheum Dis 35:463, 1976

215. Webley M, Coomes EN: An assessment of penicillamine therapy in RA and the influence of previous gold therapy. J Rheumatol 6:20, 1979

216. Halla JT, Cassidy J, Hardin JG: Sequential gold and penicillamine therapy in rheumatoid arthritis. Comparative study of effectiveness and toxicity and review of the literature. Am J Med 72:423, 1982

217. Day AT, Golding JR, Lee PN et al: Penicillamine in rheumatoid disease: a long term study. Br Med J 1:180, 1974

218. Bourke B, Maini RN, Griffiths ID et al: Fatal marrow aplasia in patient on penicillamine. Lancet 2:515, 1976

219. Blasberg B, Dorey JL, Stein HB et al: Lichenoid lesions of the oral mucosa in rheumatoid arthritis patients treated with penicillamine. J Rheumatol 11:348, 1984

220. Dische FE, Swinson DR, Hamilton EBD et al: Immunopathology of penicillamine-induced glomerular disease. J Rheumatol 11:584, 1984

221. Stein HB, Schroeder M-L, Dillon AM: Penicillamine-induced proteinuria: risk factors. Semin Arthritis Rheum 15:282, 1986

222. Kay A: European League Against Rheumatism study of adverse reactions to D-penicillamine. Br J Rheumatol 25:193, 1986

223. Steen VD, Blair S, Medsgar A: The toxicity of D-penicillamine in systemic sclerosis. Ann Intern Med 104:699, 1986

224. Baum J: The use of penicillamine in the treatment of rheumatoid arthritis and scleroderma. Scand J Rheumatol 28:65, 1979

225. Førre O, Munthe E, Kass E: Side-effects and autoimmunogenicity of D-penicillamine treatment in rheumatic diseases. Adv Inflamm Res 6:251, 1984

226. Takahashi K, Ogita T, Okudaira H et al: D-penicillamine-induced polymyositis in patients with rheumatoid arthritis. Arthritis Rheum 29:560, 1986

227. Kuncle RW, Restronk A, Drachman DB et al: The pathophysiology of penicillamine-induced myasthenia gravis. Ann Neurol 20:740, 1986

228. Multicenter Trial Group: Controlled trial of D-penicillamine in severe rheumatoid arthritis. Lancet 1:275, 1973

229. Schairer H, Stoeber E: Long-term follow-up of 235 cases of juvenile rheumatoid arthritis treated with D-penicillamine. In Munthe E (ed): Penicillamine Research in Rheumatoid Disease. Fabritius and Sonner, Oslo, 1976

230. Ansell BM, Hall MA: Penicillamine. Arthritis Rheum 20:536, 1977

231. Ansell BM, Simpson C: The effect of penicillamine on growth and height of juvenile chronic polyarthritis. Proc R Soc Med 70:suppl. 3, 123, 1977

232. Ansell BM: Penicillamine, levamisole and cytotoxic drugs. In Moore TD (ed): Arthritis in Childhood. Report of the Eightieth Ross Conference in Pediatric Research. Ross Laboratories, Columbus, Ohio, 1981, p. 127

233. Ansell BM, Hall MA, Ribero S: A comparative study of gold and penicillamine in seropositive juvenile chronic arthritis (juvenile rheumatoid arthritis) (abstract). Ann Rheum Dis 40:522, 1981

234. Ansell BM, Hall MA: Penicillamine in chronic arthritis of childhood. J Rheumatol 7:112, 1981

235. Prieur A-M, Piussan C, Manigne P et al: Evaluation of D-penicillamine in juvenile chronic arthritis. A double-blind, multicenter study. Arthritis Rheum 28:376, 1985

236. VanKerckhove C, Giannini E, Lowell DJ: Temporal patterns of response to D-penicillamine, hydroxychloroquine, and placebo in juvenile rheumatoid arthritis patients. Arthritis Rheum 31:1252, 1988

237. Cassidy JT: Treatment of children with juvenile rheumatoid arthritis (editorial). N Engl J Med 314:1312, 1986

238. Perrier P, Raffoux C, Thomas P et al: HLA antigens and toxic reactions to sodium aurothiopropanol sulphonate and D-penicillamine in patients with rheumatoid arthritis. Ann Rheum Dis 44:621, 1985

239. Svartz N: Salazopyrin, a new sulfanilamide preparation. Acta Med Scand 60:577, 1942

240. Svartz N: The treatment of rheumatoid arthritis with acid azo compounds. Rheumatism 4:56, 1948

241. Sinclair RJG, Duthie JRR: Salazopyrin in the treatment of rheumatoid arthritis. Ann Rheum Dis 8:226, 1948

242. Pullar T, Hunter JA, Capell HA: Sulfasalazine in rheumatoid arthritis. A double blind comparison of sulfasalazine with placebo and sodium aurothiomalate. Br Med J 287:1102, 1983

243. Pullar T, Hunter JA, Capell HA: Effect of sulphasalazine on the radiologic progression of rheumatoid arthritis. Ann Rheum Dis 46:398, 1987

244. Pullar T, Capell HA: Sulphasalazine: a "new" antirheumatic drug. Br J Rheum 23:26, 1984

245. Neumann VC, Grindulis KA: Sulphasalazine in rheumatoid arthritis: an old drug revived. J R Soc Med 77:169, 1984

246. Neumann VC, Grindulis KA, Hubball S et al: Comparison between penicillamine and sulphasalazine in rheumatoid arthritis: Leeds-Birmingham trial. Br Med J 287:1099, 1983

247. Grindulis K, McConkey B: Outcome of attempts to treat rheumatoid arthritis patients with gold, penicillamine, sulfasalazine or dapsone. Ann Rheum Dis 43:398, 1984

248. Bax DE, Amos RS: Sulphasalazine: a safe, effective agent for prolonged control of rheumatoid arthritis. A comparison with sodium aurothiomalate. Ann Rheum Dis 44:194, 1985

249. Watkinson G: Sulphasalazine: a review of 40 years experience. Drugs 32:1, 1986

250. Kean WF (ed): Sulfasalazine in Rheumatic Disease. Proceedings of the International Rheumatology Conference. Medicöpea, Quebec, 1987

251. Proceedings. Sulfasalazine in rheumatic diseases. J Rheumatol 16:suppl. 1988

252. Williams HJ, Ward JR, Dahl DL: A controlled trial comparing sulfasalazine, gold sodium thiomalate, and placebo in rheumatoid arthritis. Arthritis Rheum 31:702, 1988

253. Amor B, Kahan A, Dougados M et al: Sulfasalazine and ankylosing spondylitis. Ann Intern Med 101:878, 1984

254. Mielants H, Veys EM: HLA-B27 related arthritis and bowel inflammation. I: Sulfasalazine (salazopyrin) in HLA-B27 related reactive arthritis. J Rheumatol 12:287, 1985

255. Schroeder H, Campbell DES: Absorption, metabolism and excretion of salicylazosulfapyridine in man. Clin Pharmacol Ther 13:539, 1972

256. Bird HA, Dixon JS, Pickup ME et al: A biochemical assessment of sulfasalazine in rheumatoid arthritis. J Rheumatol 9:36, 1982

257. Peppercorn MA: Sulfasalazine, pharmacology, clin-

ical use, toxicities and related new drug development. Ann Intern Med 101:377, 1984

258. Thayer WR, Charland C, Field CE: Effects of sulfasalazine on selected lymphocyte subpopulations in vitro and in vivo. Dig Dis Sci 24:672, 1979

259. Heickly FE, Buckley RH: Development of IgA and IgG2 subclass deficiency after sulfasalazine therapy. J Pediatr 108:481, 1986

260. Pullar T, Hunter JA, Capell HA: Which component of sulphasalazine is active in rheumatoid arthritis? Br Med J 290:1535, 1985

261. Logan ECM, Williamson LM, Ryrie DR: Sulfasalazine associated pancytopenia may be caused by acute folate deficiency. Gut 27:868, 1986

262. Prouse PJ, Shawe D, Gumpel JM: Macrocytic anaemia in patients treated with sulfasalazine for rheumatoid arthritis. Br Med J 293:1407, 1986

263. Stenson WF, Lobos E: Sulfasalazine inhibits the synthesis of chemotactic lipids by neutrophils. J Clin Invest 69:494, 1982

264. Amos RS, Pullar T, Bax DE et al: Sulphasalazine for rheumatoid arthritis: toxicity in 774 patients monitored for one to 11 years. Br Med J 293:420, 1986

265. Farr M, Scott DGI, Bacon PA: Side effect profile of 200 patients with inflammatory arthritides treated with sulfasalazine. Drugs 32:49, 1986

266. Scott DL, Dacre JE: Adverse reactions to sulfasalazine: the British experience. J Rheumatol 15:17, 1988

267. Ozdogan H, Turunc M, Deringöl B et al: Sulphasalazine in the treatment of juvenile rheumatoid arthritis: a preliminary open trial. J Rheumatol 13:124, 1986

268. Suschke HJ: Sulfasalazin bei juveniler chronishcher arthritis. Paediatr Prax 33:681, 1986

269. Wallace SL: Colchicum, the panacea. Bull NY Acad Med 40:130, 1973

270. Hench PS: The potential reversibility of rheumatoid arthritis. Mayo Clin Proc 24:167, 1949

271. Thompson EB, Lippmann ME: Mechanism of action of glucocorticoids. Metabolism 23:159, 1974

272. Fauci AS, Dale DC, Balow JE: Glucocorticosteroid therapy: mechanisms of action and clinical considerations. Ann Intern Med. 84:304, 1976

273. Axelrod L: Glucocorticoid therapy. Medicine 55:39, 1976

274. Baxter JD: Glucocorticoid hormone action. Pharmacol Ther [B] 2:605, 1976

275. Ansell BM, Bywaters EGL, Isdale IC: Comparison of cortisone and aspirin in the treatment of juvenile rheumatoid arthritis. Br Med J 1:1075, 1956

276. Schaller JG: Corticosteroids in juvenile rheumatoid arthritis (Still's disease) (editorial). J Rheumatol 1:137, 1974

277. Schaller JG: Corticosteroids in juvenile rheumatoid arthritis. Arthritis Rheum 20:537, 1977

278. Stoeber E: Corticosteroid treatment of juvenile chronic polyarthritis over 22 years. Eur J Pediatr 121:141, 1976

279. Chan L, O'Malley BW: Steroid hormone action: recent advances. Ann Intern Med 89:964, 1978

280. Parrillo JE, Fauci AS: Mechanisms of glucocorticoid action on immune processes. Annu Rev Pharmacol Toxicol 19:179, 1979

281. Claman HN: Corticosteroids and lymphoid cells. N Engl J Med 287:388, 1972

282. Fauci AS, Dale DC: Effect of hydrocortisone on the kinetics of normal human lymphocytes. Blood 46:235, 1975

283. Weston WL, Claman HN, Krueger GG: Site and action of cortisol in cellular immunity. J Immunol 110:880, 1973

284. Rinehart JJ, Balcerzak SP, Sagone AL et al: Effects of corticosteroids on human monocyte function. J Clin Invest 54:1337, 1974

285. Balow JE, Rosenthal AS: Glucocorticoid suppression of macrophage migration inhibitory factor. J Exp Med 137:1031, 1973

286. Schreiber AD, Parsons J, McDermott P et al: Effect of corticosteroids on the human monocyte IgG and complement receptors. J Clin Invest 56:1189, 1975

287. MacGregor RR: Granulocyte adherence changes induced by hemodialysis, endotoxin, epinephrine, and glucocorticoids. Ann Intern Med 86:35, 1977

288. Granelli-Piperano A, Vassali JD, Reich E: Secretion of plasminogen activator by human polymorphonuclear leukocytes. Modulation by glucocorticoids and other effectors. J Exp Med 146:1693, 1977

289. Priestly GC, Brown JC: Effects of corticosteroids on the proliferation of normal and abnormal human connective tissue cells. Br J Dermatol 102:35, 1980

290. Hirata F, Schiffman E, Venkatasubamanian K et al: A phospholipase A_2 inhibitory protein in rabbit neutrophils induced by glucocorticoids. Proc Natl Acad Sci USA 77:2533, 1980

291. Blackwell GJ, Carnuccio R, DiRosa M et al: Macrocortin: a polypeptide causing the antiphospholipase effect of glucocorticoids. Nature 287:147, 1980

292. Good RA, Vernier RL, Smith RT: Serious untoward reactions to therapy with cortisone and A.C.T.H. in pediatric practice. Pediatrics 19:95, 1957

293. Ansell BM: Problems of corticosteroid therapy in the young. Proc R Soc Med 61:281, 1968

294. Reimer LG, Morris HG, Ellis EF: Growth of asthmatic children during treatment with alternate-day steroids. J Allergy Clin Immunol 55:224, 1975

295. Lubkin VL: Steroid cataract—a review and conclusion. J Asthma Res 14:55, 1977

296. Levine SB, Leopold IH: Advances in ocular corticosteroid therapy. Med Clin North Am 57:1167, 1973

297. Hahn TJ, Hahn BJ: Osteopenia in patients with rheumatic diseases: principles of diagnosis and therapy. Semin Arthritis Rheum 6:165, 1976

298. Loeb JN: Corticosteroids and growth. N Engl J Med 295:547, 1976

299. Brouhard B: Inhibition of linear growth using alternate day steroids. J Pediatr 91:343, 1977

300. Morris HG, Jorgensen JR, Elrick H et al: Metabolic effects of human growth hormone in corticosteroid-treated children. J Clin Invest 47:436, 1968

301. Ragan C: Corticotropin, cortisone and related steroids in clinical medicine: practical considerations. Bull NY Acad Med 29:356, 1953

302. Ilowhite NT, Samuel P, Ginzler E et al: Dyslipoproteinemia in pediatric systemic lupus erythematosus. Arthritis Rheum 31:859, 1988

303. Bulkley BH, Roberts WC: The heart in systemic lupus erythematosus and the changes induced in it by corticosteroid therapy. A study of 36 necropsy patients. Am J Med 58:243, 1975

304. Ling MH, Perry PJ, Tsuang MT: Side effects of corticosteroid therapy. Arch Gen Psychiatry 38:471, 1981

305. Rogers MP: Psychiatric aspects. In Schur PH (ed): The Clinical Management of Systemic Lupus Erythematosus. Grune & Stratton, Orlando, 1983, p. 189

306. Meikle AW, Tyler FH: Potency and duration of action of glucocorticoids. Am J Med 63:200, 1977

307. Gambertoglio JG, Amend WJC Jr, Benet LZ: Pharmacokinetics and bioavailability of prednisone and prednisolone in healthy volunteers and patients. A review. J Pharmacokinet Biopharm 8:1, 1980

308. Myles AB, Schiller LF, Glass D et al: Single daily dose of corticosteroid treatment. Ann Rheum Dis 35:73, 1976

309. MacGregor RR, Sheagren JN, Lipsett MB et al: Alternate-day prednisone therapy. Evaluation of delayed hypersensitivity responses, control of disease and steroid side effects. N Engl J Med 280:1427, 1969

310. Bell MJ: Alternate day single dose prednisone therapy: a method of reducing steroid toxicity. J Pediatr Surg 7:233, 1972

311. Ansell BM, Bywaters EGL: Alternate-day corticosteroid therapy in juvenile chronic polyarthritis. J Rheumatol 1:176, 1974

312. Dale DC, Fauci AS, Wolff SM: Alternate day prednisone. Leukocyte kinetics and susceptibility to infection. N Engl J Med 291:1154, 1974

313. Dixon RB, Christy NP: On the various forms of corticosteroid withdrawal syndrome. Am J Med 68:224, 1980

314. Amatruda TT, Jr, Hollingsworth DR, D'Esopo ND et al: A study of the mechanism of the steroid withdrawal syndrome. J Clin Endocrinol Metab 20:339, 1960

315. Laaksonen A-L, Sunell JE, Westeren H et al: Adrenocortical function in children with juvenile rheumatoid arthritis and other connective tissue disorders. Scand J Rheumatol 3:137, 1974

316. Graber AL, Ney RE, Nicholson WE et al: Natural history of pituitary-adrenal recovery following long term suppression with corticosteroids. J Clin Endocrinol Metab 25:11, 1965

317. Cathcart ES, Edelson BA, Scheinberg MA et al: Beneficial effects of methylprednisolone "pulse" therapy in diffuse proliferative lupus nephritis. Lancet 1:163, 1976

318. Miller JJ: Prolonged use of large intravenous steroid pulses in the rheumatic diseases of children. Pediatrics 65:989, 1980

319. Skinner MD, Schwartz RS: Immunosuppressive therapy. N Engl J Med 287:221, 1972

320. Steinberg AD: Efficacy of immunosuppressive drugs in rheumatic diseases. Arthritis Rheum 16:92, 1973

321. Wagner L: Immunosuppressive agents in lupus nephritis. A critical analysis. Medicine 55:239, 1976

322. Hollister JR: Immunosuppressant therapy of juvenile rheumatoid arthritis. Arthritis Rheum 20:544, 1977

323. Klippel J: Immunosuppressive therapy. In Lahita RG (ed): Systemic Lupus Erythematous. Churchill Livingstone, New York, 1987, p. 931

324. Swanson MA, Schwartz RS: Immunosuppressive therapy. The relation between clinical response and immunologic competence. N Engl J Med 277:163, 1967

325. Hersh EM, Carbone PO, Freireich EJ: Recovery of immune responsiveness after drug suppression in man. J Lab Clin Med 67:566, 1966

326. Grünwald HW, Rosner F: Acute leukemia and immunosuppressive drug use: a review of patients undergoing immunosuppressive therapy for non-neoplastic diseases. Arch Intern Med 139:461, 1979

327. Calabresi P: Leukemia after cytotoxic chemotherapy—a pyrrhic victory? (editorial). N Engl J Med 309:1118, 1983

328. Hanto DW, Simmons RL: Cancer in recipients of organ allografts. In Williams GM, Burdick JF, Solez K (eds): Kidney Transplant Rejection. Diagnosis and Treatment. Marcel Dekker, New York, 1986, p. 459

329. Kahn MF, Arlet J, Bloch-Michel H et al: Le risque de leucose aiguë traitement des rhumatismes inflammatoires chronique et de connectivites par les cytotoxiques à visée immunosuppressive. Résultats d'une enquête rétrospective portant sur 2006 malades traités. Rev Rhum Mal Osteoartic 46:165, 1979

330. McDuffie FC (ed): Proceedings of a symposium.

Neoplasms in rheumatoid arthritis: update on clinical and epidemiological data. Am J Med 78:1A, 1985

331. Palmer RG, Varonos S, Doré CJ et al: Chlorambucil induced chromosome damage in juvenile chronic arthritis. Arch Dis Child 60:1008, 1985

332. Berenbaum MC: The clinical pharmacology of immunosuppressive agents. In Gell PGH, Coombs RRA, Lachmann PJ (eds): Clinical Aspects of Immunology. Blackwell Scientific Publications, Oxford, England, 1975, p. 689

333. Elion GB: Biochemistry and pharmacology of purine analogues. Fed Proc 26:898, 1967

334. Maibach HI, Epstein WL: Immunologic responses of healthy volunteers receiving azathioprine (Imuran). Int Arch Allergy Appl Immunol 27:102, 1965

335. Abdou NI, Sweiman B, Casella SR: Effects of azathioprine therapy on bone marrow-dependent and thymus-dependent cells in man. Clin Exp Immunol 13:55, 1973

336. Sharbaugh RJ, Ainsworth SK, Fitts CT: Lack of effect of azathioprine on phytohemagglutinin-induced lymphocyte transformation and established delayed cutaneous hypersensitivity. Int Arch Allergy Appl Immunol 51:681, 1976

337. Dale I: The treatment of juvenile rheumatoid arthritis with azathioprine. Scand J Rheumatol 1:125, 1972

338. Kvien TK, Høyeraal HM, Sandstad B: Azathioprine versus placebo in patients with juvenile rheumatoid arthritis: a single center double blind comparative study. J Rheumatol 13:118, 1986

339. Roberts JJ, Brent TP, Crathron AR: Evidence for the inactivation and repair of the mammalian DNA template after alkylation by mustard gas and half mustard gas. Eur J Cancer 7:515, 1971

340. Cupps TR, Edgar LC, Fauci AS: Suppression of human B lymphocyte function by cyclophosphamide. J Immunol 128:2453, 1982

341. Turk JL, Parker D: Effect of cyclophosphamide on immunological control mechanisms. Immunol Rev 65:99, 1982

342. Rudd P, Fried JF, Epstein WV: Irreversible bone marrow failure with chlorambucil. J Rheumatol 2:421, 1975

343. Skoglund RR, Schanberger JE, Kaplan JM: Cyclophosphamide therapy for severe juvenile rheumatoid arthritis. Am J Dis Child 121:531, 1971

344. Ansell BM, Eghtedari A, Bywaters EGL: Chlorambucil in the management of juvenile chronic polyarthritis complicated by amyloidosis. Ann Rheum Dis 30:331, 1971

345. Mehra R, Moore TL, Catalano JD et al: Chlorambucil in the treatment of iridocyclitis in juvenile rheumatoid arthritis. J Rheumatol 8:141, 1981

346. Walters D, Robinson RG, Dick-Smith JB et al: Poor response in two cases of juvenile rheumatoid arthritis to treatment with cyclophosphamide. Med J Aust 2:1070, 1972

347. Trampeter RS, Evans PR, Barratt TM: Gonadal function in boys with steroid-responsive nephrotic syndrome treated with cyclophosphamide for short periods. Lancet 1:1177, 1981

348. Warne GL, Fairley KF, Hobbs JB et al: Cyclophosphamide-induced ovarian failure. N Engl J Med 289:1159, 1973

349. Cameron S: Chlorambucil and leukemia (letter). N Engl J Med 296:1065, 1977

350. Plotz PH, Klippel JH, Decker JL et al: Bladder complications in patients receiving cyclophosphamide for systemic lupus erythematosus or rheumatoid arthritis. Ann Intern Med 91:221, 1979

351. DeFronzo RA, Braine H, Colvin OM et al: Water intoxication in man after cyclophosphamide therapy: time course and relation to drug activation. Ann Intern Med 78:861, 1973

352. Gubner R, August S, Ginsburg V: Therapeutic suppression of tissue reactivity. II: Effects of aminopterin in rheumatoid arthritis and psoriasis. Am J Med Sci 221:176, 1951

353. Henderson FS, Adamson RH, Oliverio VT: The metabolic rate of tritiated methotrexate. II: Absorption and excretion in man. Cancer Res 25:1018, 1965

354. Jolivet J, Cowan KH, Curt GA et al: The pharmacology and clinical use of methotrexate. N Engl J Med 309:1094, 1983

355. Bailin PL, Tindall JP, Roenigk HH et al: Is methotrexate therapy for psoriasis carcinogenic? A modified retrospective-prospective analysis. JAMA 323:359, 1975

356. Shupack JL, Webster GF: Pancytopenia following low-dose oral methotrexate therapy for psoriasis. JAMA 259:3594, 1988

357. Abel EA, Farber EM: Pancytopenia following low-dose methotrexate therapy (editorial). JAMA 259:3612, 1988

358. DiBartolomeo AG, Mayes MD, Bathon JM: Methotrexate in rheumatoid arthritis: a longitudinal study of liver biopsies. Arthritis Rheum 27:S61, 1984

359. Roenigk HH, Jr, Auerbach R, Maibach HH et al: Methotrexate guidelines revisited. J Am Acad Dermatol 6:145, 1982

360. Weinstein A, Marlowe S, Korn J et al: Low-dose methotrexate treatment of rheumatoid arthritis. Am J Med 79:331, 1985

361. Weinblatt ME, Coblyn JS, Fox DA et al: Efficacy of low-dose methotrexate in rheumatoid arthritis. N Engl J Med 312:818, 1985

362. Andersen PA, West SG, O'Dell J, Jr et al: Weekly pulse methotrexate in rheumatoid arthritis: clinical

and immunologic effects in a randomized, double-blind study. Ann Intern Med 103:489, 1985

363. Ward JR, Weinblatt ME (eds): Advances in arthritis therapy: experience with methotrexate. J Rheumatol 12:suppl. 12, 1985

364. Healy LA: The current status of methotrexate use in rheumatic diseases. Bull Rheum Dis 36:1, 1986

365. Searles G, McKendry RJR: Methotrexate pneumonitis in rheumatoid arthritis: potential risk factors. Four case reports and a review of the literature. J Rheumatol 14:1164, 1987

366. Jacobs JC: Methotrexate and azathioprine treatment of childhood dermatomyositis. Pediatrics 59:212, 1977

367. Truckenbrodt H, Häfner R: Methotrexate therapy in juvenile rheumatoid arthritis: a retrospective study. Arthritis Rheum 29:801, 1986

367a. Giannini EH, Brewer EJ for the Pediatric Rheumatology Collaborative Study Group: Methotrexate (MTX) in the treatment of recalcitrant JRA – results of the double-blind placebo (P) controlled, randomized trial (abstract). Arthritis Rheum 32:S82, 1989

368. Wallace CA, Bleyer WA, Sherry DD et al: Methotrexate levels in juvenile rheumatoid arthritis patients (abstract). Arthritis Rheum 31:S26, 1988

369. Hansten PD, Horn JR: Methotrexate and nonsteroidal anti-inflammatory drugs. Drug Interact Newsl 6:41, 1986

370. Ahern M, Booth J, Loxton A et al: Methotrexate kinetics in rheumatoid arthritis: is there an interaction with nonsteroidal antiinflammatory drugs? J Rheumatol 15:1356, 1988

371. Ruuskanen O: Levamisole and agranulocytosis. Lancet 2:958, 1976

372. Prieur A-M: Possible toxicity of levamisole in children with rheumatoid arthritis. J Pediatr 93:304, 1978

373. Borel JF, Feurer C, Gubler HU et al: Biological effects of cyclosporin A: a new antilymphocytic agent. Agents Actions 6:468, 1976

374. Bunjes D, Hardt C, Rollinghoff M et al: Cyclosporin A mediates immunosuppression of primary cytotoxic T cell responses by impairing the release of interleukin 1 and interleukin 2. Eur J Immunol 11:657, 1981

375. Navarro J, Touraine JL: Comparative study of cycloimmune cyclosporin A on human lymphocyte proliferation in vitro: the lack of an immunosuppressive effect by specific clonal deletion. Int J Immunopharmacol 5:157, 1983

376. Kronke M, Leonard WJ, Depper JM et al: Cyclosporin A inhibits T-cell growth factor gene expression at the level of mRNA transcription. Proc Natl Acad Sci USA 81:5214, 1984

377. Tugwell P, Bombardier C, Gent M et al: Low dose cyclosporin in rheumatoid arthritis: a pilot study. J Rheumatol 14:1108, 1987

378. Myers BD, Ross J, Newton L et al: Cyclosporin-associated chronic nephropathy. N Engl J Med 311:699, 1984

379. Palestine AG, Austin HA, Balow JE et al: Renal histopathologic alterations in patients treated with cyclosporin for uveitis. N Engl J Med 314:1293, 1986

380. Rodger RSC, Turney JH, Haines I et al: Cyclosporin and liver function in renal allograft recipients. Transplant Proc 15:2754, 1983

381. Ostensen M, Høyeraal HM, Kåss E: Tolerance of cyclosporine A in children with refractory juvenile rheumatoid arthritis. J Rheumatol 15:1536, 1988

4

Musculoskeletal Pain Syndromes of Nonrheumatic Origin

The art of medicine is no better exemplified than in the approach used by an experienced clinician to the differential diagnosis of a child with musculoskeletal pain. Because the list of diagnostic possibilities is extensive and many of these disorders are rare, it is the well-informed physician who, by taking a careful history, performing a meticulous physical examination, and using a minimal number of tests and procedures, will succeed in this difficult area.[1-4] There is no single pathognomonic finding for the vast majority of these disorders, and in the absence of a clear etiology, the physician must depend on memory and experience for syndrome identification.

APPROACH TO THE CHILD WHO HAS MUSCULOSKELETAL PAIN

Although the majority of childhood aches and pains are benign, a thoughtful evaluation is necessary when a child with musculoskeletal pain is referred to a physician's attention. A useful approach to the diagnosis is outlined in the discussion that follows and in Tables 4-1 to 4-3.

History

Four questions are of particular importance in evaluating the child with pain:

1. What is the character of the pain?
2. Are there other symptoms?
3. Is there a family history of musculoskeletal disease?
4. What are the social, emotional, and educational circumstances?

CHARACTER OF THE PAIN

The factors listed in Table 4-1 are potentially important diagnostic indicators. Pain that is of recent onset may indicate the effect of trauma, infection, or malignancy, the three categories of disease that must be immediately diagnosed, since prompt treatment can prevent long-term sequelae in many cases. Pain of long duration (more than a few days) may have serious import as well, but the likelihood of a septic or traumatic cause is much less. Intermittent pain, particularly if a precipitating or alleviating factor can be identified, usually has a different diagnostic sig-

Table 4-1 History of Musculoskeletal Pain: What Is the Character of the Pain?

How long has the pain been present?
Is the pain intermittent or persistent?
What makes the pain worse? What makes it better?
Is there diurnal variation in the pain?
Does the pain interfere with function?
Is the pain present at night?
Is the pain sharp, aching, deep, boring, etc?
Does the painful part look abnormal?

nificance than persisting pain. The influence of analgesics, heat, cold, or other therapeutic modalities should be noted. Diurnal variation of pain is characteristic of some disorders such as those caused by inflammation of joints. The severity of pain can be estimated from the degree to which it interferes with function, and whether it is present at night. Some pain syndromes such as growing pains, pain caused by osteoid osteoma, as well as some inflammatory or neoplastic diseases, are characteristically worse at night. The quality of the pain is usually very hard to evaluate, especially in the young child. Inflammatory joint pain is usually described as aching; enthesitic pain is more often described as sharp. Bone pain is usually described as "deep" or "boring." It is useful to know whether the child or parent believes that the affected part looks different when it is painful. Pain associated with Raynaud's phenomenon, reflex sympathetic dystrophy, or the arthritis of serum sickness may be accompanied by changes in color or temperature that may be noted by the patient.

PRESENCE OF OTHER SYMPTOMS

The presence of systemic disease may be uncovered by seeking answers to the questions listed in Table 4-2. The presence of fever and its character may provide a clue to the diagnosis of inflammatory, infectious, or malignant disease. Documented weight loss

Table 4-2 History of Musculoskeletal Pain: Are There Other Symptoms?

Is there fever?
Is there weight loss?
Is there depression?
Is there sleep disturbance?
Is there change in gastrointestinal function?

Table 4-3 History of Musculoskeletal Pain: Family and Social History

Is there a history of spondyloarthropathies or related diseases?
Is there a family history of fibromyalgia?
Is there a family history of hemophilia?
Is there an identified stressor in the family or at school?

should suggest the presence of a systemic process such as a rheumatic disease, inflammatory bowel disease, or malignancy. Psychological changes, particularly depression, may be associated with pain amplification syndromes such as fibromyalgia. Sleep disturbances may reflect the presence of night pain or fibromyalgia. Changes in gastrointestinal function or bowel habits may indicate the presence of underlying inflammatory bowel disease.

FAMILY HISTORY OF MUSCULOSKELETAL DISEASE

A history of back pain, arthritis, or diseases suggestive of the seronegative spondyloarthropathies in family members may provide useful diagnostic clues (Table 4-3). Pain amplification syndromes sometimes tend to be familial; not infrequently an aching daughter has an aching mother. The acute onset of monarthritis in a child with a family history of hemophilia should suggest that diagnosis.

SOCIAL, EMOTIONAL, AND EDUCATIONAL CIRCUMSTANCES

Stress-related musculoskeletal pain syndromes, like headache and abdominal pain, occur commonly in children. In some instances, they take the form of a school phobia. Children with reflex sympathetic dystrophy typically have a stressing environment, often self-induced.

Physical Examination

A thorough general physical examination is an essential part of the evaluation of any child with musculoskeletal pain. The musculoskeletal examination should be aimed at addressing the points in Table 4-4. Localization of the pain to soft tissue, bone, or joint helps to differentiate the bone pain of osteomyelitis, trauma, or malignancy from the soft tissue

Table 4-4 Muscoloskeletal Examination

Is the pain localized to soft tissue, bone, or joint?
Is there more than one painful site?
Is there tenderness as well as pain?
Is the appearance of the affected area normal?

Table 4-5 Limb Pain Associated with Mechanical Stress

Hypermobility syndromes
  Generalized hypermobility
  Pes planus
  Genu recurvatum
  Recurrent patellar dislocation

Overuse syndromes
  Chrondromalacia patellae
  Sinding-Larsen-Johanssen syndrome
  Plica syndromes
  Osgood-Schlatter disease
  Stress fractures
  Shin splints
  Tennis elbow
  Tenosynovitis

Trauma
  Traumatic arthritis
  Nonaccidental trauma
  Frostbite arthropathy

pain of trauma or the joint pain of arthritis. Although the child may spontaneously complain of only one painful site, the demonstration of two or more affected areas leads to a different differential diagnosis. A complaint of pain should be differentiated from the presence of tenderness. If an area is painful, but not tender, the possibility of referred pain should be considered. The appearance of the painful site provides valuable diagnostic information. The stance and gait during walking and, if possible, during running should be observed.

Laboratory Evaluation

Specific laboratory investigations depend on the presumed diagnosis and differential diagnosis. As a general approach, however, it is appropriate to attempt to document the presence or absence of inflammation by evaluating the complete blood count and differential white blood cell count, platelet count, and erythrocyte sedimentation rate (ESR). If all of these are unequivocally normal, the possibilities of acute infection or malignancy are remote, although not excluded. Radiography of the affected part is usually indicated since changes in the soft tissues as well as bone density are early signs of most inflammatory and malignant conditions. Failing the detection of diagnostic abnormalities on radiographic evaluation, bone scintigraphy is a useful tool to rule out the possibility of significant musculoskeletal disease in a child with undiagnosed musculoskeletal pain. Laboratory investigations appropriate to specific disorders are discussed in the following chapters.

LIMB PAIN ASSOCIATED WITH MECHANICAL STRESS

Some of the syndromes of limb pain attributed to mechanical stress are shown in Table 4-5. This tabulation is by no means complete, and for more information regarding musculoskeletal pain syndromes associated with specific activities, the reader is referred to standard textbooks of orthopedics and sports medicine.

Hypermobility Syndromes

GENERALIZED HYPERMOBILITY

The term *benign hypermobility syndrome* has been used to describe children in whom generalized hypermobility of the joints is associated with musculoskeletal pain.[5–7] The diagnosis of hypermobility is based on the Carter-Wilkinson criteria (Table 4-6).[8] The benign hypermobility syndrome represents an extreme variation of the normal range of joint motion. It is not associated with underlying connective-tissue disease or Marfan's or Ehlers-Danlos syndrome. Estimates of the frequency of hypermobility

Table 4-6 Criteria for Establishing a Diagnosis of Hypermobility

Ability passively to oppose the thumbs to the flexor aspect of the forearms
Ability passively to hyperextend fingers so that they are parallel to the extensor aspect of the forearms
Ability actively to hyperextend elbows or knees more than 10° beyond 180°

(From Carter and Wilkinson,[8] with permission.)

in children range from 12 percent[9] to 19.5 percent.[8] In general, girls are more commonly affected than boys (18 versus 7 percent). There is often a family history of hypermobility. In this regard, hyperextensible joints, especially at the MCP joints, have been described in boys with the fragile X syndrome. Hypermobility predisposes to injury some children who are successful gymnasts or dancers because of their flexibility.[10,11]

The term *juvenile episodic arthritis* (JEA) has been proposed to describe children who have recurrent episodes of nonspecific arthritis in the absence of an identifiable organic disease.[9] It is regarded as a benign condition with an excellent outcome. Gedalia et al. found that 66 percent of 32 children with JEA were hypermobile by the Carter-Wilkinson criteria.[9] Mitral valve prolapse occurs in some syndromes characterized by hypermobility (Marfan's, Ehlers-Danlos), but it does not appear to be a characteristic of the benign hypermobility syndrome.[11,12]

PES PLANUS

Although hypermobile flat feet are usually asymptomatic, there may be pain on weight bearing, usually localized to the medial side of the arch. The pronated flat foot is often accompanied by mild genu valgum, slight flexion at the knees and the hips, and increased lordosis. As a result of these mechanical strains, pain in the ankles, knees, hips, or lower back may accompany pes planus. In adolescence, the Achilles tendon may shorten, thereby limiting ankle dorsiflexion.[13-15]

Substantial improvement in alignment and relief of symptoms can be achieved by the use of custom-fitted hard insoles. These insoles are constructed of hard plastic and can be slipped into any good shoe with a supportive construction surrounding the heel, such as jogging shoes. The symptomatic relief provided by well-fitted insoles is often dramatic, and compliance with their use is seldom a problem.

In contrast to the hypermobile flat foot, a rigid flat foot may result from tarsal coalition, in which a bone or cartilaginous bridge is present between tarsal bones, usually the talus and calcaneus, or the navicular and calcaneus. As the bridge ossifies, motion is restricted and pain results. A high arched or cavus foot, associated with such diseases as Friedreich's ataxia or Charcot-Marie-Tooth disease, may also be a cause of foot pain.[16]

GENU RECURVATUM

Like pes planus, genu recurvatum may be part of a generalized hypermobility syndrome or may occur as an isolated phenomenon. Symptomatic genu recurvatum occurs most commonly in adolescent girls and is associated with pain at the back of the knee, and occasionally with small bland effusions in the knees. Symptoms are worse with standing or walking and are relieved by rest. Considerable symptomatic improvement can be obtained by the patient's wearing shoes with a low heel wedge, such as that found in most jogging shoes. An exercise program designed to strengthen the knee flexors and extensors may also be beneficial. As a general rule, genu recurvatum becomes less significant as the child grows older.

RECURRENT PATELLAR DISLOCATION

As part of a hypermobility syndrome, or as an isolated phenomenon, the patella may dislocate laterally. This is accompanied by a sensation of "giving way," sudden pain, and inability to straighten the leg, which is held in a position of about 25° of flexion. It may be associated with a congenital abnormality of the patella (unifaceted or bipartite patella), the femoral condyles (shallow intercondylar groove), or the patellar ligament (lateral attachment). Femoral anteversion may also predispose to this disorder. Repeated episodes of dislocation predispose to premature degeneration of the articular cartilage of the patella-femoral joint. Treatment consists of short-arc exercises to strengthen the musculature around the knee joint, especially the vastus medialis. An antidislocation orthosis may be useful. If these interventions fail, surgical realignment of the extensor system may be indicated.

Overuse Syndromes

Overuse syndromes once occurred almost exclusively in association with work-related physical activity in adults. With the increasing emphasis on participation in athletic activities at all ages, syndromes related to overuse occur with considerable frequency in the child and adolescent. They usually represent a combination of "overdoing it," insufficient training and preparation, and occasionally inadequate or inappropriate equipment. Education of families,

Table 4-7 Chondromalacia Patellae

Age at onset: adolescence to young adulthood
Sex ratio: girls > boys
Symptoms: insidious onset of exertional knee pain, difficulty descending stairs; need to sit with legs straight or "theater sign" (knee pain with prolonged flexion)
Signs: patellar tenderness on compression; quadriceps weakness; inhibition sign, joint effusion, and instability

schools, and coaches is the essential element in the prevention of this type of syndrome.

In older children and adolescents, chronic pain frequently develops in a characteristic way as a consequence of mechanical stress. At onset, pain occurs only with the stressful activity and is relieved by rest. If repetitive stress continues, pain persists for a time after cessation of activity and ultimately becomes constant with exacerbation by activity.

CHONDROMALACIA PATELLAE

A controversial topic, the chondromalacia patellae syndrome arises because of stresses on the patella by the pull of the quadriceps muscle (Table 4-7).[17] It is most common in teenage girls. There is insidious development of retropatellar knee pain. Pain occurs at first with activity that stresses the quadriceps, such as deep knee bends, climbing or descending stairs, or running, and is lessened by rest. Pain recurs with prolonged sitting with the knee flexed and can be relieved by extension of the leg. On physical examination, knee flexion may be accompanied by patellar crepitus. Pain may be elicited by compression of the patella and by palpation along its inferomedial edge. Pain may also be precipitated if the patella is restrained when the quadriceps muscle is contracted. A small knee effusion may be present. Standard radiographs and laboratory investigations are normal. Arthroscopy reveals ridging and strands of degenerating cartilage on the retropatellar surface. Chondromalacia patellae is chronic and difficult to treat. Activities that provoke pain should be avoided. Strengthening of the muscles around the knee may help prevent progression of the problem. Surgical procedures, including shaving off the patellar irregularities, may be helpful.

SINDING-LARSEN-JOHANSSEN SYNDROME

Several other disorders must be differentiated from chondromalacia patellae. Mechanical stress caused by quadriceps action can also give rise to pain and tenderness at the patellar tendon's origin in the Sinding-Larsen-Johanssen syndrome (Table 4-8) or less commonly at the insertion of the quadriceps into the patella. Radiographs may be normal or may show fine calcifications at the origin of the patellar tendon.

PLICA SYNDROMES

The plica syndromes arise from synovial bands that separate the compartments of the knee during development (Table 4-9).[18] These folds do not usually cause symptoms but may lead to mechanically induced pain in the knee when thickened. The *mediopatellar plica syndrome* is the more common and causes pain with flexion of the knee; it may eventually cause erosion of cartilage. There is often an area of tenderness over the superomedial border of the femoral condyle and locking or snapping during movement of the joint. Diagnosis is by arthroscopy; resection if necessary can be performed at the same time.

OSGOOD-SCHLATTER DISEASE

Osgood-Schlatter disease commonly occurs in athletic adolescents (Table 4-10).[19] There is a complaint of pain over the tibial tubercle exacerbated by exer-

Table 4-8 Sinding-Larsen-Johanssen Syndrome

Age at onset: adolescence
Sex ratio: boys > girls
Symptoms: pain at origin of patellar tendon exacerbated by activity (jumping)
Signs: patellar tenderness and soft tissue swelling at lower pole (6 o'clock)
Investigations: fine calcifications on radiographs at insertion of patellar tendon

Table 4-9 Mediopatellar Plica Syndrome

Age at onset: adolescent years
Symptoms: medial knee pain, intermittent aching increased with activity or motion, giving way on weight bearing
Signs: medial palpable band, snapping on motion
Investigations: fibrous band with hemorrhage and inflammation identified by arthroscopy

Table 4-10 Osgood-Schlatter Disease

Age at onset: athletic adolescents
Sex ratio: boys > girls
Symptoms: pain over the tibial tubercle exacerbated by exercise
Signs: tenderness and swelling at insertion of the patellar tendon (avulsion)
Investigations: radiographic indications of soft tissue swelling, enlarged and fragmented tubercle

cise. On examination, tenderness and often swelling of the tibial tubercle and patellar tendon insertion are present. X-ray films should be obtained to exclude other conditions and may show soft tissue swelling and an enlarged and fragmented tubercle. It is normal, however, for the tibial tubercle to appear irregular in adolescence. Laboratory studies reveal no evidence of chronic inflammation. Treatment is rest or use of a basketball knee protector.

STRESS FRACTURES

Stress fractures may occur in the weight-bearing skeleton in children and adolescents and are associated with repetitive traumatic activity.[20] Typical sites of fractures include the metatarsal shaft, navicular or calcaneus (in association with marching or dancing), and proximal tibial shaft (running). Patients with stress fractures usually have a history of lower extremity pain and limp exacerbated by exercise and somewhat relieved by rest. The onset is frequently insidious. Physical examination reveals localized bone tenderness and swelling. Early radiographs may be normal or show only soft tissue swelling. Weeks later, callus formation is evident (Fig. 4-1).

Spondylolysis is a stress fracture of the pars interarticularis of the fifth or occasionally the fourth lumbar vertebra. The affected vertebra may slip anteriorly, giving rise to *spondylolisthesis*. Either condition may cause low back pain, which may occur with activity and radiate down the posterior thigh. Occasionally, pain can be elicited by palpation of the involved vertebra, and a defect may be noted if a slip has occurred. The neurologic examination is normal, but there may be tightness and spasm of the hamstring muscles. Oblique and lateral radiographs of the lumbar spine usually reveal the diagnosis. Spondylolysis may exist asymptomatically, especially if unilateral, and the clinician must not overlook other local causes of low back pain (Ch. 6).

SHIN SPLINTS

The term *shin splints* is applied to a pain syndrome in the anterior aspect of the lower half of the shin. It is associated with running, jogging, or walking; is

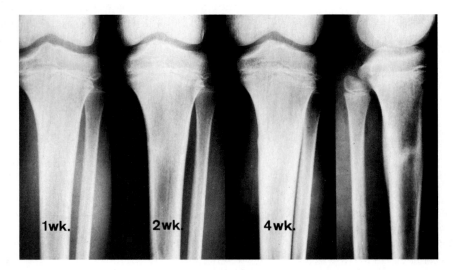

Fig. 4-1 Serial films document the radiographic evolution of a stress fracture in a 10-year-old girl who was the hopscotch champion of her block. Two weeks after the onset of leg pain, the fracture line is evident. After 4 weeks, the fracture callus is seen. (Courtesy of Dr Robert N Hensinger.)

worse with activity; and is relieved by rest. There may be numbness or anesthesia over the fourth toe. The symptoms result from overuse of the posterior tibial muscle. Rarely, an anterior compartment syndrome resulting from hemorrhage or edema, accompanied by ischemic changes in the foot, may be confused with shin splints. Shin splints are best prevented by adequate stretching and strengthening and avoidance of jogging or walking on hard surfaces. Treatment is symptomatic.

TENNIS ELBOW

Pain experienced over the lateral epicondyle, evoked by resisted supination of the wrist, is referred to as *lateral epicondylitis* or *tennis elbow*. It is believed to result from a strain or tear of the extensor aponeurosis. It may be treated by use of a "tennis elbow strap" that surrounds the forearm just distal to the painful site. Corticosteroid injections may be necessary, since the condition may persist for months.

TENOSYNOVITIS

Although tenosynovitis commonly accompanies rheumatic diseases, it may also occur as a result of unaccustomed repetitive movement, especially around the ankle (Achilles tenosynovitis, anterior tibial tenosynovitis) or at the wrist, or of stenosing tenosynovitis of the abductor pollicis longus or extensor pollicis brevis (de Quervain's disease). Treatment requires rest, with splinting if needed, and possibly injection of corticosteroid into the tendon sheath.

For a complete discussion of these and other overuse syndromes, the reader is referred to the work of Sheon, Moskowitz, and Goldberg.[21]

Trauma

TRAUMATIC ARTHRITIS

Joint swelling associated with trauma occurs in older school-age children and adolescents. An effusion arising immediately after an injury is more likely to be associated with intraarticular hemorrhage, fracture, or joint derangement than swelling that develops over several hours. In juvenile rheumatoid arthritis (JRA) a history of trauma is often elicited because a minor injury brings a swollen joint to parental attention. Trauma, especially minor trauma, is not an explanation for joint swelling in a young child (except for self-evident conditions such as "nursemaid's elbow"), and internal joint derangements (meniscal tears) are very rare. JRA is far more common than traumatic arthritis in the very young. Joint swelling can result, however, from patellar subluxation or from the repetitive trauma associated with overuse syndromes or structurally abnormal joints in older children.

NONACCIDENTAL TRAUMA

Child Abuse

An abused infant or child is sometimes initially suspected of having a rheumatic disease because of refusal to bear weight, presence of a joint effusion, or skin lesions that are thought to be vasculitic in origin. These children may be misdiagnosed as having JRA if a proper history is not documented. Beating a child, particularly over the hands and knuckles, results in brawny induration of the dorsa of the hands, as well as thickened, dense round bones and bone chips seen on radiographs. Physical abuse should be considered in a child who has a history of repeated visits to the emergency room because of poorly explained trauma, occurrence of allegedly spontaneous bruises, or hemarthrosis without an underlying bleeding disorder. Radiographic demonstration of multiple fractures and periosteal new bone formation is characteristic. The disorder termed *Munchausen's syndrome by proxy* is a bizarre form of child abuse induced by the parent in order to bring the child to medical attention for other, usually significant reasons.

PANCREATITIS WITH ARTHRITIS

Acute or chronic pancreatitis or pseudocyst formation from trauma to the pancreas may be accompanied by disseminated fat necrosis, leading to the development of subcutaneous nodules and osteolytic lesions resembling multicentric osteomyelitis or JRA.[22–24] The nodules are tender, erythematous, and widely disseminated and are similar to those of erythema nodosum. They are often accompanied by systemic illness and fever. Joint pains and effusions may develop 2 to 3 weeks after the initial insult. The rheumatic disease is self-limited in most cases and remits spontaneously.

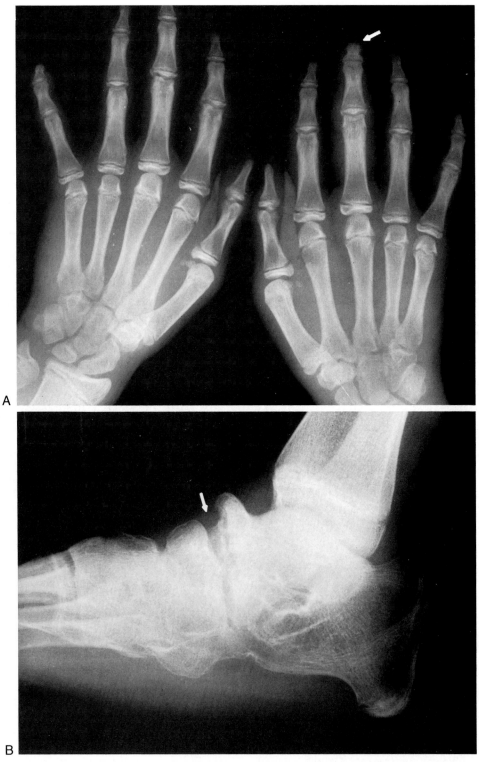

Fig. 4-2 Congenital indifference to pain. These four radiographs are from a girl with congenital indifference to pain and deafness. (**A**) She has lost the tips of several fingers (arrow). (**B**) Hypertrophic and destructive changes are seen in the calcaneus, talus, and midfoot (arrow). (*Figure continues.*)

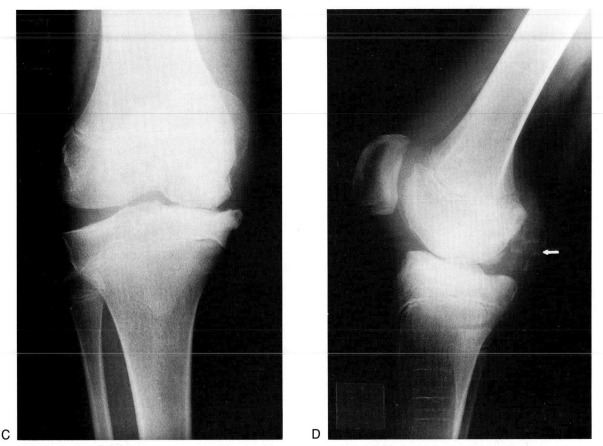

C   D

Fig. 4-2 (*Continued*). Similar changes are seen in the (**C**) anteroposterior and (**D**) lateral radiographs of the right knee joint with marked loss of the medial compartment space and posterior calcifications typical of a Charcot's arthropathy (arrow). Clinically the knees were characterized by increased warmth and large chronic effusions.

Soft tissue swelling is evident on radiographs, with multiple sites of periosteal new bone apposition and diaphyseal lytic lesions. Because the bony lesions are delayed in appearance by a few months, the initiating abdominal trauma may have been forgotten. Diagnosis is confirmed during the acute illness by elevation of the serum lipase and amylase concentrations. A bone scan may demonstrate increased uptake of isotope in the metaphyses or diaphyses because of the infarctions that have resulted from the disseminated intravascular fat.

CONGENITAL INDIFFERENCE TO PAIN

Rarely, children with congenital indifference to pain develop swollen but painless joints, associated with induration or necrosis of the toes and fingers[25] (Fig. 4-2). Such children may be deaf or have a syndrome of familial dysautonomia. This Charcot type of arthropathy results in severely damaged, often unstable joints that may eventually require arthrodesis in order to maximize function.

FROSTBITE ARTHROPATHY

Frostbite is a cold-induced necrosis of the superficial tissues that follows prolonged exposure to freezing temperatures in association with alterations in humidity. The acral or exposed areas, including the fingers, toes, nose, and ears, are predominantly affected. Immediately after exposure, the diagnosis of frostbite can be made by the characteristic appearance of swollen red fingers or toes. The history of cold exposure should be obvious, although in babies the parents may not have been aware of the increased sensitivity of the very young child to cold injury.

Vasomotor changes suggesting Raynaud's phenomenon may persist for months after injury. In the growing child, frostbite produces a characteristic stunting of growth of the small bones of the hands and feet from epiphyseal necrosis and acro-osteolysis (Fig. 4-3).[26,27] Secondary symptoms of osteoarthritis may develop in early adulthood.

PAIN AMPLIFICATION SYNDROMES

The concept of pain amplification syndromes is one that encompasses those disorders of the musculoskeletal system characterized by pain for which no organic cause can be found, or in which the patient's reaction to the pain is out of proportion to the physical findings. Syndromes that might be included in this category vary a great deal, but those in Table 4-11 will be discussed here.

Growing Pains

The use of the term *growing pains* frequently evokes a negative response, since most physicians (and many families) have experienced the diagnosis being inappropriately applied to the child who in actuality had a serious rheumatic or malignant disease. For this reason we need to restrict use of the term to a fairly narrow spectrum of complaints (Table 4-12). Deviation from this set of parameters should prompt utmost caution in attributing the child's complaint to growing pains.

Surveys of schoolchildren have indicated that as many as 10 to 20 percent of children experience the nonarticular limb pains referred to as *growing pains*.[28-30] Most growing pains occur in school-age children and young adolescents. The pain is sometimes crampy, usually localized to the lower extremities, often deep in the thigh, shin, or calf. Benign pain in the groin, back, or upper extremity is far less frequent. Growing pains may be precipitated by exercise and are usually relieved by massage. They

Table 4-11 Pain Amplification Syndromes in Childhood

Growing pains
Primary fibromyalgia syndrome
Reflex sympathetic dystrophy
Erythromelalgia

Table 4-12 Growing Pains

Age at onset: 4 to 12 years
Sex ratio: equal
Symptoms: bilateral, deep aching, cramping pain in the thighs or calves; often vague localization, usually in evening or during the night; may awaken child; never present in the morning
Signs: physical examination normal
Investigations: laboratory examination normal

occur in the evening or at night and often interrupt sleep. A few children have pain almost every night. Growing pains are never associated with a limp, and symptoms disappear by morning. Children with such pain have completely normal patterns of activity and normal findings indicated by physical examinations during and after the episode. Laboratory studies and radiographs all show normal results.

The pathophysiology of the pain is unknown. Long experience with such pains in many children, however, has proved that they do not develop into conditions that shorten life or disable. Successful management of growing pains includes education of the child and family about the benign nature of the problem. Most often the parent has already determined the most effective treatment: gentle massage with or without aspirin or acetaminophen. In children who have typical growing pains several nights a week, administration of low-dose aspirin with food at bedtime may be sufficient to prevent the pain from waking the child.

Primary Fibromyalgia Syndrome

Yunus et al. have called attention to the occurrence of fibromyalgia in the pediatric age group.[31] This is a disorder that occurs predominantly in teenage girls, rarely in boys. In a review of 50 cases, 28 percent were in children aged 9 to 15 years at onset.

Fibromyalgia is a benign syndrome characterized by diffuse, often ill-defined, musculoskeletal aching and stiffness (Table 4-13). Arthritis per se does not occur, and the child appears healthy. The patient often complains of constant fatigue, disturbed sleep patterns, anxiety, and depression. Diagnosis is based upon this history and the demonstration of multiple tender points (at least three) at characteristic, strikingly symmetric locations (insertions of tendons, bursae, epicondyles, trapezius and suboccipital mus-

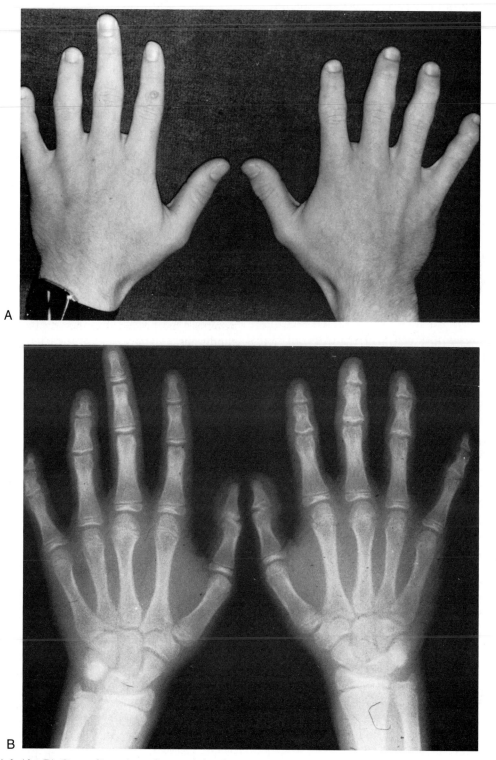

Fig. 4-3 (A&B) Gross distortion of normal development in the hands of this boy has resulted from repeated episodes of frostbite in northern Canada.

Table 4-13 Primary Fibromyalgia Syndrome

Age at onset: adolescence to adulthood
Sex ratio: girls ≫ boys
Symptoms: diffuse musculoskeletal aching and stiffness; generalized fatigue, anxiety, depression; disturbed sleep patterns
Signs: tender points at characteristic sites (3 sites for 3 months)
Investigations: laboratory examination normal

Table 4-14 Reflex Sympathetic Dystrophy

Age at onset: late childhood and adolescence to adulthood
Sex ratio: girls ≫ boys
Symptoms: exquisite superficial and deep pain in distal part of an extremity, exacerbated by passive or active movement
Signs: diffuse swelling and tenderness, evidence of autonomic dysfunction (coolness, mottling, increased sweating), bizarre posturing of affected part, refusal to move extremity
Investigations: osteoporosis, abnormal bone scintigraphy, laboratory examination normal

cles, scapulae and spine, sacroiliac joints, and iliac crests).

Fibromyalgia is a difficult disorder to treat. Diagnosis is frequently delayed because of failure to recognize the syndrome, and a high level of anxiety and skepticism in the patient and family must be dealt with as well. Assurances should be repeated that although the pain is quite real, it is not likely to represent any serious underlying disease such as arthritis. Most frequently, the child has withdrawn from most physical activities (because they appear to make the pain worse) and should be encouraged to return gradually to favorite sports and social activities. The physical therapist may be of great assistance in helping the patient establish a gradual but persistant return to normal activity, assisted by the use of physical modalities for the control of pain (ice, heat, transcutaneous nerve stimulation, ultrasound). A nonsteroidal anti-inflammatory drug (propionic acid derivative) may be helpful, as may the use of low-dose tricyclic antidepressants at bedtime.

Reflex Sympathetic Dystrophy

A number of names have been used to describe reflex sympathetic dystrophy, a pain amplification syndrome, including *reflex neurovascular dystrophy, algodystrophy, shoulder-hand syndrome, Sudek atrophy,* and *causalgia.* The syndrome is probably underrecognized in the pediatric population.[32-34] Children with reflex sympathetic dystrophy (RSD) are usually of school age or in the teenage years and have a history of constant pain and increasing disability in the distal part of an extremity that is exacerbated by even mild activity (Table 4-14).[33] It is assumed that the child has stopped using the affected limb as a response to injury although no specific trauma is identified in many children. If disuse persists long enough, any

attempt at resumption of function is painful and the child entirely abandons use of the extremity. The situation then quickly becomes a vicious cycle.

The involved extremity is characteristically tender, swollen, cool, and mottled. Even light touch may elicit severe discomfort and any attempt to move the limb passively or actively is very painful. The pain is often described as burning in character.[35] The generalized puffy appearance of the hand or foot is quite distinctive and is usually associated with purple or blue discoloration of the skin secondary to vascular dysregulation. A sudden decrease in skin temperature over the painful area may be detected clinically and confirmed by thermography. A bizarre posture (e.g., a claw hand) may be assumed. In the foot, there may be inappropriate fixed spasm of the muscles in the inverted or everted position.

Children with RSD typically present with an inappropriate affect. They often appear strangely happy—"la belle indifférence"—except when the symptomatic limb is touched or moved. They often appear to be highly motivated, overachieving individuals, who, prior to their illness, were extensively involved in school and extracurricular activities. Studies by Sherry et al. have documented abnormalities on psychological testing that may provide insights into predisposing factors.[36]

Radiographs of the affected part demonstrate soft tissue swelling, and, if 6 to 8 weeks have elapsed, generalized osteoporosis is also evident. Technetium bone scintigraphy may indicate normal findings or show a decrease or increase in uptake in the affected limb.[37-39] Care must be exercised in interpreting these studies since they are also affected by alterations in use of the limb.[34,40] Doppler studies may show changes in blood flow. The acute phase reactants are normal, and no inflammatory or infectious cause can be identified.

The treatment of RSD requires establishing a sympathetic attitude with the family and child and educating them as to the nature of the disorder. Three therapeutic approaches are followed. Control of pain is necessary if rehabilitation of the affected limb is to be successful. Pain control can often be achieved by judicious use of analgesia and transcutaneous nerve stimulation.[34,40] Physical therapy should be instituted immediately, beginning with tactile stimulation of the affected part and progressing to active and passive movement. Any form of immobilization is inappropriate and may lead to further loss of function. The use of hot packs or cooling procedures should be avoided. Sympathetic blockade with intravenous guanethidine[41] or reserpine[42] may be tried. It should be understood that the effect of the local anesthetic accompanying such procedures may be instrumental in achieving the therapeutic benefit.[41,43] Psychotherapy of the child and counseling of the family are required, especially if the episode is prolonged or if there are recurrences. Prognosis is generally excellent except for the child in whom RSD has been allowed to persist for a long period with repeated school absence and secondary gain.

Acute Transient Osteoporosis

Acute transient osteoporosis is a disorder that may resemble severe RSD. A history of trauma may precede by a few weeks the onset of debilitating pain with loss of range of motion, often in the hip. Acute phase reactants show normal findings, but radiographic studies demonstrate dramatic regional osteoporosis.[44,45] The relationship of this disorder to RSD and phantom bone disease is not clear. (See also Ch. 14.)

Erythromelalgia

A rare disorder of episodic erythema, increased heat, and burning pain in the feet (rarely in the hands) is known as *erythromelalgia* and has been described in a few children (Table 4-15).[46] There appear to be an equal sex distribution and no age predilection. The syndrome is often chronic, and exacerbations of pain are precipitated by heat, vasodilatation, and dependency. The affected child may regress to total disa-

---

Table 4-15 Erythromelalgia

Age at onset: no age predilection, occasionally hereditary(?)
Sex ratio: equal
Symptoms: episodic increased heat, redness, and burning pain in feet, less commonly in hands; precipitated by dependency, heat, vasodilatation; often progressive to total disability
Signs: erythema and increased heat of affected part; may be secondary to peripheral neuropathy, arterial occlusive disease, frostbite, polycythemia, hypertension, connective-tissue disease

---

bility. A primary form of the disease may be hereditary, or, in other cases, the disease may occur secondary to peripheral neuropathy, arterial occlusive disease, frostbite, polycythemia, hypertension, or an overt connective-tissue disease, especially systemic lupus erythematosus (SLE). Treatment involves avoidance of exposure to heat, elevation of the extremity, application of cold during acute attacks, and trials of agents such as epinephrine, propranolol, and aspirin.

HYPEROSTOSIS

Abnormal subperiosteal or endochondral bone deposition is a characteristic of a number of unrelated disorders. Hypertrophic osteoarthropathy is a type of hyperostosis in which there are clubbing of the fingers and toes, subperiosteal apposition of new bone along the shafts of the long bones, and occasionally arthritis. In children it may be a primary sporadic or hereditary disease, or it may result secondary to suppurative lung disease, inflammatory bowel disease, or tumor metastatic to lung, pleura, or mediastinum.[47] Asymptomatic isolated clubbing may occur in children with cyanotic congenital heart disease. Familial clubbing can occur without associated disease and is usually asymptomatic.

Radiographs show a distinctive picture of periosteal new bone apposition, soft tissue swelling, and joint effusions. Bone scintigraphy shows increased isotope uptake in the areas of new bone formation.

Pachydermoperiostosis is a rare familial disorder that is thought to be transmitted by an autosomal dominant gene. It is characterized by the onset (usually in adolescent boys) of "spadelike"' enlargement of the

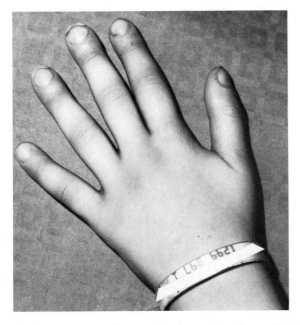

Fig. 4-4 Hypertrophic osteoarthropathy. Generalized swelling of the hand of a 13-year-old girl with pulmonary metastases from an osteogenic sarcoma.

Table 4-16 Secondary Hypertrophic Osteoarthropathy

Symptoms: deep, burning limb pain; night waking; profuse sweating

Signs: long bone tenderness, periosteal new bone formation, clubbing, joint effusions

hands and feet, sometimes accompanied by pain along the distal long bones.[48–50] In addition to cylindrical enlargement of the digits, forearms, and lower legs, there may be minimal joint effusions, coarsening of the facial features, oiliness of the skin, and occasionally gynecomastia, female hair distribution, striae, and acne.

Children with *secondary hypertrophic osteoarthropathy* (SHO) complain of deep, burning pain in the distal parts of the extremities that is present during the daytime and also awakens them at night (Table 4-16). The most common etiology of SHO in children is metastatic osteosarcoma,[48] although other causes have been reported (Figs. 4-4 and 4-5).[51,52]

A small proportion (5 percent) of children with cystic fibrosis develop SHO.[53,54] The concurrence of cystic fibrosis and JRA has been noted in several re-

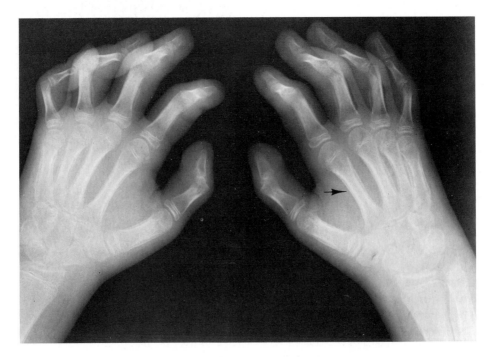

Fig. 4-5 Radiographs of the child in Fig. 4-4 showing marked periosteal new bone apposition.

ports, including of children with rheumatoid-factor-positive disease. In one teenage boy, typical rheumatoid nodules were noted at the olecranon processes.[55] Episodic arthritis has also been reported in children with cystic fibrosis.[56] In one study, three boys and two girls, age 2 to 20 years, had episodes of arthritis lasting from 1 to 10 days that occurred at intervals of weeks to months. One or more joints were affected during each episode. A pruritic nodular rash occurred in all five children. Results of serologic studies for rheumatoid factor (RF) and antinuclear antibody (ANA) were negative, and x-ray films revealed no abnormalities. The etiology of this self-limited arthropathy is unknown unless it is reactive.

Infantile Cortical Hyperostosis

Infantile cortical hyperostosis or Caffey's disease is an increasingly rare disease of the infant who presents before 4 months of age with fever, irritability, abnormal acute phase indices, and swelling, tenderness, erythema, or altered contour of the mandible, shoulder girdles, and long bones (Fig. 4-6).[57–59] Bony involvement tends to be asymmetrical. The calvarium is never affected. The ribs and clavicles are often involved by marked cortical thickening with altered bone shape. This disease is of unknown etiology although it appears to be inflammatory and is usually self-limited with a course of weeks to months. It then subsides generally without sequelae. Short-term treatment with corticosteroids may be considered in the infant with severe disease with marked systemic symptoms. There appears to be a familial but nongenetic basis for this disorder.

In diaphyseal dysplasia, progressive cortical thickening of the diaphyses of the long bones that begins between the ages of 3 and 5 years is diagnostic.[60] The lower extremities are principally affected, and there is a marked loss of muscle mass. The child experiences pain and weakness and may fail to thrive. Difficulty in walking dominates the clinical presentation. The alkaline phosphatase concentration may be increased. This disorder must be differentiated from secondary hypertrophic osteoarthropathy.

Melorheostosis leri, a rare disorder that develops after the neonatal period, commonly affects only one limb. Clinically there may be intermittent swelling and pain around joints, with loss of range of motion and development of contractures at the wrists, elbows, hips, and knees.[61,62] Skin changes may precede contractures and include tense, red, shiny skin with edema of the subcutaneous tissues.

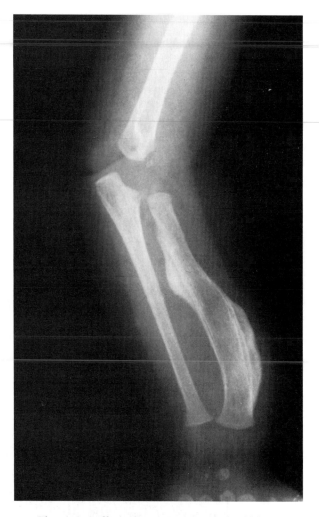

Fig. 4-6 Caffey's disease in a 5-month-old boy.

Radiographs show cortical hyperostosis in a "dripping candle wax" pattern, sometimes with endosteal hyperostosis and prominent soft tissue calcification.

The *Goldbloom syndrome* is another form of idiopathic periosteal new bone formation associated with fever, constitutional symptoms, severe pain in the extremities, and elevated serum gamma globulins and sedimentation rate.[63] Radiographs show typical periosteal new bone apposition along the long bones. The child may develop limited motion in contiguous joints and refuse to walk if the lower extremities are involved. The disorder runs a chronic course over several months with a spontaneous recovery. Nonsteroidal anti-inflammatory agents are sometimes useful for control of symptoms. There is no etiology known, but the disorder may follow an infectious disease or viral syndrome.

Other rare forms of acquired hyperostosis have been described in children. Among those to be considered in this category along with the preceding disorders are *cherubism* and *leontiasis ossei.*[64]

PAIN SYNDROMES AFFECTING THE THORAX

Chest pain in children may arise from a variety of causes, including cardiac and intra-abdominal disease. Those causes related to the musculoskeletal system are briefly outlined in this section.

Slipping Rib Syndrome

The slipping rib syndrome is produced by trauma to the costal cartilages of the eighth to tenth ribs. These cartilages attach to each other, rather than to the sternum, by fibrous tissue. Interruption of this fibrous tissue by trauma permits a rib to impinge upon the adjacent rib, causing a click and sharp pain under the ribs. Symptoms may be precipitated in a number of ways, including forward flexion, deep breathing, and raising of the arm on the affected side. The physician can reproduce the symptoms by hooking fingers under the inferior margins of the affected ribs and pulling anteriorly. Treatment consists of injection of local anesthetic or surgical excision of the subluxing cartilaginous rib tip.[65]

Costochondritis

Costochondritis, characterized by anterior chest wall pain that is reproduced by palpation of one or more costal cartilages, has been reported to be quite common in adolescents, constituting the reason for 4 percent of outpatient visits to one adolescent clinic.[66] No specific treatment is required except occasional analgesia and reassurance that there is no serious underlying disease.

Tietze's Syndrome

A number of terms have been applied to a syndrome characterized by anterior chest wall pain arising from the costal cartilages. Tietze's syndrome is one such disorder that is accompanied by swelling of the affected costal cartilage. It may result from trauma or idiopathic inflammation.[67] Onset is generally during adolescence. One and occasionally two or more costochondral junctions (usually the second or third) are painful, tender, and enlarged. The associated pain is usually acute and stabbing, often related to position or deep breathing. The syndrome may be self-limited or chronic and intermittent, lasting from a few months to a few years. Local anesthetic injections and nonsteroidal anti-inflammatory drugs may provide symptomatic relief.

MISCELLANEOUS DISORDERS

Torticollis

Torticollis, or wryneck, may accompany JRA as a manifestation of cervical spine disease or occur secondary to a neurologic abnormality or idiopathic shortening of a sternocleidomastoid muscle. Squints, if uncorrected surgically, may lead to a head tilt that can become permanent, with asymmetry of the facial structures. Acute torticollis is transient if associated with trauma or cervical adenitis. The phenothiazine group of drugs and psychogenic disorders may also lead to torticollis.[68] The therapeutic approach is through intensive physiotherapy before consideration of surgical release.

Aneuralgic Amyotrophy

Aneuralgic amyotrophy presents as an acute onset of pain in a shoulder, followed by muscle wasting but not by restricted range of motion. It is often bilateral and may follow a vaccination or infection. Some cases are familial.[69] It tends to occur in the older child. Recovery requires many months of intensive physical therapy. Brachial neuritis follows a similar pattern but is accompanied by paralysis of the affected part.

Fluorosis

Fluorosis is endemic in certain areas of the world and can cause chronic rheumatic complaints in children. High levels of fluoride are found naturally in the water supply or result from industrial pollution. Knee pain is often an early symptom, followed by limb, hand, or spinal abnormalities that mimic those of JRA or JAS. Bone density is increased on radiographs, and later severe disease develops with calcification of the spinal ligaments, intervertebral discs, and entheses. Cord compression can result from narrowing of the spinal canal.

REFERENCES

1. Passo MH: Aches and limb pain. Pediatr Clin North Am 28:209, 1982
2. Bowyer SL, Hollister JR: Limb pain in childhood. Pediatr Clin North Am 31:1053, 1984
3. Brewer EJ, Jr: Pitfalls in the diagnosis of juvenile rheumatoid arthritis. Pediatr Clin North Am 33:1015, 1987
4. Cassidy JT: Miscellaneous conditions associated with arthritis in children. Pediatr Clin North Am 33:1033, 1987
5. Kirk JA, Ansell B, Bywaters EGL: The hypermobility syndrome. Ann Rheum Dis 26:419, 1967
6. Jessee EF, Owen DS, Jr, Sagar KB: The benign hypermobile joint syndrome. Arthritis Rheum 23:1053, 1980
7. Biro F, Gewanter HC, Baum J: The hypermobility syndrome. Pediatrics 72:701, 1983
8. Carter C, Wilkinson J: Persistent joint laxity and congenital dislocation of the hip. J Bone Joint Surg 46B:40, 1964
9. Gedalia A, Person DA, Brewer EJ, Jr et al: Hypermobility of the joints in juvenile episodic arthritis/arthralgia. J Pediatr 107:873, 1985
10. Goldberg MJ: Gymnastic injuries. Orthop Clin North Am 11:717, 1980
11. Klemp P, Stevens JE, Isaacs S: A hypermobility study in ballet dancers. J Rheumatol 11:692, 1984
12. Marks JS, Sharp J, Brear SG et al: Normal joint mobility in mitral valve prolapse. Ann Rheum Dis 42:54, 1983
13. Giannestras NJ: Other problems of the forepart of the foot. In Giannestras NJ (ed): Foot Disorders. Lea & Febiger, Philadelphia, 1973, p. 410
14. Giannestras NJ: Problems of the tarsal portion of the foot in the adolescent and the adult. In Giannestras NJ (ed): Foot Disorders. Lea & Febiger, Philadelphia, 1973, p. 565
15. Harris RI, Beath T: Hypermobile flat-foot with short tendo achillis. J Bone Joint Surg 30A:116, 1948
16. Gross RH: Foot pain in children. Pediatr Clin North Am 24:813, 1977
17. Radin EL: Chondromalacia of the patella. Bull Rheum Dis 34:1, 1984
18. Reid GD, Glasgow M, Gordon DA et al: Pathological plicae of the knee mistaken for arthritis. J Rheumatol 7:573, 1980
19. Smith JB: Knee problems in children. Pediatr Clin North Am 24:841, 1977
20. Devas MB: Stress fractures in children. J Bone Joint Surg 45B:528, 1963
21. Sheon RP, Moskowitz RW, Goldberg VM: Soft Tissue Rheumatic Pain: Recognition, Management and Prevention. Lea & Febiger, Philadelphia, 1982
22. Shackleford PG: Osseous lesions and pancreatitis. Am J Dis Child 131:731, 1977
23. Goluboff N, Cram R, Ramgotra B et al: Polyarthritis and bone lesions complicating traumatic pancreatitis in two children. Can Med Assoc J 118:924, 1978
24. Buntain WL, Wood JB, Wolley MM: Pancreatitis in childhood. J Pediatr Surg 13:143, 1978
25. Nellhaus G: Neurogenic arthropathies (Charcot's joints) in children. Clin Pediatr 14:647, 1975
26. Carrera GF, Kozin F, McCarty D: Arthritis after frostbite injury in children. Arthritis Rheum 22:1082, 1979
27. Dreyfuss JR, Glimcher MJ: Epiphyseal injury following frostbite. N Engl J Med 253:1065, 1955
28. Øster J, Nielson A: Growing pains. A clinical investigation of a school population. Acta Paediatr Scand 61:328, 1972
29. Apley J: Limb pains with no organic disease. Clin Rheum Dis 2:487, 1976
30. Peterson H: Growing pains. Pediatr Clin North Am 33:1365, 1986
31. Yunus MB, Masi AT: Juvenile primary fibromyalgia syndrome: a clinical study of thirty-three patients and matched normal controls. Arthritis Rheum 28:138, 1985
32. Fermaglich DR: Reflex sympathetic dystrophy in children. Pediatrics 60:881, 1977
33. Bernstein BH, Singsen BH, Kent JT et al: Reflex neurovascular dystrophy in childhood. J Pediatr 93:211, 1978
34. Laxer RM, Allen RC, Malleson PN et al: Technetium 99-m-methylene diphosphonate bone scans in children with reflex neurovascular dystrophy. J Pediatr 106:437, 1985
35. Roberts J: A hypothesis on the physiological basis for causalgia and related pains. Pain 24:297, 1986
36. Sherry DD, Weisman R: Psychologic aspects of childhood reflex neurovascular dystrophy. Pediatrics 81:572, 1988
37. Nickerson RW, Person DA, Brewer EJ et al: Value of scintigraphy and vasodilaton medication in reflex neurovascular dystrophy (RND). Pediatr Res 16:166, 1982
38. Kozin F, Ryan LM, Carrera GF et al: The reflex sympathetic dystrophy syndrome. III: Scintigraphic studies, further evidence for the therapeutic efficacy of systemic corticosteroids and proposed diagnostic criteria. Am J Med 70:23, 1981

39. Holder LE, Mackinnon SE: Reflex sympathetic dystrophy in the hands: clinical and scintigraphic criteria. Radiology 152:517, 1984

40. Richlin DM, Carron H, Rowlingson JC et al: Reflex sympathetic dystrophy: successful treatment by transcutaneous nerve stimulation. J Pediatr 93:84, 1978

41. Holland AJC, Davies KH, Wallace DH: Sympathetic blockade of isolated limbs by intravenous guanethidine. Can Anaesth Soc J 24:597, 1977

42. Benzon HT, Chomka CM, Brunner EA: Treatment of reflex sympathetic dystrophy with regional intravenous reserpine. Anesth Analg 59:500, 1980

43. Christensen K, Henriksen O: The reflex sympathetic dystrophy syndrome. Scand J Rheumatol 12:263, 1983

44. Lequesne M, Kerboull M, Bensasson M et al: Partial transient osteoporosis. Skeletal Radiol 2:1, 1977

45. Heyden G, Kindblom L-G, Nielsen JM: Disappearing bone disease. J Bone Joint Surg 59A:57, 1977

46. Babb RR, Alarcon-Segovia D, Fairbairn JF: Erythromelalgia: review of 51 cases. Circulation 29:136, 1964

47. Cavanaugh JJA, Holman GH: Hypertrophic osteoarthropathy in childhood. J Pediatr 66:27, 1965

48. Vogl A, Goldfisher S: Pachydermoperiostosis. Primary or idiopathic hypertrophic osteoarthropathy. Am J Med 33:166, 1962

49. Rimoin DL: Pachydermoperiostosis (idiopathic clubbing and periostosis). Genetic and physiologic considerations. N Engl J Med 272:923, 1965

50. Calabro JE, Marchesano JM, Abruzzo JL: Idiopathic hypertrophic osteoarthropathy (pachydermoperiostitis): onset before puberty. Arthritis Rheum 9:496, 1966

51. Petty RE, Cassidy JT, Heyn R et al: Secondary hypertrophic osteoarthropathy. An unusual cause of arthritis in childhood. Arthritis Rheum 19:902, 1976

52. Neale G, Kelsall AR, Doyle FH: Crohn's disease and diffuse symmetrical periostitis. Gut 9:383, 1968

53. Athreya BH, Borns P, Rosenlund ML: Cystic fibrosis and hypertrophic osteoarthropathy in children. Am J Dis Child 129:634, 1973

54. Nathanson I, Riddlesberger MM, Jr: Pulmonary hypertrophic osteoarthropathy in cystic fibrosis. Radiology 135:649, 1980

55. Sagransky DM, Greenwald RA: Seropositive rheumatoid arthritis in a patient with cystic fibrosis. Am J Dis Child 134:319, 1980

56. Newman AJ, Ansell BM: Episodic arthritis in children with cystic fibrosis. J Pediatr 94:594, 1979

57. Caffey J: Infantile cortical hyperostosis: a review of the clinical and radiographic features. Proc R Soc Med 50:347, 1957

58. Caffey J: Infantile cortical hyperostosis. J Pediatr 29:541, 1946

59. Caffey J, Silverman WA: Infantile cortical hyperostosis: preliminary report on a new syndrome. Am J Roentgenol 54:1, 1945

60. Poznanski AK: The Hand in Radiologic Diagnosis. WB Saunders, Philadelphia, 1974, p. 588

61. Léri A, Joanny J: Une affection non décrite des os: hyperostose "en coulée" sur toute la longueur d'un membre ou "mélorhéostose." Bull Med Soc Hop Paris 46:1141, 1922

62. Beauvais P, Fauré C, Montagne JP et al: Léri's melorheostosis: three pediatric cases and a review of the literature. Pediatr Radiol 6:153, 1977

63. Goldbloom RB, Stein PB, Eisen A et al: Idiopathic periosteal hyperostosis with dysproteinemia. A new clinical entity. N Engl J Med 27:873, 1966

64. Jaffee HL: Various hyperostoses of obscure origin. In Jaffee HL (ed): Metabolic, Degenerative, and Inflammatory Diseases of the Bones and Joints. Lea & Febiger, Philadelphia, 1972, p. 272

65. Porter GE: Slipping rib syndrome: an infrequently recognized entity in children: a report of three cases and review of the literature. Pediatrics 76:810, 1985

66. Brown RT: Costochondritis in adolescents. J Adolescent Health Care 1:198, 1981

67. Calabro JJ, Marshesano JM: Tietze's syndrome: report of a case with juvenile onset. J Pediatr 68:985, 1966

68. Boltshauser E: Differential diagnosis of torticollis in childhood. Schweiz Med Wochenschr 106:1261, 1976

69. Lane RJM, Dewar JA: Bilateral neurologic amyotrophy. Br Med J 1:895, 1978

5

Juvenile Rheumatoid Arthritis

DEFINITION AND CLASSIFICATION

Juvenile rheumatoid arthritis (JRA) is the most common rheumatic disease in children. It is one of the more frequent chronic illnesses of childhood and an important cause of disability and blindness. JRA may not represent a single disease but a syndrome of diverse etiologies. A number of closely related series of host responses that are characterized predominantly by idiopathic peripheral arthritis are probably grouped under the classification term of JRA. Current evidence implicates an immunoinflammatory pathogenesis, activated by contact with an external antigen or antigens, in a child with a specific immunogenetic predisposition.

Classification Criteria

Numerous sets of criteria for diagnosis and classification of children with JRA have evolved during the past two decades. The criteria proposed by the American Rheumatism Association (ARA) are most frequently used in North America (Table 5-1).[1-3] In the absence of a known etiology for JRA, these criteria define the age group under discussion, conditions for a diagnosis of arthritis, duration of disease necessary for a reasonable certainty of diagnosis, type of onset, and necessity of exclusions. It is not possible to construct criteria that delimit the protean manifestations of JRA without excluding all similar diseases. Unfortunately, classification criteria for all of the other pediatric rheumatic diseases are not systematized.

The presence of one or more of the ancillary characteristics of the disease helps to support a preliminary impression of JRA (Table 5-2).[7] In U.S. studies, pericarditis was found to be of little value as a selectivity item, since it occurred in five of the non-JRA diagnoses and in four of the JRA diagnoses.[1]

Defining age of onset at 15 years or less is arbitrary and based more on practice patterns in the United States than on biologic variation in disease during the adolescent years. Furthermore, although arthritis in one or more joints for 6 weeks may be sufficient for a diagnosis, a duration of arthritis of at least 3 months provides even more assurance that JRA is the correct diagnosis. Objective arthritis must be continuous and persistent and be distinguished from arthralgia or simple pain in the joints.

The early diagnosis of JRA has been materially strengthened by the recognition of the three types of onset of disease (Table 5-3).[4-9] Although these types of onset had been popularized by the 1970s, they were recognized as early as the studies of Sury in the 1950s and were in common use by investigators in the 1960s. The type of onset is defined by a constellation of clinical signs during the first 6 months of illness.[1-3] Polyarticular JRA begins in five or more joints, usually the knees, ankles, wrists, elbows, or small joints

Table 5-1 Criteria for the Classification of Juvenile Rheumatoid Arthritis

1. Age of onset < 16 years
2. Arthritis in one or more joints defined as swelling or effusion, or presence of two or more of the following signs: limitation of range of motion, tenderness or pain on motion, and increased heat
3. Duration of disease ≥ 6 weeks
4. Type of onset of disease during the first 6 months classified as:
   a. Polyarthritis: 5 or more joints
   b. Pauciarticular disease (oligoarthritis): 4 or fewer joints
   c. Systemic disease: arthritis with intermittent fever
5. Exclusion of other forms of juvenile arthritis

(Modified from Cassidy et al.,[3] with permission.)

Table 5-2 Ancillary Manifestations of JRA

Morning stiffness
Rheumatoid rash
Intermittent fever
Pericarditis
Chronic uveitis
Cervical spondylitis
Rheumatoid nodules
Tenosynovitis
Antinuclear antibodies
Rheumatoid factors

of the hands and feet. Oligoarticular or pauciarticular JRA is defined as onset of disease in four or fewer joints, usually of the lower extremities. Monarthritis (a single involved joint) is a subtype of this onset group. Systemic onset is characterized by a daily spiking fever to greater than 39°C for 2 weeks in association with arthritis of one or more joints. The majority of these children also have a characteristic erythematous, nonpruritic rash and other evidence of extra-articular involvement such as leukocytosis or prominent visceral disease, including lymphadenopathy, hepatosplenomegaly, and pericarditis.

There is no uniform worldwide agreement on the use of diagnostic terms in JRA.[10–12] In England *juvenile rheumatoid arthritis* refers only to children who are rheumatoid factor (RF) seropositive. The larger number of children with seronegative arthritis, including those who have diseases such as juvenile ankylosing spondylitis and psoriatic arthritis, and other children with connective-tissue diseases such as systemic lypus erythematosus (SLE), are referred to as having *juvenile chronic (poly)arthritis* (Table 5-4). In general, terms used in the Scandinavian countries, Germany, and France are similar to those in the United States.

A committee of the World Health Organization is presently studying the problem of international nomenclature.[13] The EULAR/WHO Workshop Criteria were developed at the Conference on the Care of Rheumatic Children in Oslo in 1977. It was pro-

Table 5-3 Classification of the Types of Onset of Juvenile Rheumatoid Arthritis

	Polyarthritis	Oligoarthritis (Pauciarticular Disease)	Systemic Disease
Frequency of cases	40%	50%	10%
Number of joints involved	≥5	≤4	Variable
Age of onset	Throughout childhood; peak at 1–3 years	Early childhood; peak at 1–2 years	Throughout childhood; no peak
Sex ratio (F:M)	3:1	5:1	1:1
Systemic involvement	Moderate involvement	Not present	Prominent
Occurrence of chronic uveitis	5%	20%	Rare
Frequency of seropositivity			
Rheumatoid factors	10% (increases with age)	Rare	Rare
Antinuclear antibodies	40–50%	75–85%[a]	10%
Prognosis	Guarded to moderately good	Excellent except for eyesight	Moderate to poor

[a] In girls with uveitis.

Table 5-4 Classification of Juvenile Chronic Arthritis, Taplow[a]

Polyarthritis with ankylosing spondylitis	12%
JRA—adult type with IgM rheumatoid factors	11%
Still's disease	70%
Systemic disease	
Polyarticular disease	
Pauciarticular disease	
Psoriatic arthropathy	5%
Arthritis associated with ulcerative colitis or regional enteritis	2%
Polyarthropathies associated with other disorders, such as SLE, familial Mediterranean fever, etc.	—

[a] Total number of children: 647.
(From Ansell,[7] with permission.)

posed that the term *juvenile chronic arthritis* (JCA) would be the preferred English language designation for the heterogeneous group of disorders that present as juvenile arthritis. The onset types of JCA would be distinguished as systemic, pauciarticular, and polyarticular. The diagnosis of JCA required onset of disease before 16 years of age, disease duration of more than 3 months, and careful exclusion of a list of diagnoses including infectious arthritis, specific nonrheumatologic abnormalities such as familial Mediterranean fever and sarcoidosis, hematologic disorders and neoplastic disease, the other major connective-tissue diseases and forms of vasculitis, and specific diseases singled out for difficulty in diagnostic discrimination such as acute rheumatic fever, SLE, and postinfectious arthropathies including Reiter's syndrome. Within the group labeled JCA it was judged possible to diagnose eventually juvenile ankylosing spondylitis, psoriatic arthropathy, and arthropathies associated with inflammatory bowel disease.

Various sets of diagnostic criteria were reexamined in a Norwegian report in 1982.[14] The North American criteria were preferred with emphasis or modifications to include a disease onset before 16 years of age, persistent arthritis for more than 3 months, and performance of a synovial biopsy in monarticular cases except in those children who had chronic uveitis.

HISTORICAL REVIEW

The suggestion that an inflammatory polyarthritis occurred in children was first made by Cornil in 1864 in a description of a 29-year-old woman with chronic inflammatory arthritis from the age of 12.[15] During the years that followed, a number of other reports were published, chiefly from France. Diamantberger reviewed this subject in 1890 and included 35 previously published cases and 3 of his own.[16] He commented on the acute onset of disease, predominant involvement of large joints, a course characterized by exacerbations and remissions, frequent disturbances of normal growth, and generally good prognosis.

Still presented the classic description of both the acute and chronic forms of JRA in 1897 while a medical registrar at the Hospital for Sick Children, Great Ormond Street, London.[17] On the basis of marked differences between the disease in children and adults, Still suggested that JRA might have a different etiology from rheumatoid arthritis or might include more than one disease. He pointed out that the disease almost always began before the second dentition, was more frequent in girls, and was usually of insidious onset.

In his report, an acute onset of disease was described in detail and distinguished from chronic inflammatory enlargement of the joints in the absence of erosions of the cartilage. Twelve patients who had lymphadenopathy, splenomegaly, and fever were singled out for emphasis. Serositis characterized by pleuritis and pericarditis was common in these children. The rash of JRA was not noted. Still indicated that there was often no articular pain and that children exhibited a marked tendency to early contracture and muscle atrophy. The cervical spine was affected in the majority of cases, often during the early stages of the disease. This report became the classic description of the disease and an outstanding example of bedside observation. Today the acute systemic onset of JRA is often referred to as *Still's disease*.

Johannessen in 1899 described three Norwegian children with JRA, none of whom had lymphadenopathy or splenomegaly.[18] Two patients came to necropsy and showed the typical changes of rheumatoid arthritis that had been described in adults. In 1922 a number of additional cases were described from Sweden.[19] Other children from Norway were reported by Frøhlich in 1930,[20] Hajkis in 1936,[21] and Sundt in 1936.[22] The last publication included a detailed review of the literature on Still's disease and added 27 new cases. Other patients were described from Denmark by Ellermann in 1914,[23] Monrad in 1919,[24] Bentzon in 1930,[25] Svendsgård in 1933,[26] Moltke in 1933,[27] Keiding in 1943,[28] and Harving in 1944.[29]

Hirschsprung in 1901 confirmed Still's observations that

a chronic articular disease was associated in young children with lymphadenopathy and splenomegaly and also described hepatomegaly.[30] Ibrahim in 1914 collected additional cases from the literature,[31] and Atkinson in 1939 published a review of 118 cases of Still's disease, 86 of whom showed severe arthritis, lymphadenopathy, and splenomegaly.[32]

Few other large series were published before the 1950s. Those that are well documented include studies by Colver in 1937,[33] Holzmüller in 1942,[34] Coss and Boots in 1946,[35] Edstrøm in 1947,[36] Bille in 1948,[37] Pickard in 1947,[38] and Lockie and Norcross in 1948.[39] Monographs on the subject were published by Wissler in 1942[40] and Françon in 1946.[41] French authors, such as Françon, have often used the term *syndrome de Chauffard-Still* for children with chronic arthritis, lymphadenopathy, and splenomegaly. In the excellent review of Edstrøm, only 3 of 65 children showed marked lymphadenopathy and splenomegaly, and Bille[37] found no examples of Still's disease among his 65 cases.

Coss and Boots in 1946[35] were the first in the United States to stress that Still's disease did not represent an independent clinical entity in children and that the term *juvenile rheumatoid arthritis* should be used to refer to all cases of idiopathic inflammatory arthritis. Dawson in 1946[42] corroborated this view and stressed that differences between children and adults were certainly underscored in the severity and frequency of the systemic symptoms (fever, splenomegaly, and leukocytosis) and an interference with normal growth and development. Many of these early authors stressed, however, that JRA could begin as a monarthritis that most frequently affected the knee and could persist in one joint for the duration of the illness or for several years before other joints were involved.[34,36–38]

Until Colver in 1937 published the first follow-up examinations of JRA,[33] the prognosis in this disease was considered to be very poor.[43,44] Extended periods of observation of patients with onset in childhood led some early authors to the conclusion that severe destruction of cartilage occurred in many children, and ankylosis would supervene in most.[45,46] Pickard found a mortality rate of 9 percent and complete recovery in 40 percent of his patients.[38] Lockie and Norcross reported a recovery rate of 40 percent and a mortality rate of 7 percent.[39] Edstrøm's series of 65 patients included 3 who had had Still's disease who were severely disabled and indicated that 35 of 52 children treated with gold salts were in full remission.[36] Of patients seen early in the course of their disease, 87 percent had good functional recovery, and even 65 percent of those seen after the first or second year had a good prognosis. Only 39 percent of children seen later than 2 years after onset had a return of function. A long, uninterrupted period of active disease was significantly associated with a poor prognosis; only 6 percent of children whose disease became quiescent within the first 4 years developed severe disability.

Sury identified 151 patients from 1920 to 1948 who had a chronic form of JRA with onset before age 15.[47] Thirty-nine percent of referred children and 19 percent of the children from Copenhagen were severely disabled at the time of the review. The peak age of onset in 100 girls was between ages 2 and 4 years. Of 51 boys, 8 had onset during the first year of life. Of 41 patients whose disease began with monarthritis, 23 had persistent disease in only one joint for at least the first year. On necropsy, 12 children showed a verrucous endocarditis. Sury reached the conclusion that it was not entirely possible to attempt a classification of children into well-defined clinical groups. He had observed an even transition between the various forms of the disease and concluded that separation of Still's disease according to that author's original criteria was not possible.

EPIDEMIOLOGY

JRA is not a rare disease, but its true prevalence is not known (Ch. 1). It has been described in all races and geographic areas. A number of estimates of its frequency have been attempted. One approach that has been used was to determine the proportion of adults in whom onset of rheumatoid arthritis (RA) occurred in childhood. Of all patients with RA, from 2.7 percent[48] to 5.2 percent[49] experienced onset of arthritis before the age of 15 years.

Incidence

Data collected on children in the state of Michigan in 1973 suggested a minimal incidence rate for JRA of 9.2 cases per 100,000 children at risk per year.[50] More recent data from the Mayo Clinic provided an incidence of 13.9 cases per 100,000 per year with 95 percent confidence limits of 9.9 to 18.7.[51] Two studies from Finland, one published in 1966[51] and another in 1986,[52] estimated that the incidence of JRA was six to eight new cases per 100,000 per year in the first study, and 19.6 per 100,000 per year in the second.

Prevalence

The prevalence of JRA in the Mayo Clinic survey was 113.4 cases per 100,000 children with 95 percent confidence limits of 69.1 to 196.3.[53] Bywaters found the prevalence of Still's disease in English schoolchildren to be 65 cases per 100,000.[12] Since some cases of JRA are undiagnosed, the figures cited undoubtedly represent minima.[54,55] In the Tecumseh Community Health Survey of 2,000 children between the ages of 6 and 15 years,[56] 10 percent complained of joint pain, just under 10 percent related a history of previous joint swelling, and 5 percent had morning stiffness, although only 2 children were found to have probable or definite JRA, a prevalence close to that estimated by Bywaters. Clearly, rheumatic symptoms, past or present, are not uncommon in children and far exceed the prevalence of JRA when objective criteria are used.

Age of Onset

JRA is defined arbitrarily as arthritis beginning before the age of 16 years.[1-3] Among the rheumatic diseases, JRA is characteristically a disease of young children. Although onset before 6 months of age is distinctly unusual, the age of onset of JRA is often quite young, with the highest frequency occurring at 1 to 3 years of age.[35,36,39,47,50,51,57-61] This age distribution is most pronounced in girls and in children with oligoarthritis. Systemic onset appears to have no increased frequency of occurrence at any particular age.

The distribution of ages at onset is shown in Figure 5-1[50] in a study of 300 children in whom the definition of JRA conformed to that of the ARA. The peak age at onset is between 1 and 3 years of age for the total group and for girls, but for boys this relationship is much less impressive. As shown in Figures 5-2, 5-3, and 5-4[50] the early peak is largely accounted for by girls with oligoarticular and polyarticular disease. Figure 5-3 shows a second, somewhat broader peak centered at 9 years of age. The contribution of boys and girls to this peak is approximately equal, in contrast to the earlier peak, in which girls greatly outnumber boys. The relatively high proportion of boys in the second peak raises the question of whether this group represents in part another disease such as early ankylosing spondylitis. Whatever the correct answer, the heterogeneity of distribution of age at onset points to the probability that JRA includes at least three fairly distinct entities.

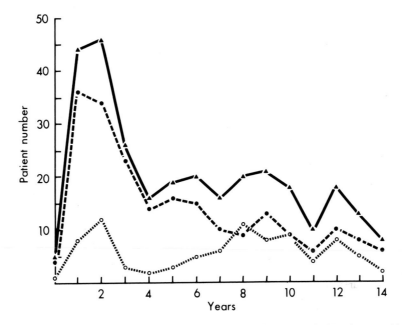

Fig. 5-1 Age of onset of 300 children with juvenile rheumatoid arthritis (JRA). Total group (▲—▲), girls (●–––●), and boys (○···○). For the total group and girls, a large peak at 1 to 2 years is observed. A bimodal distribution is clearer for boys, with the first peak at 2 years and the second at 9 years. No accentuation in frequency of onset was observed for either sex at 10 to 14 years. (From Sullivan et al.,[50] with permission.)

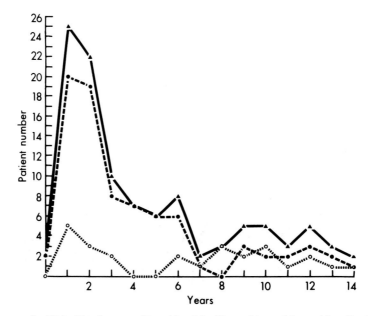

Fig. 5-2 Age of onset for JRA. Total group (▲—▲), girls (●---●), and boys (○···○). Polyarthritis. (From Sullivan et al.,[50] with permission.)

Sex Ratio

If JRA is regarded as a single entity, girls are affected twice as often as boys with a ratio of almost 2 to 1.[62] In children with uveitis accompanying JRA, the ratio of girls to boys is much higher: 5:1 to 6.6:1.[63–65] In children with polyarticular onset, girls outnumber boys in a ratio of 2.8 to 1. In striking contrast, systemic onset occurs with almost equal frequency in boys and girls.

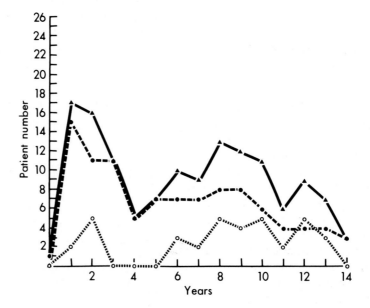

Fig. 5-3 Age of onset for JRA. Total group (▲—▲), girls (●---●), and boys (○···○). Oligoarthritis. (From Sullivan et al.,[50] with permission.)

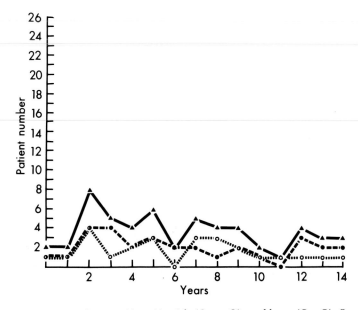

Fig. 5-4 Age of onset for JRA. Total group (▲—▲), girls (●---●), and boys (○···○). Systemic disease. (From Sullivan et al.,[50] with permission.)

These differences in sex ratios between the three onset types suggest either that there are three (or more) different diseases or that the disease expression is modified by differing genetic predispositions or environmental factors. Either or both possibilities are potentially valid.

Geographic and Racial Distribution

The incidence and prevalence data outlined previously were derived from North American or European white populations.[62–65] There are no comparable data for children of other geographic or racial groups.[66–68] Nonetheless, suggestions of disparity in frequency exist. The observations by Hanson et al. and our own suggest that there are proportionately fewer black than white children with JRA, although this impression may reflect referral pattern differences.[4] Some reports suggest that JRA and RA are less frequent in African than in European populations; in the former the proportion of all patients with onset of disease in childhood may be somewhat higher.[66] JRA may be significantly less common in North Americans of Chinese ancestry than in whites living in the same geographic area.[67] A report of increased

frequency of JRA in the North American Indian population is difficult to interpret because of the probability of inclusion of patients with B27-associated spondyloarthropathy.[67] An analysis of white and North American Indian children seen in the same rheumatology clinic suggests that although JRA occurs in Indian children, its frequency is not higher than that of the white population, whereas B27-associated arthritis is appreciably more frequent in the native Indian group (Table 5-5).

Table 5-5 Arthritis in North American Indian (NAI) Children

	Racial Origin		
	White	NAI	Total
Total number with arthritis	50	15	65
Number with clinical JRA	38	5	43
Number with HLA-B27	3	1	4
Number with clinical "seronegative spondyloarthropathy"	9	10	19
Number with HLA-B27	9	10	19

(Data from Pediatric Rheumatology Clinic, Children's Hospital, Winnipeg, Canada, Petty RE, Schroeder M-L, Oen K et al: Unpublished observations.)

ETIOLOGY AND PATHOGENESIS

The cause of JRA is unknown. There may be multiple etiologic events resulting in the similar arthritic diseases that we group under the classification of juvenile rheumatoid arthritis, or JRA may result from a single pathogenic vector with multiple clinical patterns evolving from interactions with the host. Among possible causes are infection, autoimmunity, trauma, stress, and immunogenetic predisposition.

An inflammatory arthritis of humans has been observed with infections from both mycoplasma and viruses (rubella and parvovirus).[69,70] Certain viral illnesses of childhood such as rubella may result in a self-limited arthritis. Persistent rubella virus infection has been demonstrated in the synovia of children with JRA by Chantler et al.[69] In this study, virus was isolated from peripheral blood or synovial fluid mononuclear cells in none of 16 controls and in 7 of 19 children with chronic rheumatic disease (JRA: 2 of 2 with polyarticular, 2 of 6 with pauciarticular, and 1 of 5 with systemic onset; JAS: 2 of 6). The prodrome to hepatitis B is characterized by fever, malaise, urticarial rash, and polyarthritis. Chronic inflammation may be perpetuated by immune complexes formed from autoantibodies such as antinuclear antibody (ANA) or rheumatoid factor (RF) induced by infections. Chronic arthritis is especially common in children who have impaired defense mechanisms and overt forms of immunodeficiency such as selective IgA deficiency, hypogammaglobulinemia, or C2 complement component deficiency (Ch. 11).

It is observed frequently that onset of JRA may follow physical trauma to an extremity such as a fall or an ankle sprain. Such trauma may serve as a localizing factor, may simply call attention of the family to an already involved and weakened joint, or may play a role in precipitating the disease. It is also well documented that psychological stress appears to be particularly common in families of children with JRA.[71]

Recent studies have suggested that aberrations in suppressor T-lymphocyte function may be instrumental in the immunopathogenesis of JRA.[72-79] It was noted in several of these investigations that serum antibodies from patients with JRA were directed at T-4 cells.[72,77] Lymphocytes eluted from the synovial membranes of children with JRA were shown in one study to consist of 71 percent T lymphocytes and 4 percent B lymphocytes.[80]

Autoimmune responses to collagen have been investigated in children with JRA, and antibodies to types I, II, and IV collagen have been demonstrated in recent studies.[81-83] Antibodies to streptococcal peptidoglycan were present in children with oligoarthritis and uveitis and in those with juvenile ankylosing spondylitis.[84] Antibody responses to new antigens may be defective.[85]

Peripheral blood lymphocytes from children with JRA display altered responsiveness to mitogens in vitro.[86-92] In one study, lymphocytes from children with oligoarthritis responded normally, whereas those from patients with polyarthritis or systemic disease had a diminished response.[88]

Investigators at the Rheumatism Hospital in Oslo have indicated that the presence of C-reactive protein in the sera of children with JRA was not responsible for the diminution of delayed hypersensitivity responses in children with JRA.[93] Cell-mediated immunity was assessed in our clinic in 97 children with JRA by using two in vitro assays: (1) lymphocyte transformation (LT) and (2) generation of leukocyte migration inhibition factor (LMIF).[90] LT was normal in children with JRA with the exception of patients with systemic onset. Significantly subnormal responses in LMIF generation were seen in children with pauciarticular and systemic onsets.

GENETIC BACKGROUND

Familial Juvenile Rheumatoid Arthritis

There are very few reported instances in which JRA has been observed in more than one family member. These reports are summarized in Table 5-6. Although the cases are few in number, it is striking that within any one family JRA tends to be of the same type of onset.[94] This observation suggests that each onset type may represent a different disease or the same disease occurring in children of different genetic predisposition. Early studies of Ansell et al. reported that female relatives of children with JRA showed an increased frequency of seronegative erosive polyarthritis and that male relatives had an increased prevalence of sacroiliac arthritis.[95]

Studies of identical twins have shown a remarkable concordance for JRA.[96,97] Ansell et al. reported that two of five pairs of identical twins were concordant for arthritis[98]; in one pair of twin boys, however, a

Table 5-6 Reports of JRA in Families

Reference	Type of Onset[a]	Relationship
Baum & Fink[96]	O	Monozygotic twins
Kapusta et al.[97]	O	Mother and monozygotic twin sons
Yodfat et al.[101]	S	4 siblings
Cekovský et al.[102]	O	3 brothers
Rosenberg and Petty[94]	O	2 sisters
	P	Sister and brother
	P	Mother and daughter
Clemens et al.[99]	O	3 pairs (brother/ sister)
	O	6 pairs of sisters
	O	2 brothers
	P	2 sisters
	O/P	2 sisters
Delgado et al.[103]	P	Sister and brother
Cassidy et al. (unpublished observations)	O/P	Sister and brother
	O/P	2 sisters
	P	Sister and brother

[a] Type of onset: P = polyarthritis; O = oligoarthritis; S = systemic disease.

Table 5-7 Twin Studies in Children with Oligoarticular JRA

Characteristic	No. Concordant (12 Sibling Pairs)
Sex	9
Age of onset (within 3 years)	11
Type of onset	
Oligoarthritis	10
Polyarthritis	1
Course of disease	
Oligoarthritis	9
Polyarthritis	2
ANA seropositivity	7 +/+; 3 −/−
Chronic uveitis	4 +/+; 5 −/−

(Adapted from Clemens et al.,[100] with permission.)

later diagnosis of ankylosing spondylitis (AS) was made. In the second pair of twin girls the disease remitted in both, and although they may have satisfied the criteria for a diagnosis of JRA, a viral infection may also have played a causative role.[95,98] Six nonidentical twins were discordant for this disease.

Studies by Clemens et al. showed remarkable concordance for onset of disease, clinical manifestations, and disease course (Table 5-7).[99,100] In nine twins who were concordant for type of onset, both siblings had two DR antigens and two shared one DR antigen. These findings confirmed a genetic predisposition to develop oligoarticular JRA and suggested a disease susceptibility HLA gene(s). An examination of the time of onset of arthritis in families in which two or more children were affected indicated that the intervals between onset of arthritis in each of the siblings varied from 7 months to 11 years. In no instance was there simultaneous onset of disease, although in most cases the age of onset was similar.

Three sibling pairs with JRA were identified in the University of Michigan clinic among 300 consecutive children seen between 1963 and 1972.[101] Ages of onset for these pairs were 5, 10, and 2 years. The intervals of time between onset of arthritis in the first and the second sibling were 2, 5, and 3 years.

One further association bears attention: the occurrence of JRA and adult rheumatoid arthritis (RA) in the same family. Very little documentation of this event exists, and it must be concluded that JRA and RA only occasionally occur in the same family. Rossen et al. studied, however, four families with multiple cases of RA and JRA and concluded from histocompatibility data that susceptibility to arthritis was influenced by a dominant allele with variable penetrance and expressivity.[104]

HLA Relationships

Although JRA has been rarely observed to occur in siblings or in families in which first-degree relatives have another connective-tissue disease, recent studies of histocompatibility antigens point clearly to a possible hereditary predisposition to the disease (Table 5-8).[105-126] These investigations provide evidence of fundamental distinctions between RA and JRA and its subtypes. HLA-DR4 is associated with seropositive RA in adults and in children with a more adult type of onset and course of disease and RF seropositivity. A decrease in Dw4[107] and DR4[118] has been noted principally in young girls with persistent oligoarthritis and ANA seropositivity. Increases in frequency of DR5[108,109] and of DRw8[108-118] have been

Table 5-8 HLA Relationships in Children with JRA

Type of Onset	Class I	Class II
Oligoarthritis (early onset ≤6 yrs)	A2 B44, 35, 16 Cw4	Dw7, ↓DR4
With uveitis		Dw/DR5 Dw/DRw8 Dw6 DRw52, w62 DPw2
Without uveitis ANA +	A2	DR5, w8 DR5, w6, w8 DQw1
Polyarthritis RF +	B8, 15	Dw14 Dw/DR4
Systemic disease	B8, 35	DR4 Dw7

(Modified from Howard et al.,[116] with permission.)

associated with pauciarticular disease in young girls with ANA seropositivity and chronic uveitis. Others have found normal frequencies for DR5.[111]

HLA associations in children with JRA are evolving in complexity with delineation of additional polymorphisms at the DR region and more centromeric gene loci, such as DQ and DP.[123,127] In a recent study by Hoffman et al., there was a significantly increased frequency of HLA-DPw2 in a population of children with oligoarthritis and uveitis compared to that of control subjects (67 percent versus 34 percent).[123] This finding was independent of the known association of JRA with A2 that has been identified in girls and is probably also separate from the relationships with DR5 or DRw8 cited earlier.

HLA typing has added an important dimension to the laboratory delineation of juvenile arthritis in selected cases, as the presence of HLA-B27 is characteristic of the spondyloarthropathies.[128–135] The apparently increased prevalence of HLA-B27 that was initially described in children with JRA was postulated by Schaller et al.[132] to be related to an increased frequency in two subgroups of children: those whose arthritis had progressed to juvenile ankylosing spondylitis and boys with lower extremity arthritis of later age of onset who might have early but not yet diagnosed ankylosing spondylitis.

CLINICAL MANIFESTATIONS

Constitutional Signs and Symptoms

A child's ability to communicate symptoms of illness varies according to age. In the young child with JRA there may be increased irritability, anorexia, a posture of guarding the joints, a limp, or absolute refusal to crawl or walk. The child may regress to more infantile patterns of adaptation. Increased fatigue and fever are common at onset in polyarticular and systemic disease. Weight loss and failure to grow are observed in many children; however, extreme degrees of malnutrition or muscle atrophy are seldom encountered. Frequent symptoms that may not be expressed directly include morning stiffness, gelling

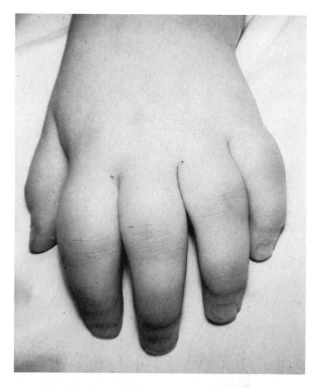

Fig. 5-5 Hand of a 2½-year-old boy with systemic onset of JRA. The hand and wrist were diffusely swollen, and the small joints were warm and painful. The distal and proximal interphalangeal joints were erythematous. Moderate flexion contractures were present in the digits, and there was swelling of the flexor tendon sheaths and digits between the phalangeal joints.

following inactivity, and night pain. Their presence may be suspected only by careful observation of the child or questioning of the parent.

Joint Pain and Pattern of Involvement

The cardinal signs of inflammation indicate the presence of objective arthritis as opposed to simple arthralgia (Fig. 5-5). Swelling results from periarticular soft tissue inflammation and edema and from intra-articular effusion. Involved joints are warm but usually not erythematous. Although tenderness or pain on motion of a joint may be present, the child often does not complain of pain at rest.[136] Studies of children with JRA have shown that they probably perceive pain as less severe than normal children or adults with RA, and complaints correlate poorly with other measures of activity or severity of the disease.[137–140]

The large joints such as the knees, ankles, wrists, elbows, and shoulders are most frequently involved. The small joints of the hands and feet may also be affected. Except in pauciarticular disease, the pattern of the arthritis is usually symmetric (Fig. 5-6). The distal interphalangeal (DIP) joints of the hands are involved in approximately 10 percent of the children and are more frequently affected in polyarthritis and much less so in oligoarthritis (Figs. 5-7 and 5-8, Table 5-9). Radial deviation at the metacarpophalangeal (MCP) joints is more characteristic than ulnar drift. Temporomandibular joint (TMJ) arthritis is relatively common and contributes to the development of micrognathia and inability to open the mouth normally. Ankylosis of these joints is, however, uncommon.[141,142] The acromioclavicular, sternoclavicular, and manubriosternal joints are infrequently affected. Cricoarytenoid arthritis is unusual in JRA but may cause acute airway obstruction.[143,144]

Disease in the apophyseal joints of the cervical spine is uncommon in JRA at onset, but approximately 60 percent of children eventually develop involvement of this area of the axial skeleton.[145–147] The neck is often painful and stiff, and a rapid loss of extension and rotation may result (Fig. 5-9). At-lantoaxial subluxation may occur early, making a

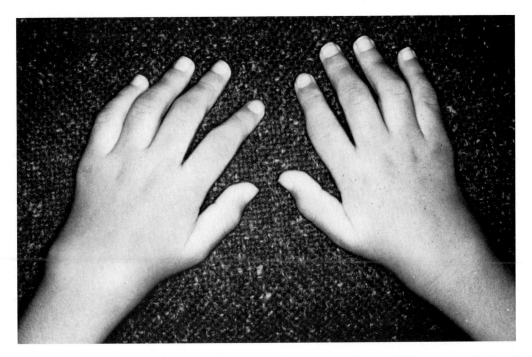

Fig. 5-6 Hands of a 6-year-old boy showing marked swelling of the PIP, IP, MCP, and carpal joints. Polyarticular onset of severe and unremitting JRA began at 1 year of age.

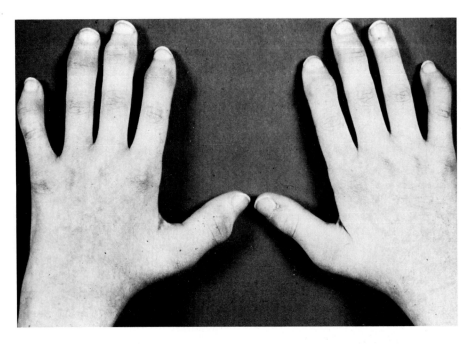

Fig. 5-7 Hands of a 7-year-old girl showing soft tissue swelling and erythema of the distal interphalangeal joints. Systemic onset of JRA began at 5½ years of age.

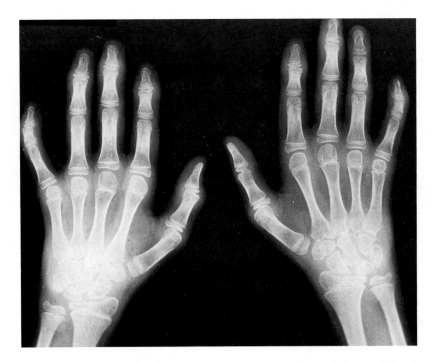

Fig. 5-8 Radiographs of the hands shown in Fig. 5-7. Soft tissue swelling of the DIP joints is present. Except for osteoporosis, the bony structure of these joints is normal. Extensive soft tissue and bony disease is present in the other small joints of these hands and wrists.

Table 5-9 Arthritis of Distal Interphalangeal (DIP) Joints in Children with JRA

Type of Onset of Disease	Number	Number with DIP Involvement	%
Polyarthritis	38	17	45
Polyarthritis → oligoarthritis	2	0	0
Oligoarthritis	33	1	3
Oligoarthritis→ polyarthritis	6	3	50
Systemic disease	17	3	18
Systemic → polyarthritis	4	0	0
Total	100	24	24

child at risk to injury in an accident or at the time of attempted intubation prior to general anesthesia. Rarely, a child develops torticollis, which may be associated with unilateral apophyseal joint disease. Involvement of the thoracolumbar apophyseal joints is generally not appreciated clinically. However, scoliosis was increased in frequency by as much as 30 times in children with JRA in one European study.[148,149] Low-grade inflammation of the sacroiliac joints may be seen in a small number of children with JRA and is to be distinguished from the more pronounced disease observed in JAS. The sacroiliac joints may eventually fuse in JRA, particularly in children who have been bedridden.

Small outpouchings of synovium are not uncommon in JRA and are particularly evident at the extensor hood of the PIP joints and around the wrist or ankle. Large synovial cysts are an unusual complication. These may appear in the popliteal space and dissect into the calf, the so-called Baker's cyst (Fig. 5-10).[150-153] Less commonly, they may develop in the antecubital area or anterior to the shoulder. Occasionally, these cysts may rupture and cause inflammation in the contiguous muscles and tissues. Contrast studies or ultrasound echograms may aid in their correct diagnosis. Synovial cysts may be the initial

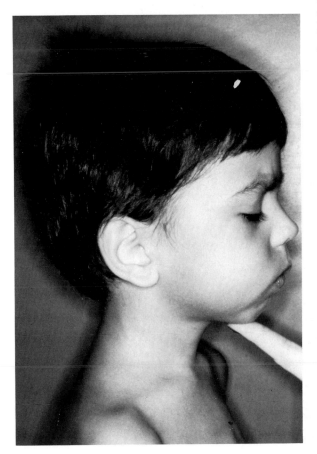

Fig. 5-9 Marked involvement of the cervical spine in a boy with polyarticular JRA. The photograph shows the maximum extension that this child could achieve.

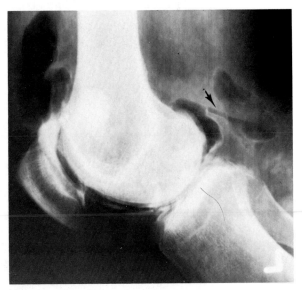

Fig. 5-10 Popliteal cyst (Baker's cyst). This arthrogram with contrast shows the communication (arrow) between the synovial space and the dissecting cyst in an 18-year-old boy who has had JRA since he was 9 years old.

or sole presentation of JRA and, when unilateral, may be misinterpreted as a tumor (Fig. 5-11).

Tenosynovitis is probably more common in JRA than is usually appreciated, since it is generally not a striking or sole clinical complaint. Except on the dorsum of the wrist and the anterior part of the ankle and foot, inflammation of the tendon sheaths is generally minimal. Unusual manifestations may occur, however, as in tenosynovitis of the superior oblique muscle.[153,154] Loss of extension of the fingers may result from a stenosing synovitis of the flexor tendon sheaths and may be responsible, in part, for a claw-hand deformity.[155] Clinically recognized carpal tunnel syndrome appears to be uncommon in children with involvement of the wrists.

POLYARTHRITIS

The onset of polyarthritis is characterized by arthritis in five or more joints (Fig. 5-12). This pattern is established within the first 6 weeks to 4 months of the disease in the majority of cases. Onset may be acute but is more often insidious, with the gradual development of progressive joint involvement. The arthritis may be remittent or indolent and generally involves the large joints of the knees, wrists, elbows, and ankles. Small joint disease involving the hands or feet may occur early or late in the course of the disease. Three-fourths of affected children have symmetric disease; however, the arthritis may be asymmetric, affecting only one side of the body. The cervical spine is often involved in this type of onset. TMJ disease is relatively common in children with polyarthritis.

In polyarthritis, an important subtype of onset includes children, predominantly girls, who have onset of disease late in childhood or adolescence in association with classic RF seropositivity. These children may develop more of the adult pattern of RA with rheumatoid nodules, erosive synovitis, and a chronic course persisting well into adulthood. They are often HLA-DR4 positive.

Systemic manifestations in children with polyarthritis are variable but usually not as acute or persistent as in systemic onset of JRA. Low-grade fever, rheumatoid rash, slight to moderate hepatosplenomegaly, or lymphadenopathy may be present. Small pericardial effusions may be detected on echocardio-

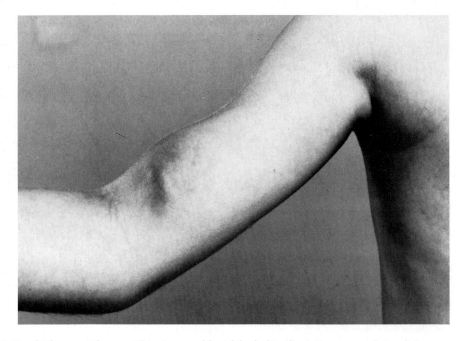

Fig. 5-11 Brachial synovial cyst. This 6-year-old girl had this dissecting cyst of the right arm as her first manifestation of JRA. A biopsy of the mass was done after a diagnosis of tumor had been made. The pathologic specimen and aspirated fluid were typical of synovitis. Later, bilateral effusions of the knees developed.

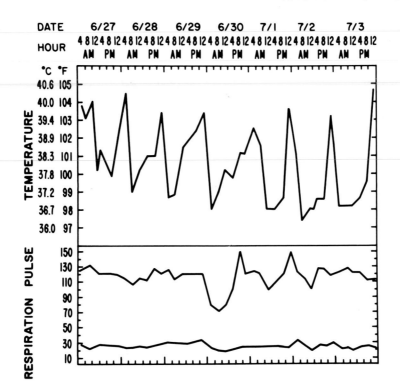

Fig. 5-15 Intermittent fever of systemic onset in a 3-year-old girl. The febrile spikes usually occurred in the late evening to early morning and were accompanied by severe malaise, tachycardia, and rash.

cally ill or may appear regularly with each systemic exacerbation. Although this rash is a diagnostic feature of systemic onset JRA, it also occurs rarely in children with polyarthritis but is probably never observed in those with classic oligoarthritis. Because the rash is transient and usually occurs late in the day with the fever, it may be missed by physicians investigating a child with fever of unknown origin (FUO) unless the child is examined at the time of the fever. Individual lesions may be precipitated at other times by rubbing or scratching the skin, the so-called Koebner's phenomenon or isomorphic response, or by a hot bath or psychological stress. The rash is occasionally pruritic,[164,165] particularly in the older patient.

Other visceral disease consists of hepatosplenomegaly, lymphadenopathy, pericarditis, or other evidence of serositis. Hepatosplenomegaly and lymphadenopathy occur in most children with active systemic disease.

Extra-Articular Manifestations of Disease

GENERALIZED GROWTH RETARDATION

Although a variety of extra-articular manifestations of the disease have been documented in JRA (Table 5-10),[166] abnormalities of growth and development are cardinal features of these children. Linear growth is retarded during periods of active systemic disease.[167,168] Full development of stature is not attained if severe chronic inflammatory activity persists for a few years. The appearance of secondary sexual characteristics is also delayed. Accelerated growth may occur with suppression of the active disease by therapy or during a remission. It is unusual, however, for a child who has suffered significant arrest or slowing of growth to regain development within the previous channel.

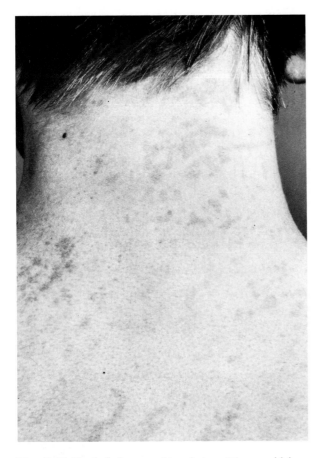

Fig. 5-16 Typical rheumatoid rash in a 15-year-old boy with systemic onset of disease. This rash is faintly erythematous (salmon-colored), macular, and nonpruritic. The individual lesions are transient, occur in crops, and conform to a linear distribution. They are located characteristically over the trunk and extremities.

Many early studies commented upon the general arrest of development, retardation of linear growth, asymmetry of development, or persistence of infantile proportions.[17,35] Ansell and Bywaters in 1956 published an extensive study of growth and development in 119 children with JRA.[167] They found that the long duration of active disease was a significant factor in reduction of linear growth in children who had not received corticosteroid drugs. During remission, height returned to normal in 2 to 3 years if premature epiphyseal fusion had not occurred. Severe stunting was found only in long-standing, active disease. Similar findings were reported in the extensive prognostic study by Laaksonen of 544 children with JRA.[51]

Corticosteroid medication also results in measurable growth retardation or may intensify that initiated by the disease.[169–171] It has been estimated that growth retardation is evident in children treated with prednisone in a dosage equal to or greater than 5 mg/M^2/day for a period of 6 months. Laaksonen et al. found that corticosteroids in this dose range did not produce growth retardation when used for shorter periods.[172]

In a study from Los Angeles, height was measured at 6-month intervals in 31 children with JRA.[168] Impairment of growth was greatest in children with systemic disease. About half of the children were below the third percentile for age and sex at the 5- to 7.5-year follow-up interval. However, 3 of 9 children were below the third percentile at onset of disease. Undetected disease of some duration may have accounted for this finding.

In another report, 20 patients with JRA and growth failure were treated with human growth hormone.[173] Five children did not respond, and in the remainder the mean growth rate accelerated during 1 to 2 years of treatment. In 6 patients, growth velocity decreased when anti-inflammatory therapy was discontinued. Onset of puberty may also accelerate growth in the child with JRA.

Table 5-10 Estimated Frequency of Extra-Articular Manifestations in JRA

	Polyarthritis (%)	Oligoarthritis (%)	Systemic Disease (%)
Fever	30	0	100
Rheumatoid rash	2	0	95
Rheumatoid nodules	10	0	5
Hepatosplenomegaly	10	0	85
Lymphadenopathy	5	0	70
Chronic uveitis	5	20	<1
Pericarditis	5	0	35
Pleuritis	1	0	20
Abdominal pain	1	0	10

LOCALIZED GROWTH DISTURBANCES

A striking example of localized growth retardation is the development of micrognathia (Figs. 5-17 and 5-18). Mandibular hypoplasia is caused by inflammatory disease of the TMJ growth centers, sometimes in association with disease of the cervical spine.[174–179] Extreme micrognathia results from unabated arthritis of long duration with onset before 4 years of age. Lesser developmental delay can be seen with onset of JRA up to the age of 12 years. In a study of 13 girls and 3 boys, aged 7 to 19 years, with radiographic evidence of TMJ disease, only 9 had a history of pain affecting those joints.[142] Bilateral disease occurred in 8 patients, 7 of whom had micrognathia. Unilateral disease was present in 8 and was characterized by mandibular asymmetry, absence of a palpable condyle, and deviation to the affected side on opening the mouth (Figs. 5-19 to 5-21).

Other secondary growth deformities are frequent in JRA. Early during active disease, development of

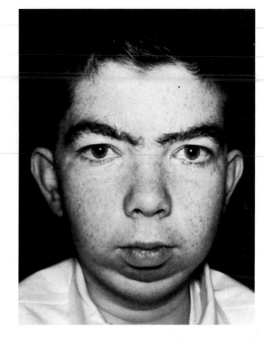

Fig. 5-18 Frontal view of micrognathia in the boy in Fig. 5-17.

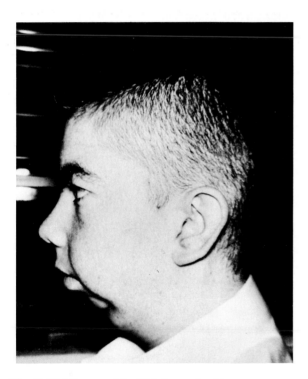

Fig. 5-17 Micrognathia. JRA began in this young man at 2½ years of age as an unremitting polyarthritis. Cervical spine disease was present. The incisor distance was preserved at 2 inches.

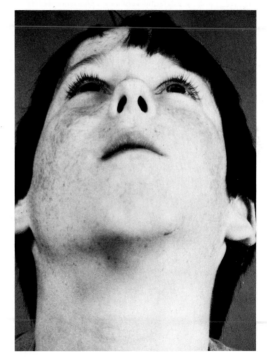

Fig. 5-19 Unilateral TMJ disease on the left with underdevelopment of the left side of the mandible and face.

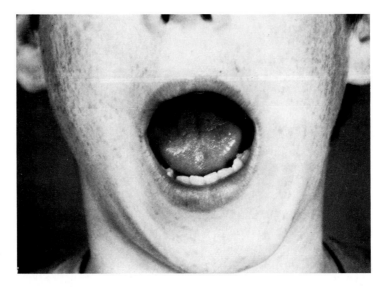

Fig. 5-20 Same boy as in Fig. 5-19 showing asymmetric opening of the mouth due to unilateral TMJ disease.

the ossification centers is accelerated, and later stunting or premature fusion of the involved bones may result.[59,61,180,181] Brachydactyly results from premature epiphyseal closure (Fig. 5-22). Small hands or feet may result, or isolated metacarpals or metatarsals may be affected.

Asymmetric arthritis of the lower limb, especially of the knee, frequently causes accelerated growth and epiphyseal maturation. As a result, a discrepancy of leg length may occur.[180,182,183] Although accurate clinical measurement of leg length is difficult,[184] a comparative difference in the distance from the superior anterior iliac spine to the medial malleous of greater than 0.5 cm is probably significant. Differences of 5 cm or greater occasionally occur. Often, simple clinical estimation of leg-length discrepancy by noting differences in the medial malleolar or calcaneal positions in the supine, straight child is suf-

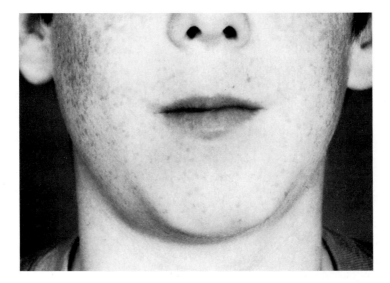

Fig. 5-21 Frontal view showing underdevelopment of the left side of the chin.

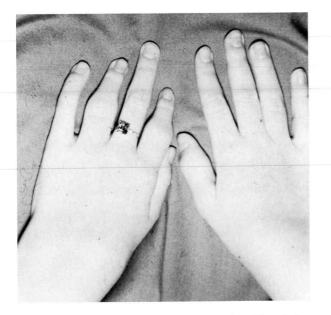

Fig. 5-22 Brachydactyly of the left second and fourth fingers. The PIP joints are involved, as well as the IP joints of the thumbs and the wrists.

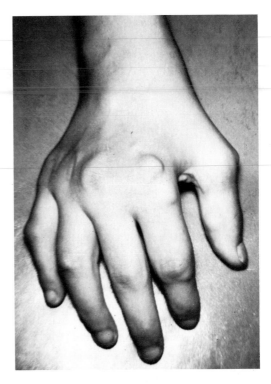

Fig. 5-23 Rheumatoid nodules. Multiple rheumatoid nodules were a constant feature of this girl's JRA and appeared over joints, pressure points (as under the nosepieces of her glasses), and tendon sheaths. Note also the flexion contractures and radial deviation at the MCP joints.

ficient. Rarely premature epiphyseal fusion results in shortening of the affected leg. As the child grows and the skeleton matures, inequalities of minimal to moderate degree may disappear, but up to two-thirds persist. In some reports surgical epiphyseal arrest of the opposite leg was judged to be necessary in approximately one-third of the patients.[185,186]

SUBCUTANEOUS NODULES

Rheumatoid nodules are not as common in JRA as in adult RA (Fig. 5-23). They occur in 5 to 10 percent of cases, usually in conjunction with polyarthritis.[187–189] They are almost always associated with RF seropositivity and in this respect are generally regarded as a poor prognostic sign. Nodules are most frequently attached to the periosteum below the olecranon process but may also be found at other pressure points and on the digital flexor tendon sheaths, Achilles tendons, occiput, and bridge of the nose in the child who wears glasses.

Typical rheumatoid nodules are firm or hard, usually mobile and nontender. The overlying skin may be erythematous. A solitary nodule as multiple nodules may be present; each nodule will usually disappear after a period of months to years. Rheumatoid nodules must be distinguished from those of rheumatic fever and the so-called benign rheumatoid nodules that are not associated with objective arthritis.

MUSCLE DISEASE

Atrophy of muscles around inflamed joints is characteristic of children with JRA and is often accompanied by a shortening of muscle and tendon that gives rise to flexion contractures, muscle weakness, and fatigue. A nonspecific myositis occurs in children with JRA and may account for some of the associated fatigue and muscle weakness. This myositis does not have a characteristic distribution, and histopathologic studies are sparse. Data from adults with RA suggest that it is characterized by a perivasculitis and lymphocytic infiltrates. Serum muscle enzyme elevations do not occur. A rare child may develop large, tender erythematous areas of epidermal and dermal inflammation and myositis as part of acute systemic disease.

A few children experience profound progressive muscle atrophy with acute systemic disease.[49] Such children have not been seen at our clinics in recent years, principally because of early diagnosis and prompt treatment.

CARDIAC INVOLVEMENT

Pericarditis

Pericarditis and pericardial effusions are especially common in children with systemic onset (Fig. 5-24).[190–195] Pericarditis tends to occur in the older child but is not related to sex or age at onset or severity of joint disease.[191] In a British study, amyloidosis was frequent.[191] The majority of the pericardial effusions are subclinical, although some children have obvious symptoms, such as precordial pain, friction rub, tachycardia, cardiomegaly, or dyspnea (Table 5-11).[193] Rarely a child progresses to tamponade; chronic constrictive pericarditis is virtually undescribed.[196–198] In general, children with pericarditis do not fare worse than others in outcome, and this complication should not necessarily be regarded as a poor prognostic sign, although pericarditis is frequently present in children with JRA who die.[191,193]

Pericarditis may precede the development of arthritis, or it may occur at any time during the course of the disease, usually accompanied by a systemic exacerbation. Each episode generally persists for 1 week to 2 months. Pericarditis may recur more frequently in poorly controlled disease. Many cases of pericardial effusion develop insidiously, are not accompanied by obvious cardiomegaly or electrocardiographic changes, and escape recognition. Echocardiography is a valuable diagnostic technique to document small accumulations of fluid.[192,194]

In a study from Los Angeles, 55 children with JRA and 38 age-matched control subjects were studied by echocardiography.[194] An effusion or pericardial thickening was present in 36 percent of the patients; 81 percent of those children who had active systemic manifestations at the time of the study had abnormal echocardiogram findings. Four children had friction rubs, and eight had abnormal electrocardiograms. Nine had an enlarged cardiac silhouette. In more than half of these children the diagnosis of pericarditis would not have been made by standard clinical methods.

Myocarditis

Myocarditis is much less common than pericarditis and may result in congestive heart failure and cardiomegaly.[199–201] In three children reported by Miller and French,[199] failure occurred in the absence of overt pericardial effusions and on a background of severe active systemic disease. One child at necropsy showed diffuse myocardial changes typical of congestive cardiomyopathy.

Endocarditis

Valvular disease has been documented in at least 10 children with JRA (Table 5-12).[103,193,195,200–204] Eight had aortic insufficiency, and two mitral insufficiency. Sudden deterioration in cardiac function may occur in such children. Valve replacement has been necessary in some of these patients.

PULMONARY DISEASE

Pulmonary disease is rare in children with JRA. Diffuse interstitial pulmonary fibrosis occurs in a small number of children with JRA[205–208] and may precede other evidence of JRA.[209] Athreya et al. noted interstitial disease in 8 of 191 children with JRA, all of whom had systemic onset.[208] Pulmonary function studies in 16 children with JRA revealed abnormalities in 10.[209] Pneumonitis or pleural effusions may occur with carditis or may be asymptomatic and be detected only as incidental findings on chest radiographs. One child observed by us had idiopathic

Table 5-11 Clinical Manifestations of Pericarditis in Children with JRA

Finding	%
Symptoms	
Precordial pain	38
Dyspnea	20
Signs	
Tachycardia	83
Friction rub	67
Tachypnea	60
Radiographs	
Cardiomegaly	71
Straightened left cardiac border	50
Globular heart	50
Electrocardiogram	
Elevation of ST segment	31
T-wave abnormality	77

(Modified from Brewer,[193] with permission.)

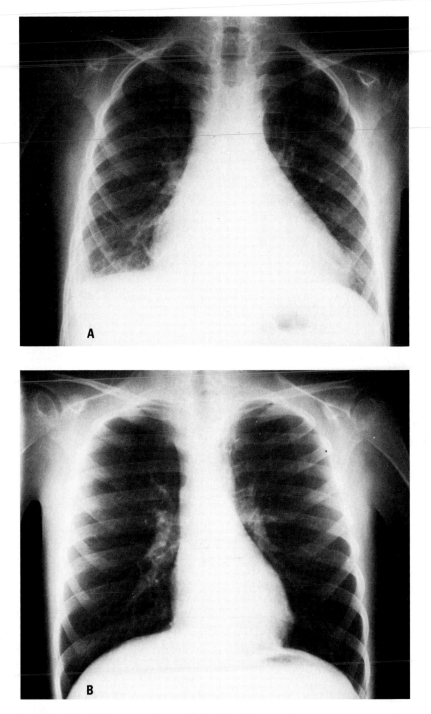

Fig. 5-24 Acute pericardial effusion in a 9-year-old girl with systemic onset at 3 years of age. This effusion persisted for 1 month and was accompanied by fever, precordial discomfort, and dyspnea. (**A**) Chest x-ray film showing pericardial effusion and a pleural reaction at both bases with fluid on right. (**B**) Radiograph taken 1 month later.

Table 5-12 Children with JRA and Valvular Heart Disease

Author (Ref.)	Sex	Arthritis				Valvular Disease		Treatment	Outcome
		Age of Onset (Years)	Type of Onset[a]	RF	Type	Age of Onset (Years)			
Brewer[193]	—	—	O	—	MI	After 11 mos. of arthritis	—	—
	—	—	—	—	MI	After long-standing disease	—	—
Leak et al.[202]	F	9.5	P	Pos	AI	12	Prosthesis, chlorambucil	Good
	F	10	P	Pos	AI	16	Prosthesis	Good
	F	8	P	Pos	AI	15	—	Died
	F	8	P	Pos	AI	18	None	Stable
Svantesson et al.[195]	—	—	—	—	AI	—	—	—
Kramer et al.[203]	F	2	S	—	AI	27	Prosthesis	Good
Hull et al.[204]	F	0.6	O	—	AI	8	Chlorambucil	Improved
Delgado et al.[103]	F	1.5	O	Pos	AI	9.7	Prosthesis	Good

[a] Type of onset: P = polyarthritis, O = oligoarthritis, S = systemic disease.
(Modified from Delgado et al.,[103] with permission.)

pulmonary hemosiderosis as the first sign of JRA. Pulmonary rheumatoid nodules as described in adult RA are rare in childhood. In one study, the pathologic findings in a child who died of pulmonary fibrosis were described in detail.[205]

LYMPHADENOPATHY

Marked symmetric lymphadenopathy is particularly common in the anterior cervical, axillary, and inguinal areas, and in a child it may suggest the occurrence of lymphoma. Mesenteric lymphadenopathy may cause abdominal pain or distention and lead to an erroneous diagnosis of an acute surgical abdomen. This is most common in children with acute systemic onset and may present a diagnostic dilemma before a correct diagnosis of JRA is made.

SPLENOMEGALY

Splenomegaly occurs in at least a fourth of the children and is generally most prominent within the first years after onset. The degree of splenomegaly may be extreme, but it is uncommonly associated with

Felty's syndrome (splenic neutropenia).[210] We have studied, however, an 11-year-old girl with polyarticular JRA, nodules, and RF seropositivity who had splenomegaly and marked neutropenia that responded to treatment with corticosteroids.

HEPATIC DISEASE

Hepatomegaly is less common than splenomegaly. Moderate to severe enlargement of the liver is often associated with only mild derangement of functional studies and relatively nonspecific histopathologic changes.[211] This type of hepatitis is most common at the onset of JRA and generally diminishes with time. Chronic liver disease is not seen. Massive enlargement of the liver is usually accompanied by abdominal distention and pain. Progressive hepatomegaly is characteristic of secondary amyloidosis. Unexplained acute yellow atrophy has been recorded.[212] Occasionally, a fatty liver is associated with corticosteroid administration, or hepatitis (transaminasemia) related to salicylate therapy may occur (Ch. 3).

A rare but serious hepatic complication of systemic JRA, particularly in boys, has been reported by Hadchouel et al.[213] The etiology of this disorder is unknown but in some children has appeared to be associated with a change in medications. It is characterized by the rapid development of hepatic failure with encephalopathy, purpura, and bleeding associated with disseminated intravascular coagulation (DIC), and sometimes renal failure with hematuria and proteinuria.[214] The hepatic enzymes and bilirubin are elevated. Death has occurred in 2 of 14 reported cases. Jacobs et al. noted 4 similar patients who died after a second gold salt injection with DIC, jaundice, and other systemic disease.[215] Subclinical coagulation abnormalities characterized by prolonged prothrombin time (PT), partial prothrombin time (PTT), and increased fibrin degradation products, fibrinopeptide A, and factor VIII–related antigen have been reported to be common in systemic onset JRA, but not in polyarticular disease.[216]

Other, very rare complications of JRA include intestinal pseudo-obstruction, which we have also observed in one girl, and peritonitis that has been documented in two children.[217] Polyserositis has been described infrequently.

CENTRAL NERVOUS SYSTEM DISEASE

Involvement of the central nervous system (CNS) during the course of JRA is often related to complicating factors such as metabolic derangements, salicylate toxicity, high fever, embolism, and other systemic disease.[218–221] In some children CNS disease has been so overwhelming as to suggest a primary relationship to JRA.[222] Calabro described 5 of 20 children with acute systemic onset of arthritis who had marked irritability, pronounced drowsiness in 3 cases, seizures in 1, and meningismus in another.[223] These reports may represent unrecognized instances of Reye's syndrome.

RENAL DISEASE

Intermittent hematuria or proteinuria is an occasional finding in some children with JRA. Problems in differential diagnosis arise when these abnormalities occur with the administration of analgesic or anti-inflammatory drugs or the use of gold salt or D-penicillamine therapy. Abnormal urinary findings also raise the possibility that one is dealing with overt vasculitis or intravascular coagulation,[224] a disease such as SLE, or, rarely, amyloidosis. Renal papillary necrosis has been described in a number of children with JRA and is believed to be related in part to NSAID use (Ch. 3). Hypercalciuria has been iden-

tified as an additional cause of hematuria in children with JRA.[225] It should be noted that low-grade proteinuria and hematuria occasionally occur in normal children.[226]

In Anttila's large study of 165 children with JRA, transient microscopic hematuria was observed in 23 percent, leukocyturia in 25 percent, and low-grade proteinuria in 42 percent.[227,228] Recurrent or persistent hematuria (4 percent) leukocyturia (6 percent), and proteinuria (2 percent) were uncommon. Hematuria and leukocyturia were more frequent during the initial observation period. Creatinine clearance was decreased in 10 percent of the children, and concentration ability was impaired in 31 percent. Proteinuria was associated with the presence of extra-articular disease, prolonged duration of active disease, and amyloidosis, which was found in 40 percent of the children who died. Chronic pyelonephritis was a common finding at necropsy. Interstitial nephritis and gold-induced nephrotic syndrome were rare.

Renal biopsy was performed in 35 percent of the children and showed minimal glomerular changes in 22 percent and tubular atrophy in 13 percent. The frequency of the histopathologic changes increased with the duration and severity of disease. Anttila concluded from these studies that the primary lesion in many of these children was a minimal glomerulitis. Most of the urinary abnormalities in this study were judged to be of little clinical significance, since they tended to be minimal and transient. Many of these findings had been documented before drug therapy was started. Markedly abnormal urinary findings were typical of children with systemic disease, ANA seropositivity, and active, severe disease.

There has been no other study to support or refute these observations of Anttila, but it is our experience that renal disease, except for transient hematuria or proteinuria associated with systemic onset disease, is uncommon in children with JRA. When persistent urinary sediment changes are observed, they are most frequently related to medications (NSAIDs, gold salts) or to the evolution of JRA to SLE.

VASCULITIS

Rheumatoid polyvasculitis has been described in a few children with acute systemic disease and may result in the death of the child (Fig. 5-25, Table 5-13).[229,230] It occurs most often in the older child who has polyarthritis and is RF seropositive. This devastating type of widespread small- to medium-size vessel involvement is to be distinguished from benign

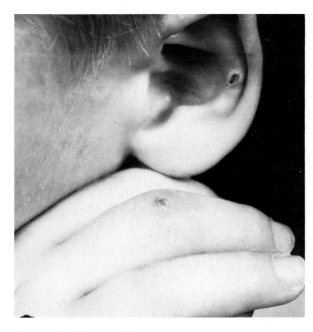

Fig. 5-25 Rheumatoid systemic necrotizing vasculitis. This unfortunate 6-year-old boy with systemic JRA developed widespread cutaneous and visceral vasculitis that led to his death 1 year after onset of disease.

Table 5-13 Clinical Features of Rheumatoid Vasculitis (Polyarteritis)

Fever
Peripheral neuropathy
Cutaneous ulcers
Digital arteritis
Raynaud's phenomenon
Gastrointestinal perforation and hemorrhage
Mesenteric thrombosis
Myocardial infarction
Nephritis

digital vasculitis, which is somewhat more frequent and may be associated with vascular calcification that is seen on radiographs along the course of the digital arteries (Fig. 5-26).[180,231,232]

PATHOLOGY

The pathologic features of JRA are similar to those described in adult RA (Ch. 2).[46,233] Electron microscopic studies have also confirmed the similarities of the juvenile

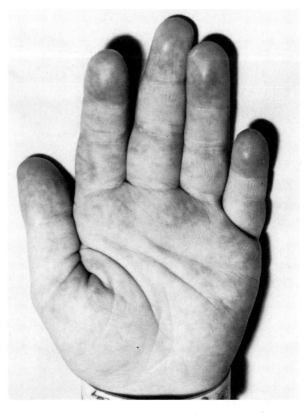

Fig. 5-26 Benign cutaneous rheumatoid vasculitis. Punctate erythema of the palms and finger pads was the sole manifestation of perivasculitis in this 5-year-old girl. The lesions were not raised or tender. She did well on aspirin therapy alone and entered a partial remission with clearing of these lesions.

and adult synovial responses to inflammation.[234,235] In routine biopsy specimens, there is villous hypertrophy and hyperplasia of the synovial lining layer (Fig. 5-27). The subsynovial tissues are hyperemic and edematous. Vascular endothelial hyperplasia is often prominent, along with infiltration by lymphocytes and plasma cells. Fibrin may be layered onto the superficial surface of the synovium or incorporated within it. An exuberant synovial inflammatory process in JRA eventually leads to pannus formation that results in progressive erosion and destruction of articular cartilage and later of contiguous bone. In our experience, rheumatoid nodules and necrotizing vasculitis have not been observed in synovial biopsy specimens from children with JRA. Oligoarthritis and polyarthritis cannot be separated on the basis of their synovial histopathology.[157,236]

End-stage disease, when it occurs, is characterized by deformity, subluxation, and fibrous or bony ankylosis. Joint destruction usually occurs much later in the course of

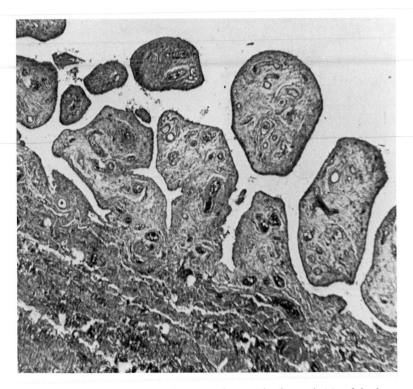

Fig. 5-27 Synovial tissue from the left knee of a young boy with oligoarthritis of the knees and ankles. The classic histopathologic changes of JRA, villous hyperplasia and hypertrophy, edema and proliferation of new blood vessels, and infiltration by round cells, are present.

JRA than in adult disease. Permanent joint damage is not seen in many children with JRA even after years of chronic inflammation. The greater thickness of juvenile cartilage may offer some protection in this regard.

Rice bodies consist primarily of amorphous fibrous material, fibrin, and small amounts of collagen (Fig. 5-28).[237,238] Viable cells are incorporated within this matrix and appear more normal than the synovial cells of the inflammatory foci. The majority of these cells resemble type B synovial lining cells, although a few type A cells are also seen. Residual blood vessels in some of these bodies attest to their former attachment to the synovial membrane.

The rash of JRA is one of the most characteristic clinical hallmarks of this disease. There is minimal perivascular infiltration of mononuclear cells around capillaries and venules in the subdermal tissues.[163,164] A neutrophilic perivasculitis resembling that seen in the rash of rheumatic fever may accompany the more flagrant lesions.

Subcutaneous nodules may be histopathologically typical of rheumatoid nodules (Fig. 5-29), or they may have a looser connective-tissue framework resembling that of the nodules of rheumatic fever.[187,239] The central area of fi-

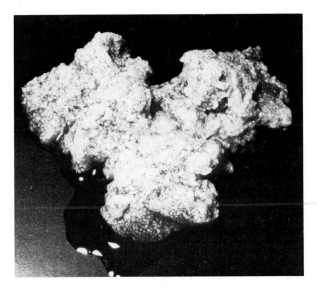

Fig. 5-28 Rice bodies from the left knee of a 15-year-old boy who went on to develop a persistent arthritis of the knees and left ankle.

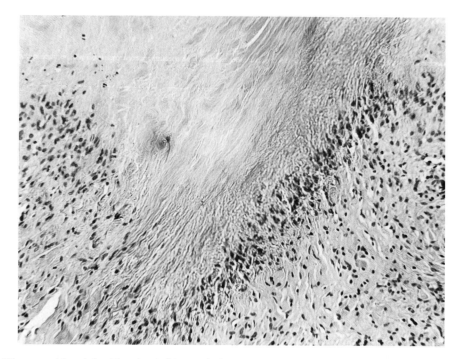

Fig. 5-29 Rheumatoid nodule. The classic histopathologic zones, a central area of fibrinoid necrosis, palisade of epithelioid cells, and peripheral fibroblastic proliferation, are present.

brinoid necrosis and the epithelioid pallisades around it may be absent or less structured.

The serosal lining surfaces of the pleural, pericardial, and peritoneal cavities of the body may exhibit a nonspecific fibrous serositis that is characterized clinically by effusion and pain. Enlargement of the lymph nodes is related to a nonspecific follicular hyperplasia that in rare instances may closely resemble lymphoma. Hepatic histopathology is characterized by a nonspecific collection of periportal inflammatory cells and hyperplasia of the Kupffer cells.

DIFFERENTIAL DIAGNOSIS

JRA is often a diagnosis of exclusion.[240,241] Certain clinical observations are especially helpful in the differential diagnosis of JRA. In the child with oligoarthritis, the affected joint is swollen and often warm but is generally not very painful, tender, or red. The child is not systemically ill.

If a child with oligoarthritis has an acutely painful and erythematous joint or systemic signs, septic arthritis or another process such as acute rheumatic fever is more likely the correct diagnosis.[242,243] Joint aspiration is always indicated in such a patient in order to exclude infectious arthritis or osteomyelitis. Synovial biopsy with a Parker-Pearson needle or by arthroscopy is useful in children with monarthritis in whom granulomatous or malignant disease is suspected.[157,244,245] It should not be done simply to make a diagnosis of JRA. Culture of synovial tissue removed at biopsy is sometimes more rewarding in the case of specific granuloma (tuberculosis) than culture of the fluid only. A negative purified protein derivative (PPD) skin test in a child virtually excludes the diagnosis of active tuberculosis. Tuberculous rheumatism (Poncet's disease) has been described in childhood.[246] Other types of infection must be considered, particularly acute hematogenous osteomyelitis, gonorrhea, and salmonella infection in a black child with sickle cell anemia. Septic arthritis usually affects a single joint, although some infections such as gonorrhea may have an initial migratory phase. Bacterial infections may be suppressed or short-lived if treated promptly with an antibiotic, and diagnosis may be especially difficult in these cases. Tenosynovitis may accompany pyogenic infections and is also prominent in granulomatous forms of arthritis such as tuberculosis. Lyme arthritis presents an important differential diagnosis of arthritis and neurologic and cardiac disease.[247,248] Monarthritis of short duration may be caused by trauma or rarely associated with an internal structural abnormality such as a discoid meniscus.[249] The monarthritis seen in hemophilia results from bleeding into a major joint that is often initiated by even minor trauma.

Ophthalmologic and slit-lamp examinations in children with limited joint disease are useful diagnostically. The finding of a nongranulomatous uveitis almost always indicates a diagnosis of JRA. Other rare causes of uveitis such as sarcoidosis must be considered, however.

JRA almost never begins in the hip, although hip involvement becomes increasingly common in children with severe polyarthritis of prolonged duration. In our experience with 145 children with oligoarthritis seen early in their course, only 1 girl had initial involvement of the hip. Onset of arthritis in the hip in a very young child should be considered first as a septic process or a congenital dislocation.[250] In the older child, osteonecrosis of the femoral head (Legg-Calvé-Perthes disease) is a diagnostic consideration, and in the adolescent age group, a slipped capital femoral epiphysis may initially mimic JRA, particularly in the obese boy. Osgood-Schlatter disease of a tibial tubercle can usually be easily differentiated from involvement of the knee.[251]

Transient synovitis of the hip is an obscure condition of uncertain origin.[252,253] Pain is minimal and the disease is self-limited, lasting no more than one to a few weeks. The results of all laboratory and radiologic studies are normal (Ch. 12).

Neuroblastoma is often the most difficult malignancy to exclude in young children with complaints of arthritis of uncertain cause.[254] Osseous infiltration in this disease causes bone pain and tenderness. The presence of bone pain on weight bearing is an important clue to the presence of a malignancy. A bone scan and urinary catecholamine determination may aid in diagnosis. Acute leukemia may present as an arthritis because of infiltration of the metaphyseal bone marrow, periosteum, and joint capsule. Leukemia causes a characteristic swelling about the joint, and the child often has generalized lymphadenopathy, splenomegaly, and constitutional signs such as fever. Many children with hematologic malignancies have moderate to severe anemia or elevation of the erythrocyte sedimentation rate (ESR) out of keeping with other features of their disease. The white blood cell count may be low or normal, whereas systemic onset of JRA would be expected to be associated with leukocytosis.[255] Examination of the bone marrow is usually diagnostic. Radiographs of the affected joints may be diagnostic in these disorders; however, the correct diagnosis in some children may be delayed for 3 to 6 months. Arthritis as a manifestation of hematologic malignancy becomes increasingly uncommon during late adolescence as red marrow ceases to occupy the ends of the long bones.

Sickle cell anemia in the very young child causes a dactylitis (hand-foot syndrome) that may mimic a true arthritis and in other children causes microinfarcts that give rise to periostitis and periarthritis.[256] Pigmented villonodular synovitis and histiocytosis are other rare causes of joint disease in children.

Occasionally, the hypermobility syndrome or a variant of the Ehlers-Danlos syndrome may present with arthritis.[257] We have also seen two children who had an isolated joint contracture that was eventually diagnosed as myositis ossificans progressiva. This diagnosis was not evident in either child until later in the course when typical ossifications in muscle were observed radiographically.

Jacobs et al.[258] and Athreya et al.[259] published studies of a series of children with familial hypertrophic synovitis who developed characteristic flexion contractures of the fingers that occurred during the first few months of life and were accompanied by joint effusions. A bent thumb is often noted soon after birth as the first diagnostic sign of the disorder. Effusions are symmetric and involve large joints (such as the knees, ankles, hips, and wrists). Minimal progressive limitation of motion of the joints develops with age. There is usually no pain or systemic manifestation of fever or inflammation.

An autosomal dominant type of inheritance has been suggested in some families. The frequency of this condition is unknown; it is not thought to be rare. Synovial biopsy has shown hypertrophic villi with giant cells but no other inflammatory infiltrate. The synovial lining cells are hyperplastic, but vascular endothelial proliferation is not prominent. Radiographs may demonstrate some proximal flattening of the femoral ossification centers in the hips. Chondrocalcinosis has been reported to occur later in life; this disorder is, however, distinct from the familial chondrocalcinosis reported from Chile.

Although children with JRA may have generalized soft tissue swelling of the extremities, such as over the dorsa of the hands or feet, this must be differentiated from a number of disorders, including lymphedema praecox, reflex sympathetic dystrophy, Noonan syndrome in boys, and Turner's syndrome.[260] Rarely a child with a mucopolysaccharidosis, particularly in Morquio's or Scheie's syndrome, may have joint stiffness or bony enlargement.

Children with systemic onset of JRA may appear to have an acute infectious disease or septicemia. Documenting the presence of arthritis or a rheumatoid rash helps the physician to consider more directly a diagnosis of JRA. Infectious mononucleosis may mimic systemic onset of JRA. Most of the arthropathies secondary to viral infections are transient.[261,262]

Fever in children with infectious diseases is of the septic type. It generally does not return to the baseline in a predictable fashion each day as does the fever of JRA, and the child remains ill even during a relatively afebrile interval. A sustained fever is characteristic of acute rheumatic fever and should respond dramatically to salicylates. Although many children with systemic JRA have an isolated pericarditis, finding a pericardial effusion along with evidence of endocarditis such as a diastolic murmur would lead the clinician toward a diagnosis of rheumatic fever or bacterial endocarditis.

Onset of rheumatic fever in the developed countries of the world generally occurs between the ages of 5 and 15 years. The arthritis in this condition in children is characteristically acute and painful, migratory, and asymmetric, involving the peripheral joints without sequelae. The initial episode generally lasts no longer than 6 weeks and rarely as long as 3 months. Evidence of a prior infection with beta-hemolytic group A streptococci is present; however, the antistreptolysin O (ASO) titer may be chronically increased to a moderate degree in one-third of children with JRA as a manifestation of their inflammatory disease and not as evidence of recent or concurrent streptococcal infection.[263] During the acute course of rheumatic fever, a two-tube rise or fall in titer should be documented.

Any of the connective-tissue diseases of childhood may present with arthritis. Up to one-third of children with dermatomyositis or scleroderma have an arthropathy at onset of the disease. The associated features of these diseases generally lead promptly to a correct diagnosis. In childhood, inflammatory myositis is almost invariably associated with a characteristic skin rash, and isolated polymyositis is uncommon. Scleroderma, on the other hand, may begin insidiously, and subtle subcutaneous calcifications may be misinterpreted as rheumatoid nodules.

Mixed connective-tissue disease[264-266] and the sicca complex or Sjögren's syndrome[267,268] are very uncommon in childhood. Raynaud's phenomenon in the child should always suggest a diagnosis such as scleroderma or SLE. In our experience, it is probably never associated with JRA.[269] Although anemia is common in severe JRA, it is not Coombs' positive. A hemolytic anemia would indicate another connective-tissue disease, usually SLE.

Ansell et al.[270] and Prieur and Griscelli[271] described patients with neonatal-onset multisystem inflammatory disease (NOMID) in which chronic arthropathy, accompanied by a severe persistent rash, occurs in the neonatal period. Distinctive epiphyseal abnormalities develop by 1 year of age that are progressive and severe and are associated with acute arthritis and flexion contractures of the knees, elbows, wrists, and ankles. The differential diagnosis includes systemic onset of JRA since fever, lymphadenopathy, and hepatosplenomegaly are also present. Affected children may develop uveitis and meningitis and become progressively retarded with frontal bossing and enlargement of the head.[565] Developmental delays and wasting illness in combination with severe arthritis lead to a chronically ill child who is confined to bed and in constant pain.

All children with NOMID have died, although survival to 17 years has been reported. Pathologic findings have shown widespread infiltration of meninges, lymphatic organs, and skin by polymorphonuclear neutrophils with evidence of a granulomatous inflammatory process and fibrinoid necrosis around small blood vessels.

A somewhat obscure, but perhaps additional differential diagnosis is the arthritis that occurs in the Ramon syndrome.[272] First described in 1967, this autosomal recessive disorder includes cherubism, gingival fibromatosis, epilepsy, mental deficiency, and stunted growth.

Three diagnostic categories have presented the most frequent problems in making the correct diagnosis of JRA in our clinic: SLE, JAS, and the arthritis of immunodeficiency (Chs. 6, 7, and 11).

The child with SLE may have arthritis that mimics JRA,[273] and the correct diagnosis may not be evident, or possible to make, until one of the more characteristic clinical findings of SLE occurs later in the course of the disease. The more specific diagnostic features of SLE include a butterfly rash, alopecia, nephritis, CNS disease, Raynaud's phenomenon, leukopenia, and hemolytic anemia. Urinalysis in most children with JRA does not show a persistent hematuria or proteinuria. The finding of an active urinary sediment in a child diagnosed as having JRA strongly suggests the alternative diagnosis of SLE.

Specific serologic tests that confirm a diagnosis of SLE should always be performed when diagnostic questions arise. A high-titer ANA reaction with a peripheral pattern, positive lupus erythematosus (LE) cell tests, high titers of anti-dsDNA antibodies, or hypocomplementemia strongly suggests active immune complex disease.[274] In this consideration, it should be noted that the type of onset of JRA that most closely resembles acute SLE, systemic disease, is the one least likely to have ANA seropositivity. Ragsdale et al. have presented the course of 10 children who developed SLE after an initial diagnosis of JRA (Tables 5-14, 7-43, 7-44).[269] In all cases, anti-dsDNA antibodies were detected before development of clinical disease characteristic of SLE.

Children with juvenile ankylosing spondylitis (JAS) usually have large joint arthropathy of the lower extremities at onset rather than lumbar pain and stiffness or hip disease.[275] Transient pain in the groin or buttock may be an early sign (Table 5-15). Two-thirds of these patients are boys who have onset of disease after the age of 7 to 10 years. A family history of similar disease is often suggestive of the correct diagnosis. RF and ANA are invariably absent. On the other hand, more than 92 percent of these children have HLA-B27.[135] Related to the normal distribution of this antigen in the white North American population, a negative test result occurs in approximately 8 percent of children with JAS, and a

Table 5-14 Risk Group for SLE Conversion

At onset of JRA
  Polyarthritis
  Raynaud's phenomenon
  No systemic disease
  No uveitis

Clinical approach:
  ANA may be negative at onset; if positive, or when it becomes positive, test for serum anti-dsDNA antibodies at periodic intervals

Table 5-15 Clinical Features Suggesting a Diagnosis of Juvenile Ankylosing Spondylitis

Male
Onset at 7 years of age or older
Monarticular onset, lower extremity
Sparing of hands and wrists and cervical spine
Negative serologic findings for rheumatoid factors and
  antinuclear antibodies
HLA-B27 positive

positive result in the same percentage with JRA. The finding of HLA-B27 in a child suspected of having JAS is therefore neither sufficient nor necessary for that diagnosis.

A firm diagnosis of JAS may not be possible at onset of the peripheral arthritis and depends on demonstration of characteristic radiologic features in the sacroiliac joints. In our experience, these abnormalities are present at or shortly after onset of the disease if technically adequate views of the sacroiliac joints are obtained, including angulated frontal views (30°). However, other investigators have concluded that definite radiographic changes may be delayed by years. Minimal radiologic signs of inflammation of the sacroiliac joints may be seen in a small number of children with JRA and are to be distinguished from the more pronounced changes observed in JAS.

Occult inflammatory bowel disease may present as disease of the axial or peripheral skeleton. The spondylitis of regional enteritis and ulcerative colitis is indistinguishable from that seen in JAS and may occur years before onset of the characteristic bowel symptoms.[276,277] Whipple's disease may cause peripheral arthritis in children but is very rare. The other spondyloarthropathies, such as Reiter's syndrome or psoriatic arthritis, must be differentiated diagnostically.[278] The course may be prolonged in certain children and cause residual deformities of the distal lower extremities with or without eventual development of characteristic sacroiliac arthritis. Postinfectious arthritis related to *Yersinia* or other gram-negative organisms such as *Shigella flexneri* has been common in certain areas of the world and is being increasingly reported in this hemisphere.

Children with immunologic deficiencies may develop an arthritis that mimics JRA. Common variable immunodeficiency and agammaglobulinemia[279] are generally obvious because of recurrent, severe bacterial infections, but selective IgA deficiency[280] and heterozygous C2 complement component deficiency[281] may be subtle and unrecognized unless specific assays are done. Approximately 4 percent of the children we have seen over a 15-year period with a peripheral arthritis that was clinically indistinguishable from JRA have had selective IgA deficiency. Therefore, it is important in any child with chronic arthritis to determine the concentrations of the three major serum immunoglobulins and the hemolytic complement titer.

LABORATORY EXAMINATION

Blood Indices

Hematologic abnormalities in general reflect the extent of the inflammation. Children with oligoarthritis seldom exhibit any hematologic problems beyond that of mild anemia. Children with moderately extensive JRA develop a normocytic hypochromic anemia. The anemia may be moderately severe, with a hemoglobin in the range of 7 to 10 g/dl (70 to 100 g/L), and is particularly marked in children with JRA of systemic onset.[282,283] Hypoplastic crises occur rarely[284] and in some instances may represent a virus-associated hemophagocytic syndrome.[285-287] Although the anemia in JRA is attributable to chronic disease (low serum iron, low iron binding capacity, adequate hemosiderin stores), iron deficiency may also play a role. In one study, 13 of 15 children with JRA who were anemic responded to supplemental iron therapy for a 6-month period by a rise in the hemoglobin of 1 g/dl (10 g/L) or more.[288] Elevation of the serum ferritin occurs in children with active JRA and correlates closely with systemic activity[289,290]; in that sense it does not reflect iron stores.

Leukocytosis is common in children with active disease, and strikingly high counts (30,000 to 50,000/mm^3; 30 to 50 × 10^9/L) may occur in children with systemic onset JRA. Polymorphonuclear neutrophils predominant. The platelet count may rise dramatically in severe systemic or polyarticular involvement and, in disease of long standing, may signal an exacerbation. Thrombocytopenia is rare[269,291] and may signal the evolution of the disease to SLE.

Acute Phase Reactants

ERYTHROCYTE SEDIMENTATION RATE AND C-REACTIVE PROTEIN

The ESR is a useful measure of active disease at onset and during follow-up of a child with JRA and is occasionally helpful in monitoring the therapeutic efficiency of a medication program.[292] The C-reactive protein (CRP) may be a more reliable monitor of the inflammatory response; at least, it is less often positive in the child in whom no clinical inflammatory disease can be found.[293,294] Other serum proteins respond to chronic arthritis as acute phase reactants and are elevated in children with JRA. Of particular note is the serum amyloidlike (SAA) protein that is increased in concentration in children with active disease. Cryofibrinogenemia may be associated with edema of the extremities.

SERUM IMMUNOGLOBULINS

Increases in the serum levels of the immunoglobulins are also correlated with activity of the disease.[295-299] Extreme degrees of hypergammaglobulinemia are seen in the sickest children and return toward normal with clinical improvement (Table 5-16).

Normal biologic variations in immunoglobulin levels related to age and sex can also obscure important clinical associations in children. In studies performed in our clinic[299] immunoglobulin concentrations were measured in 200 children with JRA and standardized by comparison to 695 normal children stratified by age and sex, so that individual immunoglobulin concentrations directly ex-

Table 5-16 Clinical Correlations of Serum Immunoglobulins in Children with JRA

Degree of elevation greatest in polyarthritis and systemic disease

Degree of elevation increases progressively with each functional class

Degree of elevation greatest for IgM

Degree of elevation of IgM correlates with rheumatoid factor titer

Degree of elevation of IgA greatest in children with active disease and erosions

Degree of elevation greater for boys than girls for both IgA and IgM

Table 5-17 Concentrations of Serum Immunoglobulins in Children with JRA

		Mean	SD	Range	Mean	SD	Range
Class		(mg/ml)			(Normalized Values[a])		
IgG	Total group	15.80	8.05	5.70–58.00	2.00	2.76	−1.19–13.97
	Girls	15.29	8.55	5.70–58.00	2.08	2.97	−1.19–13.97
	Boys	14.88	6.64	5.70–39.00	1.80	2.13	−0.98– 9.41
IgA	Total group	1.92	1.40	0– 8.20	1.61	2.43	−2.60–12.34
	Girls	1.72	1.31	0– 7.00	1.29	2.26	−2.60– 8.95
	Boys	2.43	1.51	0– 8.20	2.45	2.68	−1.94–12.34
IgM	Total group	1.92	1.58	0.32–13.23	2.24	3.11	−1.22–23.40
	Girls	2.05	1.70	0.32–13.23	1.93	2.67	−1.22–15.71
	Boys	1.61	1.17	0.48– 7.70	3.04	3.93	−0.73–23.40

[a] The normalized values were obtained by subtracting the matched sex-age mean from the respective serum concentrations of immunoglobulin and dividing by the sex-age SD. A standardized value of 2.00 indicates that the measured serum concentration for that immunoglobulin was two standard deviations greater than the sex-age mean. (Modified from Cassidy et al.,[300] with permission.)

pressed the extent of their deviation from normal (Figs. 5-30 to 5-32, Table 5-17).[300] Thirty-seven percent of the children with JRA expressed hypergammaglobulinemia, defined as a level greater than 1.96 standard deviations (SD) from the normal, in at least one immunoglobulin class. No relation of the immunoglobulin concentrations to age of onset or duration of disease was found. Mean immunoglobulin levels increased progressively with each deterio-ration of functional grade. The lowest values were found in children with oligoarthritis, including those who had uveitis.

IgA and IgM levels were correlated with the type of onset of the disease and with sex (Table 5-18). The mean IgA levels were significantly lower in children who were in remission than in those with active disease and were higher in children with erosive disease than in those without ero-

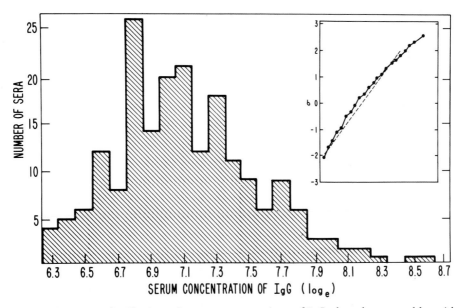

Fig. 5-30 Relative frequency distribution of serum concentrations of IgG plotted as natural logarithms against the number of sera. Cumulative distribution on a normal probability scale in the insert; the dotted line is computed from ±1.96 SD of the data (95 percent confidence limits). (From Cassidy et al.,[300] with permission.)

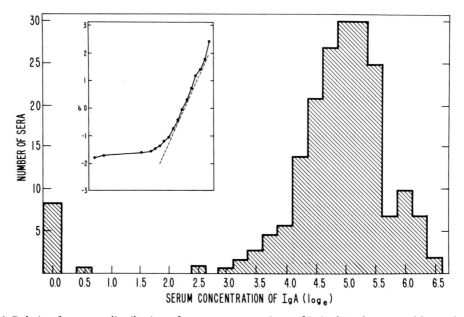

Fig. 5–31 Relative frequency distribution of serum concentrations of IgA plotted as natural logarithms against the number of sera. One (1) was added to all values before logarithmic transformation in order to include the 0 concentrations. Eight patients with undetectable IgA were essentially beyond the defined limits of the abscissa on a logarithmic scale; therefore, the indicated scale distance is only relative. Cumulative distribution on a normal probability scale in the insert; the dotted line is computed from ±1.96 SD of the data (95 percent confidence limits) with the cases of 0 concentration omitted. (From Cassidy et al.,[300] with permission.)

sions (26 percent of the study group). IgA levels were also lowest in girls even after normalization for age and sex. High RF titers were correlated with elevated serum IgM concentrations, and high ANA titers were associated with

Table 5-18 Relationship of Clinical Status to Serum Immunoglobulin Concentrations in JRA

	IgG	IgA	IgM
Type of onset of disease	NS[a]	0.004[b]	0.003
Age of onset	NS	NS	NS
Age of patient	NS	NS	NS
Duration of disease	NS	NS	NS
Sex	NS	0.003	0.01
Uveitis	NS	0.03	NS
Functional class	0.003	0.000002	0.0001
Remission	NS	0.02	NS
Activity of disease	NS	0.009	NS
Erosions	NS	0.002	0.05
Rheumatoid factors	NS	NS	0.04
Rheumatoid nodules	NS	NS	0.005
Antinuclear antibodies	NS	NS	NS

[a] NS: not significant
[b] Significance: P = or <.

decreased or normal concentrations of IgM (very likely related to their inverse relationship with RF).

Standardization of the serum immunoglobulin concentrations facilitated valid intragroup comparisons in children with JRA and permitted important associations with the clinical state of the disease to emerge. In general, persistent hypergammaglobulinemia was confirmed as being an important hallmark of a deteriorating clinical course and a poor therapeutic response. Although increases in IgG concentrations were characteristic of early disease, IgA levels appeared to be meaningfully associated with the extent of articular and systemic disease and may be a more sensitive indicator of the immunoinflammatory process in children with JRA.

In contrast, another study found that levels of immunoglobulins in 86 percent to 94 percent of children with JRA were normal.[301] IgE levels appeared, however, to correlate with an older age of the child and did not relate to activity. Significantly increased concentrations of IgG, IgA, and C4 were found in children with active disease, whereas elevated IgM levels were characteristic of the disease itself. Studies by the same authors indicated that serum antibody levels to enteric bacteria (*Escherichia coli* 055 and 086, common antigen, *Shigella* polyvalent antigen) were normal in JRA.[302] Only IgA antibodies were found in

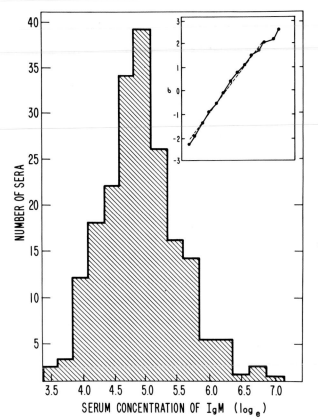

Fig. 5-32 Relative frequency distribution of serum concentrations of IgM plotted as natural logarithms against the number of sera. Cumulative distribution on a normal probability scale in the insert; the dotted line is computed from ±1.96 SD of the data (95 percent confidence limits). (From Cassidy et al.,[300] with permission.)

higher titers in these children. No abnormalities of Ig allotypes have been reported in JRA.[303]

Viral antibody titers may also be increased in specific children with JRA.[303] In our experience, antibodies to rubella and rubeola viruses are usually similar to those of appropriate control groups or are associated with a general increase in the serum immunoglobulin concentrations.[305-307] Even though recent studies do not support a direct relationship between JRA and viral antibody responses, there may be a subtle association related to type of onset or persistent viral infection (rubella, EBV).[69] As a practical matter, but without direct evidence, we advise that children with JRA not be vaccinated with attenuated rubella virus, as a postvaccination flare-up of the arthritis would complicate evaluation of the course of the disease and current therapeutic goals.

Rheumatoid Factors

The latex fixation and sensitized sheep-cell agglutination tests for the detection of classic IgM anti-IgG RF are abnormal in children with JRA less frequently than in adults with RA (Table 5-19).[292,308-316] In general, 15 to 20 percent of children with JRA are seropositive. RF tends to be found more frequently in the child of later age of onset of arthritis and in the child who is older, has subcutaneous rheumatoid nodules or articular erosions, or is in a poor functional class (Tables 5-20 and 5-21).[311] RF is unusual in the child under the age of 7 years. The diagnostic importance of RF seropositivity in a child with possible JRA is mitigated by the frequent occurrence of abnormal titers in the other connective-tissue diseases of childhood, especially SLE.

Children with high titers of RF may represent a subgroup distinct from the larger number of children with "seronegative" disease. The evidence for this hypothesis is not unequivocal, since the seropositive group is often identified in retrospect. The percentage of children with RF seropositivity rises progressively as the age of onset or the duration of disease of the cohort group under study increases (Table 5-22).[311] These observations tend to suggest that seropositivity may be the result rather than a determining event in children with JRA who go on to unremitting, disabling disease during the early adult years.

Many studies have demonstrated other types of antiglobulins in the sera in children with JRA or have reported more sensitive and specific tests for RF.[317-331] The majority of children with seronegative JRA can be shown to have IgG anti-IgG antibodies, as demonstrated by immunosorbent techniques.[318-322] Pepsin agglutinators of the IgG class are found more often in children with JRA than is classic RF.[331]

Miller et al. employed five different immunosorbents to search for occult antiglobulins in the sera of children with JRA.[321] Antiglobulins detected by binding to Sepharose-linked globulin followed by acid elution were found in eight normal children as well as in 52 children with JRA. Only four children with JRA had significantly elevated levels. These authors concluded that the presence of these antiglobulins per se was not diagnostically helpful in distinguishing children with JRA.

In the studies of Moore et al.,[323-329] 46 percent of children with JRA were shown to have hidden RF, defined as IgM 19S antiglobulins that could be detected by acid elution of IgM-containing fractions of serum from a gel filtration column. Hidden RF was found in 59 percent of children with

Table 5-19 Rheumatoid Factors in Children with JRA

Author/ No. of Children	Test Used	Percentage Positive	Sex	Age	Late Onset	Long Duration	Type of Onset	Functional Class	Stage	Activity	Nodules
Bywaters et al.[309] 142	DAT	13 45	—		+	—				—	+ + +
Toubis et al.[310] 45	SCAT LFT	40 13		+ +	—		—		—	—	—
Sievers et al.[263] 200	SCAT LFT	23 31		+ + +	+	—			—		
Laaksonen[51] 439	SCAT LFT	11 29	+ (F)		+ + +		+	+ + +	+ + +		
Cassidy and Valkenburg[311] 110	HEAT LFT	14 19	—	+	+ +	—					+ + +
Hanson et al.[312] 110	SCAT LFT	15 23	+ (F)		+ + +	—					+ + +
Petty et al.[333] 200	LFT	13	+ (F)	+ +	+ +	—	+				

(Modified from Petty et al.,[292] with permission.)

JRA who lacked classic RF by using a complement-dependent hemolytic assay, and correlated well with disease activity. Not only was hidden RF more frequent in children with JRA; it was also of higher titer than in healthy children or other disease control groups. The titers correlated with activity of the disease and did not differ significantly between polyarticular and oligoarticular children. Hidden RF could be inhibited more readily by the use of human IgG than IgG of animal origin, although the detection system continued to be a hemolytic assay employing rabbit IgG.

Antinuclear Antibodies

Tests for ANA have proved to be more useful diagnostically than those for RF in studies of children with JRA.[292,332] Results of representative investigations are summarized in Table 5-23. In some studies, RF tended to occur in a different population of chil-

Table 5-20 Clinical Associations of Rheumatoid Factors in Children with JRA

Polyarthritis
Older child
Late age of onset
Nodules
Bone erosions
Poorer functional class

Table 5-21 Relation of Functional Class to Rheumatoid Factor Seropositivity in 110 Children with JRA

Class	Number	Median Age	Median Duration	Positive RF Test Number	%
I No limitation	19	14	4	1	5
II Minimal	38	12	4	7	18
III Moderate	34	14	6	12	35
IV Severe	19	16	6	4	21

(Modified from Cassidy and Valkenburg,[311] with permission.)

Table 5-22 Relation of Rheumatoid Factor Seropositivity and Age-Dependent Parameters in 110 Children with JRA

Years	Age at Study No.	Age at Study Positive (%)	Age at Onset No.	Age at Onset Positive (%)	Duration of Disease No.	Duration of Disease Positive (%)
0–4	7	0	42	12	49	18
5–9	29	7	37	16	35	20
10–14	32	25	31	42	15	27
15–19	18	22	—	—	5	20
20–24	14	36	—	—	4	50
25 +	10	50	—	—	2	50

(Modified from Cassidy and Valkenburg,[311] with permission.)

Table 5-23 Antinuclear Antibodies in Children with JRA

Study (Ref.)	Substate	No. Studied	Serum Dilution	Positive (%) JRA	Positive (%) Normal	Correlation
Petty et al.[333]	Mouse liver	200	Undiluted	38	2	Young age Female Oligoarthritis or polyarthritis Chronic uveitis
Schaller et al.[334]	Rat liver	JCP with chronic iridocyclitis: 58	1:10	88	0	Iridocyclitis
		JCP without iridocyclitis: 133		30		
Rudnicki et al.[315]	Mouse liver	85		24		
Alsbaugh et al.[336]	Mouse kidney	77		57		
Permin et al.[337]	Rat liver; WBC	100		66		
Patel et al.[338]	HEp-2 cells	217		60		
Rosenberg et al.[339]	HEp-2 cells	61		62		
McCune et al.[340]	HEp-2 cells	207	1:40	53	6	Chronic uveitis

dren with JRA than did ANA; other studies have indicated that they occurred in the same children.[3] Our initial report indicated that approximately 40 percent of children had positive results by the fluorescent antibody technique using mouse liver as substrate.[333] The fluorescent patterns obtained were usually homogeneous or speckled, and the standardized serum dilution titers were low to moderate. Most ANA was of the IgG class, although antibodies of the IgM or IgA classes were found. In these and other studies, it was found that the frequency of ANA was highest in girls of younger age of onset and lowest in older boys and in children with systemic disease (Table 5-24).[331,343] ANA reached its highest prevalence in children who had oligoarthritis and uveitis: 65 to 85 percent.[333,334] Thus, determination of ANA positivity became critically important in diagnosis of a child suspected of having JRA and in selection of children most at risk for the development of chronic uveitis. ANA seropositivity was not frequently present in

Table 5-24 Clinical Associations of Antinuclear Antibodies in Children with JRA

Oligoarthritis and polyarthritis
Female sex
Young age
Chronic uveitis
No bone erosions

control groups of other childhood illnesses except for SLE, scleroderma, and acute viral illness.

At the present time, tests for ANA are more often performed on HEp-2 cells than on mouse liver. The frequency of ANA positivity in children with JRA is increased on this substrate compared to mouse liver, as is background positivity in normal children.[338–340] The most commonly observed patterns are homogeneous and speckled. In addition, a specific pattern of nuclear fluorescence of mitotic figures has been described in children with oligoarthritis and chronic uveitis.[340] Recent evaluation of the specificities of ANA in JRA using a Western blotting technique has revealed extensive heterogeneity of reactivity of sera with preparations of HEp-2 cell nuclei.[344]

The appearance of lupus erythematosus (LE) cell positivity during the course of JRA should be recognized as a forewarning of a potential transition to SLE. Antibody to double-stranded DNA measured by a Farr technique is normal in children with JRA.[274] The finding of significantly elevated DNA binding indicates the supervention of active immune complex disease of the lupus type.

Other types of ANA have been described, but there have been no consistent clinical correlations with these autoantibodies and the type of JRA.[337,345,346] In the studies of Permin et al., the prevalence of IgG granulocyte-specific ANA increased with the number of joints affected.[337] This type of ANA was not found with acute systemic onset. ANA of the IgG class was present in the sera of all children with chronic uveitis. Høyeraal studied granulocyte-specific ANA in 34 children with JRA and age- and sex-matched children with other diseases.[346] ANA was not found in any of the control sera. The majority of the granulocyte-specific ANA were of the IgG class; 50 percent were capable of fixing complement and tended to correlate with active disease.

Another study examined the sera of 77 children with JRA for ANA specific for distinctive nuclear antigens (Sm, RNP, DNA, RNA, RAP, SS-A, and SS-B).[336] The most common pattern was speckled in the 49 percent of the sera that were ANA seropositive. The frequency of positive tests for the defined antigens was only 13 percent; too low to enable correlations to be made. However, the authors noted a small group of girls with polyarthritis and late onset of disease who had an increased frequency of RF or RAP. These two antibodies were not associated with each other, as they were in adult disease. These studies suggested that these patients might be infected with the Epstein-Barr virus and that this virus might play a role in the pathogenesis of JRA.

Serum Complement and Immune Complexes

Serum concentration of the third component of complement (C3) and titers of hemolytic complement are often elevated as acute phase reactants in children with active JRA.[347] Soluble immune complexes can be detected in the sera of certain children with JRA and are particularly related to systemic onset of disease and polyarthritis.[348–351] Intravascular coagulation has been described.[213–216,352]

Miller et al. studied the presence of activation products of C3 in the sera of children with JRA.[353–355] Abnormal concentrations of C3c,d were found in 7 of 10 children with systemic JRA, 16 of 29 with active polyarthritis, and 7 of 20 with active oligoarthritis. Activation products were found in only 2 of 20 children with inactive joint disease. In the study by Rynes et al.[356] 4 children showed isolated depression of serum C2 activity, suggesting an immunogenetic basis for their disease. These authors also found that immunoglobulin levels, particularly of IgA, correlated with complement measurements and the ESR as evidence for active disease.

In one study immune complexes were detected by a C1q binding technique in 11 of 51 consecutive children with JRA (22 percent), most often in children who were RF seropositive.[348] On the basis of these studies, it was suggested that children with systemic onset JRA might have a relative defect in antibody forming capacity or in fixed mononuclear phagocytic cell function that resulted in decreased clearance of circulating immune complexes.

Synovial Fluid Analysis

Synovial fluid in JRA is usually a group II or inflammatory fluid (see Appendix)[157]; however, the level of the white blood cell (WBC) count does not always correlate with the degree of clinical activity (Table 5-25).[157] Very low counts, for example, 600 cells per cubic millimeter (0.6×10^9/L), have been observed in fluids from joints clinically involved by intensely active and symptomatic disease. Conversely, counts in the range of septic arthritis, for example, 100,000 cells per cubic millimeter (100×10^9/L), have been found in children with otherwise classic JRA.[357,358] Synovial levels of glucose may be intrinsically low in JRA, as in adult RA. Complement levels are not as uniformly depressed as in adult disease.[356,359,360] Rynes et al. found intra-articular activation of the complement cascade in certain children with JRA.[356] In their studies there was evidence for activation of the classic pathway in all types of disease onset. Assays for properdin and kininogen failed to support involvement of these pathways in the genesis of synovial inflammation. Three joint fluids from children with oligoarthritis did not have detectable complement activation products in the study by Miller et al.[355]

Although one might expect to find no RF in joint fluid from children with JRA and few ragocytes indicative of immune complex phagocytosis,[361–364] neither of these characteristics has been sufficiently investigated in children with JRA to enable one to be

Table 5-25 Synovial Fluid Analyses in Children with Oligoarticular Onset of JRA

Gross Characteristics	Yellow, clear to opalescent
Total white cell count (mm³)	
Range	150–41,600
Median	10,000
Average	11,400
Polymorphonuclear neutrophils (%)	
Range	18–88
Median	52
Average	56
Mucin clot test (%)	
Excellent	20
Good	20
Fair	15
Poor	45

(Modified from Cassidy JT et al.,[157] with permission.)

unequivocal about conclusions. Complexes of IgG, IgG RF, and complement components along with hidden RF have been described in both synovial tissue and eluates.

RADIOLOGIC CHANGES

Early radiographic changes consist of soft tissue swelling about the joints, widening of the joint space (Fig. 5-33), juxta-articular osteoporosis, and, less frequently, periosteal new bone formation.[59,61,180,365–367] Periosteal new bone apposition occurs most commonly in the phalanges, metacarpals, and metatarsals but occasionally involves the long bones as well (Fig. 5-34). Widening of the midportions of the phalanges from periosteal new bone apposition is another characteristic radiologic feature of children with JRA.

Later radiologic changes include marginal erosions and thinning of the cartilage (joint space narrowing) (Fig. 5-35).[365] These changes generally do not occur before 2 years of active disease even in a child with polyarthritis. Indeed, in some children with limited joint disease, erosions may not be seen even after one or two decades of constant effusion and swelling of a joint (Figs. 5-36 to 5-38). Erosion and enlargement

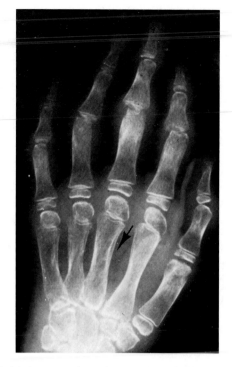

Fig. 5-34 Severe arthritis in an 8-year-old girl. Demineralization is marked, along with epiphyseal compression and swelling about the PIP joints. Periosteal new bone apposition (arrow) is present on the metacarpals.

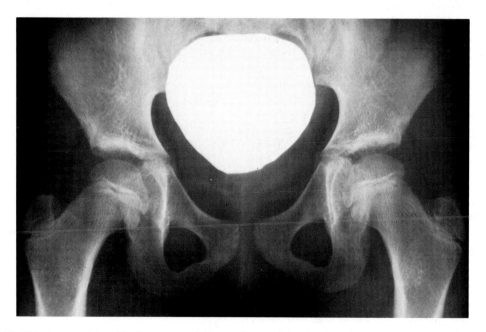

Fig. 5-33 This 8-year-old girl had an unusual onset of JRA with slight pain and restricted range of motion in the right hip. There are subtle widening of the joint space on that side and slight osteoporosis involving the femoral head and neck.

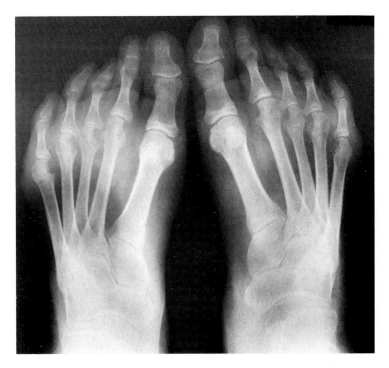

Fig. 5-35 Feet showing extensive classic rheumatoid erosions involving the medial undersurfaces of the metatarsals.

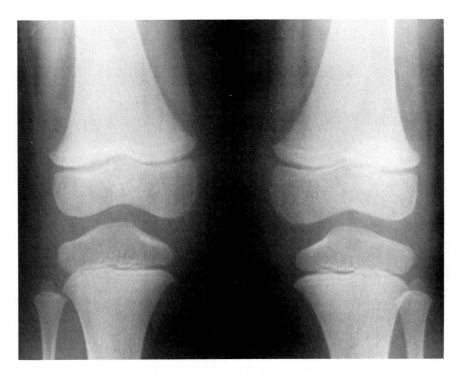

Fig. 5-36 Knees of a 4-year-old girl with JRA. Figures 5-36, 5-37, and 5-38 illustrate the usual signs of progression of arthritis in large growing joints. A duration of disease of 2 years was present when this radiograph was taken. Minimal epiphyseal enlargement and osteoporosis are present.

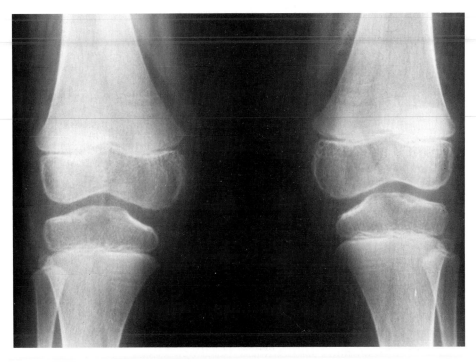

Fig. 5-37 Knees at 4 years' duration of disease, showing increased prominence of the trabecular architecture, narrowing of the joint spaces, and remodeling of the normal contours of the articulating surfaces.

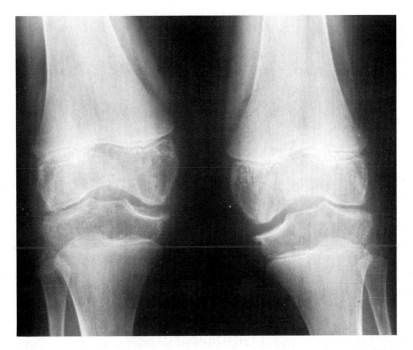

Fig. 5-38 Knees at 5 years' duration. Marked narrowing of the joint spaces is present, tibial plateaus and femoral condyles show advanced flattening, and degenerative hypertrophic changes are beginning to appear. (Note sharpening of the tibial tubercles.) The child at this time had a pronounced valgus deformity of the legs with weight bearing.

of the intercondylar notch of the femur are seen in JRA. These changes have been also reported in hemophilia and tuberculosis.

In the young child, the ossifying blood vessel buds that grow out from the epiphyseal center tend to be irregular and should not be misinterpreted as destructive changes. Growth arrest lines may result from temporary cessation of growth in the area of provisional calcification of the hyaline cartilage.

Bony ankylosis occurs more promptly in children than in adults and may be particularly pronounced in the carpal and tarsal joints (Fig. 5-39). Multiple loose cartilage-covered bony bodies, or "loose bodies," may mechanically interfere with the movement of a joint.

In children, subluxation involves large as well as small joints (Fig. 5-40). Because many of these children have an early age of onset of arthritis, subluxation of a hip may be confused with congenital dislocation; protrusio acetabuli may also develop (Fig. 5-41). The hyaline cartilage of the hip is destroyed in progressive stages during the course of severe JRA, and during healing it may be replaced by a fibrocar-

tilaginous layer.[368] Aseptic necrosis is seldom observed in children with JRA, even in those treated with high-dose corticosteroids for long periods.

Fractures related to JRA or severe generalized osteoporosis are reported frequently in some studies.[369] They are particularly seen in young children who have had severe disease and long periods of immobilization or corticosteroid therapy. The supracondylar area of the femur is a characteristic site of a fracture that follows manipulation for contracture of the knee (Fig. 5-42).[370] Destruction or microfractures of the growth plates may be related to abnormal mechanical stress in JRA (Fig. 5-43). The normally balanced muscle forces about the joints are altered by severe joint deformities, erosion, and subluxation, and by inflammation of the periarticular connective tissue. Abnormal compression forces on the growth plates result.

Growth disturbances are among the most remarkable skeletal changes seen in JRA. There are early nonspecific accelerated maturation and enlargement of the epiphyseal ossification centers (Fig. 5-44).[157] This finding is often most striking at the knee.[371,372]

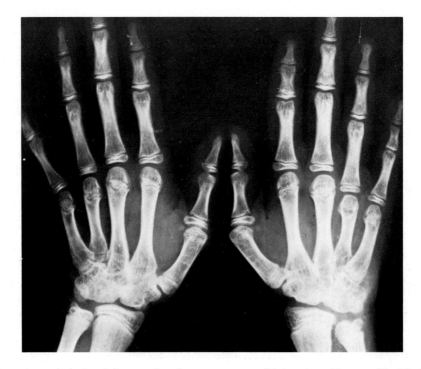

Fig. 5-39 Extensive ankylosis of the carpal and carpometacarpal joints in a 12-year-old girl. These changes were first evident after only 2 years of active arthritis. The small joints of the hands were not involved.

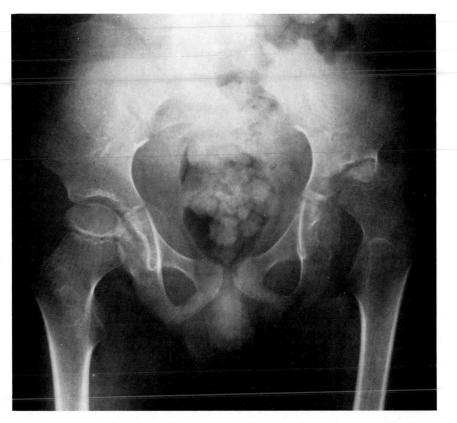

Fig. 5-40 Marked subluxation of the left hip in a 5½-year-old boy with onset of severe unremitting JRA at the age of 1½ years. This child was still able to walk with a marked limp but little pain.

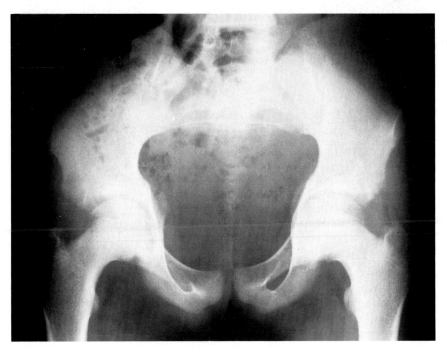

Fig. 5-41 Protrusio acetabuli of the left hip in a girl with long-standing JRA. She developed pain in the left hip with a marked reduction in range of motion. At that time her general disease activity was minimal.

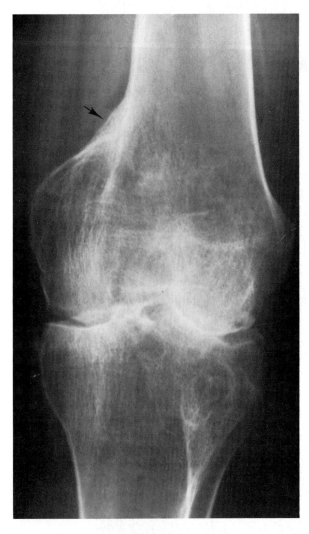

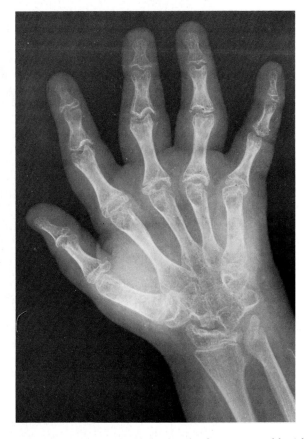

Fig. 5-43 Radiograph of the hand of a 15-year-old girl taken shortly before her death. Severe polyarthritis was present, with marked bony overgrowth and enlargement of the epiphyses. Erosions and destruction of the small joints were evident with invagination of the abutting bones. The DIP joints were also involved, and partial ankylosis of the carpus was present.

Fig. 5-42 Radiograph of the left knee of a 21-year-old woman with JRA who sustained a condylar fracture of the femur (arrow) after minor trauma at 14 years of age. There have been a marked loss of the cartilaginous space and sclerosis of the weight-bearing surfaces. (From Cassidy et al.,[370] with permission.)

Accelerated maturation of the patella may occur. A radiographic picture of marked bony overgrowth and enlargement of the epiphyses may also occur at the interphalangeal joints.

Failure of growth of small tubular bones results in brachydactyly. This condition is occasionally but not always related to premature epiphyseal fusion, especially when selective stunting of one or two bones occurs. A common site for this finding is in the fourth metatarsal bones (Fig. 5-45). Asymmetric fusion may

Table 5-26 Radiologic Characteristics of Oligoarticular JRA

Late appearance of bone erosions
Local growth abnormalities
   Increased size of epiphyseal ossification centers
   Accelerated epiphyseal maturation
   Longitudinal overgrowth of long bones
   Diminished size of small round and tubular bones
Secondary regional atrophy
   Osteoporosis
   Reduction in bone diameter
   Bone remodeling
   Soft tissue atrophy

(Modified from Cassidy et al.,[157] with permission.)

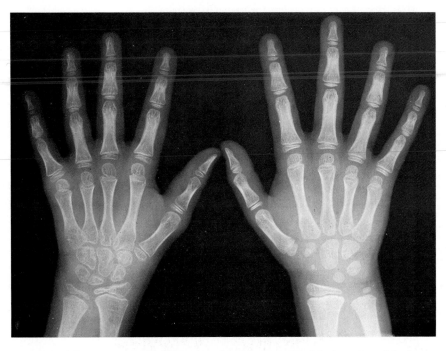

Fig. 5-44 Arthritis persisted for 7 years in the left wrist of this 9-year-old girl. Atrophy of the bones and a small hand are present on the left. There have been accelerated maturation of the bones of the left carpus and arrested development before full growth was attained. (From Cassidy et al.,[157] with permission.)

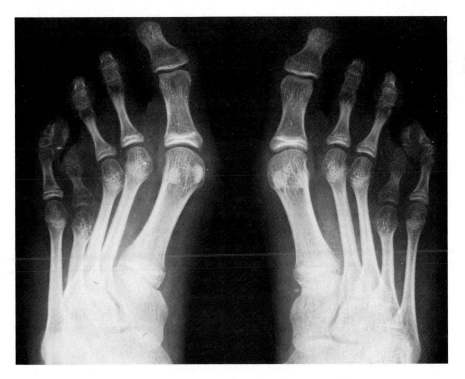

Fig. 5-45 Brachydactyly of the fourth metatarsal bones.

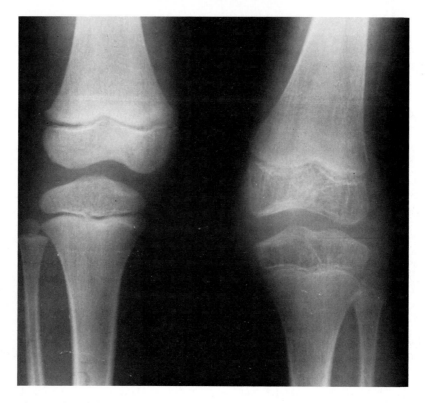

Fig. 5-46 Monarthritis of the left knee has persisted for 8 years in this 14-year-old girl. On the left, there are regional osteoporosis, accentuation of the trabecular pattern, enlargement of the epiphyseal ossification centers, and radial atrophy of the long bones. Remodeling of the distal femur is retarded compared to that of the right side. Erosive disease is absent. (From Cassidy et al.,[157] with permission.)

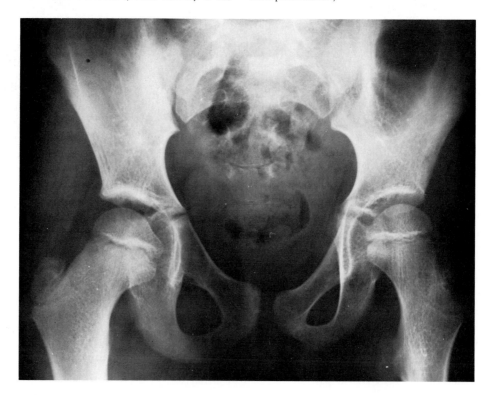

Fig. 5-47 Pelvis of the girl in Fig. 5-46. Regional osteoporosis and miniaturization of the ipsilateral pelvis are present, along with marked coxa valga. Arthritis is not present in the left hip. These changes are secondary to inflammatory disease of the left knee. (From Cassidy et al.,[157] with permission.)

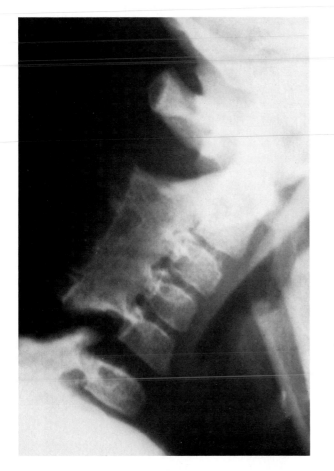

Fig. 5-48 Unusually severe pseudoarticulation and destructive changes at the C5-C6 junction in a 7-year-old boy. Apophyseal joints above and below this area of movement were fused. No neurologic symptoms or signs were present. Clinical disease was stabilized by fitting this child with a cervical collar and beginning gold salt therapy.

occur when only a portion of the epiphyseal plate is affected. When adjacent bones are not involved equally, one may become bowed; this finding is particularly common in the radius.

Frequent abnormalities in an involved extremity in oligoarticular disease are generalized demineralization, reduction in the diameters of the long bones, and atrophy of the soft tissue (Table 5-26).[157] Radial atrophy is often accompanied by linear overgrowth of the long bones (Figs. 5-46 and 5-47).[157] The entire extremity may be affected by osteoporosis. The ipsilateral pelvis may show stunting of growth with coxa valga even though the arthritis is confined clinically to the knee.

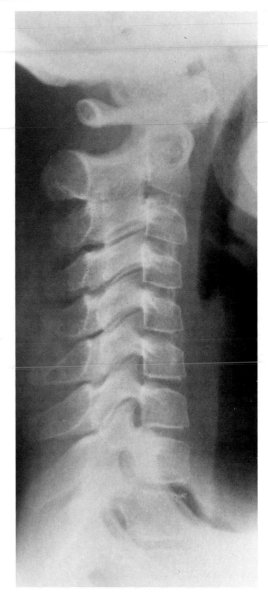

Fig. 5-49 Fusion of the C2-C3 apophyseal joint in a teenage girl with early onset of JRA.

In RF-seronegative children, predominant radiologic and clinical involvement is often centered on the knees, ankles, wrists, and hips. The smaller joints (MCP, PIP, and MTP) become involved during the course of the disease rather than at the onset. In a long-term study of children with JRA, erosive changes of the small joints of the hands and feet were present at 5 years in 67 of 70 children with seropositive disease.[373]

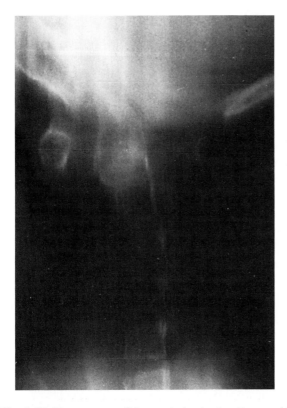

Fig. 5-50 Tomograms of the cervical spine in a 7-year-old girl. Marked atlantoaxial subluxation is present.

Characteristic radiologic abnormalities of the axial skeleton occur in JRA; cervical spine involvement is particularly characteristic.[180,374] The predominant changes are within the upper cervical segments. Here, apophyseal joint disease is especially common and bony fusion is frequent, often observed first at the C2-C3 level (Figs. 5-48, 5-49). Fusion of adjacent posterior spines may be observed. A single lateral film of the cervical spine may not be sufficient to determine the presence of ankylosis in this location. The distance between flexion and extension should be measured at the corresponding neurospines to confirm that fusion has occurred.

Atlantoaxial subluxation is a common abnormality in children with JRA involving the cervical spine (Fig. 5-50). The upper limit of the atlanto-odontoid space in children is approximately 4 mm measured on a lateral film taken in flexion with a 40-inch tube to film distance. Locke et al. studied the expected distraction in this space in 200 normal children aged 3 to 15 years.[375] When this space was measured at

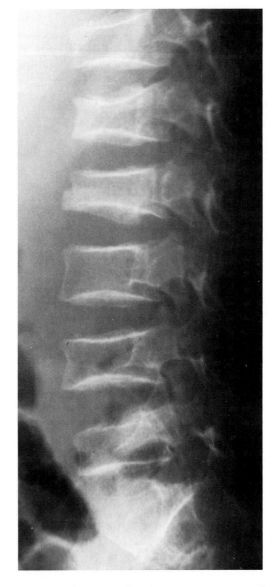

Fig. 5-51 Lumbar spine showing numerous areas of vertebral compression in this 12-year-old girl with severe debilitating JRA. Corticosteroid therapy had been used for many years.

greater than 4 mm in the neutral position, an atlantoaxial subluxation was usually confirmed. Age and sex were not significant factors in evaluating these measurements. Other signs of atlantoaxial subluxation were found to be an increased tissue density anterior to the cervical spine, flexion greater than 10° between the atlas and the axis, compensatory curve of the lower cervical spine, and narrowing of the at-

Table 5-27 Clinicoradiologic Correlations in Children with JRA

	Types of Onset		
	Polyarthritis (%)	Oligoarthritis (%)	Systemic Disease (%)
Early changes			
Soft tissue swelling or osteoporosis	45	75	45
Periosteal new bone apposition	30	—	50
Metaphyseal rarefaction	5	—	5
Advanced changes			
Cartilage destruction	55	25	50
Bone destruction	35	25	20
Bony ankylosis	25	5	15
Large-joint subluxation	15	5	20
Epiphyseal fractures	5	—	40
Vertebral compression	20	—	25
Growth abnormalities			
Long bones: under- or overgrowth	30	50	15
Brachydactyly	20	5	30
Micrognathia	15	5	40
Accelerated epiphyseal maturation	5	35	20
Spondylitis			
Cervical	35	10	20
Atlantoaxial subluxation	15	—	5
Dorsolumbar	5	—	5
Sacroiliac	5	5	—

(Modified from Cassidy et al.,[365] with permission.)

lantovertebral foramen. There is normally a small amount of displacement between the bodies of C2 and C3 in the young child (2 to 12 years of age); this change should not be misinterpreted as early subluxation.

Narrowing of an intervertebral disc associated with atrophy or maldevelopment of adjacent thoracic vertebral bodies probably reflects fusion of an apophyseal joint even though it may not be well delineated radiologically. Vertebral bodies at areas of fusion fail to grow normally and are smaller and narrower than contiguous vertebral bodies (an altered ratio of height to width). The corresponding intervertebral spaces are also reduced, and calcification of the disc is occasionally seen. Vertebral compression fractures are often seen in affected children, especially those who have been treated with corticosteroids (Fig. 5-51).[180,376]

Sacroiliac arthritis with JRA is not characterized by the degree of reactive sclerosis that is seen in JAS (Fig. 5-52).[180,377] The sacroiliac joints in JRA rarely show changes that could be confused with those of JAS. In long-standing disease there may be subchondral sclerosis and secondary cartilage space narrowing. Late fusion may occur, however, in children with severe disease who have been immobile.[180]

Presently, there is interest in the use of objective ancillary techniques other than classic radiographs to document the presence of inflammation in joints.[378] Computed tomography (CT) and magnetic resonance imaging (MRI) add information in specific instances (Fig. 5-53).[379] The enormous potential of MRI in evaluating cartilage and soft tissues is just beginning to be exploited. Bone scans with radionuclides such as ^{133}Xe and ^{99m}Tc,[380–382] as well as sonography,[383] have been evaluated. Thermography has the advantage of not employing an isotope in children and can be repeated at intervals to follow a difficult case.[384] It has been shown to correlate with the presence of other clinical parameters of active inflammation in the joints.

Sequential radiologic changes have been examined in relation to the type of onset of the disease (Table 5-27).[365]

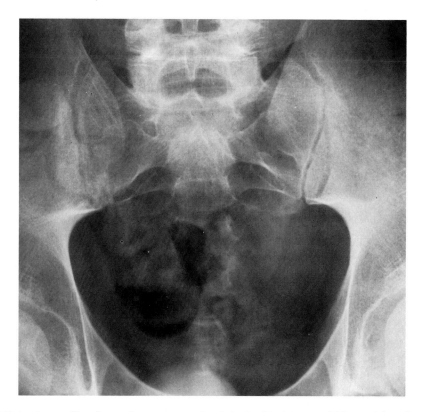

Fig. 5-52 Minimal sacroiliac disease is present on the right in this 14-year-old boy with polyarticular JRA.

Early findings of soft tissue swelling or osteoporosis were seen in 45 percent of children with polyarthritis or systemic onset and in 75 percent of those with oligoarthritis. Periosteal new bone formation and striking metaphyseal rarefaction were found only in children with polyarthritis and systemic onset (Fig. 5-54). The metaphyseal bands were thought to be related to focal osteoporosis and hyperemia of the zone of ossification of the epiphyseal plate. Periosteal new bone formation occurred adjacent to involved joints, but was not seen in children with monarthritis or oligoarthritis in spite of a subsequent polyarticular course in some of these patients.

Advanced radiologic changes were also related to the type of onset of disease. Destruction of cartilage and bone was marked in children with polyarticular or systemic onset and was less frequent and usually less severe in those with oligoarthritis who subsequently developed polyarthritis (Fig. 5-55). Bony ankylosis was a late change when it occurred. In this study,[365] large joint subluxation, especially at the hip, was particularly characteristic. Fractures of the epiphyses and vertebral compression fractures occurred only in children with severe, long-standing disease. The increased frequency of these findings in children with systemic disease was probably related to extended use of cor-

ticosteroid drugs in this group, since fractures were rarely seen when these agents had not been employed. Fractures were not observed in children who had oligoarthritis.

Growth abnormalities were particularly marked in children with monarticular or oligoarticular disease. Longitudinal overgrowth was the rule, although the affected bones were generally smaller than normal in radial diameter. Generalized growth abnormalities, such as brachydactyly and micrognathia, occurred predominantly in children with systemic disease and to a lesser extent in those with polyarthritis. Accelerated epiphyseal maturation during active disease could lead to temporary overgrowth of the round bones of joints such as the wrist, and in some cases this development was associated with future stunting of full growth of the affected bones. This change was surprisingly uncommon in children with polyarthritis.

A spondylitis typical of JRA was noted in all regions of the axial skeleton. Cervical spine disease was, of course, the most characteristic abnormality, and a few children actually presented with arthritis of the cervical spine. Atlantoaxial subluxation and disease of the thoracolumbar spine did not develop in children with monarthritis of long duration. Dwarfing or remodeling of the dorsolumbar vertebral bodies, probably attributable to arthritis of the apo-

Table 5-28 Objectives of the Conservative Management of JRA

Relief of discomfort
Arrest of the inflammatory process
Correction or control of complications
Maintenance of good nutrition and development
Maintenance of joint function
Prevention of deformities
Rehabilitation

Table 5-30 Emotional and Psychosocial Adjustment in JRA

Acceptance of goals of management of the disease
Understanding of fluctuations in disease activity
Realistic career planning
Balance of activity/rest
Regular school program
Peer group interaction

physeal joints of that region, was observed in a few patients. Characteristic sacroiliac arthritis, both with and without coincident cervical disease, was present in four children.

TREATMENT

Because the therapeutic program in children with JRA is supportive and not curative, a program of conservative management should attempt to control the clinical manifestations of the disease, preserve function, and prevent deformity (Table 5-28).[385-388] This program should stress family-centered, community-based, coordinated care.[389,390] Our approach involves a multidisciplinary team that consists of a pediatric rheumatologist, social worker, physical therapist, occupational therapist, and nurse clinician. Consultation with a physiatrist, psychiatrist, orthopedic surgeon, or dentist is sought when indicated. Regular ophthalmologic consultation is mandatory.

The treatment program in most children is prolonged, since JRA is characterized by chronic and recurrent inflammation of the joints and varying systemic manifestations. Both the child and the family must ultimately accept the long duration of therapy,

and the approach that is chosen in discussions with them must be weighed carefully to lead to compliance and an appropriate therapeutic benefit (Table 5-29). Although the outcome is excellent in the majority of children with JRA, at the onset of the disease the pediatric rheumatologist is not able to predict with certainty which child will recover promptly and which will have unremitting disease. Therefore, the initial therapeutic approach must be vigorous in all children and aimed at suppression of articular inflammation, prevention of secondary deformities, maintenance of muscle strength, and control of systemic disease. Appropriate social and educational development of the child must be encouraged during the entire course of the disease (Table 5-30).

Our philosophy of management of JRA is to begin with the safest, simplest, and most conservative measures (Table 5-31). If the treatment program proves inadequate after an appropriate interval of time, other

Table 5-29 Treatment in JRA: Compliance

Compliance is increased by
  Shared goals (patient/family/physician)
  Understanding the disease and treatment
  Positive reinforcement
Compliance is decreased by
  Numerous different medications or treatments
  Long-term management program
  Adverse side effects
  Remissions and asymptomatic periods

Table 5-31 Outline of the Management of JRA

Basic program
  Acetylsalicylic acid
  Balanced rest/exercise
  Physical and occupational therapy
  Education of patient and family
  Involvement of school and community agencies

Nonsteroidal anti-inflammatory drugs
Intra-articular steroids
Hospitalization

Hydroxychloroquine
Gold salts
Penicillamine
Sulfasalazine

Systemic corticosteroid medications
Prophylactic surgery

Reconstructive surgery
Immunosuppressive drugs and experimental therapy

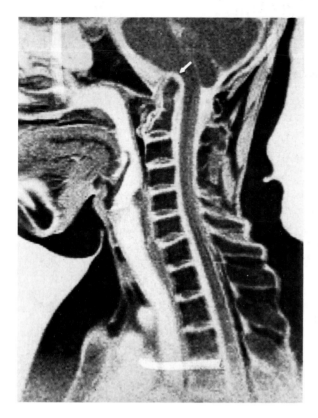

Fig. 5-53 Magnetic resonance imaging of the cervical spine in a 26-year-old woman with systemic onset of JRA at age 11. Note impingement of odontoid on upper cervical cord (arrow). (Courtesy of Dr. W. J. McCune.)

therapeutic modalities are selected in an orderly and systematic fashion (Ch. 3). Acute inflammation in JRA leads to transient disability, swelling, and pain and necessitates a different approach to the child than chronic articular inflammation, which leads progressively to increasing degrees of deformity and destruction of cartilage and bone. Potentially dangerous or experimental regimens should be chosen only for children with life-threatening disease, in approved protocols, with a full explanation of their risk/benefit ratio, and with consent of the parents and child, where appropriate.

Aspirin

Aspirin is the single most important drug in the treatment of JRA and is of indispensable value (Table 5-32).[391] Aspirin suppresses inflammation and fever in the majority of cases and has a proven record of long-term safety. It should be given 4 times a day with meals and at bedtime with milk to minimize gastrointestinal (GI) irritation and to ensure therapeutic blood levels.[392–394] A child should not chew aspirin tablets as this drug will cause gingival inflammation and erosions with destruction of the biting surfaces of the teeth.[395–396] Awakening the child at night to administer aspirin is not necessary because the serum half-life of salicylate is prolonged once therapeutic levels have been achieved.

Treatment with aspirin is started at 75 to 90 mg/kg/day in divided doses. The higher dosages are tolerated best by younger children of less than 25 kg of body weight. Salicylate blood levels are occasionally useful as a guide to correct doses in the preverbal child or when signs of toxicity such as tinnitus are not likely to be communicated to the parents or physician. The appropriate serum level varies from child to child but is usually 20 to 25 mg/dl (1.45 to 1.8 mmol/L) measured 2 h after the morning dose. It may be difficult to reach therapeutic levels in children with acute systemic disease, but increasing the dose beyond 130 mg/kg often results in salicylism. If high doses in this range are required initially for control, they should be reduced gradually to maintenance levels as the systemic manifestations of the disease subside. Intermittent fever may not respond to adequate salicylate dosage until after 1 to 4 weeks of therapy.

Treatment with aspirin is satisfactory in approximately 30 to 50 percent of children with JRA. An unanswered question is when to stop salicylate therapy if the disease appears to have entered a remission. Because limited remissions of active disease are common, we have generally continued aspirin for 1 to 2 years after all manifestations of activity have abated.

SALICYLATE HEPATITIS

Salicylate hepatitis may develop in some children but is often not clinically appreciated, since overt manifestations of liver disease appear to be uncommon (Ch. 3). Hepatitis occurs most often when the serum salicylate concentration is in the toxic range (>25 mg/dl [1.8 mmol/L]), although the transaminase enzymes, AST, aspartate transaminase (serum glutamic-oxaloacetic transaminase [SGOT]) and ALT, alanine transaminase (serum glutamic-pyruvic transaminase [SGPT]), may be intermittently increased in

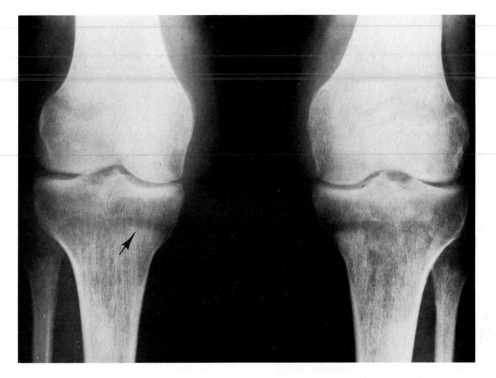

Fig. 5-54 Zones of metaphyseal rarefaction in both tibias. These abnormalities were early radiologic changes and were later replaced by growth arrest lines.

Table 5-32 Drug Therapy for JRA

Medication	Dose	Indication	Toxicity
Aspirin	75–90 mg/kg/day	Control of pain, stiffness, and inflammation	Salicylism (lethargy, hyperpnea, tinnitus), gastrointestinal irritation, bleeding, hepatitis
Nonsteroidal anti-inflammatory agent	Varies with drug	Control of pain, stiffness, and inflammation	Gastrointestinal irritation, hepatitis, decreased renal function
Hydroxychloroquine	7 mg/kg/day	Selective use for arthritis	Dermatitis, keratopathy, retinopathy
Gold salt	0.75 mg/kg/month	Polyarthritis unresponsive to nonsteroidal anti-inflammatory agents	Dermatitis, nephritis, stomatitis, bone marrow suppression
D-Penicillamine	10 mg/kg/day	Polyarthritis unresponsive to other regimens	Dermatitis, nephritis, lupuslike syndrome
Sulfasalazine	40–60 mg/kg/day	Polyarthritis unresponsive to other regimens	Bone marrow suppression, dermatitis, gastrointestinal irritation
Corticosteroid drug			
Systemic	Prednisone, 1 mg/kg/day (as low a dose as possible)	Life-threatening systemic disease, chronic uveitis	Growth retardation, infection, Cushing's syndrome
Ophthalmic	4 drops/day	Chronic uveitis	Cataracts, glaucoma
Intra-articular	30 mg prednisolone-TBA	Selective use for arthritis	Infection
Immunosuppressive agent	Varies with drug	Life-threatening systemic disease	Infection, bone marrow suppression, sterility, oncogenesis

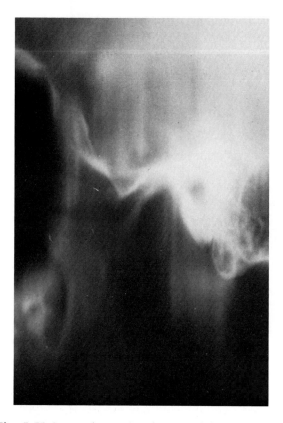

Fig. 5-55 Severe destructive changes of the TMJ in this 20-year-old woman who had had JRA since the age of 1½ years. The vertical ramus is short and small and the condyle is miniature, but the normal acetabular configuration is maintained. There was no history of pain or disability in the TMJs.

as many as 50 percent of the children receiving therapeutic doses of salicylate.[397–404] Transient elevation of these enzymes in a child who is otherwise not showing signs of salicylism is not an indication for stopping aspirin. If the levels remain increased or are very high, for example, if the AST is more than 5 times normal, the dosage should be reduced abruptly by 20 percent or the aspirin should be stopped temporarily until the enzyme concentrations return to normal.[399] Treatment may be reinstituted cautiously at that time at a lower dose than can often be gradually increased in many children without recurrence of the transaminasemia.

A rare and apparently benign transient elevation of serum alkaline phosphatase has been noted in several children with JRA.[405] (Petty RE, unpublished observations.) This ab-

normality presumably does not result from hepatotoxicity, although it may be confused with it.

The potential association between Reye's syndrome and aspirin administration has been emphasized by recent data and in the United States by directives from the Centers for Disease Control.[406–411] Our current strategy for varicella exposure is as follows:

1. If the child has had varicella, there is no need to stop salicylates if the child has been exposed to the disease.
2. If the child has had only casual contact with varicella, we stop salicylates if pox occur.
3. If the child has household, day care, or equivalent intimate contact with varicella, we stop salicylates until the disease occurs or until the incubation period (approximately 21 days) is over.
4. We will vaccinate children with JRA for varicella as soon as that vaccine is released for general use.

Our influenza strategy is as follows:

1. Since influenza is difficult to identify clinically, we stop salicylates in any child with vomiting or diarrhea until GI symptoms have ceased.
2. We vaccinate all children with JRA for the current recommended strains of influenza as an added precaution but emphasize that such vaccination should not give rise to a false sense of security since immunity is not guaranteed.

ANALGESIC NEPHRITIS

The relation between indiscriminate use of certain analgesics for long periods and nephritis was first reported more than three decades ago.[412] Interstitial nephritis and renal papillary necrosis were the two most characteristic lesions. The most common association was with phenacetin plus aspirin. The evidence for renal toxicity of aspirin used alone is insufficient to alter our opinion that it is a drug of choice in the treatment of children with JRA (Ch. 3).

A few children with JRA may seemingly develop signs of analgesic nephropathy when taking aspirin alone.[413,414] In one study, three children with JRA developed papillary necrosis while receiving long-term, high-dose aspirin therapy (Table 5-33).[413] Common characteristics of these children included severe disabling disease and dependency on others for aid in using the toilet and in drinking fluids. Chronic mild dehydration, inactivity, and poor urine output may have contributed to the eventual development of renal disease. A second study documented renal papillary necrosis in five children with JRA by intravenous pye-

Table 5-33 Analgesic Nephritis and Renal Papillary Necrosis in Children with JRA

Reference	Age (Years)	Drugs
Wortman et al.[413]	12	Aspirin
	15	Aspirin, ibuprofen, tolmetin
	12	Aspirin, tolmetin, acetaminophen
Allen et al.[414]	15	Aspirin, indomethacin, tolmetin, steroid, gold thiomalate
	4	Aspirin
	15	Aspirin, steroid, gold thiomalate, hydroxychloroquine
	11	Aspirin, indomethacin
	12	Aspirin, tolmetin

lography.[414] Each had received a nonsteroidal anti-inflammatory drug (NSAID) or acetaminophen or two or more drugs in combination and developed recurrent episodes of microhematuria. Complications such as azotemia or hypertension did not occur, but the dose of NSAID had to be reduced or stopped. All of these children, in contrast to those in the previous report, had mild or no functional disability. It is estimated that this complication may occur in approximately 1 percent of children with JRA.

Other Analgesics

Although it is not an anti-inflammatory drug, acetaminophen given 2 to 3 times a day may be useful for control of pain or fever in the systemically ill child

with JRA. This drug should not be used for long-term basic management of the disease, since its safety from the viewpoint of interstitial nephritis has been questioned.

Other Nonsteroidal Anti-Inflammatory Drugs

Most of the newer NSAIDs have not been approved for use in children (Ch. 3).[415–418] When approved, they will be indicated for the control of pain, stiffness, and inflammation in selected children who have been unresponsive to salicylates or as initial treatment of the disease. Tolmetin, 30 mg/kg/day, has been shown to be effective as an anti-inflammatory drug in JRA.[419,420] Administration of this medication does not interfere with salicylate efficacy. Naproxen, 10 to 15 mg/kg/day, has also been widely used in treatment.[421–423]

Slow Acting Antirheumatic Drugs

The slow acting antirheumatic drugs consist of the antimalarials (hydroxychloroquine), the injectable and oral gold salts, D-penicillamine, and sulfasalazine (Tables 5-34 and 5-35).[428] Use of one or more of these agents is indicated for progressive polyarthritis that has been unresponsive to the NSAIDs. Hydroxychloroquine or a gold salt is often employed initially, added to the NSAID that the child is taking at that time. If hydroxychloroquine is used first, a gold salt can be added after 3 to 6 months if the clinical re-

Table 5-34 Drug Toxicity in Children with JRA Treated with Slow-Acting Antirheumatic Drugs

Toxicity	Antimalarial Drugs	Gold Salts	Penicillamine	Sulfasalazine
No. of patients	242	340	467	28
Toxicity (%)	24	41	23	37
Toxicity requiring drug discontinuation	7	21	9	10
Type of toxicity				
Bone marrow	10	35	16	23
Kidney	28	20	21	0
Skin	8	20	16	23
GI	3	–	20	31
Mouth	–	5	3	8
Miscellaneous	51	20	24	15

(Modified from Grondin et al.,[428] with permission.)

Table 5-35 Disease Outcome in Children with JRA Treated with Slow-Acting Antirheumatic Drugs

Drug (No. of Patients)	Improvement (%)	Remission (%)
Antimalarial drugs (242)	40	27
Gold (340)	47	16
Penicillamine (467)	64	2
Sulfasalazine (28)	61	4

(Modified from Grondin et al.,[428] with permission.)

sponse is not adequate. D-penicillamine or sulfasalazine may be used alone or in combination with a NSAID. None is contraindicated in the presence of a corticosteroid drug. Each of these agents has its own toxicity and improvement has varied in reported studies.

ANTIMALARIAL DRUGS

Hydroxychloroquine is a useful adjunctive agent for treatment of the older child with JRA (Tables 5-36 and 5-37).[424–428] The initial dose of hydroxychloroquine should be 6 to 7 mg/kg/day ($\geq$600 mg).[429] After approximately 8 weeks, most rheumatologists would reduce this dose to 5 mg/kg/day. An ophthal-

Table 5-36 Comparative Trials of Antimalarial Drugs in JRA

Series (Ref.)	Study Design	Other Drugs Used
1. Stillman[424]	Retrospective	
2. Kvien et al.[425]	Open, comparative, randomized	Penicillamine Gold salts
3. Manners et al.[426]	Retrospective	a. 4 treated during systemic phase b. 15 treated after systemic phase
4. Brewer et al.[427]	Prospective, randomized, double-blind, placebo	Penicillamine
5. Grondin et al.[428]	Retrospective	

(Modified from Grondin et al.,[428] with permission.)

Table 5-37 Comparative Trials of Antimalarial Drugs in JRA

Series	1	2	3a	3b	4	5
Patients (No.)	125	25	4	15	57	19
Male/female	—	10/15	—	—	—	5/14
Type of onset (No.)						
Polyarthritis	57	12	0	0	—	7
Oligoarthritis	52	13	0	0	—	9
Systemic disease	16	0	4	15	—	0
Dose (mg/kg/wk)	7.7	5	4–7	4–7	6	5–6
Duration of treatment						
Mean (yrs)	—	0.96	2.4	2.4	1.0	1.16
Range	0.06–5.3	—	—	—	—	0.17–2.33
Outcome						
Improvement (%)	32	20	75	47	74	16
Remission (%)	45	44	0	0	0	5
Toxicity						
Total (%)	15	8	0	7	61	11
Drug stopped (%)	10	0	0	7	4	0

(Modified from Grondin et al.,[428] with permission.)

mologic examination including testing of color vision and visual fields must be performed before therapy is started and every 4 to 6 months thereafter. Although retinal toxicity is rare at this dose level, hydroxychloroquine should be discontinued at the first suspicion of retinopathy because the effects of this drug are cumulative.[430] It is stored for long periods in the pigmented tissues of the body, and total duration of treatment with this agent should probably be limited. Stillman noted that 125 of 204 children followed in Boston were treated with antimalarial drugs.[424] Three children developed a nonprogressive retinopathy (macular pigmentation) that was attributable to these medications. Corneal deposition may also occur and is usually accepted as an indication for lowering the dose of the drug rather than discontinuing it. Hydroxychloroquine has not been officially approved for use in JRA. Acute toxicity due to ingestion of large doses of the drug may be fatal in the very young child, and there is no antidote for the respiratory suppression.

Hydroxychloroquine is useful as an adjunct to NSAIDs, is relatively nontoxic, and principally requires ophthalmologic examinations to monitor toxicity. Its therapeutic effect in JRA is usually subtle, rarely dramatic. If after treatment for 6 months no advantage to its use is demonstrated, it should be discontinued.

PARENTERAL GOLD SALTS

Parenteral administration of gold salts (gold sodium thiomalate and aurothioglucose) provides an effective slower acting therapeutic program for children with JRA.[431-440] Their use is indicated in children with polyarthritis who have been unresponsive to a conservative program of management for 6 months. The basic anti-inflammatory regimen with aspirin or other NSAIDs is continued during the administration of gold salts. Before gold salt therapy is started, it should be determined that the child's hematologic, renal, and hepatic functions are normal (complete blood count, urinalysis, creatinine clearance, and liver function tests). A test dose of approximately 5 mg should be given intramuscularly and weekly doses thereafter gradually increased to a level of approximately 0.75 mg to 1 mg/kg/week ($\leq$50 mg). If objective, satisfactory improvement or a remission is achieved in 6 months, therapy is main-

tained at the same dose level with injections every 2 weeks for approximately 3 months, then every 3 weeks for 3 months. If signs of improvement have continued during this interval, the child should continue to receive gold injections every 4 weeks thereafter, adjusted periodically on the basis of growth and body weight.

In general, serum gold concentration has not correlated with the clinical response. Levels were monitored in 66 children with JRA who were treated with gold sodium thiomalate.[440] These studies showed that the dose of gold salt should be approximately 0.7 mg/kg or 20 mg/M^2 to achieve a peak serum level of approximately 500 to 600 μg/dl. It was also concluded that the maximum single dose should never exceed 27 mg/M^2.

Before each administration of gold salt, the child should be assessed for any associated toxicity, for example, stomatitis, dermatitis, pruritis, depression of any of the elements of the blood, hematuria, or proteinuria. A decrease in the WBC count below 4,500/mm^3 (4.5×10^9 L), fall in the absolute neutrophil count by 50 percent, development of thrombocytopenia or eosinophilia, hematuria, or clinical symptoms or signs of gold toxicity are an indication for at least a temporary interruption of therapy. In selected cases, gold salt therapy may be cautiously resumed at a lower dose after the child's symptoms or signs of toxicity disappear. Contraindications to reinstitution are severe leukopenia or neutropenia, proteinuria, exfoliative dermatitis, significant oral ulceration, or consumptive coagulopathy.[215]

It is estimated that approximately 25 percent of children receiving gold salts develop serious toxicity and are unable to complete a course of treatment, 25 percent do not improve objectively while receiving the initial course of gold salts, and the remaining 50 percent experience substantial relief or complete remission and should continue receiving gold salts for a longer period. In our experience, the most common toxicities are hematuria and dermatitis.

We are reluctant to discontinue use of gold salts in children who have had a satisfactory response. There is no convincing evidence of long-term cumulative toxicity, at least in adult RA. Perhaps after many years of remission, the use of gold salts may be cautiously discontinued. Relapses, if they occur, are generally delayed by 3 to 4 months after cessation of therapy.

Table 5-38 Comparative Trials of Gold Salts in JRA

Series (Ref.)	Study Design	Other Drugs Used
1. Sairanen et al.[430,431]	Open, comparative	Sulfasalazine, chloroquine, phenylbutazone
2. Hicks et al.[433]	Retrospective	
3. Debendetti et al.[434]	Retrospective	
4. Levinson et al.[435]	Retrospective	
5. Brewer et al.[436]	Retrospective	
6. Ansell et al.[437]	Open, comparative, randomized	Penicillamine
7. Ansell et al.[438]	Open, comparative, randomized	Penicillamine
8. Kvien et al.[425,426]	Open, comparative, randomized	Penicillamine, antimalarials used previously
9. Manners et al.[426]	Retrospective	a. 24 treated during systemic phase b. 24 treated after systemic phase
10. Grondin et al.[428]	Retrospective	

(Modified from Grondin et al.,[428] with permission.)

Early reports of the efficacy of gold salt therapy in children with JRA include those of Sairanen,[431,432] Coss and Boots,[35] and Edstrøm[57] (Tables 5-38 and 5-39).[428] Debendetti et al. treated 14 children with JRA for an average of 143 weeks.[434] The total average dose of gold salt was 3.3 g; 6 patients showed improvement, 3 developed dermatitis, and 3 exhibited proteinuria. Ansell et al. found that 54 percent of 65 children with JRA showed improvement at the 1-year evaluation while receiving gold salt therapy.[437,438] A 50 percent reduction in the corticosteroid dose was possible in 17 children, and in 9 steroids were stopped entirely.

Levinson et al. conducted a trial of gold salt therapy in 44 children with JRA.[435] There was improvement in arthritis and systemic manifestations of the disease in 73 percent of the group; the other 27 percent were classified as therapeutic failures.

Brewer et al. reported a trial of 6 months of gold salt therapy in 51 children with JRA.[436] The dosage was 1 mg/kg/week for 20 weeks and then 1 mg/kg every 2 to 4 weeks for years. Of these children, 63 percent had a decrease in severity of the arthritis (Table 5-40).[435] In general, children who had the most favorable response had more severe joint

Table 5-39 Comparative Trials of Gold Salts in JRA

Series	1	2	3	4	5	6	7	8	9a	9b	10
Patients (No.)	54	40	14	52	63	10	24	39	24	24	28
Male/female	22/32	12/28	6/8	—	20/43	—	9/15	11/28	—	—	5/23
Type of onset (No.)											
Polyarthritis	—	—	5	—	20	10	—	17	—	—	20
Oligoarthritis	—	—	3	—	14	—	—	22	—	—	5
Systemic disease	—	30	6	—	29	—	—	0	24	24	3
Dose (mg/kg/wk)	—	1	1	1	—	—	—	0.7	—	—	1
Duration of treatment											
Mean (yrs)	—	1.75	2.75	—	0.5	—	—	0.96	1.8	3.8	1.95
Range	0.25–3.0	—	0.23–7.6	0.5–1.0	—	1.0–3.0	—	—	—	—	0.08–8.0
Outcome											
Improvement (%)	78	52	43	32	49	70	50	46	0	42	18
Remission (%)	4	18	57	41	0	10	13	13	8	0	29
Toxicity											
Total (%)	50	48	43	52	21	20	—	23	—	—	43
Drug stopped (%)	30	20	7	—	8	20	17	13	58	25	25

(Modified from Grondin et al.,[428] with permission.)

Table 5-64 Secondary Generalized Amyloidosis

Organ distribution
  Parenchymal tissues: liver, kidney, spleen, adrenal glands

Predisposing causes
  Inflammatory: juvenile rheumatoid arthritis, ankylosing spondylitis, Reiter's syndrome, psoriatic arthritis, dermatomyositis, scleroderma, systemic lupus erythematosus, Behçet's syndrome, inflammatory bowel diseases
  Infectious: tuberculosis, leprosy, paraplegia, bronchiectasis, osteomyelitis, chronically infected burns
  Neoplastic: Hodgkin's disease; lymphomas; hypernephroma; carcinomas of gastrointestinal tract, lungs, and urogenital tract; malignant melanoma

Table 5-65 Classification of Amyloidosis

Terminology	Clinical Features	Probable Origin
AL	Primary, myeloma	Light chains
AA	Secondary, FMF	SAA
AF	Familial	Transthyretin
AS	Senile, heart, brain	Transthyretin, gamma-trace
AE	Endocrine	Thyrocalcitonin
AD	Dermal	?

2. Amyloidosis secondary to another disease, such as JRA, familial Mediterranean fever, chronic suppurative pulmonary disease, or osteomyelitis (Table 5-64)

The first type of amyloid deposition is characterized principally by disease involving the skin and GI tract. The patient may present with macroglossia, carpal tunnel syndrome or arthritis, neuropathy, congestive heart failure or arrhythmia, malabsorption or GI tract bleeding. The onset of secondary amyloidosis is usually heralded by the appearance of proteinuria and nephrotic syndrome, diarrhea, hepatosplenomegaly, or unexplained anemia in a child with profound hypergammaglobulinemia (Fig. 5-76).

Although there is considerable overlap in the tissue distribution of the amyloid deposits from patient to patient, consideration of amyloidosis into primary and secondary forms has been strengthened by studies indicating that there are precise biochemical differences in the types of amyloid deposited (Table 5-65). Electron microscopic studies indicate that amyloid is not a homogeneous, undifferentiated material, but consists of fibrils that are thin, nonbranching,

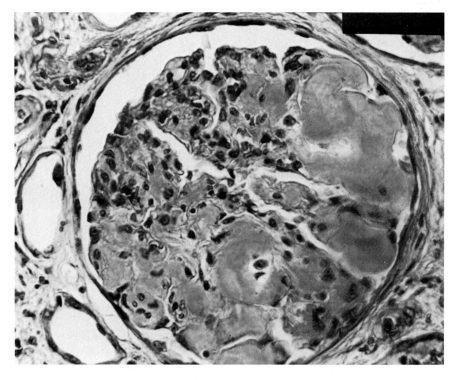

Fig. 5-78 Amyloid disease of the kidneys. The glomerular tufts are infiltrated with a homogeneous material birefringent with the Congo red stain.

and rigid. In primary amyloidosis, these fibrils assume a beta-pleated sheet configuration by x-ray diffraction. They consist of amino acid chains homologous with the NH_2-terminal end of the variable portion of light chains. In the case of adults who develop amyloidosis and multiple myeloma, the amyloid fibrils are homologous with the light chain type of the patient's myeloma protein. In these patients there is also a P component that consists of an alpha$_1$-glycoprotein that has been adsorbed onto the fibrils. It is assumed that an abnormal plasma cell clone in these patients secretes amyloidogenic light chains that circulate as polymers. These are phagocytized by mononuclear phagocytic cells and are degraded to peptides consisting of the variable region of the immunoglobulin light chain. Exocytosis occurs, and these amino acid chains aggregate as fibrils, assuming a beta-pleated sheet conformation.

In secondary amyloidosis, the major fibrillar protein is not homologous with light chains. Its amino acid sequence has been virtually identical in all patients studied. A circulating serum amyloid component (SAA) that cross-reacts immunologically with amyloid fibrils has been present in high concentrations in these patients. SAA may be the precursor to the fibrillar amyloid protein and behaves as an acute phase reactant, in part explaining the occurrence of amyloidosis as a complication of inflammatory diseases.[642] SAA circulates normally in small amounts and increases in acute inflammatory disease.

The diagnosis of amyloidosis is confirmed by biopsy (Fig. 5-78). The single most useful histologic technique is to examine tissue sections stained by Congo red dye for birefringence under a polarizing microscope. Congo red is a sensitive indicator of amyloid, and under the polarizing microscope the deposits assume a green color that is virtually pathognomonic of these fibrillar proteins.

FAMILIAL MEDITERRANEAN FEVER

Familial Mediterranean fever (FMF) is a periodic disease inherited as an autosomal recessive trait that is particularly frequent in Sephardic and Iraqi Jews, Armenians, and Levantine Arabs (Table 5-66).[643] Symptoms generally appear between the ages of 5 and 15 years but may begin earlier. Each exacerbation of FMF is characterized by fever, abdominal or pleuropericardial pain, arthritis, or cutaneous erythema about the ankles. An attack begins abruptly and lasts for up to 1 week before slowly subsiding.

Joint symptoms include arthralgias, recurrent oligoarthritis, and prolonged chronic arthritis.[644-646] Swelling and pain are prominent, erythema and increased heat are absent, and the knees are most commonly affected. Residual damage is not characteristic except in the hips, where secondary degenerative arthritis may develop. Radiographs show juxtaarticular osteoporosis and occasionally indicate sacroiliac involvement.

Table 5-66 Familial Mediterranean Fever

Autosomal recessive trait: Sephardic and Ashkenazi Jews, Armenians, Levantine Arabs, Turks, Greeks, Italians, Irish

Acute, self-limited febrile episodes with peritonitis, pleuritis, arthritis, and dermatitis

Onset in two-thirds <15 years

Generalized amyloidosis before age 40 years; deposits in renal glomeruli and blood vessels throughout body

Protein AA in deposits: fluctuating levels of SAA

Spontaneous remissions unknown

Effective prophylaxis for periodic attacks with colchicine; may influence favorably the course of the amyloidosis

Amyloidosis develops in many children with FMF and results in death from renal failure.[647,648] Like JRA, amyloidosis is uncommon in children with FMF in North America.

No form of treatment in FMF is universally successful. Analgesics, colchicine, and estrogens have all been tried. Colchicine has been reported to be effective in treating or aborting the acute, recurrent exacerbations of the disease and in preventing amyloidosis from developing.[649-652] The prognosis for FMF is good except for involvement of the kidneys from amyloidosis. Other forms of periodic disease have been described by Reimann.[653] Their relationship to FMF is unclear.

REFERENCES

1. Brewer EJ, Bass JC, Cassidy JT et al: Criteria for the classification of juvenile rheumatoid arthritis. Bull Rheum Dis 23:712, 1972
2. Brewer EJ, Bass J, Baum J et al: Current proposed revision of JRA criteria. Arthritis Rheum 20:195, 1977
3. Cassidy JT, Levinson JE, Bass JC et al: A study of classification criteria for a diagnosis of juvenile rheumatoid arthritis. Arthritis Rheum 29:274, 1986
4. Hanson V, Kornreich HK, Bernstein B et al: Three subtypes of juvenile rheumatoid arthritis (correlations of age at onset, sex, and serologic factors). Arthritis Rheum 20:184, 1977
5. Schaller JG: Juvenile rheumatoid arthritis. Series 1. Arthritis Rheum 20:165, 1977
6. Stillman JS, Barry PE: Juvenile rheumatoid arthritis. Series 2. Arthritis Rheum 20:171, 1977
7. Ansell BM: Juvenile chronic polyarthritis. Series 3. Arthritis Rheum 20:176, 1977
8. Fink CW: Patients with JRA. A clinical study. Arthritis Rheum 20:183, 1977
9. Allen RC, Ansell BM: Juvenile chronic arthritis—

clinical sub-groups with particular relationship to adult patterns of disease. Postgrad Med J 62:821, 1986

10. Bywaters EGL: Categorization in medicine. A survey of Still's disease. Ann Rheum Dis 26:185, 1967

11. Ansell BM, Bywaters EGL: Diagnosis of "probable" Still's disease and its outcome. Ann Rheum Dis 21:253, 1962

12. Bywaters EGL: Diagnostic criteria for Still's disease (juvenile RA). In Bennett PH, Wood PHN (eds): Population Studies of the Rheumatic Diseases. Excerpta Medica, Amsterdam, 1968, p. 235

13. European League against Rheumatism (EULAR) Bulletin 4. Nomenclature and Classification of Arthritis in Children. National Zeitung AG, Basel, 1977

14. Kvien TK, Høyeraal HM, Kåss E: Diagnostic criteria of rheumatoid arthritis in children. Scand J Rheumatol 11:187, 1982

15. Cornil MV: Mémoire sur les coincidences pathologiques du rhumatisme articulaire chronique. C R Mém Soc Biol (Paris) Series 4, 3:3, 1864

16. Diamantberger M-S: Du Rhumatisme Noueux (Polyarthrite Déformante) Chez Les Enfants. Lecrosnier et Babé, Paris, 1891. (Reprinted by Editions Louis Parente, Paris in 1988)

17. Still GF: On a form of chronic joint disease in children. Med Chir Trans 80:47, 1897. (Reprinted in Arch Dis Child 16:156, 1941)

18. Johannessen A: Om kronisk ledrheumatisme og arthritis deformans i barnealderen. Norsk Mag F Laegevidensk, 1899, p. 1417

19. Johannsen N: Ein Beitrag zur Kenntnis der Still'schen Krankheit. Acta Paediatr 2:354, 1922

20. Frøhlich T: Om Still's Sygdom. Nord Med Tidskr 1930, p. 337

21. Hajkis M: Om Still's Sygdom. Norsk Mag F Laegevidensk 97:173, 1936

22. Sundt H: Stillsche Krankheit mit Tuberkulose. Acta Orthop Scand 7:205, 1936

23. Ellermann V: Om Svulst af Kubitalglandlerne ved Polyarthroitis chronica rheumatica. Ugeskr Laeger 76:1938, 1914

24. Monrad S: Arthroitis multiplex chronica infantilis. Ugesk Laeger 81:1472, 1919

25. Bentzon K: The ultimate invalidism in a case of Still's disease. Acta Orthop Scand 1:340, 1930

26. Svendsgård E: Et Tilfaelde af Still's Sygdom. Ugesk Laeger 95:1073, 1933

27. Moltke O: Still's Sygdom hos Voksne. Acta Med Scand 80:427, 1933

28. Keiding KK: En Patient med Mobus Still. Ugeskr Laeger 105:911, 1943

29. Harving F: Multipel, kronisk, infektiøs Ledsygdom i barnealderen. Et atypisk Tilfaelde af Mobus Still. Nord Med 24:1821, 1944

30. Hirschsprung H: Multipel, kronisk, infektiøs Ledsygdom i Barnealderen. Hospitalstid 1901, p. 421

31. Ibrahim J: Die chronische Arthritis im Kindesalter. Z Orthop Chir 15:213, 1914

32. Atkinson FRB: Still's disease. Br J Child Dis 36:100, 1939

33. Colver T: The prognosis in rheumatoid arthritis in childhood. Arch Dis Child 12:253, 1937

34. Holzmüller G: Beitrag zur Frage der Pathogenese und Therapie der primär-chronischen Gelenkerkrankungen im Kindesalter. Z Rhemaforsch 5:57, 1942

35. Coss JA, Jr., Boots RH: Juvenile rheumatoid arthritis. A study of fifty-six cases with a note on skeletal changes. J Pediatr 29:143, 1946

36. Edstrøm G: Rheumatoid arthritis in children. Acta Paediatr 34:334, 1947

37. Bille BSV: Kronisk polyartrit hos barn och dess guldbehandling. Nord Med 37:307, 1948

38. Pickard NS: Rheumatoid arthritis in children. A clinical study. Arch Intern Med 80:771, 1947

39. Lockie LM, Norcross BM: Juvenile rheumatoid arthritis. Pediatrics 2:694, 1948

40. Wissler H: Der Rheumatismus im Kindesalter. Teil 2: Die chronishce Polyartritis des Kindes. Der Rheumatismus. Bd. 24. Steinkopff, Dresden und Leipzig, 1942, p. 152

41. Françon F: Conférences Cliniques De Rhumatologie Pratique. Paris, 1946, p. 386

42. Dawson MH: Rheumatoid arthritis in children (Still's disease). In Palmer WW (ed): Nelson Loose-Leaf Medicine. Vol. 5. T Nelson & Sons, New York, 1946, p. 626

43. Spitzy H: Ueber das Vorkommen multipier chronischer deformierende Glenkentzündungen im Kindesalter. Jahrb Kinderheilk 49:286, 1899

44. Chevallier P: La maladie de Chauffard-Still et les syndromes voisins. Rev Méd Paris 47:77, 1930

45. Sundt H: Om arthritis deformans i Barnealderen. Med Rev Bergen 38:145, 1921

46. Portis RB: Pathology of chronic arthritis of children (Still's disease). Am J Dis Child 55:1000, 1938

47. Sury B: Rheumatoid Arthritis in Children. A Clinical Study. Munksgaard, Copenhagen, 1952

48. Norcross BM: Juvenile rheumatoid arthritis. Minn Med 42:1760, 1959

49. Barkin RE: Clinical course of juvenile rheumatoid arthritis. Bull Rheum Dis 3:19, 1952

50. Sullivan DB, Cassidy JT, Petty RE: Pathogenic implications of age of onset in juvenile rheumatoid arthritis. Arthritis Rheum 18:251, 1975

51. Laaksonen A-L: A prognostic study of juvenile rheumatoid arthritis. Analysis of 544 cases. Acta Paediatr Scand suppl., 166:1, 1966

52. Kunnmo I, Kallio P, Pelkonen P: Incidence of arthritis

in urban Finnish children. Arthritis Rheum 29:1232, 1986

53. Towner SR, Michet CJ, Jr, O'Fallon WM et al: The epidemiology of juvenile arthritis in Rochester, Minnesota. Arthritis Rheum 26:1208, 1983

54. Gäre BA, Fasth A, Andersson J et al: Incidence and prevalence of juvenile chronic arthritis: a population survey. Ann Rheum Dis 46:277, 1987

55. Prieur A-M, Le Gall E, Karman F et al: Epidemiologic survey of juvenile chronic arthritis in France. Comparison of data obtained from two different regions. Clin Exp Rheumatol 5:217, 1987

56. Mikkelson WM, Dodge HJ, Duff IF et al: Clinical and serological estimates of the prevalence of rheumatoid arthritis in the population of Tecumseh, Michigan, 1959–60. In Kellgren J (ed): The Epidemiology of Chronic Rheumatism. FA Davis, Philadelphia, 1963, p. 239

57. Edstrøm G: Rheumatoid arthritis and Still's disease in children. A survey of 161 cases. Arthritis Rheum 1:497, 1958

58. Ansell BM: Heberden oration, 1977. Chronic arthritis in childhood. Ann Rheum Dis 37:107, 1978

59. Sairanen E: On rheumatoid arthritis in children. A clinicoroentgenological study. Acta Rheum Scand suppl., 2:1, 1958

60. Schlesinger BE, Forsyth CC, White RH et al: Observations on the clinical course and treatment of one hundred cases of Still's disease. Arch Dis Child 36:65, 1961

61. Grokoest AW, Synder AL, Schlaeger R: Juvenile Rheumatoid Arthritis. Little, Brown, Boston, 1962

62. Aaron S, Fraser PA, Jackson JM et al: Sex ratio and sibship size in juvenile rheumatoid arthritis kindreds. Arthritis Rheum 28:753, 1985

63. Cassidy JT, Sullivan DB, Petty RE: Clinical patterns of chronic iridocyclitis in children with juvenile rheumatoid arthritis. Arthritis Rheum 20:224, 1977

64. Chylack JT, Jr: The ocular manifestations of juvenile rheumatoid arthritis. Arthritis Rheum 20:217, 1977

65. Schaller J, Kupfer C, Wedgwood RJ: Iridocyclitis in juvenile rheumatoid arthritis. Pediatrics 44:92, 1969

66. Greenwood BM: Polyarthritis in Western Nigeria. II: Still's disease. Ann Rheum Dis 28:617, 1969

67. Hill RH: Juvenile arthritis in various racial groups in British Columbia. Arthritis Rheum 20:162, 1977

68. Haffejee IE, Raga J, Coorada HM: Juvenile chronic arthritis in black and Indian South African children. S Afr Med J 65:510, 1984

69. Chantler JK, Tingle AJ, Petty RE: Persistent rubella virus infection associated with chronic arthritis in children. N Engl J Med 313:1117, 1985

70. Schwarz TF, Rossendorf M, Suschke H et al: Human parvovirus B19 infection and juvenile chronic polyarthritis (letter). Infection 15:264, 1987

71. Henoch MJ, Batson JW, Baum J: Psychosocial factors in juvenile rheumatoid arthritis. Arthritis Rheum 21:229, 1978

72. Strelkauskas AJ, Callery RT, McDowell J et al: Direct evidence for loss of human suppressor cells during active autoimmune disease. Proc Natl Acad Sci USA 75:5150, 1978

73. Morimoto C, Reinherz EL, Borel Y et al: Autoantibody to an immunoregulatory inducer population in patients with juvenile rheumatoid arthritis. J Clin Invest 67:753, 1981

74. Barron KS, Lewis DE, Brewer EJ et al: Cytotoxic anti-T cell antibodies in children with juvenile rheumatoid arthritis. Arthritis Rheum 27:1272, 1984

75. Williams RC, Froelich CJ, Kilpatrick K et al: T cell subset specificity of lymphocyte reactive factors in juvenile rheumatoid arthritis and systemic lupus erythematosus sera. Arthritis Rheum 24:585, 1981

76. Oen K, Wilkins JA, Krzekotowska D: OKT4:OKT8 ratios of circulating T cells and in vitro suppressor cell function of patients with juvenile rheumatoid arthritis (JRA). J Rheumatol 12:321, 1985

77. Alpert SD, Turek PJ, Foung SK et al: Human monoclonal anti-T cell antibody from a patient with juvenile rheumatoid arthritis. J Immunol 138:104, 1987

78. Murata H, Yata J: Defect of suppressor cell induction in patients with juvenile rheumatoid arthritis. Asian Pac J Allerg Immunol 4:95, 1986

79. Thoen J, Förre O, Waalen K et al: Phenotypes of T lymphocytes from peripheral blood and synovial fluid of patients with rheumatoid arthritis and juvenile rheumatoid arthritis. Evidence in favour of normal helper and suppressor functions of T lymphocytes from patients with juvenile rheumatoid arthritis. Scand J Rheumatol 16:247, 1987

80. Abrahamsen TG, Frøland SS, Natvig JB et al: Lymphocytes eluted from synovial tissue of juvenile rheumatoid arthritis patients. Arthritis Rheum 20:772, 1977

81. Rosenberg AM, Hunt DWC, Petty RE: Antibodies to native type I collagen in childhood rheumatic diseases. J Rheumatol 11:421, 1984

82. Rosenberg AM, Hunt DWC, Petty RE: Antibodies to native and denatured type II collagen in children with rheumatic diseases. J Rheumatol 11:425, 1984

83. Petty RE, Hunt DWC, Rosenberg AM: Antibodies to type IV collagen in rheumatic diseases. J Rheumatol 13:246, 1986

84. Burgos-Vargas R, Howard A, Ansell BM: Antibodies to peptidoglycan in juvenile onset ankylosing spondylitis and pauciarticular onset juvenile arthritis as-

sociated with chronic iridocyclitis. J Rheumatol 13:760, 1986

85. Ilowite NT, Wedgwood RJ, Rose LM et al: Impaired in vivo and in vitro antibody responses to bacteriophage OX 174 in juvenile rheumatoid arthritis. J Rheumatol 14:957, 1987

86. Panush RS, Bianco NE, Schur PH et al: Juvenile rheumatoid arthritis. Cellular hypersensitivity and selective IgA deficiency. Clin Exp Immunol 10:103, 1972

87. Höyeraal HM: Impaired delayed hypersensitivity in juvenile rheumatoid arthritis. Ann Rheum Dis 32:331, 1973

88. Gershwin ME, Haselwood D, Dorshkind K et al: Altered responsiveness to mitogens in subgroups of patients with juvenile rheumatoid arthritis. J Clin Lab Immunol 1:293, 1979

89. Tsokos GC, Mavridis A, Inghirami G et al: Cellular immunity in patients with systemic juvenile rheumatoid arthritis. Clin Immunol Immunopathol 42:86, 1987

90. Ellsworth JE, Stein LD, Thebert PJ et al: Abnormalities of lymphokine generation in children with juvenile rheumatoid arthritis. Pediatric Res 16:221A, 1982

91. Oen K: Defects in pokeweed mitogen (PWM) induced immunoglobulin (Ig) synthesis by lymphocytes of patients with juvenile rheumatoid arthritis. J Rheumatol 12:728, 1985

92. Martini A, Ravelli A, Notarangelo LD et al: Enhanced interleukin 1 and depressed interleukin 2 production in juvenile arthritis. J Rheumatol 13:598, 1986

93. Mellbye OJ, Høyeraal HM, Frøland SS: C-reactive protein and delayed hypersensitivity in juvenile rheumatoid arthritis. Scand J Rheumatol 7:90, 1978

94. Rosenberg AM, Petty RE: Similar patterns of juvenile rheumatoid arthritis within families. Arthritis Rheum 23:951, 1980

95. Ansell BM, Bywaters EGL, Lawrence JS: A family study in Still's disease. Ann Rheum Dis 21:243, 1962

96. Baum J, Fink C: Juvenile rheumatoid arthritis in monozygotic twins: A case report and review of the literature. Arthritis Rheum 11:33, 1968

97. Kapusta MA, Metrakos JD, Pinsky L et al: Juvenile rheumatoid arthritis in a mother and her identical twin sons. Arthritis Rheum 12:411, 1967

98. Ansell BM, Bywaters EG, Lawrence JS: Familial aggregation and twin studies in Still's disease. Juvenile chronic polyarthritis. Rheumatology 2:37, 1969

99. Clemens LE, Albert E, Ansell BM: HLA studies in IgM rheumatoid factor positive arthritis of childhood. Ann Rheum Dis 42:431, 1983

100. Clemens LE, Albert E, Ansell BM: Sibling pairs affected by chronic arthritis of childhood: evidence for a genetic predisposition. J Rheumatol 12:108, 1985

101. Yodfat Y, Yossipovitch Z, Cohen I et al: A family with a high incidence of juvenile rheumatoid arthritis. Ann Rheum Dis 31:92, 1972

102. Cekovský L, Pavkovćekova O, Veréb J et al: Juveniéna reumatoidna artritida u troch susodencov. Čs Pediatr 33:400, 1978

103. Delgado EA, Petty RE, Malleson PN et al: Aortic valve insufficiency and coronary artery narrowing in a child with polyarticular juvenile rheumatoid arthritis. J Rheumatol 15:144, 1988

104. Rossen RD, Brewer EJ, Sharp RM et al: Familial rheumatoid arthritis. Linkage of HLA to disease susceptibility locus in four families where the proband presented with juvenile rheumatoid arthritis. J Clin Invest 65:629, 1980

105. Hall A, Ansell BM, James DCO et al: HL-A antigens in juvenile chronic polyarthritis (Still's disease). Ann Rheum Dis, suppl., 34:36, 1975

106. Gershwin ME, Opelz G, Tersaki PL et al: Frequency of HLA-Dw3 in juvenile rheumatoid arthritis. Tissue Antigens 10:330, 1977

107. Stastny P, Fink CW: Different HLA-D associations in adult and juvenile rheumatoid arthritis. J Clin Invest 63:124, 1979

108. Glass D, Litvin DA, Wallace K et al: Early-onset pauciarticular juvenile arthritis associated with HLA-DRw5, iritis and antinuclear antibody. J Clin Invest 66:426, 1980

109. Suciu-Foca N, Godfrey M, Jacobs J et al: Increased frequency of DRw5 in pauciarticular juvenile rheumatoid arthritis. In Terasaki P (ed): Histocompatibility Testing 1980. University of California Press, Los Angeles, 1980, p. 953

110. Glass DN, Litvin DA: Heterogeneity of HLA associations in systemic onset juvenile rheumatoid arthritis. Arthritis Rheum 23:796, 1980

111. Morling N, Hellensen C, Jakobsen BK et al: HLA-A, B, C, D, DR antigens and primed lymphocyte typing (PLT) defined DP-antigens in JCA. Tissue Antigens 17:434, 1981

112. Førre Ø, Dobloug JH, Høyeraal HM et al: HLA antigens in juvenile arthritis. Genetic basis for the different subtypes. Arthritis Rheum 26:35, 1983

113. Ansell BM, Albert ED: Juvenile chronic arthritis, pauciarticular type. Histocompatibility Testing, 1984:368, 1984

114. Moore TL, Oldfather JW, Osborn TG et al: HLA antigens in black and white patients with juvenile arthritis: associations with rheumatoid factor, hidden rheumatoid factor, antinuclear antibodies and immune complex levels. J Rheumatol 11:188, 1984

115. Nepom BS, Nepom GT, Mickelson E et al: Specific HLA-DR4 associated histocompatibility molecules characterize patients with seropositive juvenile rheumatoid arthritis. J Clin Invest 74:287, 1984

116. Howard JF, Sigsbee A, Glass DN: HLA genetics and inherited predisposition to JRA. J Rheumatol 12:7, 1985

117. Morling N, Friis J, Heilmann C et al: HLA antigen frequencies in juvenile chronic arthritis. Scand J Rheumatol 14:209, 1985

118. Sher MR, Schultz JS, Ragsdale CG et al: HLA-DR and MT associations with the clinical and serologic manifestations of pauciarticular onset juvenile rheumatoid arthritis. J Rheumatol 12:114, 1985

119. Miller ML, Aaron S, Jackson J et al: HLA gene frequencies in children and adults with systemic onset juvenile rheumatoid arthritis. Arthritis Rheum 28:146, 1985

120. Brautbar C, Mukamel M, Yaron M et al: Immunogenetics of juvenile chronic arthritis in Israel. J Rheumatol 13:1072, 1986

121. Manners PJ, Dakins RL, McCluskey J et al: An immunogenetic study of juvenile chronic arthritis. Aust Paediatr J 22:317, 1986

122. Hall PJ, Burman SJ, Laurent MR et al: Genetic susceptibility to early onset pauciarticular juvenile chronic arthritis: a study of HLA and complement markers in 158 British patients. Ann Rheum Dis 45:464, 1986

123. Hoffman RW, Shaw S, Francis LC et al: HLA-DP antigens in patients with pauciarticular juvenile rheumatoid arthritis. Arthritis Rheum 29:1057, 1986

124. Nepom BS, Palmer J, Kim SJ et al: Specific genomic markers for the HLA-DQ subregion discriminate between DR4+ insulin-dependent diabetes mellitus and DR4+ seropositive juvenile rheumatoid arthritis. J Exp Med 164:345, 1986

125. Stastny P: HLA and the role of T cells in the predisposition to disease. Rheum Dis Clin North Am 13:1, 1987

126. Oen K, Petty RE, Schroeder M-L: An association between HLA-A2 and juvenile rheumatoid arthritis in girls. J Rheumatol 9:916, 1982

127. Odum N, Morling N, Friis J et al: Increased frequency of HLA-DPw2 in pauciarticular onset juvenile chronic arthritis. Tissue Antigens 28:245, 1986

128. Rachelefsky GS, Terasaki PI, Katz R et al: Increased prevalence of W27 in juvenile rheumatoid arthritis. N Engl J Med 290:892, 1974

129. Edmonds J, Morris RI, Metzger AL et al: Follow-up study of juvenile chronic polyarthritis with particular reference to histocompatibility antigen W27. Ann Rheum Dis 33:289, 1974

130. Woodrow JL, Mapsone R, Anderson J et al: HL-A27 and anterior uveitis. Tissue Antigens 6:116, 1975

131. Gibson DJ, Carpenter CB, Stillman JS et al: Re-examination of histocompatibility antigens found in patients with juvenile rheumatoid arthritis. N Engl J Med 293:636, 1975

132. Schaller JG, Ochs HD, Thomas ED et al: Histocompatibility antigens in childhood-onset arthritis. J Pediatr 88:926, 1976

133. Ohno S, Char DH, Kimura SJ et al: HLA antigens and antinuclear antibody titres in juvenile chronic iridocyclitis. Br J Ophthalmol 61:59, 1977

134. Arnett FC, Bias WB, Stevens MB: Juvenile-onset chronic arthritis. Am J Med 69:369, 1980

135. Friis J, Morling N, Pederson FK et al: HLA-B27 in juvenile chronic arthritis. J Rheumatol 12:1, 1985

136. Laaksonen A-L, Laine V: A comparative study of joint pain in adult and juvenile rheumatoid arthritis. Ann Rheum Dis 20:386, 1961

137. Scott PJ, Ansell BM, Huskisson EC: Measurement of pain in juvenile chronic polyarthritis. Ann Rheum Dis 36:186, 1977

138. Varni JW, Thompson KL, Hanson V: The Varni/Thompson Pediatric Pain Questionnaire. I: Chronic musculoskeletal pain in juvenile rheumatoid arthritis. Pain 28:27, 1987

139. Thompson KL, Varni JW, Hanson V: Comprehensive assessment of pain in juvenile rheumatoid arthritis: an empirical model. J Pediatr Psychol 12:241, 1987

140. Varni JW, Wilcox KT, Hanson V et al: Chronic musculoskeletal pain and functional status in juvenile rheumatoid arthritis: an empirical model. Pain 32:1, 1988

141. Martis CS, Karakasis DT: Ankylosis of the temporomandibular joint caused by Still's disease. Oral Surg 35:462, 1973

142. Blasberg B, Lowe AA, Petty RE et al: Temporomandibular joint disease in children with juvenile rheumatoid arthritis. Arthritis Rheum 30:S27, 1987

143. Jacobs JC, Hui RM: Cricoarytenoid arthritis and airway obstruction in juvenile rheumatoid arthritis. Pediatrics 59:292, 1977

144. Malleson P, Riding K, Petty R: Stridor due to cricoarytenoid arthritis in pauciarticular onset juvenile rheumatoid arthritis. J Rheumatol 13:952, 1986

145. Grancher M: Du rhumatisme cervical chez l'enfant. Bull Med (Paris) 2:283, 1988

146. Barkin RE, Stillman JS, Potter TA: The spondylitis of juvenile rheumatoid arthritis. N Engl J Med 253:1107, 1955

147. Ziff M, Contreras V, McEwen C: Spondylitis in post-

pubertal patients with rheumatoid arthritis of juvenile onset. Ann Rheum Dis 15:40, 1956

148. Rombouts JJ, Rombouts-Lindemans C: Scoliosis in juvenile rheumatoid arthritis. J Bone Joint Surg 56B:478, 1974

149. Ross AC, Edgar MA, Swann M et al: Scoliosis in juvenile chronic arthritis. J Bone Joint Surg 69B:175, 1987

150. Baldassare AR, Auclair RJ, Carls GL et al: Dissecting popliteal cyst in a child with juvenile rheumatoid arthritis. J Rheumatol 4:186, 1977

151. Bamzai A, Krieger M, Kretschmer RR: Synovial cysts in juvenile rheumatoid arthritis. Ann Rheum Dis 37:101, 1978

152. Rennebohm RM, Towbin RB, Crowe WE et al: Popliteal cysts in juvenile rheumatoid arthritis. AJR 140:123, 1983

153. Moore AT, Morin JD: Bilateral acquired inflammatory Brown's syndrome. J Pediatr 106:617, 1985

154. Kaufman LD, Sibony PA, Anand AK et al: Superior oblique tenosynovitis (Brown's syndrome) as a manifestation of adult Still's disease. J Rheumatol 14:625, 1987

155. Ansell BM, Bywaters EGL: Finger contractures due to tendon lesions as a mode of presentation of rheumatoid arthritis. Ann Rheum Dis 12:283, 1953

156. Ansell BM: Joint manifestations in children with juvenile chronic polyarthritis. Arthritis Rheum 20:204, 1977

157. Cassidy JT, Brody GL, Martel W: Monarticular juvenile rheumatoid arthritis. J Pediatr 70:867, 1967

158. Bywaters EGL, Ansell BM: Monoarticular arthritis in children. Ann Rheum Dis 24:116, 1965

159. Schaller J, Wedgwood RJ: Pauciarticular juvenile rheumatoid arthritis. Arthritis Rheum 12:330, 1969

160. McMinn FJ, Bywaters EGL: Differences between the fever of Still's disease and that of rheumatic fever. Ann Rheum Dis 18:293, 1959

161. Calabro JJ, Marchesano JM: Fever associated with juvenile rheumatoid arthritis. N Engl J Med 276:11, 1967

162. Brewer EJ: A comparative evaluation of indomethacin, acetaminophen and placebo as antipyretic agents in children. Arthritis Rheum 11:645, 1968

163. Isdale IC, Bywaters EGL: The rash of rheumatoid arthritis and Still's disease. Q J Med 25:377, 1956

164. Calabro JJ, Marchesano JM: Rash associated with juvenile rheumatoid arthritis. J Pediatr 72:611, 1968

165. Schaller J, Wedgwood RJ: Pruritus associated with the rash of juvenile rheumatoid arthritis. Pediatrics 45:296, 1970

166. Sury B, Vesterdal E: Extra-articular lesions in juvenile rheumatoid arthritis. A survey based upon a study of 151 cases. Acta Rheumatol Scand 14:309, 1968

167. Ansell BM, Bywaters EGL: Growth in Still's disease. Ann Rheum Dis 15:295, 1956

168. Bernstein BH, Stobie D, Singsen BH et al: Growth retardation in juvenile rheumatoid arthritis (JRA). Arthritis Rheum 20:212, 1977

169. Blodgett FM, Burgin L, Iezzoni D et al: Effects of prolonged cortisone therapy on statural growth, skeletal maturation and metabolic status of children. N Engl J Med 254:636, 1956

170. Ward DJ, Hartog M, Ansell BM: Corticosteroid-induced dwarfism in Still's disease treated with human growth hormone. Clinical and metabolic effects including hydroxyproline excretion in two cases. Ann Rheum Dis 25:416, 1966

171. Sturge RA, Beardwell C, Hartog M et al: Cortisol and growth hormone secretion in relation to linear growth: patients with Still's disease on different therapeutic regimens. Br Med J 3:547, 1970

172. Laaksonen A-L, Sunell JE, Westeren H et al: Adrenocortical function in children with juvenile rheumatoid arthritis and other connective tissue disorders. Scand J Rheumatol 3:137, 1974

173. Butenandt O: Rheumatoid arthritis and growth retardation in children: treatment with human growth hormone. Eur J Pediatr 130:15, 1979

174. Sairanen E: On the etiology of growth disturbance of the mandible in juvenile rheumatoid arthritis. Acta Rheumatol Scand 16:136, 1970

175. Björk A, Skieller V: Contrasting mandibular growth and facial development in long face syndrome, juvenile rheumatoid polyarthritis, and mandibulofacial dysostosis. J Craniofac Genet Dev Biol 1:127, 1985

176. Ganik R, Williams FA: Diagnosis and management of juvenile rheumatoid arthritis with TMJ involvement. Cranio 4:254, 1986

177. Stabrun AE: Mandibular morphology and position in juvenile rheumatoid arthritis. A study on postero-anterior radiographs. Eur J Orthod 7:288, 1985

178. Stabrun AE, Larheim TA, Rvsler M et al: Impaired mandibular function and its possible effect on mandibular growth in juvenile rheumatoid arthritis. Eur J Orthod 9:43, 1987

179. Ogus H: Rheumatoid arthritis of the temporomandibular joint. Br J Oral Surg 12:275, 1975

180. Martel W, Holt JF, Cassidy JT: Roentgenologic manifestations of juvenile rheumatoid arthritis. Am J Roentgenol 88:400, 1962

181. Poznanski AK, Hernandez RJ, Guire KE et al: Carpal length in children—a useful measurement in the diagnosis of rheumatoid arthritis and some congenital malformation syndromes. Radiology 129:661, 1978

182. Bünger C, Bülow J, Tøndevold E et al: Microcirculation of the juvenile knee in chronic arthritis. Clin Orthop 204:294, 1986

183. Vostrejs M, Hollister JR: Muscle atrophy and leg length discrepancies in pauciarticular juvenile rheumatoid arthritis. Am J Dis Child 142:343, 1988

184. Woerman AL, Bender-Macleod SA: Leg length discrepancy assessment: accuracy and precision of five clinical methods of evaluation. J Orthop Sports Phys Ther 5:230, 1984

185. Simon S, Whiffen J, Shapiro F: Leg-length discrepancies in monarticular and pauciarticular juvenile rheumatoid arthritis. J Bone Joint Surg 63A:209, 1981

186. Rydholm U, Brattström H, Bylander B et al: Stapling of the knee in juvenile chronic arthritis. J Pediatr Orthop 7:63, 1987

187. Bywaters EGL, Glynn LE, Zeldis A: Subcutaneous nodules of Still's disease. Ann Rheum Dis 17:278, 1958

188. Bywaters EGL, Cardoe N: Multiple nodules in juvenile chronic polyarthritis. Ann Rheum Dis 31:421, 1972

189. Kaye BR, Kaye RL, Bobrove A: Rheumatoid nodules. Review of the spectrum of associated conditions and proposal of a new classification, with a report of four seronegative cases. Am J Med 76:279, 1984

190. Martel W, Cassidy JT, Brody GL et al: Spinal cord lesions in juvenile rheumatoid arthritis. J Can Assoc Radiol 20:32, 1969

191. Lietman PS, Bywaters EGL: Pericarditis in juvenile rheumatoid arthritis. Pediatrics 32:855, 1963

192. Bernstein B, Takahashi M, Hanson V: Cardiac involvement in juvenile rheumatoid arthritis. J Pediatr 85:313, 1974

193. Brewer E, Jr: Juvenile rheumatoid arthritis-cardiac involvement. Arthritis Rheum 20:231, 1977

194. Bernstein B: Pericarditis in juvenile rheumatoid arthritis. Arthritis Rheum 20:241, 1977

195. Svantesson H, Bjorkhem G, Elbough R: Cardiac involvement in juvenile rheumatoid arthritis. A follow-up study. Acta Paediatr Scand 72:345, 1983

196. Scharf J, Levy J, Benderly A et al: Pericardial tamponade in juvenile rheumatoid arthritis. Arthritis Rheum 19:760, 1976

197. Majeed HA, Kvasnicka J: Juvenile rheumatoid arthritis with cardiac tamponade. Ann Rheum Dis 37:273, 1978

198. Yancey CL, Doughty RA, Cohlan BA et al: Pericarditis and cardiac tampanade in juvenile rheumatoid arthritis. Pediatrics 68:369, 1981

199. Miller JJ, III, French JW: Myocarditis in juvenile rheumatoid arthritis. Am J Dis Child 131:205, 1977

200. Miller JJ, III: Carditis in juvenile rheumatoid arthritis. Arthritis Rheum 20:243, 1977

201. Calabro JJ: Myocarditis in juvenile rheumatoid arthritis (letter). Am J Dis Child 131:1306, 1977

202. Leak AM, Millar-Craig MW, Ansell BM: Aortic regurgitation in seropositive juvenile arthritis. Ann Rheum Dis 40:229, 1981

203. Kramer PH, Imboden JB, Waldman FM et al: Severe aortic insufficiency in juvenile chronic arthritis. Am J Med 74:1088, 1983

204. Hull RG, Hall MA, Prasad AN: Aortic incompetence in pauciarticular juvenile chronic arthritis. Arch Dis Child 61:409, 1986

205. Brinkman GL, Chaikof L: Rheumatoid lung disease. Report of a case which developed in childhood. Am Rev Respir Dis 80:732, 1959

206. Jordan JD, Snyder CH: Rheumatoid disease of the lung and cor pulmonale. Observations in a child. Am J Dis Child 108:174, 1964

207. Lovell D, Lindsley C, Langston C: Lymphoid interstitial pneumonia in juvenile rheumatoid arthritis. J Pediatr 105:947, 1984

208. Athreya B, Doughty RA, Bookspan M et al: Pulmonary manifestations of juvenile rheumatoid arthritis: a report of eight cases and review. Clin Chest Med 1:361, 1980

209. Wagener JS, Taussig LM, Debenedetti C et al: Pulmonary function in juvenile rheumatoid arthritis. J Pediatr 99:108, 1981

210. Toomey K, Hepburn B: Felty syndrome in juvenile arthritis. J Pediatr 106:254, 1985

211. Schaller J, Beckwith B, Wedgwood RJ: Hepatic involvement in juvenile rheumatoid arthritis. J Pediatr 77:203, 1970

212. Boone JE: Hepatic disease and mortality in juvenile rheumatoid arthritis. Arthritis Rheum 20:257, 1977

213. Hadchouel M, Prieur A-M, Griscelli C: Acute hemorrhagic, hepatic, and neurologic manifestations in juvenile rheumatoid arthritis: possible relationship to drugs or infection. J Pediatr 106:561, 1985

214. Silverman ED, Miller JJ, Bernstein B et al: Consumptive coagulopathy associated with systemic juvenile rheumatoid arthritis. J Pediatr 103:872, 1983

215. Jacobs JC, Gorin LJ, Hanissian AS et al: Consumption coagulopathy after gold therapy for JRA. J Pediatr 105:674, 1984

216. Scott JP, Gerber P, Maryjowski MC et al: Evidence for intravascular coagulation in systemic onset, but not polyarticular, juvenile arthritis. Arthritis Rheum 28:256, 1985

217. Bhettay E, Thomson AJ: Peritonitis in juvenile chronic arthritis. A report of 2 cases. S Afr Med J 68:605, 1985

218. Russell AS: Cerebral complications in juvenile rheumatoid arthritis. Can Med Assoc J 108:19, 1973

219. Lang H, Anttila R, Svkus A et al: EEG findings in juvenile rheumatoid arthritis and other connective tissue diseases in children. Acta Paediatr Scand 63:373, 1974

220. Brown GL, Wilson WP: Salicylate intoxication and the CNS. With special reference to EEG findings. Dis Nerv Syst 32:135, 1971

221. Sievers K, Nissil M, Sievers UM: Cerebral vasculitis visualized by angiography in juvenile rheumatoid arthritis simulating brain tumor. Acta Rheumatol Scand 14:222, 1968

222. Jan JE, Hill RH, Low MD: Cerebral complications in juvenile rheumatoid arthritis. Can Med Assoc J 107:623, 1972

223. Calabro JJ: Other extraarticular manifestations of juvenile rheumatoid arthritis. Arthritis Rheum 20:237, 1977

224. von Kemp K, Dehaen F, Huybrechts M et al: Hematuria as presenting sign in Wissler-Fanconi syndrome. J Rheumatol 14:145, 1987

225. Stapleton FB, Hanissian AS, Miller LA: Hypercalciuria in children with juvenile rheumatoid arthritis: association with hematuria. J Pediatr 107:235, 1985

226. Dodge WF, West EE, Smith EH et al: Proteinuria and hematuria in school children: epidemiology and early natural history. J Pediatr 88:327, 1976

227. Anttila R, Laaksonen A-L: Renal disease in juvenile rheumatoid arthritis. Acta Rheumatol Scand 15:99, 1969

228. Anttila R: Renal involvement in juvenile rheumatoid arthritis. A clinical and histopathological study. Acta Paediatr Scand, suppl., 227:3, 1972

229. Cullen B, Mongey AB, Molony J: Juvenile chronic arthritis associated with systemic vasculitis. Ir Med J 79:72, 1986

230. Hall S, Nelson AM: Takayasu's arteritis and juvenile rheumatoid arthritis. J Rheumatol 13:431, 1986

231. Forsyth CC: Calcification of the digital arteries in a child with rheumatoid arthritis. Arch Dis Child 35:296, 1960

232. Reid MM, Fannin TF: Extensive vascular calcification in association with juvenile rheumatoid arthritis and amyloidosis. Arch Dis Child 43:607, 1968

233. Bywaters EGL: Pathologic aspects of juvenile chronic polyarthritis. Arthritis Rheum 20:271, 1977

234. Wynne-Roberts CR, Anderson C: Light- and electron-microscopic studies of normal juvenile human synovium. Semin Arthritis Rheum 7:279, 1978

235. Wynne-Roberts CR, Anderson C, Turano AM et al: Light- and electron-microscopic findings of juvenile rheumatoid arthritis synovium. Comparison with normal juvenile synovium. Semin Arthritis Rheum 7:287, 1978

236. Fletcher MR, Scott JT: Chronic monarticular synovitis. Diagnostic and prognostic features. Ann Rheum Dis 34:171, 1975

237. Berg E, Wainwright R, Barton B et al: On the nature of rheumatoid rice bodies. An immunologic, histochemical, and electron microscope study. Arthritis Rheum 20:1343, 1977

238. Wynne-Roberts CR, Cassidy JT: Juvenile rheumatoid arthritis with rice bodies: light and electron microscopic studies. Ann Rheum Dis 38:8, 1979

239. Bennett GA, Zeller JW, Bauer W: Subcutaneous nodules of rheumatoid arthritis and rheumatic fever. A pathologic study. Arch Pathol 30:70, 1970

240. Brewer EJ, Jr: Pitfalls in the diagnosis of juvenile rheumatoid arthritis. Pediatr Clin North Am 33:1015, 1986

241. Cassidy JT: Miscellaneous conditions associated with arthritis in children. Pediatr Clin North Am 33:1033, 1986

242. Fink CW, Dick VQ, Howard J, Jr et al: Infections of bones and joints in children. Arthritis Rheum 20:578, 1977

243. Kornreich HK, Bernstein BH, Key KK et al: The rheumatic presentation of osteomyelitis. Arthritis Rheum 22:631, 1979

244. Jacobs JC, Phillips PE, Johnston AD: Needle biopsy of the synovium of children. Pediatrics 57:696, 1976

245. Konttinen YT, Bergroth V, Kunnamo I et al: The value of biopsy in patients with monarticular juvenile rheumatoid arthritis of recent onset. Arthritis Rheum 29:47, 1986

246. Southwood TR, Hancock EJ, Petty RE et al: Tuberculous rheumatism (Poncet's disease) in a child. Arthritis Rheum 31:1311, 1988

247. Steere AC, Gabofsky A, Hardin JA et al: Lyme arthritis: immunologic and immunogenetic markers. Arthritis Rheum 22:662, 1979

248. Schned ES: Epidemiology of juvenile arthritis in Rochester, Minnesota (letter). Arthritis Rheum 28:239, 1985

249. Rush PJ, Shore A, Wilmot D et al: Discoid meniscus presenting as juvenile rheumatoid arthritis. J Rheumatol 13:1173, 1986

250. Cooperman DR, Emery H, Keller C: Factors relating to hip joint arthritis following three childhood diseases—juvenile rheumatoid arthritis, Perthes disease, and postreduction avascular necrosis in congenital hip dislocation. J Pediatr Orthop 6:706, 1986

251. Robinson RP, Franck WA, Carey EJ et al: Familial polyarticular osteochondritis dissecans masquerading

as juvenile rheumatoid arthritis. J Rheumatol 5:190, 1978

252. Hellström B: The diagnosis and course of rheumatoid arthritis and benign aseptic arthritis in children. Acta Paediatr Scand 50:529, 1961

253. Jacobs BW: Synovitis of the hip in children and its significance. Pediatrics 47:558, 1971

254. Schaller J: Arthritis as a presenting manifestation of malignancy in children. J Pediatr 81:793, 1972

255. Fink CW, Windmiller J, Sartain P: Arthritis as the presenting feature of childhood leukemia. Arthritis Rheum 15:347, 1972

256. Weinberg AG, Currarino G: Sickle cell dactylitis: histopathologic observations. Am J Clin Pathol 58:518, 1972

257. Gedalia A, Person DA, Brewer EJ, Jr et al: Hypermobility of the joints in juvenile episodic arthritis/ arthralgia. J Pediatr 107:873, 1985

258. Jacobs JC, Downey JA: Juvenile rheumatoid arthritis. In Downey JA, Low NL (eds): The Child with Disabling Illness, WB Saunders, Philadelphia, 1974, p. 5

259. Athreya BH, Schumacher HR: Pathologic features of a familial arthropathy associated with congenital flexion contractures of fingers. Arthritis Rheum 21:429, 1978

260. Balestrazzi P, Ferraccioli GF, Ambanelli U et al: Juvenile rheumatoid arthritis in Turner's syndrome. Clin Exp Rheumatol 4:61, 1986

261. Sauter SVH, Utsinger PD: Viral arthritis. Clin Rheum Dis 4:225, 1978

262. Thompson GR, Weiss JJ, Shillis JL et al: Intermittent arthritis following rubella vaccination. A three year follow-up. Am J Dis Child 125:526, 1973

263. Sievers K, Ahvonen P, Aho K et al: Serological patterns in juvenile rheumatoid arthritis. Rheumatism 19:88, 1963

264. Singsen BH, Bernstein BH, Kornreich HK et al: Mixed connective tissue disease in childhood. J Pediatr 90:893, 1977

265. Peskett SA, Ansell BM, Fizzman P et al: Mixed connective tissue disease in children. Rheumatol Rehabil 17:245, 1978

266. Rosenthal M: Sharp-syndrome (mixed connective tissue disease) bei kindren. Helv Paediatr Acta 33:251, 1978

267. Jackson J, Anderson L, Schur PH et al: Sjögren's syndrome in juvenile rheumatoid arthritis (JRA). Arthritis Rheum 16:122, 1973

268. McLaughlin WS: Sjögren's syndrome and juvenile rheumatoid arthritis. Proc Br Soc Dent Maxillofac Radiol 1:17, 1986

269. Ragsdale CG, Petty RE, Cassidy JT et al: The clinical progression of apparent juvenile rheumatoid arthritis to systemic lupus erythematosus. J Rheumatol 7:50, 1980

270. Ansell BM, Bywaters EGL, Elderkin FM: Familial arthropathy with rash, uveitis and mental retardation. Proc R Soc Med 68:584, 1975

271. Prieur A-M, Griscelli C: Arthropathy with rash, chronic meningitis, eye lesions, and mental retardation. J Pediatr 99:79, 1981

272. Pina-Neto JM, Moreno AF, Silva LR et al: Cherubism, gingival fibromatosis, epilepsy, and mental deficiency (Ramon syndrome) with juvenile rheumatoid arthritis. Am J Med Genet 25:433, 1986

273. Martini A, Ravelli A, Viola S et al: Systemic lupus erythematosus with Jaccoud's arthropathy mimicking juvenile rheumatoid arthritis. Arthritis Rheum 30:1062, 1987

274. Cassidy JT, Walker SE, Soderstrom SJ et al: Diagnostic significance of antibody to native deoxyribonucleic acid in children with juvenile rheumatoid arthritis and connective tissue diseases. J Pediatr 93:416, 1978

275. Ladd JR, Cassidy JT, Martel W: Juvenile ankylosing spondylitis. Arthritis Rheum 14:579, 1971

276. Lindsley CB, Schaller JG: Arthritis associated with inflammatory bowel disease in children. J Pediatr 84:16, 1974

277. Passo M, Brandt K, Fitzgerald J: Arthritis associated with inflammatory bowel disease in children: relationship between arthritis and activity of the inflammatory bowel disease (abstract). Arthritis Rheum 22:645, 1979

278. Shore A, Ansell BM: Juvenile psoriatic arthritis—an analysis of 60 cases. J Pediatr 100:529, 1982

279. Petty RE, Cassidy JT, Tubergen DG: Association of arthritis with hypogammaglobulinemia. Arthritis Rheum 20:441, 1977

280. Cassidy JT, Petty RE, Sullivan DB: Occurrence of selective IgA deficiency in children with juvenile rheumatoid arthritis. Arthritis Rheum 20:181, 1977

281. Glass D, Raum D, Gibson D et al: Inherited deficiency of the second component of complement. J Clin Invest 58:853, 1976

282. Harvey AR, Pippard MJ, Ansell BM: Microcytic anaemia in juvenile chronic arthritis. Scand J Rheumatol 16:53, 1987

283. Prouse PJ, Harvey AR, Bonner B et al: Anaemia in juvenile chronic arthritis: serum inhibition of normal erythropoiesis in vitro. Ann Rheum Dis 46:127, 1987

284. Rubin RN, Walker BK, Ballas SK et al: Erythroid aplasia in juvenile rheumatoid arthritis. Am J Dis Child 132:760, 1978

285. Heaton DC, Moller PW: Still's disease associated with

Coxsackie infection and haemophagocytic syndrome. Ann Rheum Dis 44:341, 1985

286. Morris JA, Adamson AR, Holt PJ et al: Still's disease and the virus-associated haemophagocytic syndrome. Ann Rheum Dis 44:349, 1985

287. Prieur A-M, Fischer A, Griscelli C: Still's disease and haemophagocytic syndrome. Ann Rheum Dis 44:806, 1985

288. Koerper MA, Stempel DA, Dallman PR: Anemia in patients with juvenile rheumatoid arthritis. J Pediatr 92:930, 1978

289. Craft AW, Eastham EJ, Bell JI et al: Serum ferritin in juvenile chronic polyarthritis. Ann Rheum Dis 36:271, 1977

290. Pelkonen P, Swanljung K, Siimes MA: Ferritinemia as an indicator of systemic disease activity in children with systemic juvenile rheumatoid arthritis. Acta Paediatr Scand 75:64, 1986

291. Sherry DD, Kredich DW: Transient thrombocytopenia in systemic onset juvenile rheumatoid arthritis. Pediatrics 76:600, 1985

292. Petty RE, Cassidy JT, Sullivan DB: Serologic studies in juvenile rheumatoid arthritis. A review. Arthritis Rheum 20:260, 1977

293. Hussein A, Stein J, Ehrich JH: C-reactive protein in the assessment of disease activity in juvenile rheumatoid arthritis and juvenile spondyloarthritis. Scand J Rheumatol 16:101, 1987

294. Gianinni EH, Brewer EJ: Poor correlation between the erythrocyte sedimentation rate and clinical activity in juvenile rheumatoid arthritis. Clin Rheumatol 6:197, 1987

295. Höyeraal HM, Mellbye OJ: Humoral immunity in juvenile rheumatoid arthritis. Ann Rheum Dis 33:248, 1974

296. Houba V, Bardfeld R: Serum immunoglobulins in juvenile rheumatoid arthritis. Ann Rheum Dis 27:55, 1968

297. Salmi TT, Schmidt E, Laaksonen A-L et al: Levels of serum immunoglobulins in juvenile rheumatoid arthritis. Ann Clin Res 5:395, 1973

298. Goel KM, Logan RW, Barnard WP et al: Serum immunoglobulin and beta 1C-beta 1A globulin concentrations. Ann Rheum Dis 33:35, 1974

299. Cassidy JT: Clinical correlations of serum immunoglobulin concentrations in juvenile chronic arthritis. In Munthe E (ed): The Care of Rheumatic Children. EULAR, Basle, 1978, p. 141

300. Cassidy CT, Petty RE, Sullivan DB: Abnormalities in the distribution of serum immunoglobulin concentrations in juvenile rheumatoid arthritis. J Clin Invest 52:1931, 1973

301. Gutowska-Grzegorczyk G, Baum J: Serum immu-noglobulin and complement interrelationships in juvenile rheumatoid arthritis. J Rheumatol 4:179, 1977

302. Gutowska-Grzegorczyk G, Baum J: Antibody levels to enteric bacteria in juvenile rheumatoid arthritis. Arthritis Rheum 20:779, 1977

303. Hall PJ, de Lange GG, Ansell BM: Immunoglobulin allotypes in families with pauciarticular-onset juvenile chronic arthritis. Tissue Antigens 25:212, 1985

304. Ogra PL, Chiba Y, Ogra SS et al: Rubella-virus infection in juvenile rheumatoid arthritis. Lance 1:1157, 1975

305. Cassidy JT, Shillis JL, Brandon FB et al: Viral antibody titers to rubella and rubeola in juvenile rheumatoid arthritis. Pediatrics 54:239, 1974

306. Linnemann CC, Jr, Levinson JE, Buncher CR et al: Rubella antibody levels in juvenile rheumatoid arthritis. Ann Rheum Dis 34:354, 1975

307. Schnitzer TJ, Ansell BM, Hawkins GT et al: Significance of rubella virus infection in juvenile chronic polyarthritis. Ann Rheum Dis 36:468, 1977

308. Bywaters EGL, Carter ME, Scott FET: Differential agglutination titre (D.A.T.) in juvenile rheumatoid arthritis. Ann Rheum Dis 18:225, 1959

309. Bywaters EGL, Carter ME, Scott FET: Comparison of differential agglutination titre (D.A.T.) in juvenile and adult rheumatoid arthritis. Ann Rheum Dis 18:233, 1959

310. Toumbis A, Franklin EC, McEwen C et al: Clinical and serologic observations in patients with juvenile rheumatoid arthritis and their relatives. J Pediatr 62:463, 1963

311. Cassidy JT, Valkenburg HA: A five year prospective study of rheumatoid factor tests in juvenile rheumatoid arthritis. Arthritis Rheum 10:83, 1967

312. Hanson V, Drexler E, Kornreich H: The relationship of rheumatoid factor to age of onset in juvenile rheumatoid arthritis. Arthritis Rheum 12:82, 1969

313. Bluestone R, Goldberg LS, Katz RM et al: Juvenile rheumatoid arthritis: a serologic survey of 200 consecutive patients. J Pediatr 77:98, 1970

314. Bianco NE, Panush RS, Stillman JS et al: Immunologic studies of juvenile rheumatoid arthritis. Arthritis Rheum 14:685, 1971

315. Rudnicki RD, Ruderman M, Scull E et al: Clinical features and serologic abnomalities in juvenile rheumatoid arthritis. Arthritis Rheum 17:1007, 1974

316. Eichenfield AH, Athreya BH, Doughty RA et al: Utility of rheumatoid factor in the diagnosis of juvenile rheumatoid arthritis. Pediatrics 78:480, 1986

317. Prieur A-M, Bach JF, Griscelli C et al: Rheumatoid rosette in juvenile rheumatoid arthritis. Arch Dis Child 49:438, 1974

318. Torrigiani G, Ansell BM, Chown EEA et al: Raised

IgG antiglobulin factors in Still's disease. Ann Rheum Dis 28:424, 1969

319. Florin-Christensen A, Arana RM, Morteo OG et al: IgG, IgA, IgM, and IgD antiglobulins in juvenile rheumatoid arthritis. Ann Rheum Dis 33:32, 1974

320. Schur PH, Bianco NE, Panush RS: Antigammaglobulins in normal individuals and in patients with adult and juvenile rheumatoid arthritis and osteoarthritis. Rheumatology 6:156, 1975

321. Miller JJ, III, Olds-Arroyo L, Akasaka T: Antiglobulins in juvenile rheumatoid arthritis. Arthritis Rheum 20:729, 1977

322. Schlump U, Howard A, Ansell BM: IgG-anti-IgG antibodies in juvenile chronic arthritis. Scand J Rheumatol 14:65, 1985

323. Moore T, Dorner RW, Zuckner J: Hidden rheumatoid factor in seronegative juvenile rheumatoid arthritis. Ann Rheum Dis 33:255, 1974

324. Moore TL, Dorner RW: 19S IgM Forssman-type heterophile antibodies in juvenile rheumatoid arthritis. Arthritis Rheum 23:1262, 1980

325. Emancipator K, Moore TL, Dorner RW et al: Hidden and classical 19S IgM rheumatoid factor in a juvenile rheumatoid arthritis patient. J Rheumatol 12:372, 1985

326. Speiser JC, Moore TL, Weiss TD et al: Hidden 19S IgM rheumatoid factor in adults with juvenile rheumatoid arthritis onset. Ann Rheum Dis 44:294, 1985

327. Moore TL, Osborn TG, Dorner RW: 19S IgM rheumatoid factor-7S IgG rheumatoid factor immune complexes isolated in sera of patients with juvenile rheumatoid arthritis. Pediatr Res 20:977, 1986

328. Moore TL, Dorner RW: Separation and characterization of complement-fixing immune complexes in juvenile rheumatoid arthritis patients. Rheumatol Int 6:49, 1986

329. Moore TL, El-Najdawi E, Dorner RW: IgM rheumatoid factor plaque-forming cells in juvenile rheumatoid arthritis. Arthritis Rheum 30:335, 1987

330. Massaam J, Ferjencik P, Tempels M et al: A new method for the detection of hidden IgM rheumatoid factor in patients with juvenile rheumatoid arthritis. J Rheumatol 14:964, 1987

331. Munthe E: Anti-IgG and antinuclear antibodies in juvenile rheumatoid arthritis. Scand J Rheumatol 1:161, 1972

332. Haynes DC, Gershwin ME, Robbins DL et al: Autoantibody profiles in juvenile arthritis. J Rheumatol 13:358, 1986

333. Petty RE, Cassidy JT, Sullivan DB: Clinical correlates of antinuclear antibodies in juvenile rheumatoid arthritis. J Pediatr 83:386, 1973

334. Schaller JG, Johnson GD, Holborow EJ et al: The association of antinuclear antibodies with the chronic iridocyclitis of juvenile rheumatoid arthritis (Still's disease). Arthritis Rheum 17:409, 1974

335. Miller JJ, Henrich VL, Brandstrup NE: Sex difference in incidence of antinuclear factors in juvenile rheumatoid arthritis. Pediatrics 38:916, 1966

336. Alspaugh MA, Miller JJ: A study of specificities of antinuclear antibodies in juvenile rheumatoid arthritis. J Pediatr 90:391, 1977

337. Permin H, Hørbov S, Wiik A et al: Antinuclear antibodies in juvenile chronic arthritis. Acta Paediatr Scand 67:181, 1978

338. Patel NJ, Osborn TG, Moore TL et al: Antinuclear antibodies in juvenile arthritis using the HEp-2 cell substrate. Arthritis Rheum 26:S57, 1983

339. Rosenberg AM, Cordeiro DM, Knaus RP: Studies on the specificity of antinuclear antibodies in juvenile rheumatoid arthritis. Arthritis Rheum 26:S57, 1983

340. McCune WJ, Wise PT, Cassidy JT: A comparison of antibody tests in children with juvenile rheumatoid arthritis on HEp-2 cell and mouse liver substrates. J Rheumatol 13:980, 1986

341. Kornreich HK, Drexler E, Hanson V: Antinuclear factors in childhood rheumatic diseases. J Pediatr 69:1039, 1966

342. Osborne TG, Moore TL: Speckled pattern antinuclear antibodies in juvenile rheumatoid arthritis. Arthritis Rheum 28:S56, 1985

343. Leak AM, Ansell BM, Burman SJ: Antinuclear antibody studies in juvenile chronic arthritis. Arch Dis Child 61:168, 1986

344. Malleson PN, Fung M, Petty RE: Antigenic heterogeneity of antinuclear antibodies (ANA) in juvenile rheumatoid arthritis (JRA) determined by immunoblotting (I-B). Arthritis Rheum 30:S126, 1987

345. Rosenberg JN, Johnson GD, Holborow EJ et al: Eosinophil-specific and other granulocyte-specific antinuclear antibodies in juvenile chronic polyarthritis and adult rheumatoid arthritis. Ann Rheum Dis 34:350, 1975

346. Høyeraal HM: Granulocyte reactive antinuclear factors in juvenile rheumatoid arthritis. Scand J Rheumatol 5:84, 1976

347. Høyeraal HM, Mellbye OJ: High levels of serum complement factors in juvenile rheumatoid arthritis. Ann Rheum Dis 33:243, 1974

348. Rossen RD, Brewer EJ, Person DA et al: Circulating immune complexes and antinuclear antibodies in juvenile rheumatoid arthritis. Arthritis Rheum 20:1485, 1977

349. Moran H, Ansell BM, Mowbray JF et al: Antigen-

antibody complexes in the serum of patients with JCA. Arch Dis Child 54:120, 1979

350. Miller JJ, III, Osborne CL, Hsu Y-P: C1q binding in serum in juvenile rheumatoid arthritis. J Rheumatol 7:665, 1980

351. Moore TL, Dorner RW: Separation and characterization of complement-fixing immune complexes in juvenile rheumatoid arthritis patients. Rheumatol Int 6:49, 1986

352. Sbarbaro JA, Bennett RM: Aspirin hepatotoxicity and disseminated intravascular coagulation. Ann Intern Med 86:183, 1977

353. Miller JJ, III, Hsu Y-P, Moss R et al: The immunologic and clinical associations of the split products of C3 in plasma in juvenile rheumatoid arthritis. Arthritis Rheum 22:502, 1979

354. Miller JJ, III, Olds LC, Silverman ED et al: Different patterns of C3 and C4 activation in the varied types of juvenile arthritis. Pediatr Res 20:1332, 1986

355. Miller JJ, III, Olds LC, Huene DB: Complement activation products and factors influencing phagocyte migration in synovial fluids from children with chronic arthritis. Clin Exp Rheumatol 4:53, 1986

356. Rynes RI, Ruddy S, Spragg J et al: Intraarticular activation of the complement system in patients with juvenile rheumatoid arthritis. Arthritis Rheum 19:161, 1976

357. Zuckner J, Baldassare A, Chang F et al: High synovial fluid leukocyte counts of noninfectious etiology. Arthritis Rheum 20:270, 1977

358. Baldassare AR, Chang F, Zuckner J: Markedly raised synovial fluid leucocyte counts not associated with infectious arthritis in children. Ann Rheum Dis 37:404, 1978

359. Hedberg H: The total complement activity of synovial fluid in juvenile forms of arthritis. Acta Rheumatol Scand 17:279, 1971

360. Mollnes TE, Paus A: Complement activation in synovial fluid and tissue from patients with juvenile rheumatoid arthritis. Arthritis Rheum 29:1359, 1986

361. Panush RS, Biancho NE, Schur PH: Serum and synovial fluid IgG, IgA and IgM anti-gamma globulins in rheumatoid arthritis. Arthritis Rheum 14:737, 1971

362. Munthe E: Complexes of IgG and IgG rheumatoid factor in synovial tissues of juvenile rheumatoid arthritis. Scand J Rheumatol 1:153, 1972

363. Martin CL, Pachman LM: Synovial fluid in seronegative juvenile rheumatoid arthritis: Studies of immunoglobulins, complement, and α2-macroglobulin. Arthritis Rheum 23:1256, 1980

364. Egeskjold EM, Høyeraal HM, Permin H et al: Immunoglobulins, anti-IgG antibodies and antinuclear antibodies in paired serum and synovial fluid samples. A comparison between juvenile and adult rheumatoid arthritis. Scand J Rheumatol 14:51, 1985

365. Cassidy JT, Martel W: Juvenile rheumatoid arthritis: clinicoradiologic correlations. Arthritis Rheum 20:207, 1977

366. Ansell BM, Kent PA: Radiological changes in juvenile chronic polyarthritis. Skeletal Radiol 1:129, 1977

367. Pettersson H, Rydholm U: Radiologic classification of joint destruction in juvenile chronic arthritis. Acta Radiol 26:719, 1985

368. Bernstein B, Forrester D, Singsen B et al: Hip joint restoration in juvenile rheumatoid arthritis. Arthritis Rheum 20:1099, 1977

369. Badley BWD, Ansell BM: Fractures in Still's disease. Ann Rheum Dis 19:135, 1960

370. Cassidy JT: Juvenile rheumatoid arthritis. In Kelly WN, Harris ED, Jr, Ruddy S, Sledge CB (eds): Textbook of Rheumatology, WB Saunders, Philadelphia, 1989, p. 1289

371. Brattström M, Sundberg J: Juvenile rheumatoid gonarthritis. I: Clinical and roentgenological study. Acta Rheumatol Scand 11:266, 1965

372. Sundberg J, Brattström M: Juvenile rheumatoid gonarthritis. II. Disturbance of ossification and growth. Acta Rheumatol Scand 11:279, 1965

373. Williams RA, Ansell BM: Radiological findings in seropositive juvenile chronic arthritis (juvenile rheumatoid arthritis) with particular reference to progression. Ann Rheum Dis 44:685, 1985

374. Hensinger RN, DeVito PD, Ragsdale CG: Changes in the cervical spine in juvenile rheumatoid arthritis. J Bone Joint Surg 68A:189, 1986

375. Locke GR, Gardner JI, Van Epps EF: Atlas-dens interval (ADI) in children. A survey based on 200 normal cervical spines. Am J Roentgenol 97:135, 1966

376. Varonos S, Ansell BM, Reeve J: Vertebral collapse in juvenile chronic arthritis: its relationship with glucocorticoid therapy. Calcif Tissue Int 41:75, 1987

377. Hall MA, Burgos Vargos R, Ansell BM: Sacroiliitis in juvenile chronic arthritis. A 10-year follow-up. Clin Exp Rheumatol 1:S65, 1987

378. Poznanski AK, Conway JJ, Shkolnik A et al: Radiological approaches in the evaluation of joint disease in children. Rheum Dis Clin North Am 13:57, 1987

379. Yulish BS, Lieberman JM, Newman AJ et al: Juvenile rheumatoid arthritis: assessment with MR imaging. Radiology 165:149, 1987

380. Shuler SE, Helvie WW: Peripheral joint imaging in juvenile rheumatoid arthritis. South Med J 67:789, 1974

381. Gomez E, Green FA, Hays MT: New techniques for identification of synovitis and evaluation of joint disease. Bull Rheum Dis 25:786, 1974

382. Weiss TE, Schuler SE: Joint imaging as a clinical aid in diagnosis and therapy of arthritic and related diseases. Bull Rheum Dis 25:791, 1974

383. Rydholm U, Wingstrand H, Egund N et al: Sonography, arthroscopy, and intracapsular pressure in juvenile chronic arthritis of the hip. Acta Orthop Scand 57:295, 1986

384. Viitanen S-M, Laaksonen A-L: Thermography in juvenile rheumatoid arthritis. Acta Rheumatol Scand 16:91, 1970

385. Ansell BM: Treatment of juvenile chronic arthritis. Clin Rheum Dis 1:443, 1975

386. Levinson JE: The ideal program for juvenile arthritis. Arthritis Rheum 20:607, 1977

387. Brewer EJ, Giannini EH, Person DA: Juvenile Rheumatoid Arthritis. 2nd Ed. WB Saunders, Philadelphia, 1982

388. Orozco-Alcala JJ, Baum J: Treatment of juvenile rheumatoid arthritis—a world survey. J Rheumatol 1:187, 1974

389. Hobbs N, Perrin JM (eds): Issues in the Care of Children with Chronic Illness. A Source Book on Problems, Services, and Policies. Jossey-Bass, San Francisco, 1985

390. Hobbs N, Perrin JM, Ireys HT: Chronically Ill Children and Their Families. Problems, Prospects, and Proposals From the Vanderbilt Study. Jossey-Bass, San Francisco, 1985

391. Hollister JR: Aspirin in juvenile rheumatoid arthritis (editorial). Am J Dis Child 139:866, 1985

392. Pachman LM, Olufs R, Procknal JA et al: Pharmacokinetic monitoring of salicylate therapy in children with juvenile rheumatoid arthritis. Arthritis Rheum 22:826, 1979

393. Poe TE, Mutchie KD, Saunders GH et al: Total and free salicylate concentrations in juvenile rheumatoid arthritis. J Rheumatol 7:717, 1980

394. Kvien TK, Olsson B, Høyeraal HM: Acetylsalicylic acid and juvenile rheumatoid arthritis. Effect of dosage interval on the serum salicylic acid level. Acta Paediatr Scand 74:755, 1985

395. Weaver AL, Sullivan RE, Kramer WS: Iatrogenic tooth erosions in juvenile rheumatoid arthritis patients. Clin Res 30:810A, 1982

396. Tanchyk AP: Prevention of tooth erosion from salicylate therapy in juvenile rheumatoid arthritis. Gen Dent 34:479, 1986

397. Kornreich H, Malouf NN, Hanson V: Acute hepatic dysfunction in juvenile rheumatoid arthritis. J Pediatr 79:27, 1971

398. Rich RR, Johnson JS: Salicylate hepatotoxicity in patients with juvenile rheumatoid arthritis. Arthritis Rheum 16:1, 1973

399. Athreya BH, Moser G, Cecil HS et al: Aspirin-induced hepatotoxicity in juvenile rheumatoid arthritis. A prospective study. Arthritis Rheum 18:347, 1975

400. Zucker P, Daum F, Cohen MI: Aspirin hepatitis. Am J Dis Child 129:1433, 1975

401. Miller JJ, III, Weissman DB: Correlations between transaminase concentrations and serum salicylate concentration in juvenile rheumatoid arthritis. Arthritis Rheum 19:115, 1976

402. Rachelefsky GS, Kar NC, Coulson A et al: Serum enzyme abnormalities in juvenile rheumatoid arthritis. Pediatrics 58:730, 1976

403. Bernstein BH, Singsen BH, King KK et al: Aspirin-induced hepatotoxicity and its effect on juvenile rheumatoid arthritis. Am J Dis Child 131:659, 1977

404. Schaller JG: Chronic salicylate administration in juvenile rheumatoid arthritis. Aspirin "hepatitis" and its clinical significance. Pediatrics 62:916, 1978

405. Jacobs JC: JRA and hyperphosphatasemia (letter). J Pediatr 107:828, 1985

406. Ulshen MH, Grabd RJ, Crain JD et al: Hepatotoxicity with encephalopathy associated with aspirin therapy in rheumatoid arthritis. J Pediatr 93:1034, 1978

407. Rennebohm RM, Heubi JE, Daugherty CC et al: Reye's syndrome in children receiving salicylate therapy for connective tissue disease. J Pediatr 107:877, 1985

408. Remington PL, Shabino CL, McGee H et al: Reye syndrome and juvenile rheumatoid arthritis in Michigan. Am J Dis Child 139:870, 1985

409. Kauffman RE, Roberts RJ: Aspirin use and Reye syndrome. Pediatrics 74:1049, 1987

410. Arrowsmith JB, Kennedy DL, Kuritsky JN et al: National patterns of aspirin use and Reye syndrome reporting, United States 1980–1985. Pediatrics 79:858, 1987

411. Hurwitz ES, Barrett MJ, Bregman D et al: Public Health Service study on Reye's syndrome and medications. JAMA 257:1905, 1987

412. Spuehler O, Zollinger HU: Die chronisch-interstitielle nephritis. Z Klin Med 151:1, 1953

413. Wortmann DW, Kelsch RC, Kuhns L et al: Renal papillary necrosis in juvenile rheumatoid arthritis. J Pediatr 97:37, 1980

414. Allen RC, Petty RE, Lirenman DS et al: Renal papillary necrosis in children with chronic arthritis. J Pediatr 140:16, 1986

415. Brewer EJ, Jr, Arroyo I: Use of nonsteroidal anti-inflammatory drugs in children. Pediatr Ann 15:575, 1986

416. Pediatric Rheumatology Collaborative Study Group: Methodology and studies of children with juvenile rheumatoid arthritis. J Rheumatol 9:107, 1982

417. Lovell DJ, Giannini EH, Brewer EJ, Jr: Time course of response to nonsteroidal antiinflammatory drugs in juvenile rheumatoid arthritis. Arthritis Rheum 27:1433, 1984

418. Barron KS, Person DA, Brewer EJ: The toxicity of nonsteroidal antiinflammatory drugs in juvenile rheumatoid arthritis. J Rheumatol 9:149, 1982

419. Levinson JE, Baum J, Brewer E, Jr et al: Comparison of tolmetin sodium and aspirin in the treatment of juvenile rheumatoid arthritis. J Pediatr 91:799, 1977

420. Gewanter HL, Baum J: The use of tolmetin sodium in systemic onset juvenile rheumatoid arthritis. Arthritis Rheum 24:1316, 1981

421. Mäkelä A-I: Naproxen in the treatment of JRA. Scand J Rheumatol 6:193, 1977

422. Moran H, Hanna DB, Ansell BM et al: Naproxen in juvenile chronic polyarthritis. Ann Rheum Dis 38:152, 1979

423. Nicholls A, Hazelman B, Todd RM et al: Long-term evaluation of naproxen suspension in juvenile chronic arthritis. Curr Med Res Opin 8:204, 1982

424. Stillman JS: Antimalarials in the treatment of juvenile rheumatoid arthritis. In Moore TD (ed): Arthritis in Childhood, Ross Laboratories, Columbus, Ohio, 1981, p. 125

425. Kvien TK, Høyeraal HM, Sandstad B: Slow acting antirheumatic drugs in patients with juvenile rheumatoid arthritis—evaluated in a randomized, parallel 50-week clinical trial. J Rheumatol 12:533, 1985

426. Manners PJ, Ansell BM: Slow-acting antirheumatic drug use in systemic onset juvenile chronic arthritis. Pediatrics 77:99, 1986

427. Brewer EJ, Giannini EH, Kuzmina H et al: Penicillamine and hydroxychloroquine in the treatment of severe juvenile rheumatoid arthritis: results of the U.S.A.—U.S.S.R., double-blind placebo–controlled trial. N Engl J Med 314:1269, 1986

428. Grondin C, Malleson P, Petty RE: Slow acting antirheumatic drugs in chronic arthritis of childhood. Semin Arthritis Rheum 18:38, 1988

429. Laaksonen A-L, Koskiahde V, Juva K: Dosage of antimalarial drugs for children with juvenile rheumatoid arthritis and systemic lupus erythematosus. A clinical study with determination of serum concentrations of chloroquine and hydroxychloroquine. Scand J Rheumatol 3:103, 1974

430. Sassaman FW, Cassidy JT, Alpern M et al: Electroretinography in patients with connective tissue diseases treated with hydroxychloroquine. Am J Ophthalmol 70:515, 1970

431. Sairanen E, Laaksonen A-L: The toxicity of gold therapy in children suffering from rheumatoid arthritis. Ann Paediatr Fenn 8:105, 1962

432. Sairanen E, Laaksonen A-L: The results of gold therapy in juvenile rheumatoid arthritis. Ann Paediatr Fenn 10:274, 1963

433. Hicks RM, Hanson V, Kornreich HK: The use of gold in the treatment of juvenile rheumatoid arthritis. Arthritis Rheum 13:323, 1970

434. Debenedetti C, Tretbar H, Corrigan JJ: Gold therapy in juvenile rheumatoid arthritis. Ariz Med 33:373, 1976

435. Levinson JE, Balz GP, Bondi S: Gold therapy. Arthritis Rheum 20:531, 1977

436. Brewer EJ, Jr, Giannini EH, Barkley E: Gold therapy in the management of juvenile rheumatoid arthritis. Arthritis Rheum 23:404, 1980

437. Ansell BM, Hall MA, Ribero S: A comparative study of gold and penicillamine in seropositive juvenile chronic arthritis (juvenile rheumatoid arthritis). Ann Rheum Dis 40:522, 1981

438. Ansell BM, Hall MA: Penicillamine in chronic arthritis of childhood. J Rheumatol 7:112, 1981

439. Kvien TK, Høyeraal HM, Sandstad B: Gold sodium thiomalate and D-penicillamine. A controlled, comparative study in patients with pauciarticular and polyarticular juvenile rheumatoid arthritis. Scand J Rheumatol 14:346, 1985

440. Mäkelä A-L, Peltola O, Mäkelä P: Gold serum levels in children with juvenile rheumatoid arthritis. Scand J Rheumatol 7:161, 1978

441. Brewer EJ, Jr, Giannini EH, Person DA: Early experiences with auranofin in juvenile rheumatoid arthritis. Am J Med 75:152, 1983

442. Giannini EH, Brewer EJ, Person DA: Auranofin in the treatment of juvenile rheumatoid arthritis. J Pediatr 102:138, 1983

443. Giannini EH, Brewer EJ, Person DA et al: Long-term auranofin therapy in patients with juvenile rheumatoid arthritis. J Rheumatol 13:768, 1986

444. Brewer EJ, Giannini EH: Oral gold (auranofin) in juvenile rheumatoid arthritis—results of the double-blind, placebo controlled trial. Arthritis Rheum 30:S31, 1987

445. Kvien TL, Høyeraal HM, Sandstad B et al: Auranofin therapy in juvenile rheumatoid arthritis: a 48-week phase II study. Scand J Rheumatol 63:79, 1986

446. Schairer H, Stoeber E: Long-term follow-up of 235 cases of juvenile rheumatoid arthritis treated with D-penicillamine. In Munthe E (ed): Penicillamine Research in Rheumatoid Disease. Fabricius and Sonner Publisher Oslo, 1977, p. 279

447. Ansell BM, Simpson C: The effect of penicillamine

on growth and height of juvenile chronic polyarthritis. Proc R Soc Med 70:suppl. 3, 123, 1977

448. Prieur A-M, Piussan C, Manigne P et al: Evaluation of D-penicillamine in juvenile chronic arthritis. A double-blind, multicenter study. Arthritis Rheum 28:376, 1985

449. Wooley PH, Griffin J, Panayi GS: HLA-DR antigens and toxic reaction to sodium aurothiomalate and D-penicillamine in patients with rheumatoid arthritis. N Engl J Med 303:300, 1980

450. Cassidy JT: Treatment of children with juvenile rheumatoid arthritis (editorial). N Engl J Med 314:1312, 1986

451. Ozdogan H, Turunc M, Deringöl B et al: Sulphasalazine in the treatment of juvenile rheumatoid arthritis: a preliminary open trial. J Rheumatol 13:124, 1986

452. Miller JJ: Prolonged use of large intravenous steroid pulses in the rheumatic diseases of children. Pediatrics 65:989, 1980

453. Ansell BM, Bywaters EGL, Isdale IC: Comparison of cortisone and aspirin in the treatment of juvenile rheumatoid arthritis. Br Med J 1:1075, 1956

454. Good RA, Vernier RL, Smith RT: Serious untoward reactions to therapy with cortisone and A.C.T.H. in pediatric practice. Pediatrics 19:95, 1957

455. Lindbjerg IF: Juvenile rheumatoid arthritis. A follow-up of 75 cases. Arch Dis Child 39:576, 1964

456. Ansell BM: Problems of corticosteroid therapy in the young. Proc R Soc Med 61:281, 1968

457. Laaksonen A-L, Sunell JE, Westeren H et al: Adrenocortical function in children with juvenile rheumatoid arthritis and other connective tissue disorders. Scand J Rheumatol 3:137, 1974

458. Schaller JG: Corticosteroids in juvenile rheumatoid arthritis (Still's disease) (editorial). J Rheumatol 1:137, 1974

459. Schaller JG: Corticosteroids in juvenile rheumatoid arthritis. Arthritis Rheum 20:537, 1977

460. Stoeber E: Juvenile Chronic Polyarthritis and Still's Syndrome. Doc Geigy 1, 1977

461. Ansell BM, Bywaters EGL: Alternate-day corticosteroid therapy in juvenile chronic polyarthritis. J Rheumatol 1:176, 1974

462. Allen RC, Gross KR, Laxer RM et al: Intraarticular triamcinolone hexacetonide in the management of chronic arthritis in children. Arthritis Rheum 29:997, 1986

463. Cassidy JT, Bole GG: Cutaneous atrophy secondary to intra-articular corticosteroid administration. Ann Intern Med 65:1008, 1966

464. Hollister JR: Immunosuppressant therapy of juvenile rheumatoid arthritis. Arthritis Rheum 20:544, 1977

465. Kvien TK, Høyeraal HM, Sandstad B: Azathioprine versus placebo in patients with juvenile rheumatoid arthritis: a single center double blind comparative study. J Rheumatol 13:118, 1986

466. Ansell BM, Eghtedari A, Bywaters EGL: Chlorambucil in the management of juvenile chronic arthritis complicated by amyloidosis. Ann Rheum Dis 30:331, 1971

467. Giannini EH, Boesver EJ: Methotrexate (MTX) in the treatment of recalcitrant JRA-results of the double-blind, placebo (P) controlled, randomized trial. Arthritis Rheum 32:S82, 1989

468. Truckenbrodt H, Häfner R: Methotrexate therapy in juvenile rheumatoid arthritis: a retrospective study. Arthritis Rheum 29:801, 1986

469. Høyeraal HM, Frøland SS, Salvesen CF et al: No effect of transfer factor in juvenile rheumatoid arthritis by double-blind trial. Ann Rheum Dis 37:175, 1978

470. Ruuskanen O: Levamisole and agranulocytosis. Lancet 2:958, 1976

471. Prieur A-M: Possible toxicity of levamisole in children with rheumatoid arthritis. J Pediatr 93:304, 1978

472. Field EH, Strober S, Hoppe RT et al: Sustained improvement of intractable rheumatoid arthritis after total lymphoid irradiation. Arthritis Rheum 29:934, 1983

473. Johanssen U, Portinsson S, Akesson A et al: Nutritional status in girls with juvenile chronic arthritis. Hum Nutr Clin Nutr 40:57, 1986

474. Donovan WH: Physical measures in the treatment of juvenile rheumatoid arthritis. Arthritis Rheum 20:553, 1977

475. Emery HM, Kucinski J: Management of Juvenile Rheumatoid Arthritis. A Handbook for Occupational and Physical Therapists. LaRabida Children's Hospital and Research Center, Chicago, 1987

476. Schull SA, Dow MB, Athreya BH: Physical and occupational therapy for children with rheumatic diseases. Pediatr Clin North Am 33:1053, 1986

477. Lechner DE, McCarthy CF, Holden MK: Gait deviations in patients with juvenile rheumatoid arthritis. Phys Ther 67:1335, 1987

478. Arden GP, Ansell BM (eds): Surgical Management of Juvenile Chronic Polyarthritis. Academic Press, London, 1978

479. Arden GP: Surgical treatment of Still's disease. Ann R Coll Surg Engl 53:288, 1973

480. Arden GP: Surgical treatment of juvenile rheumatoid arthritis. Ann Chir Gynaecol 198:103, 1985

481. Fink CW, Baum J, Paradies LH et al: Synovectomy in juvenile rheumatoid arthritis. Ann Rheum Dis 28:612, 1969

482. Eyring EJ, Longert A, Bass JC: Synovectomy in juvenile rheumatoid arthritis. Indications and short-term results. J Bone Joint Surg 53A:638, 1971

483. Granberry EM, Brewer EJ, Jr: Results of synovectomy in children with rheumatoid arthritis. Clin Orthop 101:120, 1974

484. Granberry WM: Synovectomy in juvenile rheumatoid arthritis. Arthritis Rheum 20:561, 1977

485. Jacobsen ST, Levinson JE, Crawford AH: Late results of synovectomy in juvenile rheumatoid arthritis. J Bone Joint Surg 67A:8, 1985

486. Rydholm U, Elborgh R, Ranstam J et al: Synovectomy of the knee in juvenile chronic arthritis. A retrospective, consecutive follow-up study. J Bone Joint Surg 68B:223, 1986

487. Kvien TK, Pahle JA, Høyeraal HM et al: Comparison of synovectomy and no synovectomy in patients with juvenile rheumatoid arthritis. A 24-month controlled study. Scand J Rheumatol 16:81, 1987

488. Swann M: Juvenile chronic arthritis. Clin Orthop 219:38, 1987

489. Rydholm U, Brattström H, Lidgren L: Soft tissue release for knee flexion contracture in juvenile chronic arthritis. J Pediatr Orthop 6:448, 1986

490. Swann M, Ansell BM: Soft-tissue release of the hips in children with juvenile chronic arthritis. J Bone Joint Surg 68B:404, 1986

491. Rydholm U: Arthroscopy of the knee in juvenile chronic arthritis. Scand J Rheumatol 15:109, 1986

492. Paus A, Pahle JA: The value of arthroscopy in the diagnosis and treatment of patients with juvenile rheumatoid arthritis. Ann Chir Gynaecol 75:168, 1986

493. Sledge CB: Joint replacement surgery in juvenile rheumatoid arthritis. Arthritis Rheum 20:567, 1977

494. Arden GP, Ansell BM, Hunter MJ: Total hip replacement in juvenile chronic polyarthritis and ankylosing spondylitis. Clin Orthop 84:130, 1972

495. Colvile J, Raunio P: Total hip replacement in juvenile rheumatoid arthritis. Analysis of 59 hips. Acta Orthop Scand 50:197, 1979

496. Singsen BH, Isaacson AS, Bernstein BH et al: Total hip replacement in children with arthritis. Arthritis Rheum 21:401, 1978

497. Crowe W, Hauselman C, Shear E et al: Total hip arthroplasty in children with juvenile rheumatoid arthritis. Arthritis Rheum 22:602, 1979

498. Lachiewicz PF, McCaskill B, Inglis A et al: Total hip arthroplasty in juvenile rheumatoid arthritis. Two to eleven-year results. J Bone Joint Surg 68B:502, 1986

499. Ruddlesdin C, Ansell BM, Arden GP et al: Total hip replacement in children with juvenile chronic arthritis. J Bone Joint Surg 68B:218, 1986

500. Rydholm U, Bfegard T, Lidgren L: Total knee replacement in juvenile chronic arthritis. Scand J Rheumatol 14:329, 1985

501. Carmichael E, Chaplin DM: Total knee arthroplasty in juvenile rheumatoid arthritis. A seven-year follow-up study. Clin Orthop 210:192, 1986

502. Harrison SH: Wrist and hand problems and their management. In Arden GP, Ansell BM (eds): Surgical Management of Juvenile Chronic Arthritis. Academic Press, London, 1978, p. 161

503. Dabrowski W, Fonseka N, Ansell BM et al: Shoulder problems in juvenile chronic polyarthritis. Scand J Rheumatol 8:49, 1979

504. We can: A Guide for Parents of Children with Arthritis. Arthritis Foundation, Atlanta, 1985

505. Athreya BH, McCormick MC: Impact of chronic illness on families. Rheum Dis Clin North Am 13:123, 1987

506. Stoff E, Molock SD, White PH: A needs assessment of children with rheumatic diseases. J Sch Health 57:162, 1987

507. Meenan RF: Health status assessment in pediatric rheumatology. Rheum Dis Clin North Am 13:133, 1987

508. Rapoff MA, Lindsley CB, Christophersen ER: Parent perception of problems experienced by their children in complying with treatments for juvenile rheumatoid arthritis. Arch Phys Med Rehabil 66:427, 1985

509. Morse J: Aspiration and achievement. A study of one hundred patients with juvenile rheumatoid arthritis. Rehabil Lit 33:290, 1972

510. Cleveland SE, Reitman EE, Brewer EJ, Jr: Psychological factors in juvenile rheumatoid arthritis. Arthritis Rheum 8:1152, 1965

511. King K, Hanson V: Psychosocial aspects of juvenile rheumatoid arthritis. Pediatr Clin North Am 33:1221, 1986

512. Keltikangas-Järvinen L: Body-image disturbances ensuing from juvenile rheumatoid arthritis, a preliminary study. Percept Mot Skills 64:984, 1987

513. Ungerer JA, Horgan B, Chaitwo J et al: Psychosocial functioning in children and young adults with juvenile arthritis. Pediatrics 81:195, 1988

514. Whitehouse R, Shope J, Kulik C-L et al: Implementation of Public Law 94-142 for children with juvenile rheumatoid arthritis. Arthritis Rheum 25:S11, 1982

515. Whitehouse R, Shope JT, Graham-Tomasi G et al: Educational needs of school personnel working with children with juvenile rheumatoid arthritis. Arthritis Rheum 26:S84, 1983

516. Spencer CH, Zanga J, Passo M et al: The child with arthritis in the school setting. Pediatr Clin North Am 33:1251, 1986

589. Perkins ES: Patterns of uveitis in children. Br J Ophthalmol 50:169, 1966

590. Rosenberg AM, Oen KG: The relationship between ocular and articular disease activity in children with juvenile rheumatoid arthritis and associated uveitis. Arthritis Rheum 29:797, 1986

591. Kanski JJ: Anterior uveitis in juvenile rheumatoid arthritis. Arch Ophthalmol 95:1794, 1977

592. Hollwich F, Damaske E: Augen-Symptome beim Morbus Still. Med Monatsschr 22:109, 1968

593. Hinzpeter EN, Naumann G, Bartelheimer HK: Ocular histopathology in Still's disease. Ophthalmol Res 2:16, 1971

594. Sabates R, Smith T, Apple D: Ocular histopathology in juvenile rheumatoid arthritis. Ann Ophthalmol 11:733, 1979

595. Chylack LT, Jr, Dueker DK, Pihlaja DJ: Ocular manifestations of juvenile rheumatoid arthritis: pathology, fluorescein iris angiography, and patient care patterns. In Miller JJ, III (ed): Juvenile Rheumatoid Arthritis. PSG Littleton, Mass, 1978, p. 149

596. Godfrey WA, Lindsley CB, Cuppage FE: Localization of IgM in plasma cells in the iris of a patient with iridocyclitis and juvenile rheumatoid arthritis. Arthritis Rheum 24:1195, 1981

597. Merriam JC, Chylack LT, Albert DM: Early onset pauciarticular juvenile rheumatoid arthritis. A histopathologic study. Arch Ophthalmol 101:1085, 1983

598. Epstein WF, Tan M, Easterbrook M: Serum antibody to double stranded RNA and DNA in patients with idiopathic and secondary uveitis. N Engl J Med 285:1502, 1971

599. Petty RE, Hunt DWC, Rollins DF et al: Immunity to soluble retinal antigen in patients with uveitis accompanying juvenile rheumatoid arthritis. Arthritis Rheum 30:287, 1987

600. Rahi AH, Kanski JJ, Fielder A: Immunoglobulins and antinuclear antibodies in aqueous humour from patients with juvenile "rheumatoid" arthritis (Still's disease). Trans Ophthalmol Soc UK 97:217, 1977

601. Kanski JJ: Clinical and immunological study of anterior uveitis in juvenile chronic polyarthritis. Trans Ophthalmol Soc UK 96:123, 1976

602. Person DA, Leatherwood CM, Brewer EJ et al: Immunology of the vitreous in juvenile rheumatoid arthritis. Arthritis Rheum 24:591, 1981

603. Kaplan HJ, Aalberg TM, Keller RH: Recurrent clinical uveitis: cell surface markers in vitreous lymphocytes. Arch Ophthalmol 100:585, 1982

604. Schaller JG, Hansen J: Early childhood pauciarticular juvenile rheumatoid arthritis: clinical and immunogenetic studies. Arthritis Rheum, suppl.,25:53, 1982

605. Mehra R, Moore TL, Catalano JD et al: Chorambucil in the treatment of iridocyclitis in juvenile rheumatoid arthritis. J Rheumatol 8:141, 1981

606. Palmer RG, Kanski JJ, Ansell BM: Chlorambucil in the treatment of intractable uveitis associated with juvenile chronic arthritis. J Rheumatol 12:967, 1985

607. Wizemann AJS, Wizemann V: Therapeutic effects of short-term plasma exchange in endogenous uveitis. Am J Ophthalmol 97:565, 1984

608. Nussenblatt RB, Palestine AG, Chan C-C: Cyclosporin A therapy in the treatment of intraocular inflammatory disease resistant to systemic corticosteroids and cytotoxic agents. Am J Ophthalmol 96:275, 1983

609. Olson NY, Lindsley CB, Godfrey WA: Treatment of chronic childhood iridocyclitis with nonsteroidal anti-inflammatory drugs. J Allerg Clin Immunol 79:220, 1981

610. March WF, Coniglione TC: Ibuprofen in the treatment of uveitis. Ann Ophthalmol 17:103, 1985

611. Donne JA, Jacobs N, Morrison A et al: Efficacy in anterior uveitis of two known steroids and topical tolmetin. Br J Ophthalmol 69:120, 1985

612. Smiley WK: The visual prognosis in Still's disease with eye involvement. Proc R Soc Med 53:196, 1960

613. Edström G: Band-shaped keritis in juvenile rheumatoid arthritis. Acta Rheum Scand 7:169, 1961

614. Lipton NL, Crawford JS, Greenberg ML et al: The risk of iridocyclitis in juvenile rheumatoid arthritis. Can J Ophthalmol 11:26, 1976

615. Galea P, D'Amato B, Goel KM: Ocular complications in juvenile chronic arthritis (JCA). Scott Med J 30:164, 1985

616. Leak AM, Ansell BM: The relationship between ocular and articular disease activity in juvenile rheumatoid arthritis complicated by chronic anterior uveitis. Arthritis Rheum 30:1196, 1987

617. Wolf MD, Lichter PR, Ragsdale CG: Prognostic factors in the uveitis of juvenile rheumatoid arthritis. Ophthalmology 94:1242, 1987

618. Bywaters EGL: Still's disease in the adult. Ann Rheum Dis 30:121, 1971

619. Aptekar RG, Decker JL, Bujak JS et al: Adult onset juvenile rheumatoid arthritis. Arthritis Rheum 16:715, 1973

620. Elkon KB, Hughes GRV, Bywaters EGL et al: Adult-onset Still's disease. Twenty-year follow-up and further studies of patients with active disease. Arthritis Rheum 25:647, 1982

621. Wouters JM, van Rijswijk MH, van de Putte LB: Adult onset Still's disease in the elderly: a report of two cases. J Rheumatol 12:791, 1985

and steroid treatment. Trans Ophthalmol Soc UK 85:351, 1965

553. Smiley WK: The eye in juvenile rheumatoid arthritis. Trans Ophthalmol Soc UK 94:817, 1974

554. Schaller JG: Iridocyclitis. Arthritis Rheum 20:227, 1977

555. McGill NW, Gow PJ: Juvenile rheumatoid arthritis in Auckland: a long term follow-up study with particular reference to uveitis. Aust NZ J Med 17:305, 1987

556. Rosenberg AM: Uveitis associated with juvenile rheumatoid arthritis. Semin Arthritis Rheum 16:158, 1987

557. Chadwick AJ, Rosen AS: Papillitis and Still's disease. Am J Ophthalmol 65:748, 1968

558. Chylack LT, Jr: The ocular manifestations of juvenile rheumatoid arthritis. Arthritis Rheum 20:217, 1977

559. Key SN, III, Kimura SJ: Iridocyclitis associated with juvenile rheumatoid arthritis. Am J Ophthalmol 80:425, 1975

560. Ohno S, Miyajima J, Higuchi M et al: Ocular manifestations of Kawasaki's disease (mucocutaneous lymph node syndrome). Am J Ophthalmol 93:713, 1982

561. Lambert JR, Ansell BM, Stephenson E et al: Psoriatic arthritis in childhood. Clin Rheum Dis 2:339, 1976

562. Rankin GB, Watts HD, Mielnyk CS et al: National cooperative Crohn's disease study: extraintestinal manifestations and perianal complications. Gastroenterology 77:914, 1979

563. Davies NE, Haverty JR, Boatwright M: Reiter's disease associated with shigellosis. South Med J 62:1011, 1969

564. Iveson JMI, Nanda BS, Nancock JAH et al: Reiter's disease in three boys. Ann Rheum Dis 34:364, 1975

565. Kaufman RA, Lovell DJ: Infantile onset multisystem inflammatory disease: radiologic findings. Radiology 160:741, 1986

566. Yarom A, Rennebohm RM, Levinson JE: Infantile multisystem inflammatory disease: a specific syndrome? J Pediatr 106:390, 1985

567. Hoover DL, Khan JA, Giangiacomo J: Pediatric ocular sarcoidosis. Sur Ophthalmol 30:215, 1986

568. Kanski JJ, Shun-Shin A: Systemic uveitis syndromes in childhood: an analysis of 340 cases. Ophthalmology 91:1247, 1984

569. Jose DG, Good RA: Iridocyclitis and pauciarticular juvenile rheumatoid arthritis. J Pediatr 78:910, 1971

570. Spalter HF: The visual prognosis in juvenile rheumatoid arthritis. Trans Am Ophthalmol Soc 73:554, 1975

571. Petty RE: Current knowledge of the etiology and pathogenesis of chronic uveitis accompanying juvenile rheumatoid arthritis. Rheum Dis Clin North Am 13:19, 1987

572. Ohm J: Bandförmige Hornhauttrübung bei einem neunjährigen Mädchen und ihre Behandlung mit subkonjunktivalen Jodkaliumeinspritzungen. Klin Monatsbl Augenheilkd 48:243, 1910

573. Fuchs E: Ueber gürtelförmige Hornhauttrübung. Klin Monatsbl Augenheilkd 61:10, 1918

574. Waubke H: Zur Kenntnis der bandförmigen Hornhauttrübung in sehender Augen. Klin Monatsbl Augenheilkd 69:79, 1922

575. Friedländer A: 2 Tilfaelde af kronisk septisk Polyartritis i Barnealderen med Øjenkomplikationer. Ugeskr Laeger 95:1190, 1933

576. Holm E: Iridocyclitis and ribbon-like keratitis in cases of infantile polyarthritis (Still's disease). Trans Ophthalmol Soc UK 55:478, 1935

577. Karsch J: Ueber sekundäre bandförmige Hornhauttrübünge bei der Polyarthroitis chronica leucocytotica (Still) und lympho-cytotica (Rhonheimer). Arch Augenheilkd 110:106, 1937

578. Hässler E: Augenkomplikationen bei Polyarthroitis chronica infantilis und Still'scher Krankheit mit einer kritischen Bemerkung über die Pathogenese der allgemeinen rheumatischen Infektion. Monatsschr Kinderhilkd 77:23, 1939

579. Zeemann WPC: Gordelvormige hoornvliesdegeneratie en arthritis bej kinderen. Ned Tijdschr Geneeskd 84:134, 1940

580. Bane W, Sherwood EF: Band keratitis and uveitis in polyarthritis. Am J Ophthalmol 24:701, 1941

581. Wong RT: Band-shaped opacity of the cornea associated with juvenile atrophic arthritis. Arch Ophthalmol 26:21, 1941

582. Blegvad O: Iridocyclitis and disease of the joints in children. Acta Ophthalmol 19:219, 1941

583. Kurnick N: A rare syndrome of band-shaped keratitis and arthritis. Am J Dis Child 63:742, 1942

584. Poulsen AG: Om Ledlidelse og chronisk Iridocyclitis hos Børn. Nord Med 35:1963, 1947

585. Hobbs HE: Ocular defects in Still's disease. Proc R Soc Med 42:755, 1949

586. Franceschetti A, Blum JD, Bamatter F: Diagnostic value of ocular symptoms in juvenile chronic polyarthritis (Still's disease). Trans Ophthalmol Soc UK 71: 1951

587. Smiley WK: The eye in juvenile chronic polyarthritis. Clin Rheum Dis 2:413, 1976

588. Calabro JJ, Parrino GR, Atchoo PD et al: Chronic iridocyclitis in juvenile rheumatoid arthritis. Arthritis Rheum 13:406, 1970

589. Perkins ES: Patterns of uveitis in children. Br J Ophthalmol 50:169, 1966

590. Rosenberg AM, Oen KG: The relationship between ocular and articular disease activity in children with juvenile rheumatoid arthritis and associated uveitis. Arthritis Rheum 29:797, 1986

591. Kanski JJ: Anterior uveitis in juvenile rheumatoid arthritis. Arch Ophthalmol 95:1794, 1977

592. Hollwich F, Damaske E: Augen-Symptome beim Morbus Still. Med Monatsschr 22:109, 1968

593. Hinzpeter EN, Naumann G, Bartelheimer HK: Ocular histopathology in Still's disease. Ophthalmol Res 2:16, 1971

594. Sabates R, Smith T, Apple D: Ocular histopathology in juvenile rheumatoid arthritis. Ann Ophthalmol 11:733, 1979

595. Chylack LT, Jr, Dueker DK, Pihlaja DJ: Ocular manifestations of juvenile rheumatoid arthritis: pathology, fluorescein iris angiography, and patient care patterns. In Miller JJ, III (ed): Juvenile Rheumatoid Arthritis. PSG Littleton, Mass, 1978, p. 149

596. Godfrey WA, Lindsley CB, Cuppage FE: Localization of IgM in plasma cells in the iris of a patient with iridocyclitis and juvenile rheumatoid arthritis. Arthritis Rheum 24:1195, 1981

597. Merriam JC, Chylack LT, Albert DM: Early onset pauciarticular juvenile rheumatoid arthritis. A histopathologic study. Arch Ophthalmol 101:1085, 1983

598. Epstein WF, Tan M, Easterbrook M: Serum antibody to double stranded RNA and DNA in patients with idiopathic and secondary uveitis. N Engl J Med 285:1502, 1971

599. Petty RE, Hunt DWC, Rollins DF et al: Immunity to soluble retinal antigen in patients with uveitis accompanying juvenile rheumatoid arthritis. Arthritis Rheum 30:287, 1987

600. Rahi AH, Kanski JJ, Fielder A: Immunoglobulins and antinuclear antibodies in aqueous humour from patients with juvenile "rheumatoid" arthritis (Still's disease). Trans Ophthalmol Soc UK 97:217, 1977

601. Kanski JJ: Clinical and immunological study of anterior uveitis in juvenile chronic polyarthritis. Trans Ophthalmol Soc UK 96:123, 1976

602. Person DA, Leatherwood CM, Brewer EJ et al: Immunology of the vitreous in juvenile rheumatoid arthritis. Arthritis Rheum 24:591, 1981

603. Kaplan HJ, Aalberg TM, Keller RH: Recurrent clinical uveitis: cell surface markers in vitreous lymphocytes. Arch Ophthalmol 100:585, 1982

604. Schaller JG, Hansen J: Early childhood pauciarticular juvenile rheumatoid arthritis: clinical and immunogenetic studies. Arthritis Rheum, suppl.,25:53, 1982

605. Mehra R, Moore TL, Catalano JD et al: Chorambucil in the treatment of iridocyclitis in juvenile rheumatoid arthritis. J Rheumatol 8:141, 1981

606. Palmer RG, Kanski JJ, Ansell BM: Chlorambucil in the treatment of intractable uveitis associated with juvenile chronic arthritis. J Rheumatol 12:967, 1985

607. Wizemann AJS, Wizemann V: Therapeutic effects of short-term plasma exchange in endogenous uveitis. Am J Ophthalmol 97:565, 1984

608. Nussenblatt RB, Palestine AG, Chan C-C: Cyclosporin A therapy in the treatment of intraocular inflammatory disease resistant to systemic corticosteroids and cytotoxic agents. Am J Ophthalmol 96:275, 1983

609. Olson NY, Lindsley CB, Godfrey WA: Treatment of chronic childhood iridocyclitis with nonsteroidal anti-inflammatory drugs. J Allerg Clin Immunol 79:220, 1981

610. March WF, Coniglione TC: Ibuprofen in the treatment of uveitis. Ann Ophthalmol 17:103, 1985

611. Donne JA, Jacobs N, Morrison A et al: Efficacy in anterior uveitis of two known steroids and topical tolmetin. Br J Ophthalmol 69:120, 1985

612. Smiley WK: The visual prognosis in Still's disease with eye involvement. Proc R Soc Med 53:196, 1960

613. Edström G: Band-shaped keratitis in juvenile rheumatoid arthritis. Acta Rheum Scand 7:169, 1961

614. Lipton NL, Crawford JS, Greenberg ML et al: The risk of iridocyclitis in juvenile rheumatoid arthritis. Can J Ophthalmol 11:26, 1976

615. Galea P, D'Amato B, Goel KM: Ocular complications in juvenile chronic arthritis (JCA). Scott Med J 30:164, 1985

616. Leak AM, Ansell BM: The relationship between ocular and articular disease activity in juvenile rheumatoid arthritis complicated by chronic anterior uveitis. Arthritis Rheum 30:1196, 1987

617. Wolf MD, Lichter PR, Ragsdale CG: Prognostic factors in the uveitis of juvenile rheumatoid arthritis. Ophthalmology 94:1242, 1987

618. Bywaters EGL: Still's disease in the adult. Ann Rheum Dis 30:121, 1971

619. Aptekar RG, Decker JL, Bujak JS et al: Adult onset juvenile rheumatoid arthritis. Arthritis Rheum 16:715, 1973

620. Elkon KB, Hughes GRV, Bywaters EGL et al: Adult-onset Still's disease. Twenty-year follow-up and further studies of patients with active disease. Arthritis Rheum 25:647, 1982

621. Wouters JM, van Rijswijk MH, van de Putte LB: Adult onset Still's disease in the elderly: a report of two cases. J Rheumatol 12:791, 1985

482. Eyring EJ, Longert A, Bass JC: Synovectomy in juvenile rheumatoid arthritis. Indications and short-term results. J Bone Joint Surg 53A:638, 1971

483. Granberry EM, Brewer EJ, Jr: Results of synovectomy in children with rheumatoid arthritis. Clin Orthop 101:120, 1974

484. Granberry WM: Synovectomy in juvenile rheumatoid arthritis. Arthritis Rheum 20:561, 1977

485. Jacobsen ST, Levinson JE, Crawford AH: Late results of synovectomy in juvenile rheumatoid arthritis. J Bone Joint Surg 67A:8, 1985

486. Rydholm U, Elborgh R, Ranstam J et al: Synovectomy of the knee in juvenile chronic arthritis. A retrospective, consecutive follow-up study. J Bone Joint Surg 68B:223, 1986

487. Kvien TK, Pahle JA, Høyeraal HM et al: Comparison of synovectomy and no synovectomy in patients with juvenile rheumatoid arthritis. A 24-month controlled study. Scand J Rheumatol 16:81, 1987

488. Swann M: Juvenile chronic arthritis. Clin Orthop 219:38, 1987

489. Rydholm U, Brattström H, Lidgren L: Soft tissue release for knee flexion contracture in juvenile chronic arthritis. J Pediatr Orthop 6:448, 1986

490. Swann M, Ansell BM: Soft-tissue release of the hips in children with juvenile chronic arthritis. J Bone Joint Surg 68B:404, 1986

491. Rydholm U: Arthroscopy of the knee in juvenile chronic arthritis. Scand J Rheumatol 15:109, 1986

492. Paus A, Pahle JA: The value of arthroscopy in the diagnosis and treatment of patients with juvenile rheumatoid arthritis. Ann Chir Gynaecol 75:168, 1986

493. Sledge CB: Joint replacement surgery in juvenile rheumatoid arthritis. Arthritis Rheum 20:567, 1977

494. Arden GP, Ansell BM, Hunter MJ: Total hip replacement in juvenile chronic polyarthritis and ankylosing spondylitis. Clin Orthop 84:130, 1972

495. Colvile J, Raunio P: Total hip replacement in juvenile rheumatoid arthritis. Analysis of 59 hips. Acta Orthop Scand 50:197, 1979

496. Singsen BH, Isaacson AS, Bernstein BH et al: Total hip replacement in children with arthritis. Arthritis Rheum 21:401, 1978

497. Crowe W, Hauselman C, Shear E et al: Total hip arthroplasty in children with juvenile rheumatoid arthritis. Arthritis Rheum 22:602, 1979

498. Lachiewicz PF, McCaskill B, Inglis A et al: Total hip arthroplasty in juvenile rheumatoid arthritis. Two to eleven-year results. J Bone Joint Surg 68B:502, 1986

499. Ruddlesdin C, Ansell BM, Arden GP et al: Total hip replacement in children with juvenile chronic arthritis. J Bone Joint Surg 68B:218, 1986

500. Rydholm U, Bfegard T, Lidgren L: Total knee replacement in juvenile chronic arthritis. Scand J Rheumatol 14:329, 1985

501. Carmichael E, Chaplin DM: Total knee arthroplasty in juvenile rheumatoid arthritis. A seven-year follow-up study. Clin Orthop 210:192, 1986

502. Harrison SH: Wrist and hand problems and their management. In Arden GP, Ansell BM (eds): Surgical Management of Juvenile Chronic Arthritis. Academic Press, London, 1978, p. 161

503. Dabrowski W, Fonseka N, Ansell BM et al: Shoulder problems in juvenile chronic polyarthritis. Scand J Rheumatol 8:49, 1979

504. We can: A Guide for Parents of Children with Arthritis. Arthritis Foundation, Atlanta, 1985

505. Athreya BH, McCormick MC: Impact of chronic illness on families. Rheum Dis Clin North Am 13:123, 1987

506. Stoff E, Molock SD, White PH: A needs assessment of children with rheumatic diseases. J Sch Health 57:162, 1987

507. Meenan RF: Health status assessment in pediatric rheumatology. Rheum Dis Clin North Am 13:133, 1987

508. Rapoff MA, Lindsley CB, Christophersen ER: Parent perception of problems experienced by their children in complying with treatments for juvenile rheumatoid arthritis. Arch Phys Med Rehabil 66:427, 1985

509. Morse J: Aspiration and achievement. A study of one hundred patients with juvenile rheumatoid arthritis. Rehabil Lit 33:290, 1972

510. Cleveland SE, Reitman EE, Brewer EJ, Jr: Psychological factors in juvenile rheumatoid arthritis. Arthritis Rheum 8:1152, 1965

511. King K, Hanson V: Psychosocial aspects of juvenile rheumatoid arthritis. Pediatr Clin North Am 33:1221, 1986

512. Keltikangas-Järvinen L: Body-image disturbances ensuing from juvenile rheumatoid arthritis, a preliminary study. Percept Mot Skills 64:984, 1987

513. Ungerer JA, Horgan B, Chaitwo J et al: Psychosocial functioning in children and young adults with juvenile arthritis. Pediatrics 81:195, 1988

514. Whitehouse R, Shope J, Kulik C-L et al: Implementation of Public Law 94-142 for children with juvenile rheumatoid arthritis. Arthritis Rheum 25:S11, 1982

515. Whitehouse R, Shope JT, Graham-Tomasi G et al: Educational needs of school personnel working with children with juvenile rheumatoid arthritis. Arthritis Rheum 26:S84, 1983

516. Spencer CH, Zanga J, Passo M et al: The child with arthritis in the school setting. Pediatr Clin North Am 33:1251, 1986

517. Taylor J, Passo MH, Champion VL: School problems and teacher responsibilities in juvenile rheumatoid arthritis. J Sch Health 57:186, 1987

518. White PH, McPherson M, Levinson JE: Community programs for children with rheumatic diseases. Pediatr Cl North Am 33:1239, 1986

519. Cope C, Anderson E: Special units in disabled schools. In Studies in Education. Institute of Education, University of London, London, 1977

520. McAnarney ER, Pless IB, Satterwhite B et al: Psychological problems of children with chronic juvenile arthritis. Pediatrics 53:523, 1974

521. Mozziconacci P: Pour une "prise en charge psychologique" des polyarthrites juvéniles. Ann Pediatr 23:415, 1976

522. Weil-Halpern F, Rapoport D, Hatt A et al: La polyarthrite chronique de l'enfant dans la structure hospitalière. Étude psychosociologique. I: La consultation. Ann Pediatr 22:499, 1975

523. Weil-Halpern F, Rapoport D, Hatt A et al: La polyarthrite chronique juvénile dans la structure hospitalière. Étude psycho-sociologique. II: L'hospitalisation. Ann Pediatr 23:420, 1976

524. Hatt A, Weil-Halpern F, Rapoport D et al: La polyarthrite chronique juvénile dans la structure hospitalière. Étude psycho-sociologique. III: Entretiens avec les parents. Ann Pediatr 23:429, 1976

525. Rapoport D, Hatt A, Weil-Halpern F et al: La polyarthrite chronique juvénile dans la structure hospitalière. IV: Étude psychologique des enfants atteints. Ann Pediatr 23:427, 1976

526. Tursz A: La polyarthrite chronique juvénile dans la structure hospitalière. V. Scolarité, vie sociale et familiale. Ann Pediatr 23:442, 1976

527. Pless IB, Satterwhite B, Van Vechten D: Division, duplication and neglect: patterns of care for children with chronic disorders. Child Care Health Dev 4:9, 1978

528. Edström G, Gedda PO: Clinic and prognosis of rheumatoid arthritis in children. Acta Rheumatol Scand 3:129, 1957

529. Ansell BM, Bywaters EGL: Prognosis in Still's disease. Bull Rheum Dis 9:189, 1959

530. Goel KM, Shanks RA: Follow-up study of 100 cases of juvenile rheumatoid arthritis. Ann Rheum Dis 33:25, 1974

531. Ansell BM, Wood PHN: Prognosis in juvenile chronic polyarthritis. Clin Rheum Dis 2:397, 1976

532. Hanson V, Kornreich H, Bernstein B et al: Prognosis of juvenile rheumatoid arthritis. Arthritis Rheum 20:279, 1977

533. Calabro JJ, Burnstein SL, Staley HL et al: Prognosis in juvenile rheumatoid arthritis: a fifteen year follow-up of 100 patients. Arthritis Rheum 20:285, 1977

534. Stoeber E: Prognosis in juvenile chronic arthritis. Eur J Pediatr 135:225, 1981

535. Dequecker J, Mardjuadi A: Prognostic factors in juvenile chronic arthritis. J Rheumatol 9:909, 1982

536. Michels H, Häfner R, Morhart R: Five year follow-up of a prospective cohort of juvenile chronic arthritis with recent onset. Clin Rheumatol 6 suppl., 2:87, 1987

537. Ansell BM: Still's disease followed into adult life. Proc R Soc Med 62:912, 1969

538. Jeremy R, Schaller J, Arkless R et al: Juvenile rheumatoid arthritis persisting into adulthood. Am J Med 45:419, 1968

539. Hill RH, Herstein A, Walters K: Juvenile rheumatoid arthritis: follow-up into adulthood—medical, sexual and social status. Can Med Assoc J 76:790, 1976

540. FitzGerald O, Bresnihan B: Juvenile chronic arthritis: spectrum of disease in an adult rheumatology department. Ir J Med Sci 155:266, 1986

541. Steinbrocker O, Traeger CH, Batterman RC: Therapeutic criteria in rheumatoid arthritis. JAMA 140:659, 1949

542. Medsger TA, Jr, Christy WC: Carpal arthritis with ankylosis in late onset Still's disease. Arthritis Rheum 19:232, 1976

543. Isdale IC: Hip disease in juvenile rheumatoid arthritis. Ann Rheum Dis 29:603, 1970

544. Ansell BM, Unlu M: Hip involvement in juvenile chronic poly-arthritis. Ann Rheum Dis 29:687, 1970

545. Rombouts JJ, Rombouts-Lindemans C: Involvement of the hip in juvenile rheumatoid arthritis. A radiological study with special reference to growth disturbances. Acta Rheumatol Scand 17:248, 1971

546. Blane CE, Ragsdale CG, Hensinger RN: Late effects of JRA on the hip. J Pediatr Orthop 7:677, 1987

547. Baum J, Gutowska G: Death in juvenile rheumatoid arthritis. Arthritis Rheum 20:253, 1977

548. Bernstein B: Death in juvenile rheumatoid arthritis. Arthritis Rheum 20:256, 1977

549. Bywaters EGL: Deaths in juvenile chronic polyarthritis. Arthritis Rheum 20:256, 1977

550. Arden GP: Sepsis in juvenile chronic polyarthritis. In Arden GP, Ansell BM (eds): Surgical Management of Juvenile Chronic Polyarthritis. Academic Press, London, 1978, p. 225

551. Smiley WK, May E, Bywaters EGL: Ocular presentations of Still's disease and their treatment. Iridocyclitis in Still's disease: its complications and treatment. Ann Rheum Dis 16:371, 1957

552. Smiley WK: Iridocyclitis in Still's disease. Prognosis

622. Wouters JM, Reekers P, van de Putte LB: Adult-onset Still's disease. Disease course and HLA associations. Arthritis Rheum 29:415, 1986

623. Wouters JM, van de Putte LB: Adult-onset Still's disease: clinical and laboratory features, treatment and progress of 45 cases. Q J Med 61:1055, 1986

624. Cush JJ, Medsger TA, Jr, Christy WC et al: Adult-onset Still's disease. Clinical course and outcome. Arthritis Rheum 30:186, 1987

625. Reginato AJ, Schumacher HR, Jr, Baker DG et al: Adult onset Still's disease: experience in 23 patients and literature review with emphasis on organ failure. Semin Arthritis Rheum 17:39, 1987

626. Björkengren AG, Pathria MN, Sartoris DJ et al: Carpal alterations in adult-onset Still's disease, juvenile chronic arthritis, and adult-onset rheumatoid arthritis: comparative study. Radiology 165:545, 1987

627. Pindborg S: Et tilfaelde af Still's Sygdom. Ugeskr Laeger 104:1417, 1942

628. Roberts-Thomson PJ, Southwood TR, Moore BW et al: Adult onset Still's disease or coxsackie polyarthritis? Aust NZ J Med 16:509, 1986

629. Beatty EC: Rheumatic-like nodules occurring in nonrheumatic children. Arch Pathol 68:154, 1959

630. Taranta A: Occurrence of rheumatic-like subcutaneous nodules without evidence of joint or heart disease. Report of a case. N Engl J Med 266:13, 1962

631. Altman RS, Caffrey PR: Isolated subcutaneous rheumatic nodules. Pediatrics 34:869, 1964

632. Burrington JD: "Pseudorheumatoid" nodules in children. Report of 10 cases. Pediatrics 45:473, 1970

633. Simon FER, Schaller JG: Benign rheumatoid nodules. Pediatrics 56:29, 1975

634. Schaller JG: Benign rheumatoid nodules. Arthritis Rheum 20:277, 1977

635. Mesara BW, Brody GL, Oberman HA: "Pseudorheumatoid" subcutaneous nodules. Am J Clin Pathol 45:684, 1966

636. Calabro JJ: Amyloidosis and juvenile rheumatoid arthritis. J Pediatr 75:521, 1969

637. Schnitzer TJ, Ansell BM: Amyloidosis in juvenile chronic polyarthritis. Arthritis Rheum 20:245, 1977

638. Burman SJ, Hall PJ, Bedford PA et al: HLA antigen frequencies among patients with juvenile chronic arthritis and amyloidosis: a brief report. Clin Exp Rheumatol 4:261, 1986

639. Woo P, O'Brien J, Robson M et al: A genetic marker for systemic amyloidosis in juvenile arthritis. Lancet 2:767, 1987

640. Smith ME, Ansell BM, Bywaters EGL: Mortality and prognosis related to the amyloidosis of Still's disease. Ann Rheum Dis 27:137, 1968

641. Glenner GG: Amyloid deposits and amyloidosis. The B-fibrilloses. N Engl J Med 302:1283, 1980

642. Filipowicz-Sosnowska AM, Roztropowicz-Denisiewicz K, Rosenthal CJ et al: The amyloidosis of juvenile rheumatoid arthritis-comparative studies in Polish and American children. I: Levels of serum SAA protein. Arthritis Rheum 21:699, 1978

643. Sohar E, Gafni J, Pras M et al: Familial Mediterranean fever. Am J Med 43:227, 1967

644. Heller H, Garni J, Michaeli D et al: The arthritis of familial Mediterranean fever. Arthritis Rheum 9:1, 1966

645. Herness D, Makin M: Articular damage in familial Mediterranean fever. J Bone Joint Surg 57A:265, 1975

646. Sneh E, Pras M, Michaeli D et al: Protracted arthritis in familial Mediterranean fever. Rheumatol Rehabil 16:102, 1977

647. Ludominsky A, Passivell J, Boichis H: Amyloidosis in children with familial Mediterranean fever. Arch Dis Child 56:464, 1981

648. Bakir F, Murtadha M, Issa N: Amyloidosis and periodic peritonitis (familial Mediterranean fever). West J Med 131:193, 1979

649. Lerner D, Revach M, Pras M et al: A controlled trial of colchicine in preventing attacks of familial Mediterranean fever. N Engl J Med 291:932, 1974

650. Wright DG, Wolff SM, Fauci AS et al: Efficacy of intermittent colchicine therapy in familial Mediterranean fever. Ann Intern Med 86:162, 1977

651. Levy M, Eliakim M: Long-term colchicine prophylaxis in familial Mediterranean fever. Br Med J 2:808, 1977

652. Lehman TJA, Peters RS, Hanson V et al: Long-term colchicine therapy of familial Mediterranean fever. J Pediatr 93:876, 1978

653. Reimann HR: Periodic disease: a probable syndrome including periodic fever, benign paroxysmal peritonitis, cyclic neutropenia and intermittent arthralgia. JAMA 136:239, 1948

6
Spondyloarthropathies

CLASSIFICATION

The spondyloarthropathies (SAs) consist of a group of inflammatory arthropathies that affect the joints of the axial skeleton as well as peripheral joints and that differ from juvenile rheumatoid arthritis (JRA) in many ways. A classification of the spondyloarthropathies is outlined in Table 6-1. The clinical and laboratory characteristics of this group of arthropathies are summarized in Table 6-2. There are several reasons for grouping these disorders under the heading spondyloarthropathy:

1. Inflammation of the joints of the axial skeleton (spine and sacroiliac joints) and inflammation of entheses are clinical features frequently exhibited by members of this group and seldom observed in other chronic arthritides such as JRA.

2. Relatives of children with juvenile ankylosing spondylitis (JAS) commonly have ankylosing spondylitis (AS), psoriatic arthritis, inflammatory bowel disease, or, less commonly, Reiter's syndrome. This genetic influence is related to the high frequency of HLA-B27 among patients with sacroiliitis.

3. There are extra-articular features that may be shared by several members of this group: iritis, usually acute, occurs in all members of the group; the cutaneous manifestations of psoriasis and Reiter's syndrome may be indistinguishable.

4. Rheumatoid factor is absent.

Thus, although individual members of the SA group differ from each other, they share characteristics that distinguish them from the disease complex called JRA and from other connective tissue diseases. In spite of these differences, and because of the frequent presentation of JAS and related diseases as peripheral arthropathies, it may be difficult to distinguish SA from JRA, especially early in the disease course. In addition to the extra-articular signs and symptoms listed in Table 6-2, the recognition of the syndrome of seronegativity, enthesitis, and arthritis (SEA syndrome), which is common in many of the spondyloarthropathies, may also assist in the early diagnosis of children with this group of disorders.

A SYNDROME OF SERONEGATIVITY, ENTHESOPATHY, AND ARTHROPATHY

Many children have some of the characteristics of one of the spondyloarthropathies but lack the sacroiliac (SI) joint changes needed to make a diagnosis of JAS by accepted criteria. A group of 39 such children, representing approximately 20 percent of a pediatric rheumatic disease clinic population, was described as having the SEA syndrome (Table 6-3).[1] These children were "seronegative" (lacked rheumatoid factor [RF] and antinuclear antibody [ANA]), had enthesitis (usually around the heel and the knee), and had arthritis of a few joints, particularly large and small joints of the lower extremities.

Table 6-1 Classification of Spondyloarthropathies

Juvenile ankylosing spondylitis
Psoriatic arthritis
Arthritis associated with inflammatory bowel disease
Reiter's syndrome

Table 6-3 Classification Criteria: SEA Syndrome

Onset of musculoskeletal symptoms before age 17 years
Absence of RF and ANA
Presence of enthesopathic signs
Presence of arthralgia or arthritis

(From Rosenberg and Petty,[1] with permission.)

Comparison of children with the SEA syndrome and those with JRA or JAS is shown in Table 6-4. Of the 39 children with SEA syndrome in this report, 8 had bilateral sacroiliitis, consistent with a diagnosis of JAS; 2 each had inflammatory bowel disease and reactive arthritis; and 1 had Reiter's syndrome. The remaining 26 children had idiopathic SEA syndrome, no other rheumatic disease being identified. The striking similarities of this group of patients and those with JAS with regard to age, sex, mean number of affected joints, and family history of arthritis and back symptoms suggest that SEA syndrome may be an early or mild form of JAS. The high incidence of HLA-B27 in both groups further supports this possibility.

Jacobs et al.[2] studied 58 patients selected on the basis of the presence of HLA-B27, who were seen in a pediatric rheumatology clinic. Two-thirds were boys, and most had onset of symptoms after 9 years of age. None had RF and only 7 had ANA. Although 51 of 58 had disease that satisfied the American Rheumatism Association (ARA) criteria for a diagnosis of JRA,[3] 1 had Reiter's syndrome and 6 had brief episodes of arthritis and enthesitis. In all, 75 percent of the children with HLA-B27 had enthesitis, and many had other features of one of the spondyloarthropathies.

Although the presence of exquisite, well-localized tenderness at characteristic entheses strongly suggests

Table 6-4 Comparison of JRA, JAS, and SEA Syndrome

	JRA	JAS	SEA
Male:female	1:4	7:1	9:1
Average age at onset (yr)	5	>10	10
Average number of joints	9 (may be many)	6 (rarely many)	5 (rarely many)
Family history of "arthritis"	30%	65%	65%
Back signs	2%	100%	45%
ANA-positive	30%–80%	0%	0%
RF-positive	15%	0%	0%
HLA-B27-positive	15%	90%	72%

the diagnosis of SA, it must be noted that enthesitis occurs occasionally in JRA and even in systemic lupus erythematosus (SLE) and could be confused with other noninflammatory states such as Osgood-Schlatter disease and Sever's disease. The ultimate diagnosis of a child with idiopathic SEA syndrome will not be known until the development of the full clinical syndrome over the course of time. Conceivably, the disease will remit in some children and they will never develop a diagnosable seronegative SA. Others will have JRA or SLE. It seems probable, however, that most will develop JAS (Fig. 6-1).

Table 6-2 Overlapping Characteristics of the Spondyloarthropathies

	Enthesitis	Axial Arthritis	Peripheral Arthritis	B27 Positive	RF-Negative	Iritis	Skin	MM	GI
AS	+ + +	+ + +	+ + +	+ + +	+ + +	+	−	−	−
PsA	+	+ +	+ + +	+ +	+ + +	+	+ + +	−	−
IBD	+	+ +	+ + +	+	+ + +	+	+	+	+ + +
RS	+ +	+	+ + +	+ + +	+ + +	+	+	+	+ + +

AS, ankylosing spondylitis; PsA, Psoriatic arthritis; IBD, inflammatory bowel disease; RS, Reiter's syndrome; MM, mucous membrane lesions; GI, gastrointestinal symptoms.
−, absent; +, present in up to 25%; + +, present in up to 50%; + + +, present in up to 75%; + + + +, present in up to 100%.

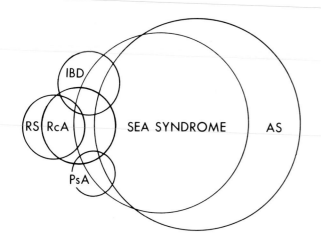

Fig. 6-1 Diagnostic considerations in children with the SEA syndrome. AS, ankylosing spondylitis; IBD, inflammatory bowel disease; PsA, psoriatic arthritis; RCA, reactive arthritis; RS, Reiter's syndrome.

JUVENILE ANKYLOSING SPONDYLITIS

Definitions

Calin defines AS as "an inflammatory arthritis that always affects the sacroiliac joints and less commonly the extra-pelvic spine and peripheral joints."[4] Such a definition does not appear to be entirely appropriate in childhood. Juvenile ankylosing spondylitis is characterized by the features listed in Table 6-4 and can be defined as a chronic inflammatory arthritis of the peripheral and axial skeleton, frequently accompanied by enthesitis, not accompanied by rheumatoid factor seropositivity, and having a genetic basis. It is likely that the sacroiliac joints are eventually affected in all children with JAS, and for the purpose of this discussion, radiologic evidence of sacroiliitis is required for the diagnosis of definite JAS. It is not entirely clear that JAS and AS are the same diseases, although they are undoubtedly closely related.

Epidemiology

INCIDENCE AND PREVALENCE

Juvenile ankylosing spondylitis is much less frequently recognized in childhood than is JRA. Early disease, in particular, is often difficult to differentiate from JRA, and therefore children with early JAS may

Table 6-5 Rome Criteria for the Diagnosis of Ankylosing Spondylitis[a]

Low back pain and stiffness for more than 3 months that is not relieved by rest
Pain and stiffness in the thoracic region
Limited motion in the lumbar spine
Limited chest expansion
History or evidence of iritis or its sequelae

[a] Ankylosing spondylitis is present if bilateral sacroiliitis on x-ray examination is associated with any of the clinical criteria listed.
(From Kellgren et al.,[7] with permission.)

be diagnosed as having JRA. The criteria for the diagnosis of AS in adults (Tables 6-5 and 6-6) are not applicable to the younger age group for a number of reasons: data for some of the physical measurements are not available in children (chest expansion), or, if available (back range),[5] have not yet been tested in a population of children with JAS. The fact that peripheral joint disease precedes axial skeleton disease by years in many children precludes an early diagnosis where abnormalities in axial skeleton motion or radiologic changes are essential diagnostic features. In adults, as well, the limitation of spine and chest motion may reflect disease duration and is therefore of limited help in facilitating early diagnosis.[6] There remains a clear need for the development and testing of diagnostic criteria for JAS in children.

Estimates of the prevalence of AS in adults range widely. Using modified New York criteria, including radiographic

Table 6-6 New York Criteria for Diagnosis of Ankylosing Spondylitis

1. Limitation of lumbar spine motion in all three planes
2. Pain or history of pain at the dorsolumbar junction or lumbar spine
3. Limitation of chest expansion to 2.5 cm or less at the level of the fourth intercostal space

Definite AS
    Grade 3–4 bilateral sacroiliitis on x-ray examination with at least one clinical criterion
    Grade 3–4 unilateral or grade 2 bilateral sacroiliitis on x-ray examination with criterion 1 or criterion 2 and 3

Probable AS
    Grade 3–4 bilateral sacroiliitis without clinical criteria

(From Bennett and Wood,[8] with permission.)

evidence of sacroiliitis, Carter et al.[9] determined a prevalence of 129 per 100,000 in an American population of northern European extraction. This number undoubtedly represents a minimum estimate. On the basis of the prevalence of HLA-B27 and the frequency of radiographic evidence of sacroiliitis in the B27-positive population, Calin[4] estimated the prevalence of AS to be 1,000 per 100,000 (1 percent). Although this estimate includes asymptomatic (disease-free) individuals, it also excludes 8 percent of the AS population who do not have HLA-B27 and may be a more accurate reflection of the prevalence of the entire spectrum of AS.

In a large retrospective study, 8.6 percent of adults with AS were found to have had onset of disease in childhood.[8] The prevalence of JAS in children could thus be extrapolated to be from 0.01 to 0.08 percent (11–86 per 100,000). If this admittedly rough estimate is near the mark, the prevalence of JAS is close to or may exceed that of JRA! This possibility is startling when one considers the relative infrequency with which the disease is recognized in childhood. Ladd et al.[10] reported 15 patients with onset of JAS prior to age 17 years seen during a 10-year period. In all patients, radiologic changes (sclerosis, erosions, fusion of SI joints) confirmed the diagnosis. During the same period, 208 children with JRA were seen in the same clinic. A greater awareness of the possibility of onset of JAS in childhood and its clinical and laboratory differentiation from JRA will result in an increase in the proportion of children with chronic arthritis in this category.

SEX RATIO

As clinically observed, JAS has a much higher frequency in boys than in girls (Table 6-7). This disproportionate representation of boys may not accurately represent the actual occurrence of the disease, however. The strong correlation between JAS and HLA-B27 and the equal distribution of this antigen in males and females suggest that JAS may be as common in girls as in boys. Furthermore, in radiographic surveys of adult blood donors with HLA-B27, sacroiliitis was as common in women as in men.[18] The manifestations in the female may be less severe,[19] and women with AS may have more peripheral and less axial disease.[20] These observations may account for the relative infrequency with which the diagnosis is made in women.

AGE AT ONSET

JAS usually has its onset in late childhood or adolescence, although instances of onset in younger children have been recorded.[21,22] Using data derived from three studies,[10,11,23] a graphic depiction of age at onset of JAS in the less-than-16-year age group is shown in Figure 6-2. The distribution appears to be homogeneous and presumably is continuous with that described in adult populations, suggesting that, at least on this basis, the disease as seen in adults is the same as that in children.

Genetic Considerations

There is often a striking familial occurrence of AS and related diseases in adults and children.[24] A pedigree documenting this occurrence is shown in Figure

Table 6-7 Sex Ratio and Frequency of HLA-B27 among Patients with JAS

Authors	Male	Female	M:F Ratio	% HLA-B27 Positive
Ladd et al.[10]	13	2	6.5:1	nd[a]
Bywaters[11]	50	11	4.5:1	nd
Kleinman et al.[12]	24	4	6.0:1	nd
Schaller[13]	18	2	9.0:1	nd
Hafner[14]	67	4	16.8:1	94
Veys et al.[15]	17	3	5.7:1	95
Sturrock et al.[16]	13	4	3.2:1	82
Edmonds et al.[17]	14	1	14.0:1	93
Overall	216	31	6.9:1	91

[a] nd, not determined.

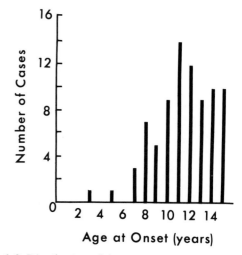

Fig. 6-2 Distribution of the age at onset in JAS. Data obtained from published series.[10,11,23]

6-3.[150] Ansell and her colleagues[25] have noted that 6 of 12 monozygous twin pairs concordant for arthritis had HLA-B27, making the diagnosis of JAS likely (although not certain). Older epidemiologic studies in adults suggest that AS occurs 10 to 20 times as frequently in all relatives of patients with AS and 50 to 80 times as frequently in their siblings.[26,27]

The studies by Brewerton et al.[26] and Schlosstein et al.[27] (and subsequently by many others) showed that the HLA-B27 was strongly associated with AS in adults. Evidence to date suggests that this association is no less strong in JAS (Table 6-7). Recent studies of HLA-B27 have demonstrated restriction fragment length polymorphisms that have even more striking associations with AS.[28,29] Although the HLA-B27 association is the strongest, there is also an increase in HLA-A2, an association that is shared with other chronic arthritides of childhood,[30] and that has been noted in adults with AS. Woodrow has calculated by meta-analysis a relative risk of spondylitis in HLA-A2-positive patients of 1.72.[31] Reports of increased HLA-A28 in HLA-B27-positive patients with AS suggest that this antigen, too, may contribute to disease susceptibility.[32,33] The reported increased frequency of Cw1 and Cw2[34,35] probably reflects a linkage disequilibrium with HLA-B27. There are no known HLA-DR or HLA-D associations with JAS (or AS), in contrast to JRA and adult RA.

There are no data specifically related to geographic and racial differences in JAS. The low incidence of AS in North American blacks[36] and in Japanese[37] and the high frequency in the Haida Indians of Pacific Canada[38] reflect, in part, the frequency of HLA-B27 in these populations. Other factors may be significant, however, since this antigen occurs in only 50 percent of American blacks with AS[39] and in from 65 to 90 percent of Japanese with AS.[37]

Etiology and Pathogenesis

There is no known cause of JAS. The strong association with HLA-B27 suggests that a genetically determined mechanism is important. The clinical, genetic, and epidemiologic similarities of JAS to diseases such as Reiter's syndrome and reactive arthritis in which enteric or genitourinary tract bacterial infections are known to play a triggering role suggest an infectious etiology, although none has been proved. Other lines of evidence also support a role for bacterial infection in the etiology of SA. The reactivity of synovial fluid lymphocytes to ureaplasmal and other microbial antigens has been shown to correlate with the specificity of bacterial isolates in some adult patients with chronic arthritis.[40] Recurring, but as yet inconclusive, reports of an association between HLA-B27 and *Klebsiella* species in adults with AS suggest a role for these organisms. Some investigators have shown increased fecal carriage of *Klebsiella pneumoniae* in patients with active AS compared to those with inactive disease or normal controls.[41-44] The mechanism known as molecular mimicry, in which an epitope is shared by some HLA-B27 molecules and some bacterial species, has been suggested as the mechanism by which this association confers a pathogenic effect (Ch. 2).

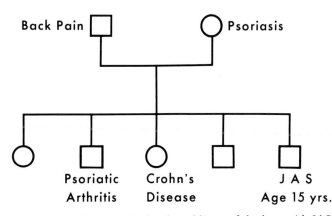

Fig. 6-3 Familial spondyloarthropathies. In this family, siblings of the boy with JAS have psoriatic arthritis and Crohn's disease. His father has back pain of unknown cause and his mother has psoriasis without arthritis. (From Petty and Malleson,[150] with permission.)

Table 6-8 Joints Affected at Onset of JAS

Authors	n	Number of Patients with Disease at Onset Affecting Peripheral Joints				
		Axial Skeleton	Proximal	Distal	Upper Limb	Lower Limb
Schaller et al.[23]	7	1	2	4	1	5
Ladd et al.[10]	15	7	0	8	1	7
Riley et al.[45]	28[a]	2	7	18	n/a	n/a
Kleinman et al.[12]	28	9	18	4	0	22
Hafner[14]	71	n/a	n/a	n/a	18	65
Total	149	19	27	34	20[b]	99[b]
(%)		(24)	(35)	(44)	(16.5)	(81.8)

[a] One patient not categorized.
[b] Out of 121.
n/a, not available.

Clinical Characteristics

ARTHRITIS

The presenting joint symptoms that have been recorded in the largest reported series of JAS are summarized in Table 6-8. The initial musculoskeletal symptoms are often difficult to localize and include pain in the buttocks, groin, thigh, and heels or around the shoulders. The vague quality and localization of the pain and its frequent spontaneous disappearance early in the disease are sources of delay and confusion in diagnosis.

In contrast to AS in adults, JAS in children seldom causes symptoms of axial skeleton disease at onset; only 24 percent of the reported children (Table 6-8) had pain, stiffness, or limitation of motion of the lumbosacral spine or SI joints. Peripheral joint symptoms occurred at onset in 79 percent of children. With the exception of one report in which hip disease was common at onset,[12] distal joints are affected more commonly than proximal joints. All reports agree that lower extremity joints are much more commonly affected at onset (82 percent) than are upper extremity joints (16 percent). In most instances, the number of joints involved is small (four or fewer), although approximately 25 percent of children have a polyarticular onset. Aside from the number and distribution of the affected joints, there is nothing to distinguish the peripheral joint disease clinically from that of JRA.

SI and lumbosacral spine tenderness may be elicited by pressure over one or both SI joints, or by compression or distraction of these joints. Pain or stiffness in the lumbar spine, often with loss of the normal lumbar lordosis, and flattening of the lumbosacral spine on forward flexion or loss of hyperextention of the spine may signify early axial skeleton disease.

The early course is remitting and frequently mild. Often only in retrospect are the musculoskeletal complaints recognized as harbingers of JAS. Almost half of the children have four or fewer joints affected during the course of the disease (Table 6-9), and even in those who exceed this number, it is uncommon to have more than six or seven inflamed joints. It should be noted that with few exceptions, patients with JAS eventually develop peripheral joint disease, if they do not have it at onset. Lower extremity predominance remains the rule throughout the disease, with hips, knees, ankles, and feet much more commonly affected than upper extremity joints. Shoulders are not uncommonly affected, however, and even the temporomandibular joint may become inflamed. The

Table 6-9 Peripheral Joints Affected during the Course of JAS

Author	n	Number of Joints Affected during Disease		
		0	1–4	>4
Schaller et al.[23]	7	0	5	2
Ladd et al.[10]	15	1	5	9
Kleinman et al.[12]	28	3	16	9
Hafner[14]	71	0	26	45
Total	121	4	52	65
(%)		(3)	(43)	(54)

least commonly affected joints are the small joints of the hand. Symptoms of pain or tenderness at the symphysis pubis, ischial tuberosities, and costochondral junctions, although infrequent, support the diagnosis of JAS. Pain at costosternal and sternoclavicular joints and sternomanubrium, often in conjunction with tenderness over the proximal clavicle, may be associated with significant impairment of chest expansion. In the series of Schaller et al.[23] five of seven patients had decreased chest expansion. Ansell noted that the mean interval from onset of symptoms to radiographic sacroiliitis was 6.5 years (range 1 to 15 years) and that back limitation was not detected until 11 to 33 years after onset of symptoms.[22]

ENTHESITIS

Enthesitis is a characteristic early manifestation of JAS. Pain and tenderness at the insertion of the Achilles tendon into the calcaneus, insertion of the patellar ligament into the tibial tuberosity or the patella, insertion of the quadriceps muscles into the patella, and insertion of the plantar fascia into the calcaneus, metatarsal heads, and base of the fifth metatarsal seem to occur with greater frequency than in adult onset AS. Inflammation at these sites frequently produces severe pain, which may be the child's single most important complaint.

SYSTEMIC DISEASE

Constitutional manifestations at onset of JAS are rare; possibly 5 to 10 percent of patients have fever. Other systemic signs, such as diarrhea or urethritis, suggest Reiter's syndrome or the arthropathy of inflammatory bowel disease.

Acute Iritis

The iritis of AS is characterized by a red, painful, photophobic eye. It frequently recurs and usually leaves no ocular residua. Iritis rarely preceeds the onset of musculoskeletal complaints. Acute iritis is said to occur in 20 percent of adults with AS, particularly in those with peripheral joint involvement, but may be less common in JAS. In the series of Ladd et al.,[10] 1 of the 15 patients developed acute iritis, and in the series of Schaller et al., 2 of 20 developed this complication.[13] However, Hafner recorded acute iritis in 14 percent of 71 patients with JAS,[14] and Ansell noted acute iritis in 27 percent of a group of 77 patients with sacroiliitis of childhood onset.[22] These higher figures may reflect a longer follow-up period.

Cardiovascular Disease

Cardiovascular disease is very uncommon in JAS, although severe aortic valve insufficiency has been reported in at least five patients,[46–49] and in one patient with sacroiliitis and Crohn's disease.[22] The apparently lower frequency of such complications in JAS may reflect the fact that follow-up has been of much shorter duration than in adults, in whom cardiac disease develops in approximately 5 percent of cases an average of 15 years after onset of spondylitis.[50]

Pulmonary Disease

Although diminished chest expansion and resultant decreased vital capacity are not infrequent, clinical parenchymal pulmonary disease is rare. In the large review of Rosenow et al.,[51] 1.3 percent of 2,080 adults with AS had pleuropulmonary disease with apical pleural thickening. No data relating to pleuropulmonary disease in JAS are available.

Nervous System Complications

Central nervous system disease rarely occurs in JAS. Subluxation of the atlantoaxial joint leading to severe cervico-occipital pain has been reported in one boy with JAS.[52] The cauda equina syndrome, caused by bony impingement on the cauda equina and characterized by weakness of the sphincters of bowel and bladder, saddle anesthesia, and leg weakness, occurs in adults with AS but has not been reported in JAS. The spinal cord may be injured as a result of fracture through the ankylosed spine after minor injury in adults with AS,[53] but such complications have not been reported in children.

Renal Disease

Renal abnormalities in JAS are very uncommon. Renal papillary necrosis, thought to be secondary to nonsteroidal anti-inflammatory drugs (NSAIDs), has been reported.[54] Immunoglobulin A (IgA) nephropathy, occasionally with uveitis,[55] has also been noted in 15 adults with AS or other seronegative spondyloarthropathies.[56] Most have elevated serum IgA; some have hypertension and impaired renal function.

Amyloidosis

Amyloidosis is extremely rare in the rheumatic diseases of childhood in North America. However, in the United Kingdom, Ansell documented amyloidosis in 3.8 percent of 77 patients with JAS and noted its association with severe peripheral arthropathy and persistently elevated ESR.[22]

Diagnosis

MUSCULOSKELETAL EXAMINATION

The diagnosis of JAS depends on careful clinical observation, often over several years. The musculoskeletal examination can be divided into three parts: (1) examination of the peripheral joints, (2) examination of the entheses, and (3) examination of the joints of the axial skeleton, including those of the pelvis, spine, and chest.

Peripheral Joint Examination

The peripheral arthropathy of JAS may be indistinguishable from that of JRA, although the number and distribution of affected joints may provide helpful clues to the differentiation of these diseases. The arthritis of JAS is often asymmetrical. Small joints of the toes are seldom affected in JRA but are not uncommonly affected in JAS. Thus, for example, the presence of arthritis in the metatarsophalangeal (MTP) joint of the first toe, the ankle, and the knee, particularly in a boy, should strongly suggest a diagnosis of JAS. In contrast, symmetric disease of the small joints of the hands or polyarticular disease, particularly in a girl, is more likely to be the result of JRA.

Enthesitis

The most helpful feature in differentiating JAS and JRA is the presence of enthesitis, inflammation at the site of attachment of ligament, tendon, fascia, or capsule to bone.[57] A careful history and thorough, but gentle palpation of entheses may reveal evidence of past or present inflammation. The enthesitis is often remarkably discrete and painful. Marked tenderness at the 10, 2, and 6 o'clock positions at the patella, the tibial tuberosity, and the attachment of the Achilles tendon or plantar fascia to the calcaneus, or of the plantar fascia to the base of the fifth metatarsal or the heads of the first through fifth metatarsals, strongly supports a diagnosis of JAS. Tenderness is less com-

monly demonstrable at the greater trochanters of the femur, the superior anterior iliac spines, pubic symphysis, or ischial tuberosities, and seldom at entheses of the upper extremity (Figs. 6-4 to 6-6). Observation of stance and gait may indicate that the child stands or moves in such a way as to prevent pressure on inflamed entheses.

Axial Skeleton

Examination of the joints of the axial skeleton is central to the diagnosis of JAS. In patients with SI joint inflammation, pain may be elicited by direct pressure over the SI joint, compression of the pelvis, or distraction of the SI joint (Patrick's test). Examination of the back should first be directed at detecting asymmetry in the standing position. Abnormalities

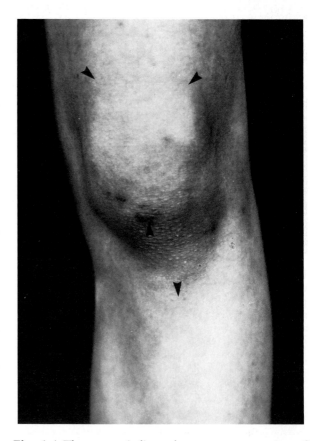

Fig. 6-4 The arrows indicate the most common sites of tenderness associated with enthesitis at the insertions of the quadriceps muscles to the patella and the insertion of the patellar ligament to the patella and to the tibial tuberosity. (From Petty and Malleson,[150] with permission.)

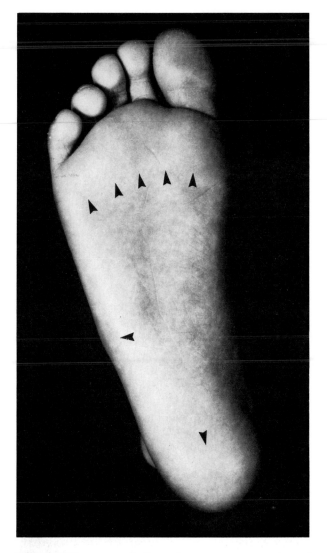

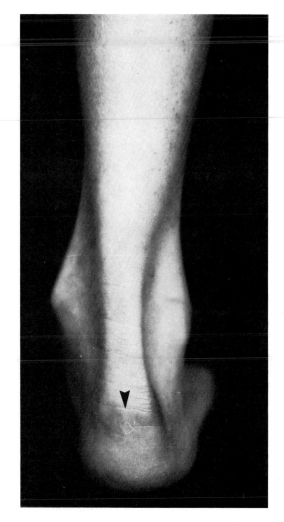

Fig. 6-5 The arrows indicate the most common sites of tenderness associated with enthesitis at the insertion of the plantar fascia to the calcaneus, base of the fifth metatarsal, and heads of the first through fifth metatarsals. (From Petty and Malleson,[150] with permission.)

Fig. 6-6 The arrow indicates the site of tenderness at the enthesis of the Achilles tendon as it inserts into the calcaneus. (From Petty and Malleson,[150] with permission.)

in contour such as loss of the normal lumbar lordosis or thoracic kyphosis are best seen while the patient is standing upright. The contour of the back on full forward flexion may show loss of the normal smooth curve in the lower part of the thoracolumbar spine (Fig. 6-7). Asymmetry of lateral flexion or rotation indicates unilateral facet joint disease, and loss of hyperextension of the spine is highly suggestive of spon-

dylitis. The rigid spine of long-standing AS is rarely seen in children.

Although observations of abnormalities of the contour of the back are often more informative than actual numerical measurements, sequential measurement of thoracolumbar spinal mobility is useful in documentating progression of disease. The Schober test as modified by Macrae and Wright[58] provides one such index (Figs. 6-8 and 6-9). With the child standing with the feet together, a line joining the dimples of Venus is used as a surface landmark for the lumbosacral junction. A mark is made 5 cm below (point *A*) and 10 cm above (point *B*) the lumbosacral junc-

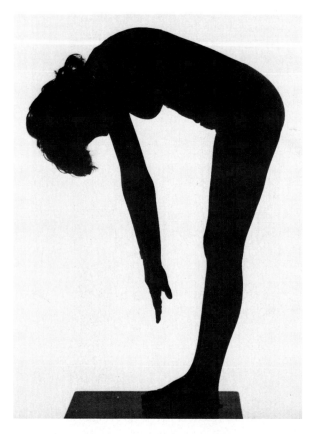

Fig. 6-7 A 15-year-old girl with a normal Schober test shown in the position of maximal forward flexion. Note the flattened back on this silhouette. Radiographs show bilateral sacroiliitis, but no abnormality of the lumbosacral spine.

tion. With the patient in maximal forward flexion and with the knees straight, the increase in distance between points *A* and *B* is used as an indicator of lumbosacral spine mobility. Normal values +1 SD are shown in Figure 6-10. Care should be exercised in application of these values since it is clear that there are large variations in normal at each age, and these measurements have not been adequately tested in children with musculoskeletal disease. In general, however, a Schober measurement of less than 6 cm (i.e., an increase from 15 to less than 21 cm) should be regarded with suspicion. Measurement of the distance from fingertips to floor on maximal forward flexion is often used to quantitate spinal motion but is poorly reproducible and does not correlate with the Schober measurement. Furthermore, finger-to-floor distance reflects hip as well as back flexion.

Pain in the costosternal and costovertebral joints may be elicited by palpation. Sternomanubrial tenderness sometimes occurs, but sternoclavicular pain is more common. Thoracic joint disease may be reflected in limitation of chest expansion. Normal thoracic excursion varies a great deal, and normal age- and sex-adjusted ranges have not been established. Sequential measurement of thoracic motion may be very useful in detecting progressive loss of range. In the adolescent, any thoracic excursion of less than 5 cm (maximum expiration to maximum inspiration, measured at the fourth intercostal space) should be regarded with caution. Even in the absence of symptoms, chest expansion in children with JAS may be restricted to 1 or 2 cm.

GENERAL PHYSICAL EXAMINATION

A complete physical examination should be an integral part of any rheumatologic evaluation and in children with JAS may provide important diagnostic information indicating the presence of complications such as iritis or cardiovascular disease. Furthermore, cutaneous, mucous membrane, gastrointestinal, or genitourinary abnormalities may influence the examiner to consider an alternative diagnosis among the other members of the SA group.

Laboratory Investigations

INFLAMMATORY INDEXES

There are few distinguishing laboratory features in JAS, although the indexes of inflammation are frequently elevated. Anemia is usually mild and characteristic of the anemia of chronic inflammation. White blood cell (WBC) counts are usually normal or moderately elevated, with normal differential counts. The platelet count and the erythrocyte sedimentation rate (ESR) are often elevated and may remain so for years. Very high values for the ESR (>100 mm/h Westergren method) are seen occasionally in JAS but should also alert the physician to the possibility of occult inflammatory bowel disease. Conversely, a normal ESR may accompany clinically active disease. Elevated immunoglobulin levels reflect inflammation, and selective deficiency of IgA has been reported.[59,60] High serum levels of IgA and C4[61] and of circulating immune complexes[62] in adults with AS suggest the presence of an immunoreactive state.

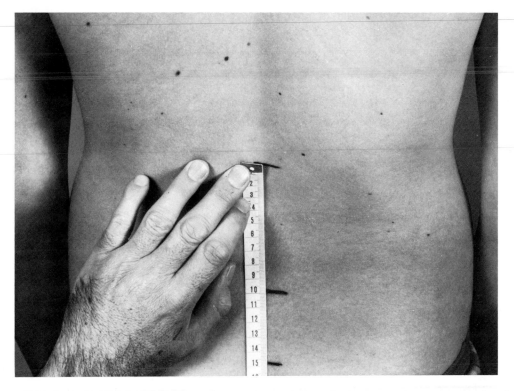

Fig. 6-8 Schober test. Measurement 10 cm above and 5 cm below the lumbosacral junction (the dimples of Venus) in the upright position.

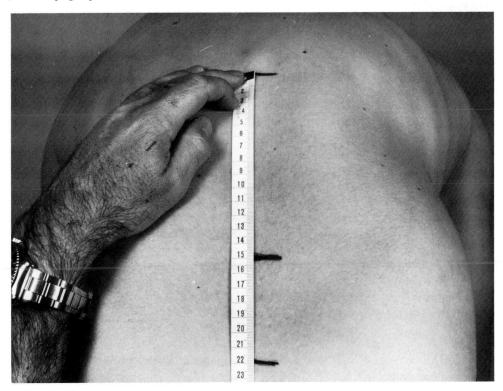

Fig. 6-9 Schober test. Measurement of the distance between the upper and lower marks when the child is bending forward.

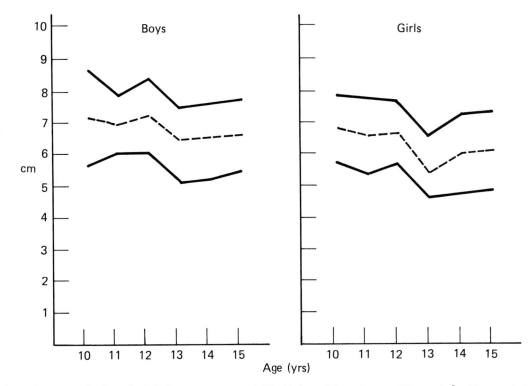

Fig. 6-10 Normal values for Schober test: mean ±1 SD. (Adapted from Moran HM et al.,[5] with permission.)

SEROLOGIC ABNORMALITIES

Characteristically, RF (IgM anti-IgG) detected by standard latex fixation techniques is always absent. IgG RF, demonstrable in some adults with AS,[63] has not been studied in JAS. ANAs do not occur in children with JAS, in marked contrast to their frequency in JRA. Occasional reports of the presence in adults with AS, of ANA reacting only with granulocytes[64] or chromosomes of *Drosophila*,[65] have not included children and have not been confirmed.

SYNOVIAL FLUID ANALYSIS

No specific studies of synovial fluid from children with JAS have been reported, but it is likely that changes are similar if not identical to those seen in AS, in which the differential is said to include more polymorphonuclear neutrophil leukocytes (PMNs) and fewer lymphocytes than in RA.[66] The predominant large mononuclear cell in AS synovial fluid is macrophage-derived, whereas in RA it is of lymphocytic origin.[67] Macrophages containing degen-erated polymorphs are more common in synovial fluid of patients with AS and related diseases such as Reiter's syndrome than in RA.[68] The biochemistry of the synovial fluid is similar to that in RA except that complement is usually normal[69] or increased.[22]

RADIOGRAPHIC EVALUATION

Radiographic demonstration of bilateral sacroiliitis is necessary to establish the unequivocal diagnosis of JAS (Table 6-10), although classic radiographic changes of bilateral sacroiliitis may not occur for several years after the onset of disease. The sacroiliac joint has some unique anatomic characteristics, an explanation of which will assist in understanding certain radiologic features. The sacral side of the joint is covered by hyaline cartilage, whereas the iliac side is protected by a thin layer of fibrocartilage. This difference may account for the higher frequency of abnormalities on the iliac side of the joint. Only the lower one-third to one-half of the SI joint is diarthrodial and enclosed in a synovial membrane; the upper portion

Table 6-10 Radiologic Characteristics of JAS

Sacroiliac arthritis (bilateral)
  Blurring of subchondral margins
  Erosions (iliac side first)
  Reactive sclerosis
  Joint space narrowing
  Late fusion
  Diffuse osteoporosis of pelvis

Enthesitis (calaneus, tibial tuberosity, etc.)
  Soft tissue edema
  Erosions at insertions
  Spur formation

Periostitis (metatarsals, proximal femur)
  Linear diaphyseal subperiosteal new bone deposition

Peripheral joints (knee, ankle, hip, etc.)
  Soft tissue swelling
  Accelerated ossification and epiphyseal overgrowth
  Joint space narrowing
  Erosion
  Bony fusion

Vertebral column[a]
  Vertebral epiphysitis (shining corners)
  Anterior vertebral squaring
  Anterior ligament calcification
  "Bamboo spine"

[a] Rare during childhood.

is a fibrous synostosis.[70] A single posteroanterior (PA) view of the pelvis may provide an adequate screening examination of the SI joints and minimizes radiation exposure, although stereoscopic, angulated (30°), or oblique views are preferred by some pediatric radiologists. Evaluation of the SI joints in children and adolescents is not easy, and a systematic approach should be used to look for pseudowidening, sclerosis, and fusion. Pseudowidening (erosions on one or both sides of the joint) occurs in the inferior, synovial portion of the joint. The lesion may appear initially as haziness of the bony margin, followed by dissolution of subchondral bone, giving a punched-out appearance. Early minimal changes may be unilateral. An osteoblastic reaction occurring on both sides of the joint results in increased density (reactive sclerosis (Fig. 6-11). Late changes may include fusion of the SI joints and generalized osteoporosis. Computed tomography of the SI joints may be very useful in documenting erosive disease,[71] especially if standard pelvic radiographic findings are inconclusive.

Tomograms at three levels through the synovial portion of the joint are sufficient to demonstrate all but the smallest erosions but should not be undertaken routinely (Fig. 6-12).

Radiographic changes in the lumbosacral spine are much less frequent and occur much later than do SI joint changes. Periostitis with deposition of new bone along the anterior margins of the vertebral border results first in the "shining corner" and then in flattening of the slightly concave anterior margin of the vertebral border. Syndesmophyte formation (Fig. 6-13), the hallmark of advanced disease in adults, is rare in children or adolescents but occurs during the adult years in those patients with juvenile onset of disease. Periostitis at the iliac crests or the inferior pubic rami and erosions at the symphysis pubis are very uncommon in children (Fig. 6-14).

Radiographic evaluation of entheses around the calcaneus and, rarely, the patella may show subtle changes in soft tissue density. Loss of the distinct margins of the Achilles tendon at its insertion, together with effacement of the triangular fat shadow, may be an early sign of inflammation. Erosion at the Achilles insertion and spur formation at the insertion of the plantar fascia into the calcaneus are best evaluated by a lateral radiograph of the calcaneus (Figs. 6-15 and 6-16).

Radionuclide scanning of the SI joints has little role in documentation of sacroiliitis in the child since the interpretation of this examination in the growing child is extremely difficult.

PATHOLOGY

Studies of the pathology of JAS have not been reported, but it is probable that there are changes similar to those of adult AS. It is generally stated that the synovitis and degree of cartilage erosion in peripheral joints are milder in AS than in adult RA.[72] The synovitis itself is virtually indistinguishable from that of RA, although there may be relatively more PMN leukocytes. Enthesitis, said by Ball et al. to be the hallmark of AS,[73] is characterized by a nonspecific inflammation. Granulation tissue, infiltrated with lymphocytes and plasma cells and causing localized osteitis, replaces the bony and cartilaginous attachment of the ligament or tendon. Repair of this lesion gives rise to a bony spur. When this process occurs at the insertion of the plantar fascia into the calcaneus,

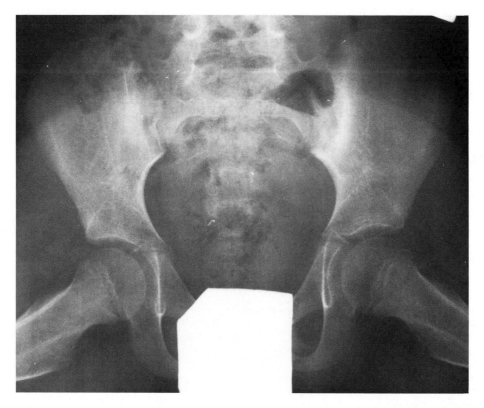

Fig. 6-11 Radiograph of the pelvis showing reactive sclerosis and irregularity of the inferior portion of the left SI joint.

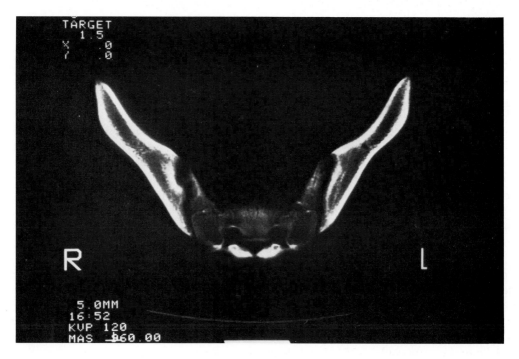

Fig. 6-12 Computed tomograph of the SI joints showing erosions ("psuedowidening") and sclerosis of the right SI joint.

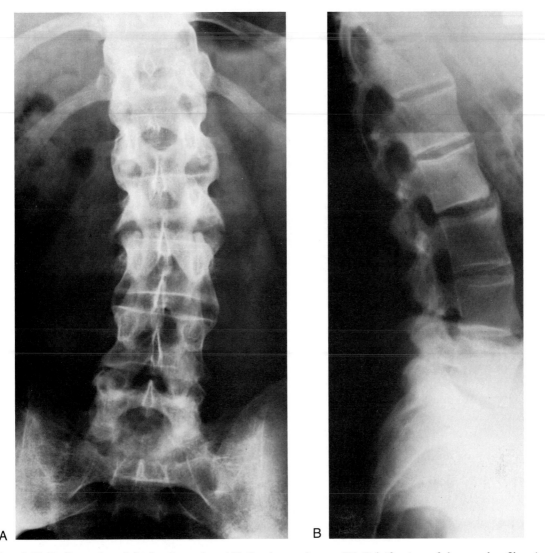

Fig. 6-13 Radiographs of the lumbar spine. (**A**) Syndesmophytes. (**B**) Calcification of the annulus fibrosis. The bamboolike appearance of the spine indicates long-standing JAS and is very uncommon in childhood.

it produces a calcaneal spur; when it occurs at the attachment of the outer fibers of the annulus fibrosus to the anterolateral aspects of the rim of the vertebral body, it gives rise to a syndesmophyte.

In the apophyseal joints and the SI joint, the characteristic pathologic changes are capsular and enchondral ossification. The early lesion in the SI joints appears to be subchondral inflammation leading to the formation of subchondral granulation tissue with few inflammatory cells. The surfaces of the SI joints appear to be only slightly affected, and pannus is not present.[74] Enchondral ossification of the iliac side of the SI joint accounts for the radiographic appearance

of erosions.[75] Ball comments: "As a rule, it seems that in any synovial joint in ankylosing spondylitis the outcome represents a balance of erosive synovitis and capsular and/or ligamentous ossification. In joints of low mobility the ossific process tends to be the dominant feature."[75]

Differential Diagnosis

The combination of peripheral joint inflammation, enthesitis, and SI or lumbosacral spine disease points strongly to a diagnosis of one of the seronegative spondyloarthritides. The presence of nonmusculo-

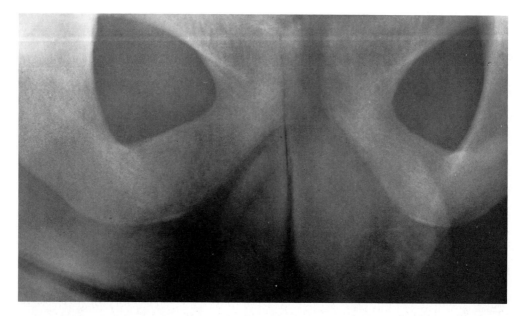

Fig. 6-14 Radiograph of the pelvis showing erosions of the symphysis pubis in a patient with early JAS.

skeletal manifestations usually indicates to which member of the group the patient belongs. In most instances, however, SI and back symptoms are absent, and the differentiation of JAS from JRA and other disorders of the entheses, back, and SI joints may be difficult (Table 6-4). To assist the reader in differentiating JAS from nonrheumatic diseases, brief descriptions of other disorders that can cause pain at the entheses, back, or SI joints are provided in the following discussion.

PAIN AT ENTHESES

The onset of pauciarticular arthritis of joints of the lower extremity together with enthesitis in an adolescent boy should always raise the possibility of JAS. Pain at entheses may arise from other causes, however, especially from excessive running or jogging. In such instances, however, the tenderness is often more diffuse than in the inflammation enthesitis of JAS. Persistent isolated pain at the Achilles insertion (Sever's disease) often follows a traction injury.

Occasionally, patients with JAS and prominent tibial tuberosity pain are regarded as having Osgood-Schlatter disease. This disorder, considered the result of an avulsion fracture of the developing tibial tubercle[76] or inflammation of the patellar tendon,[77] occurs most commonly in 10- to 15-year-old children. Boys are affected three times more commonly than girls, and the condition is bilateral in approximately 30 percent.[78] Swelling and pain over the tibial tubercle are aggravated by local pressure or running and

climbing. Radiographic studies show swelling of the soft tissue overlying the tibial tubercle. The disorder is self-limited in 90 percent of children, although a chronic condition associated with the development of a separate ossicle in the patellar ligament insertion may occur.[79] Osteochondritis of the inferior pole of the patella (Sinding-Larsen syndrome) may cause pain at that location. The co-existence of enthesitis at multiple sites usually eliminates these disorders from consideration. The absence of HLA-B27 may also be of assistance in differentiating these disorders from the inflammatory enthesitis of JAS.[80]

BONE PAIN

Pressure over bony prominences, such as the tibial tubercle and iliac crests, may produce pain in children with leukemia or bone tumors. In most instances, the pain of enthesitis is well localized, whereas the bone pain associated with infiltrative diseases is somewhat less discrete and is frequently more severe. Localized bone pain may result from osteomyelitis.

Pain in the back in the absence of an inflammatory arthropathy or enthesitis may be the presenting symptom in JAS or other spondyloarthropathies, although mechanical or inflammatory lesions may be responsible.

Spondylolysis and Spondylolisthesis

Spondylolysis, the congenital (or occasionally posttraumatic) discontinuity or elongation of the pars interarticularis of the posterior elements of the spine, may itself be

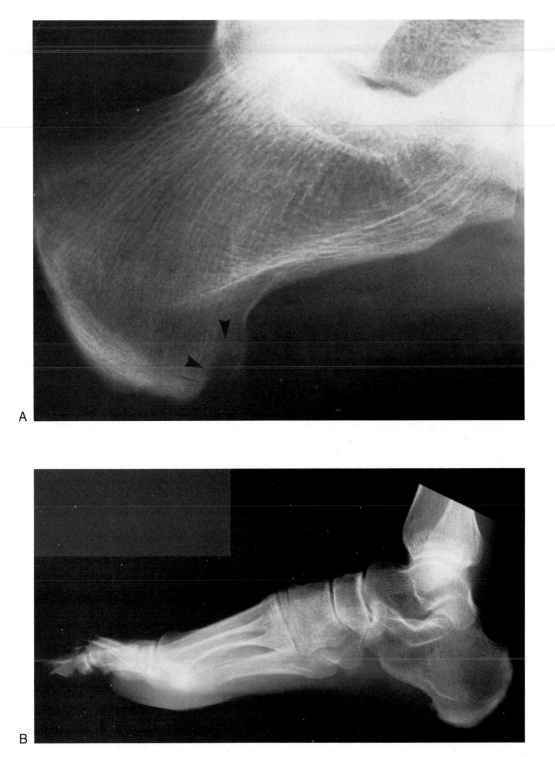

Fig. 6-15 Lateral radiograph of the calcaneus showing (**A**) erosion at the site of insertion of plantar fascia to calcaneus and (**B**) spur formation at the plantar fascia insertion to the calcaneus. (Part A from Petty and Malleson,[150] with permission.)

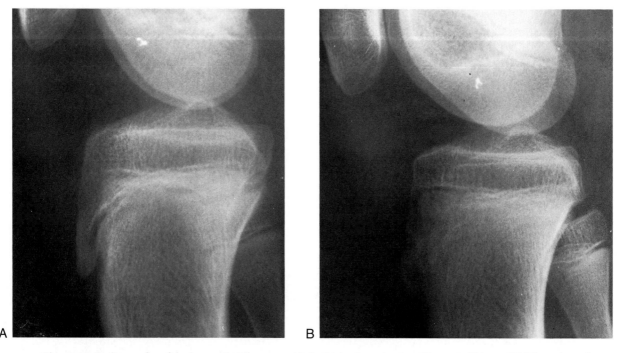

Fig. 6-16 Radiographs of the knee. (**A**) The normal left tibial tuberosity in a 15-year-old boy. (**B**) The enlarged, osteoporotic tibial tuberosity, the site of tender enthesitis in a boy with SEA syndrome.

associated with back pain in the active preadolescent child (Fig. 6-17). More commonly, however, it is asymptomatic. Spondylolysis may lead to the forward slipping of one vertebral body (usually L5) on the one below it. This condition, termed spondylolisthesis, usually causes low back pain radiating to the posterior thigh, with insidious onset in the 10- to 20-year age range. Standing or walking may aggravate the symptoms. Severe spondylolisthesis may be accompanied by impingement on the nerve roots of L5 and S1.[77]

Scheuermann's Disease

Scheuermann's disease (juvenile kyphosis) is a disorder associated with anterior wedging of one to three adjacent vertebral bodies by at least 5 degrees each[81] (Fig. 6-18). It may be somewhat more common in girls and is most frequently manifested in the 13- to 17-year age range, usually as a complaint by the patient or her parent of "round back" or poor posture. Pain is entirely absent in up to half of affected children, but in others there is aching pain with tenderness over the kyphosis. In 75 percent the kyphosis is thoracic, whereas in 25 percent it is thoracolumbar, or, rarely, lumbar.[77] A prominent fixed dorsal kyphosis with a compensatory increase in the lumbar lordosis is characteristic. Tightness of the pectoral and hamstring muscles

has been noted.[82] A standing lateral radiograph of the spine will reveal anterior vertebral wedging, irregularity of vertebral end-plates, and increased dorsal kyphosis.

Intervertebral Disc Herniation

Disc herniation is rare in childhood. A study of 17 affected children under age 16 years showed that almost three-quarters were boys.[83] Sixty percent had protrusion of L4, 35 percent of L5, and 5 percent of L3. Less than half had an abrupt onset of back or leg pain aggravated by bending, coughing, or sneezing. In over half, the onset of symptoms was insidious. Physical examination revealed gait abnormalities, limitation of straight leg raising, and, in 25 percent, weakness of the plantar flexors. Plain radiographs are seldom helpful, although the disc space is diminished in 20 percent of patients. Computed tomographic myelography with contrast MRI reveals the lesion. (See also the discussion of discitis in Ch. 12.)

SACROILIAC JOINT PAIN

Sacroiliac joint tenderness occurs in many patients with JAS, but septic sacroiliitis (Ch. 12) and familial Mediterranean fever (Ch. 14) also cause pain at this site.

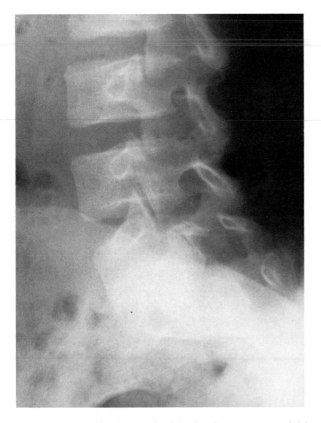

Fig. 6-17 Lateral radiograph of the lumbar spine in a child with low back pain. The discontinuity of the pars inter-articularis of L5 (the broken neck of the Scottie dog) is shown in this patient with spondylolysis.

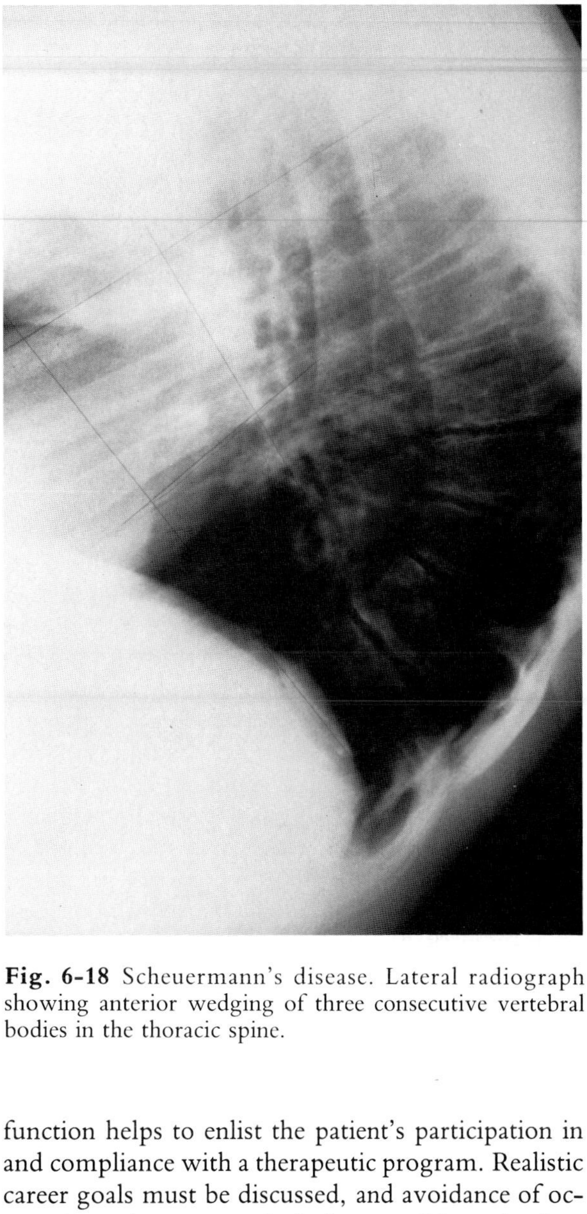

Fig. 6-18 Scheuermann's disease. Lateral radiograph showing anterior wedging of three consecutive vertebral bodies in the thoracic spine.

Treatment

GENERAL APPROACH

Children with JAS have frequently had undiagnosed symptoms for months or years or have been diagnosed as having JRA or other disorders. Careful explanation of the correct diagnosis is therefore essential so that the child and family can appreciate the chronicity of the disease, possible complications, and need for long-term anti-inflammatory medication, physical therapy, and medical follow-up. The good overall long-term prognosis should be emphasized, particularly in the adolescent, who may regard the diagnosis of JAS as the end of his or her recreational, social, educational, and career goals. An understanding of the importance of medication and exercise in preventing debilitating disease and maintaining good function helps to enlist the patient's participation in and compliance with a therapeutic program. Realistic career goals must be discussed, and avoidance of occupations that are particularly stressful to the low back and leg joints should be emphasized. At the same time, the child should be encouraged to participate as fully as possible in the social and recreational peer-group activities appropriate to his or her age. The genetic implications of JAS should be fully discussed to ensure that the patient has an accurate and balanced understanding of the risk of transmitting JAS to offspring. The overall risk that an HLA-B27 heterozygous patient with JAS will have a male child with the disease is approximately 5 percent. The risk of a female child having JAS is even lower.

ANTI-INFLAMMATORY MEDICATION

It is important to attempt to control the inflammatory disease with anti-inflammatory drugs. Aspirin in therapeutic doses is useful in some children. The drug should be given with food in three to four doses a day in amounts sufficient to ensure a blood level of at least 25 mg/dl (1.8 mmol/L) when measured 2 h after a dose is given, providing signs or symptoms of toxicity do not occur. Toxicity or therapeutic failure after 1 to 3 months of aspirin administration should prompt the addition or substitution of another NSAID. It is a clinical impression that far fewer children with JAS than JRA respond satisfactorily to aspirin. Tolmetin sodium (25 to 30 mg/kg/day) in three divided doses with food is a good alternative, and other agents such as naproxen may be worthwhile, although no studies exist to support their usefulness in JAS. Indomethacin (1 to 2 mg/kg/day) in three divided doses with food often provides remarkable improvement in many children with JAS. Toxicity to indomethacin is common, however, and the drug must be used cautiously, beginning with low doses. Headaches, epigastric pain, and changes in ability to pay attention occur in 20 to 30 percent of children and frequently necessitate cessation of therapy. Indomethacin suppositories are probably of some use as a substitute, if upper gastrointestinal (GI) tract symptoms result from oral administration of the drug. Sustained-release capsules provide good overnight analgesic effect. Phenylbutazone and oxyphenbutazone have a very limited role in pediatrics because of their toxicity and should be used only in patients with severe disease that is unresponsive to other drugs. Sulfasalazine has emerged as an option in the treatment of RA,[84,85] and preliminary studies in children with JRA indicate that it may be useful in that disease as well.[86] Anecdotal reports indicate that it has a useful role in the child with JAS. Slow-acting anti-inflammatory agents have been used very little in JAS, and, in general, gold salts and penicillamine are not recommended. Local injections of corticosteroids at sites of enthesitis may occasionally be useful, particularly at the plantar fascia-calcaneal junction. Topical steroids are used in the management of acute iritis, and occasionally oral prednisone is needed to control severe arthritis and enthesitis.

PHYSICAL AND OCCUPATIONAL THERAPY

Physical therapy should be directed toward regaining lost range in peripheral joints and preventing loss of range and poor functional positioning in the spine and chest. Careful daily active bending (forward, lateral, and backward flexion) and deep-breathing exercises will help preserve range. Many young patients with JAS breathe predominantly with the diaphragm and have to be taught to use the intercostal muscles. Strengthening of abdominal and back muscles should be undertaken cautiously. Swimming is a form of physical activity that can be used to augment these specific exercises.

Painful enthesitis may be dramatically helped by the use of custom-made insoles. Careful fitting of the insole to take pressure off the plantar aspects of the heel and MTP joints is quite useful. The insole also helps to support the fatty cushion under the heal to relieve pain at that site. If the Achilles insertions alone are painful, use of a slightly higher heel may also be of help. Trials of ultrasound or transcutaneous nerve stimulation for pain at the insertion of the plantar fascia into the calcaneous are sometimes beneficial. Enthesitis is often resistant to therapy and may be an important functionally limiting aspect of the disease.

SURGERY

There is little role for orthopedic surgery in the management of the child with JAS, although in later life, joint reconstruction and replacement are invaluable contributions to function and quality of life of the patient with severely damaged joints. After hip joint replacement, bony ankylosis can occur as a result of exuberant overgrowth of bone around the prosthesis.[22]

Course and Prognosis

Long-term follow-up is essential to the care of the child with JAS. Subtle changes in range of motion of the thorax or back should be detected as early as possible. The support and counsel of a team of health professionals, including physical and occupational therapists, nurses, social workers, and physicians, will help to provide optimal care. Accurate data on the outcome of children with JAS are not yet available, although for most the prognosis is probably good. In one study, however,[87] outcome in JAS was worse than in AS. The persistence of peripheral joint disease may be more common in children than in adults,[87,88] and hip disease in particular appears to be associated with a poor functional outcome.[86] Iritis almost never leaves significant residua. Aortitis is rare but could contribute to late morbidity and mortality.

PSORIATIC ARTHROPATHIES

Definitions

Juvenile psoriatic arthritis (JPsA) is said to occur if chronic inflammatory arthritis before the age of 16 years is preceded by, accompanied by, or followed within 15 years by psoriasis. Although there is no universally accepted definition of this disorder, that cited previously has been used by the authors of the two largest published series of psoriatic arthritis in childhood.[89,90] Lack of precision in diagnosis is inherent in such a definition, and in order to provide a more standardized framework within which to make the diagnosis of JPsA, we have used the definition outlined in Table 6-11. The classification of Moll and Wright is most frequently used to categorize patients

Table 6-11 Vancouver Criteria for the Diagnosis of Psoriatic Arthritis in Childhood[a]

Definite psoriatic arthritis
  Arthritis with typical psoriatic rash

  Arthritis with three of the four following minor criteria
    Dactylitis
    Nail pitting or onycholysis
    Psoriasislike rash
    Family history (1st- or 2nd-degree relatives) of psoriasis

Probable psoriatic arthritis
  Arthritis with 2 of the 4 minor criteria listed

[a] The clinical manifestations need not be present simultaneously.
(Adapted from Southwood et al.,[91] with permission.)

Table 6-12 Classification of Psoriatic Arthritis

Onset Type	Characteristics	Percentage
Monarticular or asymmetric pauciarticular	Fingers, toes, dactylitis; often becomes polyarticular	70
Symmetric rheumatoidlike	Polyarticular, large and small joints, including DIP joints	15
Predominant DIP[a] joint	Almost always with nail disease	5
Spondylitis	Peripheral arthritis with SIJ[b] disease	5
Arthritis mutilans	Severely deforming, often with SIJ disease and ankylosis	5

[a] DIP, distal interphalangeal.
[b] SIJ, sacroiliac joint.
(Adapted from Moll and Wright,[92] with permission.)

with psoriatic arthritis[92] (Table 6-12). The relative proportions of each type of psoriatic arthritis in the child are probably similar to those seen in the adult. By far the most commonly recognized subset consists of children with asymmetric pauciarticular disease affecting small as well as large joints, often accompanied by pitting of the nails.

Epidemiology

INCIDENCE AND PREVALENCE

Although psoriasis is a common disease, affecting 1 to 2 percent of the white population[93]; has onset in childhood in one-third of patients[94]; and, in 5 to 7 percent, is accompanied by arthritis (at least in adults),[95] psoriatic arthritis is infrequently diagnosed in childhood. Since the skin disease not uncommonly follows the articular disease, early cases may be diagnosed as JRA or JAS (Table 6-13). Sills has reported making a diagnosis of JPsA in 24 children during a 10-year period, during which JRA was diagnosed in 271 children.[96] In other studies JPsA constituted 2 percent of a group of 223 children with juvenile chronic arthritis (EULAR criteria),[97] and in Vancou-

Table 6-13 Childhood Psoriatic Arthritis: Summary of Reported Series

	Lambert[89]	Calabro[103]	Sills[96]	Shore[90]	Wesolowska[104]
No. of patients	43	12	24	60	21
Male:female	11:32	5:7	7:17	35:25	13:8
Age at onset (yr)					
Joint disease	9.3	n/a	10	11	n/a
Skin disease	10.4	12	11	8.8	n/a
Disease sequence					
Psoriasis first (%)	40	67	33	42	33
Arthritis first (%)	53	33	58	43	62
Simultaneous onset (%)	7	0	9	15	5
Pauci onset (<5 joints) (%)	55	42	58	73	86
Poly onset (>4 joints) (%)	45	58	42	27	14
DIP joints affected (%)	21	50	62	42	10
Sacroiliitis (%)	28	17	29	47[a]	100[a]
Nail changes (%)	70	92	83	77	86
Uveitis (%)	9	0	13	8	14

[a] Only selected patients had pelvic radiographs.
n/a, not available.

ver, children with arthritis and psoriasis constitute one of every seven or eight children with chronic arthritis (unpublished). On the basis of the population studies noted previously, the prevalence of JPsA would be expected to be from 10 to 15 cases per 100,000, making it approximately one-fifth as common as JRA.

SEX RATIO

JPsA is unique among the spondyloarthropathies because it is more common in girls than in boys (1.2:1) (Table 6-13), unlike adult PsA, which is slightly more common in males. These differences could reflect differences in the relative prevalences of the types of psoriatic arthritis in the two age groups.

AGE AT ONSET

JPsA can begin in children less than 1 year of age, although the onset of psoriasis is often slightly later (10 to 11 years) (Table 6-13).

Genetics

There is often a history of psoriasis, PsA, or another of the spondyloarthropathies in relatives of children with psoriatic arthritis. Lambert et al.[89] noted a family history of psoriasis in 40 percent and of ar-

thritis in 21 percent of children with psoriatic arthritis. Associations with antigens of the histocompatibility system have been demonstrated, but the relationships are much more complex than in JAS. HLA-B27 is associated with the spondylitic type of psoriatic arthritis, but not with the other forms. Lambert et al. noted that 1 of 19 children with peripheral PsA had HLA-B27, a normal prevalence, whereas 3 of 8 (37.5 percent) with psoriatic spondylitis had this antigen.[89] A number of studies of histocompatibility antigens in adult psoriatic arthritis have given somewhat inconsistent results, probably reflecting differences in subgroup composition of each study group. Psoriasis unaccompanied by arthritis is associated with HLA-B17 and HLA-Cw6, and possibly HLA-DR7.[98] In studies of PsA in adults, increases have been noted in A1,[99] Aw26, B38, and DR7.[100] The most consistent associations, however, have been with B17,[98,99] B27,[98,99,101] and Cw6.[98,101] When the HLA distribution is analyzed by subset of psoriatic arthritis, B27 is consistently associated with spondylitis,[98,99,101] B38 and B39 appear to be related to polyarthritis, and DR7 is associated with peripheral joint disease,[99,101] more severe disease in one study,[99] and milder disease in another in association with B7 and B13.[98] Symmetric peripheral arthritis is also related to HLA-B17; asymmetric pauciarthritis, enthesitis, and dactylitis are associated with HLA-B38. These data reflect adult onset PsA; there are no comparable studies for childhood onset disease. These associations should therefore be viewed as tentative.

Etiology and Pathogenesis

The etiology of psoriatic arthritis, like that of psoriasis, is unknown. The pathogenic relationship among skin, nail, and joint diseases is also unknown. A relationship to infection is suspected but unproved. Shore and Ansell[90] noted onset of arthritis immediately following chickenpox in three children; we have observed the same phenomenon in one child. Preceding streptococcal infection has also been implicated.[102]

Clinical Characteristics

ARTHRITIS

The arthropathy most commonly associated with psoriasis in children is a scattered, asymmetric oligoarthritis of large and small joints. The joints most commonly affected in JPsA are shown in Table 6-14. It may begin as arthritis in a single joint such as the knee and be indistinguishable from monarticular JRA. The onset of arthritis in a single *small* joint, in contrast, should alert the physician to the possibility of JPsA, since isolated small joint disease, particularly of the toes, is uncommon in JRA. The arthritis may be quite florid, with erythema of the overlying skin, suggesting sepsis or even gout. The characteristic dactylitis, resulting from inflammation of the flexor

Table 6-14 Joints Affected in Juvenile Psoriatic Arthritis

Joint	Initial (%)	Cumulative (%)
Knee	53	77
PIP finger	28	40
PIP/DIP toe	25	45
Ankle	21	63
Wrist	11	62
Elbow	10	43
Hindfoot	8	38
MCP	8	53
DIP finger	8	42
MTP	7	33
Cervical spine	7	32
Hip	5	38
Sternoclavicular	0	15

(Adapted from Shore and Ansell,[90] with permission.)

tendon sheath, produces a sausagelike swelling of a toe or finger and is particularly suggestive of psoriatic arthritis (Fig. 6-19). Tenosynovitis at other sites, particularly the flexors of the wrist and dorsiflexors of the ankle, is often observed.[96]

Other patterns of arthritis are seen less commonly in JPsA, and arthritis mutilans is especially rare. Predominant distal interphalangeal joint disease is also unusual, although inflammation of these joints together with other small joints of the hands is not uncommon in polyarticular JRA. Sacroiliitis occurs in 25 percent of children with JPsA,[89,90] and arthritis of the cervical spine develops less commonly.[89] As in other seronegative spondyloarthropathies, axial skeleton disease usually follows peripheral joint disease by months or years.[89] Enthesitis may be a prominent feature in some children and is clinically indistinguishable but less frequent than that seen in JAS.

SYSTEMIC MANIFESTATIONS

Skin

Typical patches of psoriasis on the face, scalp, extremities (especially the extensor surfaces of the knees, MCP joints, and elbows), umbilicus, or natal cleft occur in approximately 50 percent of children with JPsA (Fig. 6-20). The cutaneous lesions of psoriatic arthritis do not differ from those of psoriasis without arthritis. Shore and Ansell[90] reported that psoriasis vulgaris was by far the most common (83 percent); guttate lesions (32 percent) and pustular psoriasis (<2 percent) were less frequent.

The relationship of the onset of joint and skin complaints is variable, however (Table 6-13). In approximately 11 percent of children, the onset of skin and joint disease is simultaneous or occurs within a few weeks of each other. In 40 percent, psoriasis precedes arthritis, whereas in 48 percent, the reverse is true. Lambert et al.[89] documented arthritis that occurred up to 9 years after the onset of psoriasis and psoriasis that followed arthritis by as much as 14 years. These long intervals contribute significantly to the difficulty of making the diagnosis of JPsA in children. There appears to be little correlation between severity of the psoriasis and activity of joint disease.

Nails

Pitting of nails is seen in 75 percent of children with JPsA and is more common in children with distal interphalangal (DIP) joint disease than in other forms

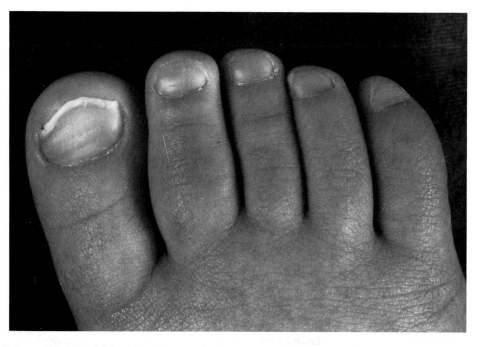

Fig. 6-19 Dactylitis in a child with psoriatic arthritis. The second and fifth toes are diffusely swollen. (From Petty and Malleson,[150] with permission.)

of arthritis or in patients with psoriasis alone (Fig. 6-21). There are no precise criteria for the assessment of nail changes in children, and scattered individual nail pits are not uncommon in healthy individuals. In one recent report it was concluded that patients

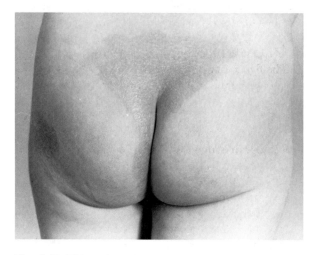

Fig. 6-20 This scaly pink rash was initially treated as diaper dermatitis. The isolated patch on the left buttock suggested the diagnosis of psoriasis.

with a total of nail pits greater than 60 were almost certain to have psoriasis.[105] The occurrence of multiple pits in a single nail, often that of the finger with the affected DIP joint or dactylitis, is highly characteristic of psoriatic arthritis, however. Vertical or horizontal ridging also occurs with some frequency, but onycholysis, although characteristic of psoriasis, is uncommon in children. Similar changes occur in eczema and fungal infections and may occur without any other disease.

Uveitis

Chronic anterior uveitis that is clinically indistinguishable from that accompanying JRA is seen in some children with JPsA. The overall frequency is probably lower than in JRA and may be relatively higher in boys than it is in JRA. However, in our series, chronic anterior uveitis occurred in 20 percent of the JPsA group and included 2 boys and 4 girls.[91]

Other Systemic Manifestations

Fever may be present, especially near the onset of the disease. Pericarditis,[90] mitral valve prolapse,[106]

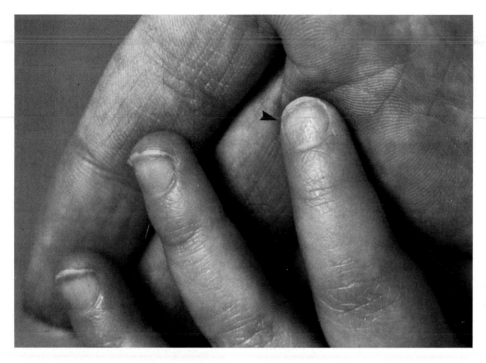

Fig. 6-21 The nail of the index finger has multiple pits characteristic of psoriasis. The digit is also swollen, suggesting dactylitis. (From Petty and Malleson,[150] with permission.)

inflammatory bowel disease,[90] and amyloidosis[96] have occasionally been noted.

Diagnosis

MUSCULOSKELETAL EXAMINATION

The diagnosis of JPsA should be suspected in any child with chronic arthritis, especially if there is dactylitis or asymmetric involvement of large and small joints, particularly the first MTP joint, or the DIP joints. The presence of enthesitis is also suggestive of this diagnosis. The criteria outlined in Table 6-11 may be helpful in classifying children with this disease.

GENERAL PHYSICAL EXAMINATION

The presence of rash or characteristic nail changes helps to confirm the diagnosis of JPsA. It is important to remember that skin and nail changes may be transient, and that they may be separated in time from the onset of the arthritis by many years. The accuracy of the dermatologic diagnosis is also critical since other diseases can mimic psoriasis.

LABORATORY EVALUATION

Inflammatory Indexes

Aside from abnormalities in the indexes of inflammation, there are no characteristic findings. RF is absent, although ANA of unknown specificity may be present in from 17 percent[90] to more than 50 percent.[91] Uric acid levels, which may be elevated in severe psoriasis per se, are usually normal in PsA.[90]

The few studies of synovial fluid in JPsA that have been reported indicate a predominance of PMNs.[90]

Radiographic Studies

Radiographs may be normal or may show juxtaarticular osteoporosis. Occasionally, extensive periostitis is seen. When erosions occur, they tend to be larger than those seen in corresponding locations in JRA, more asymmetric, often not associated with regional osteoporosis, and accompanied by periosteal new bone formation, particularly if flexor tenosynovitis is present. Periostitis eventually leads to widening of the affected bone (Fig. 6-22). Late changes at the DIP joints, although characteristic of psoriatic

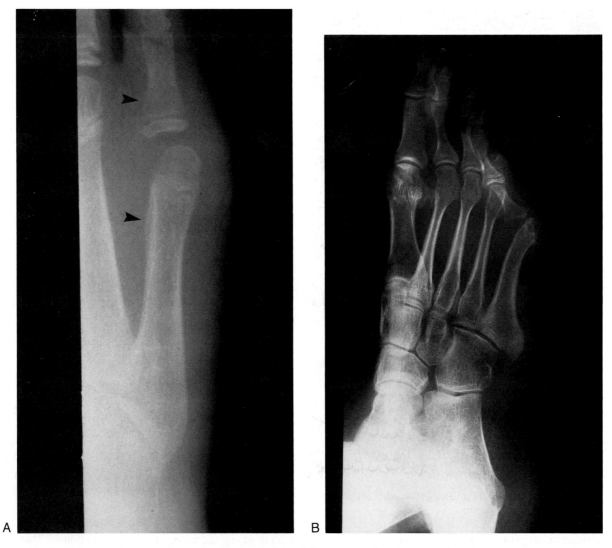

Fig. 6-22 (**A**) Radiograph showing periostitis of the fifth metatarsal and proximal phalanx of a 14-year-old boy with psoriatic arthritis of recent onset. (**B**) Radiograph of the foot of a 12-year-old girl with psoriatic arthritis of several years' duration. There is marked erosion of the head of the fifth metatarsal and the base of the proximal phalanx, with dislocation of the joint. The other joints are relatively normal. (Part A from Petty and Malleson,[150] with permission.)

arthritis, are infrequent (Fig. 6-23). Sacroiliitis is similar to that seen in other spondyloarthropathies of childhood, especially Reiter's syndrome, since both are frequently unilateral at onset. Late radiologic changes (syndesmophytes, paraspinal calcification, and atlantoaxial subluxation) rarely occur in juvenile psoriatic arthritis.

Pathology

In early disease synovial histologic findings are indistinguishable from those of JRA or RA, although the degree of synovial hyperplasia and fibrin exudate may be less in psoriatic arthritis. In chronic PsA, histologic study shows increased fibrosis of capsule and arterial walls and less prominent synovial hypertro-

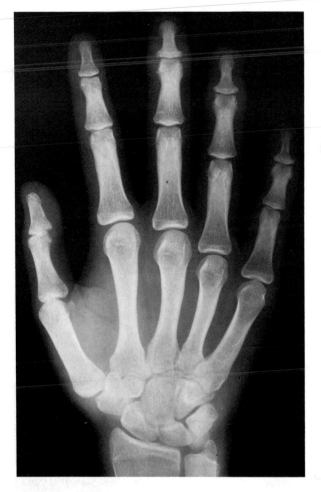

Fig. 6-23 Psoriatic arthropathy affecting the DIP joints of the second to fourth fingers.

phy, in comparison to RA.[107] Changes in the microvasculature (hypertrophy of endothelial cells with dilated rough endoplasmic reticulum and increased nucleoli, thickened arteriolar basement membranes, and increased perivascular collagen deposition) have been described as the basic ultrastructural characteristics of psoriatic arthritis in adults.[108] Synovial histology in 14 patients reported by Shore and Ansell showed hyperemia with a round cell infiltrate.[90]

Treatment

Initially, the management of this disease is like that of JRA: a careful trial of NSAIDs (aspirin, tolmetin, or naproxen), together with physical and occupa-

tional therapy. An inadequate response to these drugs should prompt the use of indomethacin or possibly sodium gold thiomalate or prednisone. Corticosteroid drugs injected into the joints or the synovial sheaths may be helpful in selected children. Although hydroxychloroquine has been said to make the skin rash worse,[89] we have used this drug with benefit to management of the joint disease and without detriment to the skin in JPsA. Methotrexate has been reported to be of benefit in one child with PsA.[109] Chlorambucil, azathioprine, and penicillamine have occasionally been used.[90] Treatment must include the guidance of a dermatologist, whose assessment of skin and nail disease is of great value. It is a clinical impression that response of the skin disease to intensive treatment may be accompanied by abatement of the peripheral joint disease. Topical management of the skin disease requires coal tar preparations and topical corticosteroids in some children. Newer approaches to management of the skin disease (PUVA, retinoic acid derivatives) have not been reported in children with PsA.

Course and Prognosis

Although it has been suggested that JPsA is a relatively mild disorder,[96,103] this is not the experience of most authors. Many children with pauciarticular onset JPsA experience progression to a polyarticular course, and some require major reconstructive surgery of hips and other joints.[90] The course may be a relapsing and remitting one, with synchronous or asynchronous flares in the skin disease. Amyloidosis has been noted in the British[90] and Polish[104] series, resulting in death in at least three children.[104]

INFLAMMATORY BOWEL DISEASE

Definitions

The arthropathies of inflammatory bowel disease may be defined as any noninfectious arthritis occurring before or during the course of either regional enteritis (Crohn's disease) or ulcerative colitis. In fact, arthritis is probably the most common systemic complication of these disorders. Two patterns of joint inflammation are seen: peripheral polyarthritis and, less commonly, sacroiliitis.

Epidemiology

INCIDENCE AND PREVALENCE

The incidence of inflammatory arthropathies in children with inflammatory bowel disease (IBD) has been estimated at from 7.5 to 21.0 percent (Table 6-15). The reasons for the wide range in reported incidences are not known, and it is not clear whether arthritis is more common in children with ulcerative colitis (UC) or those with regional enteritis (RE). It is apparent that differentiation of these two disorders is not always easy, and the conflicting data on the relative frequencies of arthritis in UC and RE reported by Hamilton et al.[111] and Lindsley and Schaller[113] may simply reflect a difference in the diagnosis of IBD. Taken together, the overall incidence of arthritis in IBD of both types is from 13 to 17 percent. Additional patients have polyarthralgia, myalgia, skeletal pain associated with corticosteroid-induced osteopenia, or secondary hypertrophic osteoarthropathy without objective arthritis.

SEX AND AGE

In their study of 136 patients with onset of IBD before the age of 20 years, Lindsley and Schaller[113] concluded that age at onset of IBD in patients with arthritis did not differ significantly from that of those without arthritis. The ratios of boys to girls in those with and without peripheral arthritis were almost identical, although all of the 5 children with spondylitis were boys.[113]

Genetic Considerations

There is a tendency for familial clustering of RE and UC. Hamilton et al.[111] reported that approximately 15 percent of children with UC and 8 percent of children with RE had first-degree relatives with IBD. Both diseases are more common in children of Jewish descent, who comprised 21 percent of the IBD population compared to 2 percent of the population as a whole in one study.[111] There has been no consistent relationship between either RE or UC and any HLA antigen. However, it is estimated that sacroiliitis is 30 times more common in patients with IBD than in the general population,[114] a fact that reflects the high frequency of HLA-B27 in such patients. Peripheral polyarthritis accompanying IBD has no known HLA association.

Etiology and Pathogenesis

The etiologies of IBD and the accompanying arthritis are obscure. The possible roles of gastrointestinal infection or allergic reactions to foods absorbed across an inflamed mucosa remain speculative. The sacroiliitis probably shares its etiology with that of ankylosing spondylitis, and the studies of *Klebsiella* species and immunity to them may be relevant. The peripheral arthropathy may involve entirely different mechanisms (immune complexes) and is more closely related to the activity of the intestinal disease.

Clinical Manifestations

ARTHRITIS

Two quite distinct patterns of joint disease are observed. The less common is sacroiliitis, which may be asymptomatic but often appears as low back, but-

Table 6-15 Arthritis in Inflammatory Bowel Disease in Children

Author	Disease	Number of Patients	Number with Arthritis	%
Farmer & Michener[110]	RE[a]	522	39	7.5
Hamilton et al.[111]	RE	58	11	18.9
Burbige et al.[112]	RE	58	6	10.3
Lindsley & Schaller[113]	RE	50	5	10.0
Lindsley & Schaller[113]	UC[a]	86	18	20.9
Hamilton et al.[111]	UC	87	8	9.2

[a] RE, regional enteritis; UC, ulcerative colitis.

tock, or thigh pain with stiffness. It is frequently accompanied by enthesitis like that seen in other forms of sacroiliitis. It may also be associated with chronic asymmetric oligoarthritis predominantly affecting the joints of the lower limbs.

The more common pattern of arthritis seen in patients with IBD is that affecting peripheral joints. Lindsley and Schaller[113] noted that of 18 children, 11 had four or fewer joints affected at onset or during the course of the illness, whereas 5 had five to nine and only 2 had more than 10 joints affected. (In these last 2 patients, small joints of the hand were involved.) Lower extremity joints, especially knees and ankles, are most frequently affected,[112,113] although upper extremity joints, occasionally including small joints of the hand and the temporomandibular joints, may be affected. Most children have two or more episodes of peripheral arthritis lasting 4 to 6 weeks, although about one-third have a single episode of several weeks' duration. Rarely, the joint inflammation lasts for months, although permanent functional loss or joint damage is most unusual. Whereas the sacroiliitis bears little relationship to the activity of the gut disease, the peripheral arthritis reflects the activity of the GI inflammation, and a flare in the arthritis is suggestive of poor control of the underlying bowel disease.

SYSTEMIC DISEASE

The extent of systemic disease in children with arthritis accompanying IBD is variable. Some children appear to have no systemic disease whatsoever, and an initial diagnosis of SEA syndrome, JAS, or JRA is likely. There are, however, a number of diagnostic clues that may lead to the correct diagnosis. In other children, the arthritis is a minor component of a severe disease dominated by GI complaints.

GASTROINTESTINAL DISEASE

Crampy abdominal pain, often with localized or generalized tenderness, anorexia, and diarrhea, sometimes occurring at night, are characteristic of IBD. Differentiation of ulcerative colitis and Crohn's disease on the basis of GI symptoms is uncertain, although bloody diarrhea is highly suggestive of ulcerative colitis, whereas perianal skin tags and fistulae are suggestive of RE (Table 6-16).

Table 6-16 Gastrointestinal and Other Systemic Disease in Children with Inflammatory Bowel Diseases

Symptom or Sign	Ulcerative Colitis	Regional Enteritis
Diarrhea	+ + + +	+ +
Hematochezia	+ +	+
Abdominal Pain	+ +	+ + +
Weight Loss	+ +	+ + + +
Fever	+	+ + +
Vomiting	+	+ +
Perianal disease	+	+ + +
Finger clubbing	+	+ +
Erythema nodosum	+	+
Oral lesions	+	+
Uveitis	(+)	(+)
Pyoderma gangrenosum	(+)	(+)

[a] + + + +, 75% or more; + + +, 50–75%; + +, 25–50%; +, <25%; (+), rare.

Relationship of Intestinal and Articular Disease

Although there are no clear-cut correlations between the extent of GI inflammation and the incidence of arthritis, most studies support the view that there is a higher incidence of arthritis in children with extensive as opposed to segmental bowel disease.[110,111] Patients with arthritis usually have active gut disease, although the onset of arthritis is not necessarily related to obvious flares in the intestinal inflammation.

Gastrointestinal tract symptoms usually precede joint disease by months or years, although occasionally both systems are affected simultaneously or joint symptoms precede intestinal disease. In the latter case, disease in a child with what appears to be JRA, JAS, or SEA syndrome whose course is punctuated by intermittent abdominal pain, low-grade diarrhea, unexplained fever, weight loss, or growth retardation out of proportion to the extent and activity of the joint disease should alert the physician to the possibility of occult IBD. Mucocutaneous lesions (erythema nodosum, oral ulcers, pyoderma gangrenosum) appear to be more common in children who also have arthritis (especially peripheral arthritis) as a complication of their IBD.

OTHER SYSTEMIC MANIFESTATIONS

Erythema Nodosum (Nodular Panniculitis)

The lesions of erythema nodosum occur most commonly in the subcutaneous fat of the pretibial region (Fig. 6-24) as erythematous, painful, slightly elevated lesions 1 to 2

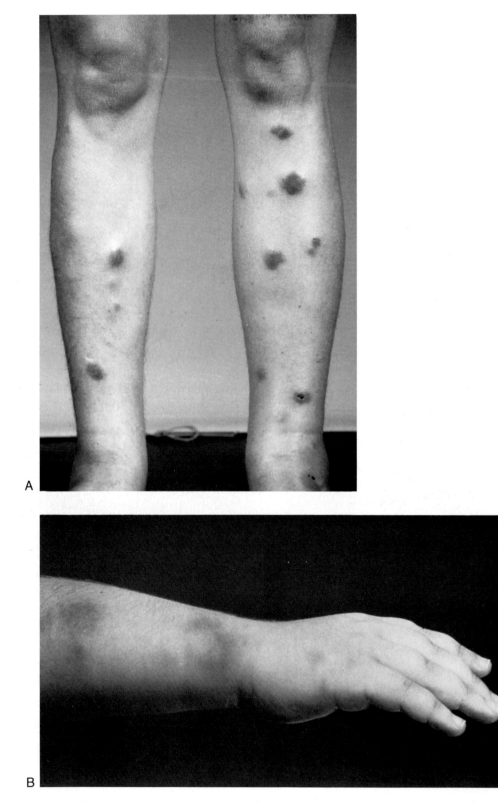

Fig. 6-24 (**A**) Erythema nodosum. This young girl had tender, circumscribed, purple-red nodules on the shins. (**B**) Lesions on forearm of a child.

cm in diameter, erupting in groups and reappearing in new areas after several days. The nodules tend to persist for several weeks and may recur in crops for several months. As they heal they frequently leave pigmented areas that persist for many months. In approximately two-thirds of instances, articular pain and synovitis are noted. Although erythema nodosum may occur as a distinct clinical syndrome, it is commonly associated with systemic illnesses or diverse cause.[115,116] (See Ch. 12.)

Pyoderma Gangrenosum

The lesions of pyoderma gangrenosum may occur alone or in concert with IBD (Fig. 6-25). They usually follow minor trauma, may be single or multiple, and usually begin as a pustule that breaks down and rapidly enlarges to form a painful, chronic, deep, undermined ulcer with a red, raised edge. They have rarely been reported in children; in adults they may accompany IBD, RA, or other diseases.[117] Jacobs reported pyoderma gangrenosum in a 2-year-old boy with joint effusions, but without IBD, associated with

enhanced leukocyte mobility induced by the so-called streaking leukocyte factor.[118]

The diagnosis of arthritis in IBD rests on recognition of the significance of the association and on a high level of suspicion. The diagnosis of IBD should be suspected in any child with arthritis accompanied by lower abdominal pain, hematochezia, weight loss, or fever. This suspicion would be supported by laboratory evidence of inflammation (high ESR and other acute-phase reactants, low serum albumin) but negative test results for RF and ANA. Synovial fluid analyses of children with IBD have not been reported, although in adults, synovial fluid WBC counts have ranged from 5,000 to 15,000/mm^3 (5 to 15 × 10^9/L) with a predominance of PMN leukocytes. Synovial fluid protein, glucose, and hemolytic complement levels have been normal.[69] There is a nonspecific synovitis with proliferation of synoviocytes and infiltration with lymphocytes, plasma cells, and histio-

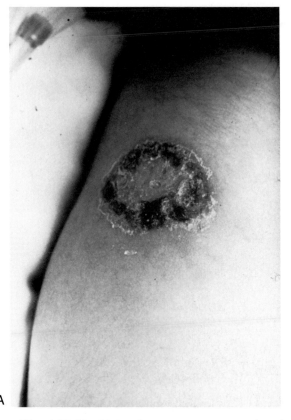

A

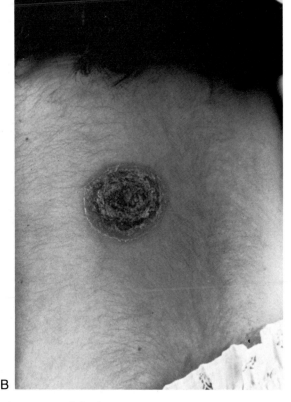

B

Fig. 6-25 (A&B) Pyoderma gangrenosum. These lesions begin as nodules but progress to ulcers with considerable tissue loss.

cytes.[119] Granulomatous synovitis occasionally occurs.[120]

Radiographs of peripheral joints show soft tissue thickening and joint effusions. Sacroiliitis, when it occurs, is not distinguishable from that seen in JAS. Spur formation is sometimes identified at the insertion of the plantar fascia into the calcaneus. Periostitis may be demonstrable by radiographs or radionuclide scanning. Burbige et al.[112] noted erosive lesions secondary to granulomatous synovitis in one patient.

Treatment

Successful management of the peripheral arthritis depends upon effective treatment of the intestinal inflammation: control of the primary disease usually results in remission in the peripheral arthritis. Peripheral arthritis is best managed by the use of therapeutic salicylate and, if indicated by the severity of the bowel disease, by sulfasalazine or corticosteroids. In spite of the potential for gastrointestinal side effects from aspirin, its administration with food usually prevents this problem, even in patients with IBD. Because of its beneficial effect in the treatment of GI inflammation, early use of sulfasalazine may have a place in the management of the arthropathy of IBD, although no therapeutic trials have been published. There is a striking remission in the peripheral joint symptoms and signs after removal of the diseased colon, although colectomy for the control of peripheral joint arthritis is not indicated.

The spondylitis of IBD is much more likely than the peripheral arthritis to persist and progress, independent of the activity of the gut disease and unaffected by procedures such as colectomy. Therapeutic salicylates or indomethacin, coupled with range of motion exercises to maintain back and chest motion (as for JAS), may help to prevent or slow the progress of the disease, although permanent changes in the spine and hips are very frequent in this group.

Course and Prognosis

The outcome of the gastrointestinal disease is the most important determinant of overall prognosis in the child with IBD and arthritis. The outcome of the peripheral joint disease is usually excellent, although the axial skeleton disease may progress independent of the severity of the GI disease. Severe, unresponsive disease may require systemic corticosteroids, sulfasalazine, and even surgery. Poor nutrition and growth retardation may be major problems.

REITER'S SYNDROME

Definitions

The term *Reiter's syndrome* (RS) is applied to a triad of inflammatory lesions occurring in the synovium, conjunctiva, and urethra that was first described in the English language literature in 1818 by Sir Benjamin Brodie.[121] Almost 100 years later, Hans Reiter, whose name is now associated with this syndrome, reported a 16-year-old boy who developed arthritis, urethritis, and conjunctivitis after dysentery.[122] RS is almost certainly a postinfectious or reactive arthritis and therefore could justifiably be included in the discussion of postinfectious arthritides (Ch. 12). It is traditionally included with the seronegative spondyloarthropathies because the clinical characteristics of the joint disease and the high frequency of HLA-B27 link it with this group of disorders.

Epidemiology

The frequency of the disease in childhood is difficult to determine with precision, since it is frequently self-limited and may be overlooked in the examination of a child with sterile monarthritis, conjunctivitis, or minimal pyuria. Wright has estimated that in 739 cases of RS, 0.67 percent occurred in children under 16 years of age.[123] Of 37 documented cases of RS in children,[124] 30 were boys, a ratio of approximately 4 boys to 1 girl. This is considerably lower than the ratio of 10 men to 1 woman in adult postdysenteric RS[125] or the ratio of 50 men to 21 women in adult venereal forms of RS.[126]

Genetic Considerations

Predisposition to RS is marked by the presence of HLA-B27, which was present in 76 percent of 33 men with RS compared to 9 percent of a similar number of men with nonspecific urethritis and 6 percent of a control population. The presence of HLA-B27 in RS correlates with the presence of sacroiliitis and spondylitis,[127] with acute anterior uveitis, a chronic relapsing course, and systemic signs such as fever and weight loss.[128] The relationship between HLA-B27 and RS in children appears to be just as strong as that in adults. In the children in whom histocompatibility antigens have been determined, 13 of 14 had B27[124,129]; a frequency of approximately 90 percent.

Etiology and Pathogenesis

The cause or causes of RS have not been firmly established. The strong relationship to sexually acquired infection or diarrhea in the adult is evidence that RS is a postinfectious or "reactive" arthritis. The studies of Paronen[125] and Noer[130] clearly established the temporal relationship of RS to infectious diarrhea (*Shigella*) in some cases of RS, although many cases follow nonspecific urethritis. In children, diarrhea precedes the onset of RS in 79 percent of cases. *Shigella flexneri*,[125,131–134] *Yersinia enterocolitica*,[135] *Salmonella enteritidis*,[136] *S. oranienburg*,[134] and *S. typhimurium*[137] have been isolated from children with postdysenteric RS. In at least two youths, sexual intercourse preceded RS and in three children, *Chlamydia trachomatis*[124] or *Mycoplasma tiny*[138] has been isolated from synovial fluid. In adults, chlamydiae have been isolated from urethra, conjunctiva, and synovial membrane and fluid[139] of patients with RS. In the same population, titers of complement-fixing antibody to chlamydia are only occasionally found. In vitro reactivity of lymphocytes from RS patients to chlamydial and ureaplasmal antigens has been noted.[140,141] Thus, although there is evidence suggesting various microbial agents as causes of RS, it is clear that the majority of persons infected with such agents do not develop RS. It has been estimated that RS follows dysentery in 0.24 to 1.5 percent of persons[125,130] and is a sequel to nonspecific urethritis in 1 to 4 percent of cases.[132,142]

Clinical Characteristics

The triad of arthritis, urethritis, and conjunctivitis may occur simultaneously or may develop over a period of 3 to 4 weeks or even longer.[123,135]

MUSCULOSKELETAL MANIFESTATIONS

Arthritis is a presenting complaint in one-quarter of children with RS. As a rule, the disease affects only a few joints, occasionally only a single joint, and is most common in joints of the lower extremities, particularly the knees and ankles. Not infrequently, however, upper extremity joints, cervical spine, and temporomandibular joints are involved. Additional joints frequently become involved during the first 2 weeks of the disease. Rarely, a flitting pattern is seen. In some patients, the amount of swelling and the severity of pain are remarkable. In most instances the joint is hot but rarely red.

Discrete pain at entheses may be a striking feature of the musculoskeletal symptoms in children with RS. In general, the most commonly affected locations are around the calcaneus and patella (as described in the discussion of SEA syndrome). Pain in the axial skeleton is not frequent in children with RS, but pain on palpation over the SI joints or on movement of the spine should suggest the presence of inflammation at those sites. Muscle atrophy and weakness may occur quickly and attest to the degree of pain and inflammation present in and around affected joints.

SYSTEMIC MANIFESTATIONS

Genitourinary Tract

The most common urinary tract complaint is dysuria. In 30 percent of children, urethritis is present at onset of the disease. In some children, a purulent urethral discharge is noted, whereas in a few, inflammation of the meatus may be the only abnormality. Not infrequently, urinary tract symptoms are mild or may be absent. In such instances, examination of the centrifuged urinary sediment may reveal pyuria. In a child with arthritis and conjunctivitis, even minimal pyuria should alert the physician to the possibility of RS. Although previous sexual exposure is apparently an infrequent event in RS in children, and diarrhea is common, urethritis nonetheless occurs in both groups. Likewise, in adults, urethritis is common in the dysenteric form of RS,[130] and diarrhea is common in sexually acquired RS.[123] Balanitis[124,134,135] and labial ulceration[134] are seen. More severe genitourinary tract disease has not been reported in children, although prostatitis and hemorrhagic cystitis occur in adults.

Ocular Symptoms

Conjunctivitis is present at the onset of disease in two-thirds of children with RS. Complaints range from a feeling of grittiness in the eye or transient redness of the bulbar conjunctivae to severe photophobia and inflammation of bulbar and palpebral conjunctivae. Blepharitis with marked edema of the eyelids and a mucopurulent discharge may ensue. Acute anterior iritis[133,136] keratitis,[131,135] corneal ulcerations,[131,135,137] and optic neuritis[143] have been reported. Corneal scarring is rare.

Mucocutaneous Manifestations

The abnormalities of skin, nails, and mucous membranes are so frequently seen with the RS triad that they are often included to form a tetrad. In children, however, mucocutaneous lesions of RS are probably less common than they are in adults. Two lesions are characteristic of RS: keratodermia blennorrhagica, and ulcers and erythema of the oral mucosa. Keratodermia blennorrhagica (Fig. 6-26) begins as a papular eruption on the soles of the feet and may progress to a pustular scaling eruption that cannot be distinguished from pustular psoriasis. It is said to occur less frequently in RS of diarrheal origin than

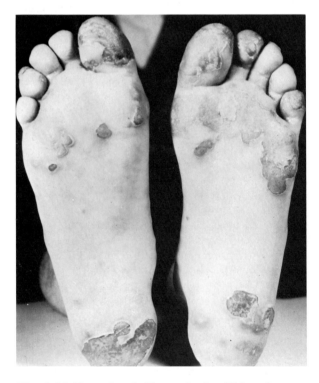

Fig. 6-26 Keratodermia blennorrhagica. This scaly eruption on the soles of the feet may be difficult to distinguish from psoriasis.

in venereal RS, a possible explanation of its rather low incidence in children. Nail changes ranging from pitting to hyperkeratosis and paronychiae can occur. Painless erythematous patches occur on the palate, tongue, and buccal mucosa and may ulcerate.[134-137] Other less specific cutaneous changes include pustules,[134] erythema nodosum,[134] and other rashes.[144]

Other Abnormalities

Low grade fever is usually present. Other systemic signs occasionally recorded include weight loss,[144,145] epistaxis, pleuritic pain with pleural effusion,[124] lymphadenopathy, and splenomegaly.[144]

Laboratory Investigations

Indexes of inflammation are usually abnormal. The ESR is almost always high during the early active disease and may remain elevated for weeks or months. ESR values range from 40 to 130 mm/h (Westergren method) but average 50 to 60 mm/h. Similarly, WBC counts are usually increased, up to 20,000/mm^3 (20 × 10^9/L), generally with a left shift and occasionally with low grade eosinophilia. Immunoglobulin levels have been normal or elevated when measured. The presence of ANA and RF has not been demonstrated, although in most instances the results of these tests have not been reported.

Synovial fluid examinations have been documented in 10 cases[124,134,135,146] and in general are characterized by a moderate increase in the WBC count (10,000 to 40,000/mm^3 [10 to 40 × 10^9/L]), mainly PMN leukocytes. Reiter's cells (large macrophages containing PMN leukocytes, lymphocytes, or plasma cells) are rare. Synovial fluid complement levels are normal or increased.[134,146] This fact may help distinguish RS synovial fluid from that of other inflammatory arthritides.

Urinalyses may be abnormal with 5 to 1,000 WBC/hpf and, frequently, small numbers of erythrocytes and low amounts of protein.

Microbiologic studies have yielded inconsistent results. Synovial fluid cultures have been negative except as noted previously. Cultures of conjunctiva and urethra have occasionally demonstrated chlamydia.[124] Stool cultures have grown *S. flexneri* in four instances[134,135] and *Salmonella* species in three instances.[133,147] In patients in whom stool cultures are negative, elevated antibody titers to *S. flexneri* or *Y. enterocolitica* are sometimes found.[135]

Radiography

Radiographs may be normal, but changes suggestive of RS include soft tissue swelling and sometimes marked juxta-articular osteoporosis. Erosions at insertions of the Achilles tendons, spur formation at the insertion of plantar ligaments, and SI joint changes (widening, erosions, sclerosis) may occur, especially with chronic disease.[124,148]

Treatment

Aspirin provides effective symptomatic relief but does not significantly influence the course of the disease. Other NSAIDs,[136] prednisone,[148] and antibiotics[131,133] have been used, but their efficacy cannot be accurately assessed on the basis of the relatively few isolated reports. Because of the frequently persistent joint involvement, aggressive physiotherapy may be necessary.

Course and Prognosis

RS in most children appears to be a self-limited condition characterized by gradual resolution of symptoms and signs over a period of months. Gough reported a child who initially had arthritis, conjunctivitis, and keratodermia and 1 year later developed arthritis, keratodermia, and urethritis.[148] One patient reported by Iveson et al. with complete RS had incomplete RS 18 months earlier.[136] Two children who have been followed for more than 5 years have had no late complications related to RS.[144,149] However, it is conceivable that RS occurring in childhood may be an early event in the natural history of seronegative spondyloarthropathies of later onset.

REFERENCES

1. Rosenberg AM, Petty RE: A syndrome of seronegative enthesopathy and arthropathy in children. Arthritis Rheum 25:1041, 1982
2. Jacobs JC, Berdon WE, Johnston AD: HLA-B27-associated spondyloarthritis and enthesopathy in childhood: clinical, pathologic and radiographic observations in 58 patients. J Pediatr 100:521, 1983
3. Brewer EJ, Bass JC, Baum JR et al: Current proposed revision of JRA criteria. Arthritis Rheum, suppl., 20:195, 1977
4. Calin A: The epidemiology of ankylosing spondylitis: a clinician's point of view. In Lawrence RC, Shulman LE (eds): Epidemiology of the Rheumatic Diseases. Gower, New York, 1984, p. 51–59
5. Moran HM, Hall MA, Barr A et al: Spinal mobility in the adolescent. Rheumatol Rehabil 18:181, 1979
6. Goei T, Steven MM, van der Linden S et al: Evaluation of diagnostic criteria for ankylosing spondylitis: a comparison of the Rome, New York and modified New York criteria in patients with a positive clinical history screening test for AS. Br J Rheumatol 24:242, 1985
7. Kellgren JH, Jeffrey MR, Ball J: The Epidemiology of Chronic Rheumatism. Blackwell Scientific Publications, Oxford, 1963, p. 326
8. Bennett PH, Wood PHN: Population Studies of the Rheumatic Diseases. Excerpta Medica, New York, 1968, p. 456
9. Carter ET, McKenna CH, Brian DD et al: Epidemiology of ankylosing spondylitis in Rochester, Minnesota, 1935–1973. Arthritis Rheum 22:365, 1979
10. Ladd JR, Cassidy JT, Martel W: Juvenile ankylosing spondylitis. Arthritis Rheum 14:579, 1971
11. Bywaters EGL: Ankylosing spondylitis in childhood. In BM Ansell (ed): Clinics in Rheumatic Diseases. Vol. 3. WB Saunders, London, p. 387, 1976
12. Kleinman P, Rivelis M, Schneider R et al: Juvenile ankylosing spondylitis. Pediatr Radiol 125:775, 1977
13. Schaller J: Ankylosing spondylitis of childhood onset. Arthritis Rheum, suppl., 20:398, 1977
14. Hafner R: Die juvenile Spondarthritis. Retrospektive Untersuchung an 71 Patienten. Monatsschr Kinderheilkunde 135:41, 1987
15. Veys EM, Coigne E, Mielants H et al: HLA and juvenile rheumatoid polyarthritis. Tissue Antigens 8:62, 1976
16. Sturrock RD, Dick HM, Henderson N et al: Association of HL-A 27 in juvenile rheumatoid arthritis and ankylosing spondylitis. J Rheumatol 1:269, 1974
17. Edmonds J, Morris RI, Metzger AL et al: Followup study of juvenile chronic polyarthritis with particular reference to histocompatibility antigen W 27. Ann Rheum Dis 33:289, 1974
18. Calin A, Fries JF: Striking prevalence of ankylosing spondylitis in "healthy" W27 positive males and females. N Engl J Med 293:835, 1975
19. Masi AT: HLA-B27 and other host interactions in spondyloarthropathy syndromes. J Rheumatol 5:359, 1978
20. Resnick D, Dwosh IL, Goergen TG et al: Clinical and

radiographic abnormalities in ankylosing spondylitis: a comparison of men and women. Radiography 119:293, 1976

21. Edstrom G, Thune S, Wittbom-Cigen G: Juvenile ankylosing spondylitis. Acta Rheumatol Scand 6:161, 1960

22. Ansell BM: Juvenile spondylitis and related disorders. In Moll JMH (ed): Ankylosing Spondylitis. Churchill Livingstone, Edinburgh, 1980, p. 120

23. Schaller J, Bitnum S, Wedgwood RJ: Ankylosing spondylitis with childhood onset. J Pediatr 74:505, 1969

24. Kellgren JH: The epidemiology of rheumatic diseases. Ann Rheum Dis 23:109, 1964

25. Ansell BM, Bywaters EGL, Lawrence JS: Familial aggregation and twin studies in Still's disease, juvenile chronic polyarthritis. Rheumatology 2:37, 1969

26. Brewerton DA, Caffrey M, Hart FD: Ankylosing spondylitis and HL-A 27. Lancet 1:904, 1973

27. Schlosstein L, Terasaki PI, Bluestone R et al: High association of an HL-A antigen W27 with ankylosing spondylitis. N Engl J Med 288:704, 1973

28. McDaniel DO, Acton RT, Barger BO et al: Association of a 9.2 kb Pvu II MHC class I restriction fragment length polymorphism with ankylosing spondylitis. Arthritis Rheum 30:897, 1987

29. McDaniel DO, Barger BO, Reveille JD et al: Analysis of restriction fragment length polymorphisms in rheumatic diseases. Rheum Dis Clin North Am 13:353, 1987

30. Oen K, Petty RE, Schroeder ML: An association between HLA-A2 and juvenile rheumatoid arthritis in girls. J Rheumatol 9:916, 1982

31. Woodrow JC: Genetics. In Moll JMH (ed): Ankylosing Spondylitis. Churchill Livingstone, Edinburgh, 1980, p. 26–41

32. Arnett FH, Schacter BZ, Hochberg MC et al: HLA-A28 in patients with B27-associated rheumatic diseases. Arthritis Rheum 20:106, 1977

33. Calin A, Porta J, Payne R: HLA-A28 in B27 positive controls and patients with ankylosing spondylitis. Arthritis Rheum 20:1428, 1977

34. Truog P, Steiger U, Contu L et al: Ankylosing spondylitis (AS): a population and family study using HL-A serology and MLR. In Kissmeyer-Nielsen F (ed): Histocompatibility Testing. Munksgaard, Copenhagen, 1975, p. 788

35. Berg-Loonen EM, van den Dekker-Saeys BJ, Meuwissen SGM et al: Histocompatibility antigen and other genetic markers in ankylosing spondylitis and inflammatory bowel disease. J Immunogenet 4:167, 1977

36. Baum J, Ziff M: The rarity of ankylosing spondylitis in the black race. Arthritis Rheum 14:12, 1971

37. Sonozaki H, Seki H, Chang S et al: Human lymphocyte antigen HL-A27 in Japanese patients with ankylosing spondylitis. Tissue Antigens 5:131, 1975

38. Gofton JP, Robinson HS, Trueman GE: Ankylosing spondylitis in a Canadian Indian population. Ann Rheum Dis 25:525, 1966

39. Good AE, Kawanishi H, Schultz JS: HLA B27 in blacks with ankylosing spondylitis or Reiter's disease. N Engl J Med 294:166, 1976

40. Ford DK, Da Roza DM, Schulzer M: Lymphocytes from the site of disease but not blood lymphocytes indicate the cause of arthritis. Ann Rheum Dis 44:701, 1985

41. Cowling P, Ebringer R, Cawdell D et al: C-reactive protein, ESR and Klebsiella in ankylosing spondylitis. Ann Rheum Dis 39:545, 1980

42. Geczy AF, Seager K, Bashir HV et al: The role of Klebsiella in the pathogenesis of ankylosing spondylitis. II: Evidence for a specific B27-associated marker on the lymphocytes of patients with ankylosing spondylitis. J Clin Lab Immunol 3:23, 1980

43. Kinsella TD, Lanteigne C, Fritzler MJ et al: Absence of impaired lymphocyte transformation to Klebsiella spp. in ankylosing spondylitis. Ann Rheum Dis 43:590, 1984

44. Cameron FH, Russell PJ, Easter JF et al: Failure of *Klebsiella pneumoniae* antibodies to cross-react with peripheral blood mononuclear cells from patients with ankylosing spondylitis. Arthritis Rheum 30:300, 1987

45. Riley MJ, Ansell BM, Bywaters EGL: Radiological manifestations of ankylosing spondylitis according to age at onset. Ann Rheum Dis 30:138, 1971

46. Stewart SR, Robbins DL, Castles JJ: Acute fulminant aortic and mitral insufficiency in ankylosing spondylitis. N Engl J Med 299:1448, 1978

47. Reid GD, Patterson MWH, Patterson AC et al: Aortic insufficiency in association with juvenile ankylosing spondylitis. J Pediatr 95:78, 1979

48. Kean WF, Anastassiades TP, Ford PM: Aortic incompetence in HLA B27 positive juvenile arthritis. Ann Rheum Dis 39:294, 1980

49. Gore JE, Vizcarrondo FE, Rieffel CN: Juvenile ankylosing spondylitis and aortic regurgitation: a case presentation. Pediatrics 68:423, 1981

50. Toone E, Johnson WL: The clinical and pathological cardiac manifestations of rheumatoid spondylitis. Virginia Med 95:132, 1968

51. Rosenow EC, Strimlan CV, Muhm JR et al: Pleuropulmonary manifestations of ankylosing spondylitis. Mayo Clin Proc 52:641, 1977

52. Reid GD, Hill RH: Atlantoaxial subluxation in juvenile ankylosing spondylitis. J Pediatr 93:531, 1978

53. Hunter T, Dubo H: Spinal fractures complicating ankylosing spondylitis. Ann Intern Med 88:546, 1978

54. Allen RC, Petty RE, Lirenman DS et al: Renal papillary necrosis in children with chronic arthritis treated with non-steroidal anti-inflammatory drugs. Am J Dis Child 140:20, 1986

55. Mustonen J: IgA glomerulonephritis and associated diseases. Ann Clin Res 16:161, 1984

56. Bruneau C, Villiaumey JH, Avouac B et al: Seronegative spondyloarthropathies and IgA glomerulonephritis: a report of four cases and a review of the literature. Semin Arthritis Rheum 15:179, 1986

57. Niepal GA, Sit'az S: Enthesopathy. Clin Rheum Dis 5:857, 1979

58. Macrae IF, Wright V: Measurement of back movement. Ann Rheum Dis 28:584, 1969

59. Barkely DO, Hohermuth HJ, Howard A et al: IgA deficiency in juvenile chronic polyarthritis. J Rheumatol 6:219, 1979

60. Cassidy JT: Selective IgA deficiency and chronic arthritis in children. In Moore TD (ed): Arthritis in Childhood. Report of the Eightieth Ross Conference in Pediatric Research. Ross Laboratories, Columbus, Ohio, 1981, p. 82

61. Kinsella TD, Espinoza L, Vasey FB: Serum complement and immunoglobulin levels in sporadic and familial ankylosing spondylitis. J Rheumatol 2:308, 1975

62. Corrigall V, Panayi GS, Unger A et al: Detection of immune complexes in serum of patients with ankylosing spondylitis. Ann Rheum Dis 37:159, 1978

63. Veys EM, Van Laere M: Serum IgG, IgM and IgA levels in ankylosing spondylitis. Ann Rheum Dis 332:493, 1973

64. Vasey FB, Kinsella TD: Increased incidence of granulocyte specific antinuclear factor in sera of patients with ankylosing spondylitis. J Rheumatol, suppl., 1:63, 1974

65. Lakomek HJ, Will H, Zech M et al: A new serologic marker in ankylosing spondylitis. Arthritis Rheum 27:961, 1984

66. Kendall MJ, Farr M, Meynell MJ et al: Synovial fluid in ankylosing spondylitis. Ann Rheum Dis 32:487, 1973

67. Traycoff RB, Pascual E, Schumacher HR: Mononuclear cells in human synovial fluid. Arthritis Rheum 19:743, 1976

68. Spriggs AI, Boddington MM, Mowat AG: Joint fluid cytology in Reiter's disease. Ann Rheum Dis 37:557, 1978

69. Bunch TW, Hunder GG, McDuffie FC et al: Synovial fluid complement determination as a diagnostic aid in inflammatory joint disease. Mayo Clin Proc 49:715, 1974

70. Bellamy N, Park W, Rooney PS: What do we know about the sacroiliac joint? Semin Arthritis Rheum 12:282, 1983

71. Carrera GF, Foley WD, Kozin F et al: CT of sacroiliitis. Am J Radiol 136:41, 1981

72. Julkunen H: Synovial inflammatory cell reaction in chronic arthritis. Acta Rheumatol Scand 12:188, 1966

73. Ball J: Enthesopathy of rheumatoid and ankylosing spondylitis. Ann Rheum Dis 30:213, 1971

74. Shichikawa K, Tsujimoto M, Nishioka J et al: Histopathology of early sacroiliitis and enthesitis in ankylosing spondylitis. Adv Inflammation Res 9:15, 1985

75. Ball J: Pathology and pathogenesis. In Moll JMH (ed): Ankylosing Spondylitis. Churchill Livingstone, Edinburgh, 1980, p. 96

76. La Zerte GD, Rapp IH: Pathogenesis of Osgood-Schlatter's disease. Am J Pathol 34:803, 1958

77. Tachdjian MO: Pediatric Orthopedics. WB Saunders, Philadelphia, 1972, p. 1244

78. Adams JA: Transient synovitis of the hip joint in children. J Bone Joint Surg 45B:471, 1963

79. Mital MA, Matza RA, Cohen J: The so-called unresolved Osgood-Schlatter lesion. J Bone Joint Surg 62A:732, 1980

80. Sherry DD, Petty RE, Tredwell S et al: Histocompatibility antigens in Osgood-Schlatter's disease. J Pediatr Orthoped 5:302, 1985

81. Sorenson KH: Scheuermann's Juvenile Kyphosis. Munksgaard, Copenhagen, 1964, p. 11

82. Moe JH, Winter RB, Bradford DS et al: Juvenile kyphosis. In Scoliosis and Other Spinal Deformities. WB Saunders, Philadelphia, 1978, p. 331

83. Nelson CL, Janecki GJ, Gildenberg PL et al: Disc protrusions in the young. Clin Orthop 88:142, 1972

84. Neumann VC, Grindulis KA, Hubball S et al: Comparison between penicillamine and sulphasalazine in rheumatoid arthritis: Leeds-Birmingham trial. Br Med J 2:1099, 1983

85. Pullar T, Hunter JA, Capell HA: Sulphasalazine in rheumatoid arthritis: a double-blind comparison of sulphasalazine with placebo and sodium aurothiomalate. Br Med J 2:1102, 1983

86. Ozdogan H, Turunc M, Deringol B et al: Sulphasalazine in the treatment of juvenile rheumatoid arthritis: a preliminary open trial. J Rheumatol 13:124, 1986

87. Garcia-Morteo O, Maldonado-Cocco JA, Suarez-Almazor ME et al: Ankylosing spondylitis of juvenile onset: comparison with adult onset disease. Scand J Rheumatol 12:246, 1983

88. Marks SH, Barnett M, Calin A: A case-control study of juvenile- and adult-onset ankylosing spondylitis. J Rheumatol 9:739, 1982

89. Lambert JR, Ansell BM, Stephenson E et al: Psoriatic arthritis in childhood. Clin Rheum Dis 2:339, 1976
90. Shore A, Ansell BM: Juvenile psoriatic arthritis—an analysis of 60 cases. J Pediatr 100:529, 1982
91. Southwood TR, Delgado EA, Wood B et al: Psoriatic arthritis in childhood. Arthritis Rheum 31:s119, 1988
92. Moll JMH, Wright V: Psoriatic arthritis. Semin Arthritis Rheum 3:55, 1973
93. Baker H: Epidemiological aspects of psoriasis and arthritis. Br J Dermatol 78:249, 1966
94. Church R: The prospect of psoriasis. Br J Dermatol 70:139, 1958
95. Espinoza LR: Psoriatic arthritis: further epidemiologic and genetic considerations. In LH Gerber, LR Espinoza (eds): Psoriatic Arthritis. Grune & Stratton, Orlando, 1985, p. 9–32
96. Sills EL: Psoriatic arthritis in childhood. Johns Hopkins Med J 146:49, 1980
97. Andersson GB, Fasth A, Andersson et al: Incidence and prevalence of juvenile chronic arthritis: a population survey. Ann Rheum Dis 46:277, 1987
98. Gladman D, Anhorn KAB, Schachter RK et al: HLA antigens in psoriatic arthritis. J Rheumatol 13:586, 1986
99. McHugh NJ, Laurent MR, Treadwell BLJ et al: Psoriatic arthritis: clinical subgroups and histocompatibility antigens. Ann Rheum Dis 46:184, 1987
100. Espinoza LR, Vasey FB, Gaylord SW et al: Histocompatibility typing in the seronegative spondyloarthropathies: a survey. Semin Arthritis Rheum 11:375, 1982
101. Armstrong RD, Panayi GS, Welsh KI: Histocompatibility antigens in psoriasis, psoriatic arthropathy, and ankylosing spondylitis. Ann Rheum Dis 42:142, 1983
102. Vasey FB, Deitz C, Fenske NA et al: Possible involvement of group A streptococci in the pathogenesis of psoriatic arthritis. J Rheumatol 9:719, 1982
103. Calabro JJ: Psoriatic arthritis in children. Arthritis Rheum, suppl., 20:415, 1977
104. Wesolowska H: Clinical course of psoriatic arthropathy in children. Mat Med Pol 55:185, 1985
105. Eastmond CJ, Wright V: The nail dystrophy of psoriatic arthritis. Ann Rheum Dis 38:226, 1979
106. Pines A, Ehrenfeld M, Fisman EZ et al: Mitral valve prolapse in psoriatic arthritis. Arch Intern Med 146:1371, 1986
107. Khan MA, Kammer GM: Laboratory findings and pathology in psoriatic arthritis. In LH Gerber, LR Espinoza (eds): Psoriatic Arthritis. Grune & Stratton, Orlando, 1985, p. 109–124
108. Espinoza LR, Vasey FB, Espinoza CG et al: Vascular changes in psoriatic synovium. Arthritis Rheum 25:677, 1982
109. Bjorksten B, Back OL: Methotrexate and prednisolone treatment of a child with psoriatic arthritis. Acta Paediatr Scand 64:664, 1975
110. Farmer RG, Michener WM: Prognosis of Crohn's disease with onset in childhood or adolescence. Dig Dis Sci 24:752, 1979
111. Hamilton JR, Bruce MD, Abdourhaman M et al: Inflammatory bowel disease in children and adolescents. Adv Pediatr 26:311, 1979
112. Burbige EJ, Shi-Shung Huang, Bayless TM: Clinical manifestations of Crohn's disease in children and adolescents. Pediatr 55:866, 1975
113. Lindsley C, Schaller JG: Arthritis associated with inflammatory bowel disease in children. J Pediatr 84:16, 1974
114. Brewerton DA, James DCO: The histocompatibility antigen HL-A 27 and disease. Semin Arthritis Rheum 4:191, 1975
115. Lorber J: The changing etiology of erythema nodosum in children. Arch Dis Child 33:137, 1958
116. Winkelmann RK, Forstrom L: New observations in the histopathology of erythema nodosum. J Invest Dermatol 65:441, 1975
117. Hurwits S: The skin and systemic disease in children. Year Book Medical Publishers, Chicago, 1985
118. Jacobs JC, Goetzl EJ: "Streaking leukocyte factor," arthritis and pyoderma gangrenosum. Pediatrics 56:570, 1975
119. Ansell BM, Wigley RAD: Arthritis manifestations in regional enteritis. Ann Rheum Dis 23:64, 1964
120. Lindstrom H, Wramsby H, Ostberg G: Granulomatous arthritis in Crohn's disease. Gut 13:257, 1972
121. Brodie BC: Pathological and surgical observations on diseases of the joints. Longman Hurst Rees, Orme and Brown, London, 1818
122. Reiter H: Ueber eine bisher unerhannte spirochaten-infektion (Spirochaetosis arthritica). Dtsch Med Wochenschr 42:1535, 1916
123. Wright V: Reiter's disease. In Scott JT (ed): Copeman's Textbook of the Rheumatic Diseases. 5th Ed. Longmans Green, London, 1978, p. 549
124. Rosenberg AM, Petty RE: Reiter's disease in children. Am J Dis Child 133:394, 1979
125. Paronen I: Reiter's disease: a study of 344 cases observed in Finland. Acta Med Scand [Suppl] 212:1, 1948
126. Oates JK, Czonka GW: Reiter's disease in the female. Ann Rheum Dis 18:37, 1959
127. Brewerton DA, Caffrey M, Nicholls A et al: Reiter's disease and HLA B27. Lancet 2:996, 1973
128. McClusky OE, Lordon RE, Arnett FC, Jr.: HL-A27 in Reiter's syndrome and psoriatic arthritis. A genetic factor in disease susceptibility and expression. J Rheumatol 1:263, 1974

129. Friis J: Reiter's disease with childhood onset having special reference to HLA B27. Scand J Rheumatol 9:250, 1980

130. Noer HR: An "experimental" epidemic of Reiter's syndrome. JAMA 198:693, 1966

131. Florman AL, Goldstein HM: Arthritis, conjunctivitis and urethritis (so-called Reiter's syndrome) in a 4 year old boy. J Pediatr 33:172, 1948

132. Czonka GW: The course of Reiter's syndrome. Br Med J 1:1088, 1958

133. Davies NE, Haverty JR, Boatwright M: Reiter's disease associated with shigellosis. South Med J 62:1011, 1969

134. Singsen BH, Bernstein BH, Koster-King KG et al: Reiter's syndrome in childhood. Arthritis Rheum, suppl., 20:471, 1977

135. Russell AS: Reiter's syndrome in children following infection with *Yersinia enterocolitica* and *Shigella*. Arthritis Rheum, suppl., 20:471, 1977

136. Iveson JMI, Nanda BS, Hancock JAH et al: Reiter's disease in three boys. Ann Rheum Dis 34:364, 1975

137. Jacobs AG: A case of Reiter's syndrome in childhood. Br Med J 2:155, 1961

138. Schachter J: Isolation of Bedsoniae from human arthritis and abortion tissues. Am J Ophthalmol 63:364, 1967

139. Kossman JC, Floret D, Renaud H et al: Syndrome de Fiessinger Leroy Reiter chez l'enfant et ureaplasma urealyticum. Pediatrie 35:237, 1980

140. Pattin S, Durosoir JL, Thabaut A et al: Le test de transformation lymphoblastique avec l'antigen bedsonien (TTL bedsonien), dans les syndromes de Fressinger-Leroy-Reiter anciens et recents et dans les spondylarthrites ankylosantes. Rev Rhum 43:407, 1976

141. Ford DK, da Roza D, Shah P et al: Cell-mediated immune responses of synovial mononuclear cells in Reiter's syndrome against ureaplasmal and Chlamydial antigens. J Rheumatol 7:751, 1980

142. Keat AC, Maini RN, Nkwazi GC et al: Role of *Chlamydia trachomatis* and HLA B27 in sexually acquired reactive arthritis. Br Med J 1:605, 1978

143. Zewi M: Morbus reiteri. Acta Ophthalmol 25:47, 1947

144. Lockie GN, Hunder GG: Reiter's syndrome in children. Arthritis Rheum 14:767, 1971

145. Corner BD: Reiter's syndrome in childhood. Arch Dis Child 25:398, 1950

146. Vergnani RJ, Smith RS: Reiter's syndrome in a child. Arch Ophthalmol 91:165, 1974

147. Jones RA: Reiter's disease after *Salmonella typhimurium* enteritis. Br Med J 1:1391, 1977

148. Gough KR: Reiter's syndrome in father and son. Ann Rheum Dis 21:292, 1962

149. Margileth AM: Reiter's syndrome in children. Case report and review of the literature. Clin Pediatr 1:148, 1962

150. Petty RE, Malleson P: Spondyloarthropathies of childhood. Pediatr Clin North Am 33:1079, 1986

7

Systemic Lupus Erythematosus

DEFINITION AND CLASSIFICATION

Systemic lupus erythematosus (SLE) is an episodic, multisystem disease characterized by widespread inflammation of the blood vessels and connective tissues. Its clinical manifestations are extremely variable, and its natural history is unpredictable; untreated, SLE is often progressive and leads to death.

SLE is regarded as a prototype of autoimmune diseases in humans.[1,2] In no other disease are there such widespread immunologic abnormalities. Many scientific observations are consistent with the hypothesis that SLE results from altered immunologic responsiveness on a background of a genetic predisposition to the disease. Through a better understanding of the pathogenesis of this disorder, great advances have been made in the treatment and diagnosis of other immunologic problems.

DIAGNOSIS

Diagnosis of SLE is clinical and is confirmed by specific laboratory abnormalities. Clinical diagnosis is suggested by three prominent features of the disease:

1. SLE is an episodic disease. Commonly older children have a previous history of intermittent symptoms such as arthritis, pleuritis, dermatitis, or nephritis.

2. SLE is a multisystemic disease (in contrast to organ-specific autoimmune diseases such as thyroiditis). Therefore, children generally present with more than one organ system involved by the small vessel vasculitis that is the basic pathologic lesion.

3. Antinuclear antibody (ANA) is usually present. Detection of ANA is one of the hallmarks of the diagnosis of SLE. A diagnosis of acute SLE cannot usually be made without a positive ANA reaction. However, ANA seropositivity alone is not grounds for a diagnosis of SLE in a child.

Criteria for the Classification of Patients with SLE

Eleven manifestations of SLE have been identified by a committee of the American Rheumatism Association (ARA) as criteria for the classification of the disease (the previous criteria contained 14 items) (Table 7-1).[3,4] In this study, the presence of four criteria in adults had a sensitivity of 96 percent and a specificity of 96 percent for a diagnosis of SLE. These criteria have proved not only to be valuable in classification of patients for study but also to delineate some of the more important clinical features of SLE. There have been a number of subsequent studies of

Table 7-1 Criteria for the Classification of Systemic Lupus Erythematosus[a]

Malar (butterfly) rash
Discoid-lupus rash
Photosensitivity
Oral or nasal mucocutaneous ulcerations
Nonerosive arthritis
Nephritis[b]
  Proteinuria >0.5 g/day
  Cellular casts
Encephalopathy[b]
  Seizures
  Psychosis
Pleuritis or pericarditis
Cytopenia
Positive immunoserology[b]
  Antibodies to nDNA
  Antibodies to Sm nuclear antigen
  Positive LE-cell preparation
  Biologic false-positive test for syphilis
Positive antinuclear antibody test

[a] Four of 11 criteria provide a sensitivity of 96% and a specificity of 96%.
[b] Any one item satisfies that criterion.
(Adapted from Tan EM et al.,[3] with permission.)

the value of these criteria in diagnosis, but none specifically in children.[5,6]

A number of other diseases are often considered by the clinician at the onset of SLE. In one study, diagnoses that were mentioned frequently were juvenile rheumatoid arthritis (JRA), acute glomerulonephritis, acute hemolytic anemia, acute leukemia, allergic dermatitis, epilepsy, infectious mononucleosis, rubella, acute rheumatic fever, infectious arthritis, traumatic arthritis, and other viral infections.[7]

HISTORICAL REVIEW

Lupus, derived from the Latin word for "wolf," was originally used in medicine from the 13th to the 19th centuries to describe a dermatitis characterized by recurrent florid facial ulcerations.[8] The acute and chronic types of the skin disease were first clarified by Kaposi in 1872.[9] In 1895, Osler recognized the systemic nature of this disease and its characteristic exacerbations and remissions and suggested that "erythema exudativum" was a form of vasculitis.[10] Cardiac involvement was described in detail by Libman and Sacks in 1924[11] and by Gross in 1940.[12] The clinical features of SLE as recognized today, however, were first delineated

by Baehr, Klemperer, and Schifrin in 1935.[13] These authors emphasized that characteristic visceral involvement could occur in the absence of the typical cutaneous lesions.

In 1948, the description of the lupus erythematosus (LE) cell by Hargraves, Richmond, and Morton at the Mayo Clinic[14] represented a major advance in interest in and knowledge of this disease. It became possible to recognize a broader spectrum of patients with SLE. Not only was the frequency with which the diagnosis was made remarkably increased, but investigation of the mechanism of the formation of LE cells led rapidly to an increased understanding of the concepts of autoimmunity, for example, the production of circulating antibodies directed against nuclear antigens.

The introduction of corticosteroid drugs into the treatment of connective-tissue diseases represented a major advance in the management of SLE. It became possible not only to prolong the life of severely afflicted patients and to control acute manifestations of the disease but also to follow the unfolding course of the disease in successfully treated patients. Later, the discovery of ANAs and the clinical application of the technique of indirect fluorescence microscopy in routine diagnostic laboratories led to more accurate diagnosis. Identification of a specific antibody to native deoxyribonucleic acid (DNA) in serum and in the pathologic lesions of patients with the disease led to the concept of toxic immune complex disease as an explanation for the pathogenesis of SLE. The mediation of inflammation invoked by soluble immune complexes through activation of complement was soon demonstrated. Later, impaired cell-mediated immunity was found in patients with active SLE, and most recently the potential role of immunogenetic predisposition and the possibility of viral "triggers" of the disease have been studied.

EPIDEMIOLOGY

Incidence and Prevalence

There have been several large studies of the incidence and prevalence of SLE (Table 7-2),[15–17] but data on children are few. The incidence of SLE in the

Table 7-2 Incidence and Prevalence of Systemic Lupus Erythematosus

	Incidence	Prevalence	Clinical Nephritis
Nobrega et al.[15] (1968)	6.4/10⁵	1/2,400	—
Fessel[16] (1974)	7.6/10⁵	1/1,969	16%
Recent estimate (1986)[a]	—	112,000	18,000

[a] Estimated numbers in the United States.

under-15 age group has been estimated at 0.6 per 100,000.[18] No accurate prevalence data are available. Meislin and Rothfield noted that of 242 patients with SLE in their series, 42 (17 percent) had onset before age 16 years.[19] In most pediatric rheumatology clinics, SLE constitutes up to 10 percent of the new diagnoses of systemic rheumatic diseases in children.

Age of Onset

Onset of disease is rare in the child younger than 5 years of age, becomes increasingly more common during adolescence, and is almost as high during these years as in any subsequent decade. The distribution of ages at onset for 345 children with SLE determined from data available in reported series is depicted in Figure 7-1.[19-26] The apparent fall in frequency in the 15- to 19-year age group almost certainly reflects referral to adult rather than pediatric clinics. In two large reviews of SLE, 3.5 percent of the patients had onset of disease at <10 years of age in one,[27] and the frequency of childhood onset was estimated at 4 to 15 percent of all cases in the other.[28] SLE in terms of frequency of onset (allowing for referral bias) is predominantly a disease of the adolescent years (Fig. 7-1). In a summary of the Los Angeles data,[29] 17 of 54 children had onset of the disease at ≥10 years of age.

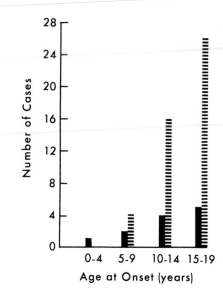

Fig. 7-2 Age by sex at onset of SLE. Boys ■. Girls ▤.

Sex Ratio

Girls are affected 4.5 times more frequently than boys; however, the overall ratio varies to some extent with age at onset.[30-33] In our Ann Arbor study,[24] the ratio of girls to boys with SLE was 4:3 in the 0- to 9-year age range, in the 10- to 14-year range 16:4, and in the 15- to 19-year range 26:5 (Fig. 7-2, Table 7-3). Three of the seven youngest patients with SLE were boys, and the youngest child was a boy with onset at the age of 3 years. Similar differences were noted by King and her colleagues, with girls outnumbering boys by 3:1 in the under-12-year onset group and by almost 10:1 in the over-12-year onset group.[25] In 101 children with a diagnosis of SLE observed at the Mayo Clinic between 1945 and 1970, 86 were girls and 15 were boys.[31] Only nine children were less than 9 years of age. There was a nearly uniform distribution of ages of onset in boys. In large

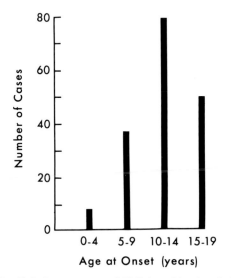

Fig. 7-1 Age at onset of SLE (combined series).

Table 7-3 Sex Distribution of Children with SLE

Publication	Number	Percentage Female	Male
Hagge et al.[33]	41	90	10
Meislin and Rothfield[19]	42	81	19
Walravens and Chase[34]	50	72	28
King et al.[25]	108	83	17
Cassidy et al.[24]	58	79	21
Total	299	81	19

Table 7-14 Correlation of Histopathologic Characteristics and Clinical State of Lupus Nephritis

Type of Renal Disease	Nephrotic Syndrome	Renal Failure	Remission	Uremic Deaths
Glomerular				
Mesangial	−	−	+	−
Focal proliferative	±	±	+ +	±
Diffuse proliferative	+ +	+ +	±	+ + +
Membranous	+ + +	+ +	+	+
Extraglomerular				
Interstitial	+	+	±	±
Necrotizing arteritis	±	+	+	±
End-stage	+ +	+ + +	−	+ + +

Absent, −; minimal, ±; moderate, +; severe, + +; very severe, + + +.

ized histopathologically on the basis of the pattern of deposition of immune complexes. The wide spectrum of renal abnormalities makes a system of classification difficult.[272–278] The subdivisions of lupus nephritis are important in determining the type and duration of therapy and in estimating prognosis. The types that will be discussed are based on classifications that have evolved empirically[272–275] and been documented in the studies of Baldwin et al. (Table 7-14),[279,280] and in the classification of the World Health Organization (Table 7-15).[281] These are mesangial nephritis, mild or focal nephritis, severe or diffuse proliferative nephritis, and membranous nephritis. In addition, interstitial nephritis, glomerular sclerosis,

necrotizing angiitis, and end-stage renal disease are discussed as representative of an additional spectrum of the renal abnormalities encountered in children with SLE.

This current classification of lupus nephritis, although an acceptable approach to categorization of the severity of the glomerular lesions, is not a wholly satisfactory answer to the problems of diagnosis, prediction of the course and outcome, and selection of a therapeutic regimen by the physician. A system based on the site of immune complex deposition, although documenting abnormalities in a patient at a specific moment in time, is arbitrary, does not reflect the direction of change or evolution of the lesions,

Table 7-15 World Health Organization Classification of Lupus Nephritis

Class I	Normal	No detectable disease ·
Class II	Mesangial	
IIA	Minimal alteration	Normal LM; mesangial deposits of immunoglobulin and complement by IFM; mesangial deposits by EM[a]
IIB	Mesangial glomerulitis	IIA plus mesangial hypercellularity (more than 3 cells per mesangial area or increased mesangial matrix); minimal tubular or interstitial disease
Class III	Focal and segmental proliferative glomerulonephritis	Focal areas of intra- and extracapillary cellular proliferation, necrosis, karyorrhexis, and leukocytic infiltration in <50% of the glomeruli; subendothelial or mesangial deposits on IFM or EM; focal tubular and interstitial disease
Class IV	Diffuse proliferative glomerulonephritis	Class III changes involving more glomerular surface area and >50% of the glomeruli; IFM and EM show abundant subendothelial deposits; marked interstitial involvement; membranoproliferative variant has prominent mesangial cell proliferation and capillary wall thickening
Class V	Membranous glomerulonephritis	No mesangial, endothelial, or epithelial cellular proliferation; diffusely and uniformly thickened capillary walls; IFM and EM show mesangial and subepithelial deposits; minimal interstitial involvement

[a] LM, light microscopy; IFM, immunofluorescent microscopy; EM, electron microscopy.

and does not take into account the complexity of combined or mixed lesions. It also principally classifies the glomerular disease and does not score the activity (intracapillary cellular proliferation, polymorphonuclear infiltrates, karyorrhexis, epithelial crescents, subendothelial fibrinoid change (wire-loops), hyaline, fibrin, or platelet thrombi, interstitial inflammation, necrotizing vasculitis) or the chronicity (segmental, global, mesangial, or vascular sclerosis, glomerular obsolescence, thickening of capillary basement membrane, fibrous adhesions or crescents, tubulointerstitial scarring) of the nephritis as reflected in other pathoanatomic changes.[281]

MESANGIAL LUPUS NEPHRITIS

Mesangial nephritis represents the most minimal glomerular lesion (Table 7-16, Figs. 7-16 and 7-17). Light microscopy reveals that all glomeruli are normal or, at the most, show a minimal increase in the number of mesangial cells and matrix. Diagnosis depends on immunofluorescent demonstration of mesangial deposition of IgG and C3. Electron micros-

Table 7-16 Mesangial Lupus Nephritis

May be initial immune complex lesion
Usually no clinical features of renal disease, or there may be minimal proteinuria or hematuria
Remission or progression of the nephritis may occur with transition to diffuse or membranous disease

copy indicates electron-dense deposits in the mesangia and along the paramesangial capillary basement membranes.

Children with mesangial nephritis almost always have a normal urinalysis or, at most, transient minimal proteinuria and hematuria. Serologically, however, anti-nDNA antibody levels may be elevated and serum complement levels somewhat depressed. Mesangial disease has been shown to progress occasionally to focal or diffuse proliferative nephritis.[282,283] It is assumed, however, that most of these children will not develop serious, life-threatening renal insufficiency. We believe this is particularly true if active systemic disease is adequately treated initially, with normalization of the serologic abnormalities.

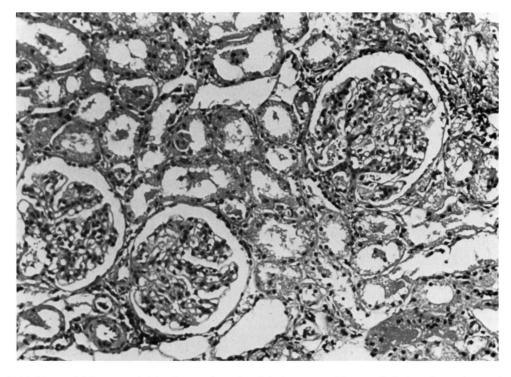

Fig. 7-16 Mesangial lupus nephritis. Except for a few lobular areas of hypercellularity, these glomeruli from a renal biopsy of a 12-year-old black girl with acute SLE appear normal.

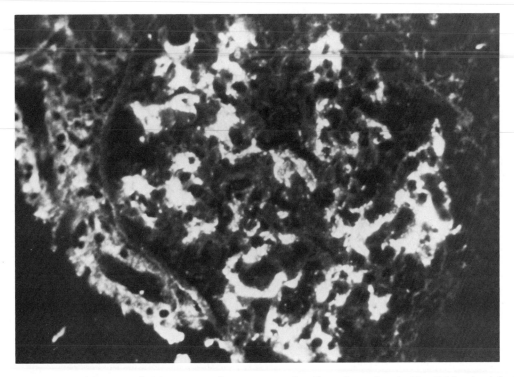

Fig. 7-17 Mesangial lupus nephritis. Immunofluorescent section from the patient in Fig. 7-16 stained for IgG. Massive deposits of immunoglobulin are identified in the mesangium, in contrast to the paucity of abnormalities shown by light microscopy.

FOCAL PROLIFERATIVE GLOMERULITIS

Mild or focal nephritis is characterized by areas of hypercellularity in less than half of the glomeruli in the renal biopsy specimen (Table 7-17 and Fig. 7-18).[284] Local lesions within each glomerulus tend to be located in the peripheral loops, as opposed to the central involvement of poststreptococcal glomerulonephritis.

Light microscopy reveals segmental proliferation of the glomerular tufts that is usually accompanied by mesangial proliferation. Immunoglobulins and complement components appear by immunofluores-

Table 7-17 Focal Proliferative Lupus Glomerulitis

Minimal proteinuria
Microscopic hematuria
Nephrotic syndrome or renal insufficiency in 20%
Responsive to corticosteroid therapy
Does not usually progress to renal failure

cence microscopy as lumpy-bumpy deposits along the basement membranes. Ultrastructural studies show subendothelial electron-dense deposits of immune complexes along the capillary basement membrane with accompanying proliferative changes. Less frequently, a few subepithelial and intramembranous deposits may be found. The characteristic endothelial myxoviruslike inclusion is seen in virtually all biopsy specimens of children with SLE. It is uncommonly observed in patients with other types of renal disease.

Clinically, proteinuria and mild hematuria may be present, but renal insufficiency is either minimal or absent, and the nephrotic syndrome is distinctly uncommon. These children are often acutely ill at presentation, however, and have severe extrarenal disease. The anti-nDNA antibody assay is elevated (75 to more than 90 percent binding), and the serum hemolytic complement activity is low to absent.

As in the mesangial form of the disease, progression of focal disease to the more severe forms of lupus nephritis has been observed.[285] Actual documentation of this progression in an individual child is un-

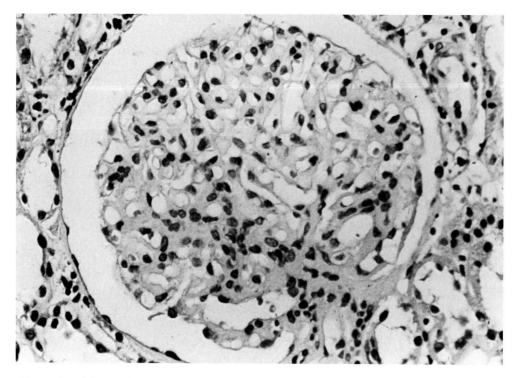

Fig. 7-18 Focal proliferative lupus nephritis. A lobular area of hypercellularity and necrosis is seen in an otherwise normal glomerulus. The majority of the glomeruli appeared normal on light microscopy.

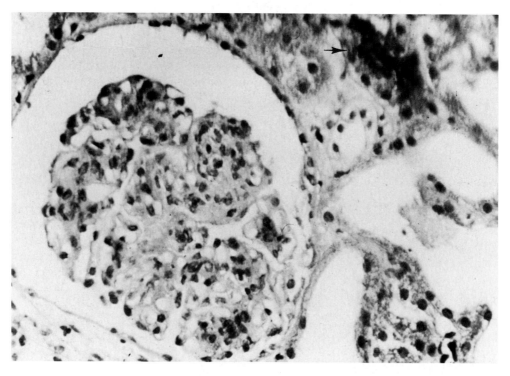

Fig. 7-19 Diffuse proliferative lupus glomerulonephritis. All glomeruli in the biopsy core were uniformly involved by the immunoinflammatory process. The outlines of many glomeruli were obliterated. Marked hypercellularity, hyaline thrombi, hematoxylin bodies, and areas of necrosis were present. An RBC cast (arrow) is present in an adjacent tubule.

common. It is probably most likely to occur with a severe, uncontrolled, and prolonged exacerbation of systemic disease. Minimal and focal glomerulitis progressed to diffuse disease in 7.4 percent of 81 cases in one series,[286] 29 percent of 31 cases in another,[283] and 35 percent of 17 cases in a third.[287]

Table 7-18 Diffuse Proliferative Lupus Glomerulonephritis

Proteinuria and hematuria
Nephrotic syndrome and renal insufficiency in 60%
Limited remissions in 50%
Death in 3–5 yr from renal failure

DIFFUSE PROLIFERATIVE GLOMERULONEPHRITIS

Severe or diffuse nephritis is characterized by a more uniform involvement of the majority (>50 percent), if not all, of the glomeruli in the biopsy specimen (Table 7-18, Figs. 7-19 to 7-21). In addition, the severity of the individual glomerular changes is usually more pronounced than in focal disease. There is a lumpy-bumpy deposition of immunoglobulin and complement along the peripheral capillary walls, as well as in the mesangium. Interstitial infiltrates and extraglomerular immune complex deposition may also be noted along the tubular basement membranes, within the walls of the peritubular capillaries, or in the interstitium. Electron microscopy shows extensive immune deposits occurring in the mesangium and subendothelial space and, to a lesser extent, in the subepithelial and intramembranous areas. Ultrastructurally, these electron-dense deposits may exhibit a fingerprint or microtubular structure. This or-

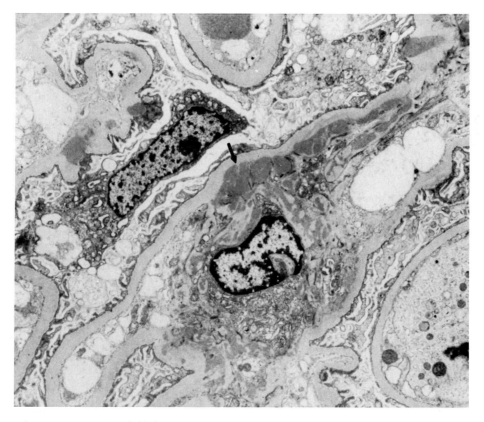

Fig. 7-20 Electron microscopic field showing subendothelial and paramesangial immune deposits (arrow) from a patient with diffuse proliferative glomerulonephritis.

ganized configuration is a result of crystallization within the immune complexes.

Clinically, these children have moderate to heavy proteinuria with or without the nephrotic syndrome. Hematuria is almost invariably present, as is mild to severe renal insufficiency. Red cell casts indicate the presence of active glomerulitis. Antibody activity to nDNA is very high, and serum complement levels are very low to undetectable. In the nephrotic syndrome, serologic markers of active disease such as anti-DNA antibodies and even ANA may be falsely low because of profuse loss of IgG in the urine. An estimate of glomerular damage may be determined by the size of the proteins that are excreted (selectivity of the proteinuria). As in the idiopathic nephrotic syndrome, more severe disease is characterized by loss of the larger molecules and an altered IgG-to-transferrin ratio.

Table 7-19 Membranous Lupus Glomerulonephritis

Persistent nephrotic syndrome
Hypertension in 30%
Remissions in 30%
Eventual renal insufficiency

MEMBRANOUS LUPUS GLOMERULONEPHRITIS

In membranous nephritis the characteristic lesion is deposition of immune complexes along the subepithelial border of the glomerular basement membrane with obliteration of the foot processes (Table 7-19, Figs. 7-22 and 7-23).[288–290] The basement membranes assume a rigid, enlarged, glassy appearance, with few proliferative changes being evident. There may be slight, irregular increases in the numerical density of

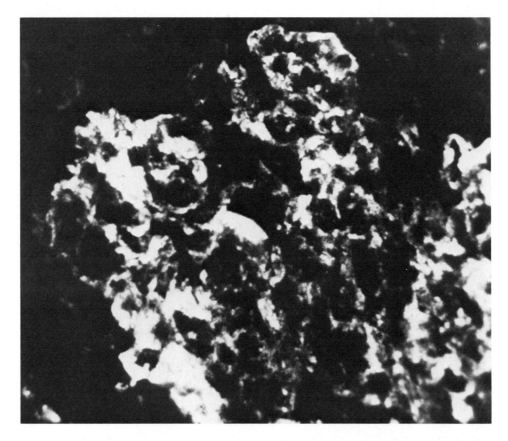

Fig. 7-21 Fluorescent microscopy of a renal biopsy section from a young girl who died with CNS lupus and the nephrotic syndrome. Deposits of IgG are shown in a lumpy-bumpy pattern (subendothelial) and a finer granular pattern (epimembranous).

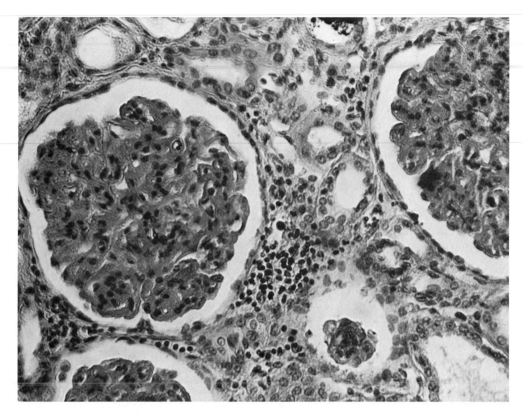

Fig. 7-22 Membranous lupus glomerulonephritis. This patient was a 17-year-old white girl who had the nephrotic syndrome and congestive heart failure. The hospital course was unusually short, and she died from an arrhythmia. Libman-Sacks endocarditis was found at necropsy (Fig. 7-7). Routine sections of kidney showed uniform glomerular involvement with prominent thickening and wire-loop changes of the endothelial walls. These had a "glassy" refractility on hematoxylin-eosin sections. There was minimal hypercellularity, and deposits of inflammatory cells were present in the tubular interstitial tissues.

the mesangial cells and in the mesangial matrix. Silver or periodic acid–Schiff (PAS) stains define a spike pattern along the basement membrane related to immune complex deposition on the capillary loops. Fluorescence microscopy shows a granular deposition of IgG and complement along the basement membrane, usually finer and smaller than the deposits found in diffuse glomerulonephritis. In addition, there may be intrabasement membrane deposits, suggesting that in certain situations immune complexes may traverse the basement membrane from the subendothelial to the subepithelial surfaces.

Patients with membranous nephritis invariably have proteinuria and often hematuria, and the nephrotic syndrome is common. If not present initially, the nephrotic syndrome supervenes shortly thereafter during the course of the disease. Serologic evidence

of disease activity may be less striking than in diffuse proliferative nephritis. This is particularly true if extrarenal systemic activity is absent at the time of presentation. However, rapidly progressive glomerulonephritis is usually superimposed on diffuse or membranous forms of lupus nephritis.

INTERSTITIAL NEPHRITIS

Approximately half of the children with significant involvement of the glomerulus also show evidence of interstitial nephritis.[291] In the early studies of Pollak et al.,[273,275] interstitial and tubular diseases were identified as poor prognostic findings. Focal or diffuse infiltrates of inflammatory cells, necrotic tubules, and interstitial fibrosis are all observed. Immunoglobulins and complement are deposited along

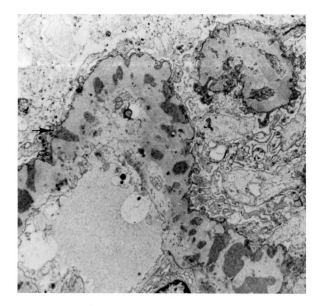

Fig. 7-23 Electron microscopic section of membranous nephritis showing epimembranous complexes (arrow).

the peritubular capillaries or the tubular basement membranes in a granular pattern and in the interstitium. The severity of the interstitial abnormalities often correlates with the severity of the glomerular changes; rarely, severe interstitial nephritis with little or no glomerular abnormalities has been noted.

Renal tubular acidosis or incomplete Fanconi's syndrome may be seen in some of these patients. In addition, others have concomitant Sjögren's syndrome, which may account in part for the interstitial nephritis. Last, analgesic nephropathy leading to interstitial inflammation and tubular damage should always be considered in patients with these changes.

GLOMERULAR SCLEROSIS

Glomerular sclerosis (WHO class VI) secondary to immune complex deposition may develop but is generally minimal. Segmental glomerulosclerosis, in the absence of extensive membranoproliferative disease or interstitial nephritis, may not be an ominous finding. Studies of sequential biopsy specimens in 40 patients with diffuse nephritis have been reported by Morel-Maroger.[286] Minimal to mild sclerosis was noted in 8 of 16 patients who had a stable course. It was also present in half of the initial biopsy specimens of patients who later progressed to diffuse nephritis.

Extensive sclerotic lesions indicated a poor prognosis. High-dose prednisone therapy in 14 of these patients did not prevent progression of the sclerosis in 8, although the activity of the individual glomerular lesions diminished. In 19 of 25 patients in whom active glomerulitis was accompanied by only moderate sclerosis, the activity of the lesions was seen to have decreased on repeat biopsy. These conclusions were similar to those reported by Striker et al.,[292] who noted an absence of correlation between the evolution of active lesions that responded to therapy and that of sclerotic lesions that progressed in spite of treatment.

NECROTIZING ANGIITIS

Some children with lupus nephritis may also demonstrate an immune complex arteriolitis in renal tissues as well as elsewhere. The vascular histopathologic features in these cases may be indistinguishable from those of other forms of necrotizing arteritis. Fibrinoid necrosis, thrombosis, and arteriolar inflammation are usually present. This type of vasculitis may be associated clinically with fulminant renal failure and malignant hypertension or renal venous thromboses.

END-STAGE RENAL DISEASE

There are a few children with seemingly inactive lupus nephritis and normal serum complement levels who have chronic progressive renal disease on the basis of prior immunologic injury (Table 7-20). In these patients, proteinuria is constant and does not in

Table 7-20 SLE Nephritis: End-Stage Disease

Clinical characteristics
Clinical inactivity
Serologic inactivity
Severe hypertension
Intermittent sepsis
Therapy
Minimal corticosteroid or immunosuppressive medication
Control of hypertension
Nephrectomy
Satisfactory hemodialysis
Infrequent recurrence in the transplanted kidney

itself indicate active glomerulitis. Treatment of these children with high-dose prednisone therapy is fraught with many hazards, and the overall prognosis for renal function is extremely poor. If a child appears to be deteriorating under these circumstances, a trial of high-dose prednisone restricted to 2 weeks or steroid-pulse therapy should be evaluated before a judgment is made on prognosis. Repeat biopsy and potential use of immunosuppression or plasmapheresis should also be considered.

It is also possible for children with severe sclerosis, inactive renal glomerular lesions, and moderate insufficiency to remain in clinical remission while taking either small doses of corticosteroids or none at all. Some of these patients have prolonged serologic and clinical remissions and do not require active treatment of the SLE. Hemodialysis or renal transplantation may be necessary in others.

EVALUATION OF LUPUS NEPHRITIS

Evaluation of the child with SLE for significant renal disease should proceed from examination of the child, urinalysis, and culture through serologic tests, measurement of creatinine clearance and protein excretion, renal ultrasound, and biopsy (Table 7-21). Renal biopsy should be considered in any child before corticosteroid therapy is started, and certainly before cytotoxic drugs are employed.

It is not possible to assess the true extent of renal involvement in children with SLE solely on the basis of clinical examination. Extensive glomerular abnormalities have been identified by biopsy of patients who have no clinical evidence of renal disease.[19,274,293–295] In two reports of 27 children in whom lupus nephritis was found at necropsy, 6 children had had no laboratory evidence of renal disease during life.[21,180]

Table 7-21 Clinical Evaluation of Lupus Nephritis

Urinalysis
Urine culture
Creatinine clearance
24-h protein excretion
Anti-nDNA antibody assay
Serum complement assay
Renal ultrasound
Renal biopsy

New data suggest that "silent" diffuse nephritis (e.g., without clinically apparent disease) may not always protend as poor a prognosis as clinically obvious disease.[296–298] Additional studies in children will be necessary in this regard.

The diagnosis of clinical lupus nephritis is confirmed by the finding of an abnormal urinary sediment. Proteinuria and microscopic hematuria with or without red blood cell casts may be present. Impaired renal function is confirmed by a fixed specific gravity, elevated blood urea nitrogen or creatinine, and decreased creatinine clearance. Children with the nephrotic syndrome have an elevated serum cholesterol and decreased serum albumin. Glomerular filtration rate and renal blood flow can also be determined by isotopic studies.

The two most important laboratory measures related to activity of the nephritis in children with SLE are an abnormally high level of anti-nDNA antibodies and depression of the serum complement level.[299–306] Conversely, it is not likely that a child with good clinical control will have persistent, moderate to severe abnormalities in these tests.

The serum complement level in active SLE is low to absent, in part because of activation of complement by immune complex deposition. Rarely a patient with seemingly active SLE has a near normal complement level. As serum complement components are increased by inflammatory disease, it may be simply lowered to normal levels by immune complex fixation, rather than being reduced to subnormal levels.

Occasionally a child with SLE may have hemolytic complement values in the subnormal range for long periods of time with no indication of clinically active disease. This observation alone is not an indication for a change of therapy, since the catabolic events associated with corticosteroid therapy, general illness, or uremia may impair the synthesis of complement components, particularly the C3 moiety.[307] Isolated deficiency of complement (especially heterozygous C2 deficiency) may also be seen in children with SLE-like disease.[141,142,147–149,156] In these children, hemolytic activity is depressed, whereas C3 or C4 assays are normal if there is no active immune complex formation.

Assays for circulating immune complexes may be useful in evaluation of disease activity. Abrass et al. showed that an abnormal C1q binding assay was significantly associated with active SLE, including arthritis and nephritis, and correctly predicted a variation in disease activity 82 percent of the time.[308] In this study, detection of serum immune complexes correlated better with disease activity than did the anti-nDNA antibody assay or serum C3 level. (This has been rarely our experience.)

LONG-TERM STUDIES

Sequential biopsies have provided some insight into the progression of the renal lesion. However, these studies must be interpreted with caution since indications for biopsy and influence of therapy undoubtedly affect the results.[309,310] In general, however, sequential biopsies in children have demonstrated progression of mesangial or focal proliferative glomerulonephritis to diffuse proliferative glomerulonephritis in months to years.[287] Similar observations have been made in the careful studies of adults and children by Baldwin et al.[279,280] and others.[25,311] Occasional progression from diffuse proliferative to membranous disease or less commonly focal proliferative to membranous disease was also documented.[280,311] In some studies improvement was noted in 15 to 20 percent of patients in whom the initial biopsy had shown diffuse proliferative or focal proliferative glomerulonephritis, but membranous disease tended to be worse on subsequent examination.

PREDICTORS OF PROGRESSIVE RENAL DISEASE

In the studies of Baldwin et al.,[279,280] focal nephritis generally followed a benign course except for the occasional transition mentioned. The majority of patients with diffuse disease and nephrotic syndrome had necrotizing renal vasculitis, severe hypertension, and accelerated renal failure. A fatal outcome often occurred within approximately 5 years. A small number of patients with diffuse nephritis went into remission, and membranous nephritis, when characterized by a persistent nephrotic syndrome, progressed slowly to renal failure. In the studies of Garin et al.,[311] chronic renal failure occurred in only one child, and the 5-year survivorship of all groups was 72 percent. Six children with diffuse disease, however, died. Children with diffuse lesions could survive for long periods, and decreased renal function

was rare in patients with focal and membranous disease. In a subsequent study,[306] these investigators found no correlation among the renal histologic changes and serum C4 or nDNA-binding levels. In the study by Zimmerman et al.,[287] the authors were unable to identify clinical features of the initial illness, and often even to determine differences on the initial renal biopsy, that would distinguish patients whose nephritis progressed from those whose remained stable. In another study,[25] renal histology did not correlate with age of onset, sex, or duration of disease. However, in general the severity of renal lesions found on the initial biopsy correlated with the clinical assessment of outcome. Minimal or focal nephritis generally did not progress to renal failure. When a change in histopathologic classification was found on repeat biopsy, it usually showed progression in the severity of the lesion. Children with diffuse proliferative disease did worse by all parameters than comparable groups; all patients who died were in this histologic classification.

Our studies in this regard are summarized in Table 7-22.[24] Clinical nephritis generally was evident at onset of SLE; in only six patients did it develop more than 2 years after onset. Renal deaths also tended to occur early. Five deaths occurred in children who had diffuse nephritis and in one with membranous disease.

Table 7-22 Lupus Nephritis in 58 Children with SLE

	1958–1966	1967–1975
Number of children with SLE	30	28
Clinical nephritis	25	25
Renal biopsies	13	22
Focal proliferative glomerulitis	—	6
Diffuse proliferative glomerulonephritis	—	9
Diffuse proliferative and membranous glomerulonephritis	—	2
Duration of clinical disease		
Range	1 mo–13 yr	2 mo–8 yr
Average	4.6 yr	3 yr
Deaths from renal failure	6	1

(Modified from Cassidy JT et al.,[24] with permission.)

LABORATORY EXAMINATIONS

Nonspecific Signs of Inflammation

Acute-phase indices of inflammation are increased in children with SLE in proportion to the activity of the systemic disease. These include an increased erythrocyte sedimentation rate, polyclonal hypergammaglobulinemia, and an increase in the α_2 globulins of the serum and C-reactive protein (CRP) levels.[312–316] It is more likely that elevation of the CRP level reflects systemic activity of the SLE and does not distinguish acute autoimmune disease from infection.

Hematologic Abnormalities

Anemia occurs in approximately one-half of the children with SLE and is usually typical of that seen in chronic disease (normocytic, hypochromic) (Table 7-23). The cause of anemia in children with SLE is often multifactorial. At the simplest, low hemoglobin and hematocrit values reflect the "iron deficiency" anemia of chronic inflammatory disease. Blood loss, including menorrhagia and hemorrhage from the GI tract related to ulceration and thrombocytopenia, may be an obvious or covert cause. Hemolysis may also play a role. The causes of hemolysis vary and are related to hypersplenism, Coombs' antibodies (IgG, complement-fixing), cold agglutinins, drug hypersensitivity, and, rarely, microangiopathy.

Leukopenia is a hallmark of acute SLE. Neutrophils predominate even in low counts (<4,000 cells/mm^3; <4.0 × 10^9/L). Children with WBC counts below 2,000 cells/mm^3 may not respond to septicemia with the degree of leukocytosis expected of normal children. White blood cell counts in the range of 8,000 to 12,000/mm^3 may represent their maximal response to infection and stress. The majority of children are leukopenic at the onset of disease, but extreme degrees of leukopenia (<2,000 cells/mm^3) are uncommon, and leukocytosis may occur.[25]

Most children with SLE have a normal platelet count, but with increased production and peripheral destruction of platelets. In one study, although the frequency of antiplatelet antibodies was 78 percent, only 14 percent of the patients were thrombocytopenic.[317] Qualitative abnormalities of platelet aggregation also occur. Some children with SLE have clinically important immune thrombocytopenic purpura. Bone marrow examination in these cases shows an increased number of megakaryocytes with poor platelet budding. Patients with thrombocytopenic purpura and hemolytic anemia (Evan's syndrome) may progress to SLE or eventually develop the features of thrombotic thrombocytopenic purpura.

Autoantibodies

Children with SLE have a wide variety of nonspecific and tissue-specific antibodies, such as antithyroglobulin (Table 7-24).[318,319] Cryoglobulinemia is often present in active SLE and may be responsible for certain expressions of the disease by precipitation in vascular endothelium or through development of the hyperviscosity syndrome (Raynaud's phenomenon, acrocyanosis, purpura, and abdominal crisis). These cryoglobulins contain ANA and DNA. Cold agglutinins are also found in some children with SLE and are directed against the I antigen of erythrocytes.

Table 7-23 Frequency of Hematologic Abnormalities in Children with SLE

Abnormality	Patients (%)
Anemia (hematocrit <30%)	50
Acute hemolytic anemia	5
Leukopenia	
<2,000 WBC/mm^3(<2 × 10^9/L)	10
<4,500 WBC/mm^3(<4.5 × 10^9/L)	40
Thrombocytopenia	
<150,000 pts/mm^3(<150 × 10^9/L)	30
<100,000 pts/mm^3(<100 × 10^9/L)	5

Table 7-24 Principal Abnormalities of Serum Antibody Activity in SLE

Antinuclear Antibodies	Other Antibodies
Anti-nDNA	Anticytoplasmic antibodies
Anti-DNP antibodies	Antilymphocytotoxic antibodies
Anti-Ro antibodies	Antitissue-specific antibodies
Anti-La antibodies	Antiviral antibodies
Anti-Sm antibodies	Anticardiolipin antibodies
Antihistone antibodies	Biologic false-positive serologic test for syphilis
	Rheumatoid factors

Table 7-25 Antibodies to Cellular Antigens in Connective-Tissue Diseases

Antigens	Antibody Specificity	Disease Specificity
Nuclear antigens		
DNA		
ds-DNA only	Deoxyribose-phosphate backbone	SLE (80%)
ds/ss-DNA		SLE (70%), rarely in other diseases
ss-DNA only	Purines and pyrimidines	SLE (90%), other connective tissue and nonrheumatic diseases
DNA-histone (DNP)	Nucleosome	SLE, JRA, other connective tissue diseases, chronic active hepatitis
Histones	H1, H2A, H2B, H3, H4	Drug-induced SLE (95%), SLE (30%), RA (20%), JRA
Nonhistone antigens		
ENA complex		
Sm	snRNP	SLE (40%)
nRNP	U1RNP	MCTD (95%), SLE (50%), DLE, scleroderma
SS-A(Ro)	snRNP	Scleroderma (60%), SLE (30%), sicca syndrome, neonatal lupus syndrome, ANA-negative lupus, C2 deficiency
SS-B (La, Ha)	snRNP	Scleroderma (50%), SLE (15%), sicca syndrome, ANA-negative lupus
Scl-70 (Scl-1)	Topoisomerase (chromatin-associated)	Scleroderma (20%)
Centromere	Inner and outer plates of kinetochore	CREST syndrome (70%)
RANA	EB-virus induced but distinct from EBNA (antigen for RAP)	RA (90%), sicca syndrome
MA antigen		SLE (20%)
PCNA	Dividing cells	SLE (10%)
PM-1	Acidic nuclear protein	Polymyositis/scleroderma overlap (85%), dermatomyositis (20%)
Mi-1		Dermatomyositis (30%)
Jo-1	Histidyl-tRNA synthetase	Polymyositis (30%)
Ku		Polymyositis/scleroderma overlap (50%)
Nucleolar Antigens		
4S-6S RNA	U3-RNA	Scleroderma (60%), overlap and sicca syndromes, Raynaud's phenomenon
RNA, RNP		Scleroderma
Cytoplasmic antigens		
Common antigens		
Mitochondria		Primary biliary cirrhosis
Microsomes		Chronic active hepatitis
RNA		SLE
Tissue-specific antigens		Organ-specific autoimmune diseases

ANTINUCLEAR ANTIBODIES

ANAs are present in the sera of a majority of children with active SLE (Table 7-25).[90–94,320,321] ANA titers have not proved very useful for following the course of the disease; however, the peripheral or shaggy nuclear fluorescent pattern is virtually diagnostic of active immune complex vasculitis and of nephritis associated with antibodies to double-stranded or native DNA (Fig. 7-24). Quantitative assays of these antibodies, along with determinations of the level of serum complement, have proved to be the most clinically accurate laboratory measures of therapeutic response.

The most important ANA historically is the LE-cell factor (Fig. 7-25).[14] This is an antideoxyribonucleoprotein (anti-DNP or anti-DNA histone). It does not appear to participate in the causation of clinical disease. It is responsible, however, for two important phenomena: the LE cell and hematoxylin bodies. LE-cell positivity is seen in active disease: 86 percent of our children had positive LE-cell

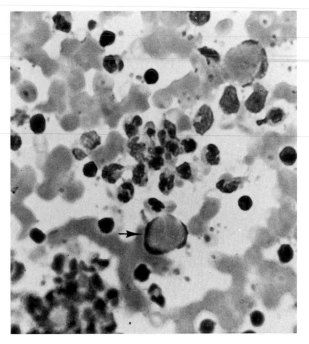

Fig. 7-25 LE-cell preparation. The patient had acute SLE with abundant LE cells identified. LE cell showing a homogeneous nuclear inclusion within a polymorphonuclear leukocyte is identified by the arrow.

preparations at onset, and all had LE-cell positivity at some time during the course of their disease. The LE cell is not pathognomonic for SLE. However, its presence always suggests that the basic underlying diathesis is SLE. When hematoxylin bodies occur in tissue sections not showing profound necrosis, they are pathognomonic of SLE.

The LE-cell test is not as sensitive a test as fluorescent ANA procedures. LE cells are most predictably found during an acute systemic exacerbation of the disease. An LE-cell test may be diagnostically helpful in a child who is thought to have an exacerbation of SLE but in whom the classic features of the disease are not present or have not recurred. Finding LE cells at that time would confirm the clinical suspicion that the current systemic illness of the child was related to an activation of the SLE. In other diagnostic dilemmas, an LE-cell test is useful, as it has a high degree of specificity. In most laboratories, assays for ANA and antibody to nDNA have superseded the LE-cell test.

Antibody to Native DNA

Antibodies to native, double-stranded DNA (nDNA) are characteristic of active immune complex disease in children with SLE and especially with active nephritis (Table 7-26).[322–324] They are rarely if

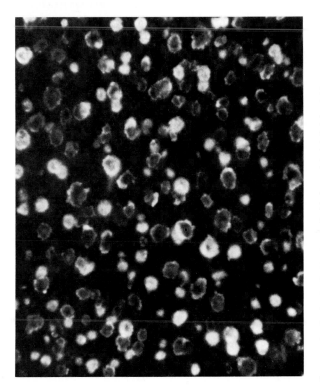

Fig. 7-24 Antinuclear antibody test on mouse liver. Fluorescent microscopy with conjugated anti-IgG antibodies was characteristic of the peripheral or shaggy pattern of anti-nDNA antibodies.

Table 7-26 Anti-nDNA Antibodies

Antigenic specificity	Native, double-stranded deoxyribonucleic acid (double-helical conformation)
Mechanism of action	Immune complex disease
Clinical correlations	Systemic lupus erythematosus, active glomerulotubular nephritis

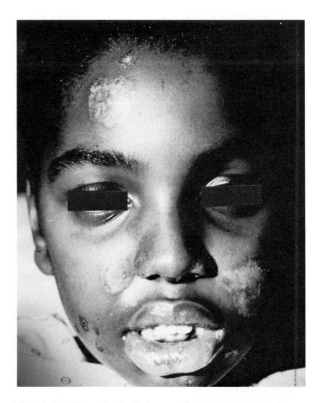

Fig. 7-26 Discoid skin lesions and mucocutaneous disease were present in this teenage boy who had anti-Ro antibody activity with a negative ANA test on mouse liver substrate.

ever associated with other rheumatic diseases. Children with active SLE also have very high values by the Farr radioimmunoassay. Normal binding is less than 3 to 10 percent.

Other methods for assaying DNA antibodies are in use in clinical laboratories and the substrate employed varies. Immunofluorescent tests using cultures of *Crithidia luciliae* provide a simple, titered semiquantitative method for detecting anti-nDNA antibodies.[325,326] This assay, however, is relatively insensitive and should not be used as a screening test.

Increased or increasing antibody to nDNA is often a clue to the onset or presence of active renal disease, particularly when accompanied by low or decreasing values for serum complement concentration. It should be noted that although anti-nDNA is very specific for a diagnosis of SLE, anti-single-stranded antibody activity is not.

Anti-Ro/La Antibodies

A rare child with SLE may have negative ANA tests ("ANA-negative lupus")[327,328] and have instead antibodies directed against nuclear antigens that are detected only with human tissue substrates by immunofluorescent or precipitin techniques. These nuclear antigens include Ro and La.[319,329,330] We have seen one such child, a teenage boy with anti-Ro antibodies, who presented with classic discoid cutaneous lesions, developed CNS disease, and died from cerebromalacia (Fig. 7-26). Another rare SLE-like disease associated with negative tests for ANA is the C1q-precipitin syndrome.[141]

Anti-Ro/SS-A antibody activity is most characteristic of the neonatal lupus syndrome previously discussed (Table 7-27). The Ro antigen was originally thought to be cytoplasmic but is predominantly a nuclear antigen[319] and is often not well detected on tissue

Table 7-27 Anti-Ro Antibodies

Antigenic specificity	Nuclear (? cytoplasmic) 60-kDa peptide-sRNA complex
Mechanism of action	? Control of RNA translation or transport (concentrated in fetal heart and brain)
Clinical correlations	Association with anti-La and RF antibodies, ANA-negative lupus, subacute cutaneous lupus, neonatal lupus syndromes, CCHB, renal and pulmonary disease in SLE, extraglandular sicca syndrome with cytopenia and vasculitis, asymptomatic normal individuals (5–15%)

Table 7-28 Anti-La Antibody

Antigenic specificity	Nuclear (? cytoplasmic) 50-kDa peptide-sRNA complex; ? induced by viral infection
Mechanism of action	? Interferes with termination of RNA polymerase III enzyme complex
Clinical correlations	Virtually always found in association with anti-Ro antibodies; neonatal lupus syndromes, sicca syndrome, SLE (? mild disease), asymptomatic normal individuals (5%)

Table 7-30 Anti-U1RNP Antibodies

Antigenic specificity	snRNP(U1)–68 kDa, A, C peptide complex (related to anti-Sm antibodies)
Mechanism of action	? Interferes with synthesis of mRNA
Clinical correlations	Mixed connective-tissue disease, SLE, scleroderma, RA

tivity have been related to CNS disease (Table 7-29).[334,335] Anti-Sm antibodies are only partially related to anti-U1RNP activity (Table 7-30), the latter being more characteristic of children with mild disease, no renal involvement, and a clinical picture suggestive of mixed connective-tissue disease.

substrates used in the fluorescent ANA procedure (e.g., mouse liver).[331,332] The majority of the Ro-positive patients, who were ANA negative on tissue sections, are positive on the HEp-2 cell substrate.

In addition to the neonatal lupus syndrome, anti-Ro antibodies have been associated with active renal disease in patients with SLE.[330] Classic ANA-positive SLE also demonstrates antibodies directed against these nuclear antigens in about one-fourth of the cases.[333] Between 5 and 15 percent of normal individuals have low levels of anti-Ro activity.[319] As many as 1 percent of normal pregnant women have been noted to have precipitating levels of this antibody. Like anti-Ro, anti-La may be present in low levels in approximately 5 percent of the normal population (Table 7-28).

Antibodies to Histones

Antihistone antibodies in drug-induced LE were delineated by Fritzler and Tan.[336] Specificities of antihistone antibodies have been found to be markedly different in spontaneous SLE and the various types of drug-induced disease (Table 7-31).[337-339] Reactivity in each of these diseases appeared to be restricted to a limited number of histone determinants. In procainamide-induced lupus, antibodies reacted with the H2A, H2B, and the H2A-H2B complex. In hydralazine-induced disease they reacted primarily with H3 and H4. The finding of antihistone antibodies in the absence of high titers of anti-nDNA antibodies is highly suggestive of drug-induced LE.

Anti-Sm Antibodies

Antibodies to the Sm antigen complex are specific for SLE and in the absence of other autoantibody ac-

ANTICARDIOLIPIN ANTIBODIES

Circulating anticoagulants in children with SLE are not rare. The *lupus anticoagulant* was described in 1952 by Conley and Hartmann as responsible for a hemorrhagic disorder that occurred in some patients with

Table 7-29 Anti-Sm Antibodies

Antigenic specificity	snRNP(U1,2,4/6,5) B′B, D peptide complex (related to anti-U1RNP antibodies)
Mechanism of action	? Interferes with RNA processing, mRNA synthesis and splicing
Clinical correlations	Specific for SLE, CNS lupus

Table 7-31 Antihistone Antibodies

Antigenic specificity	Histone complex (H2A-H2B), H1 > H2B > H2A > H3 > H4
Mechanism of action	? Interferes with nucleosome packaging of DNA
Clinical correlations	Drug-induced lupus, SLE

SLE.[340] It is a unique antibody inhibitor that acts at the junction of the intrinsic and extrinsic coagulation pathways: The conversion of prothrombin to thrombin by thromboplastin is inhibited by interference with the interaction of the prothrombin-activator complex (factors Xa and V, calcium, and phospholipid).[341] Such patients have a prolonged partial thromboplastin time and prothrombin time. These antibodies are directed at diphosphatidyl glycerol and may cross react with DNA (Table 7-32). Menorrhagia in young girls may result from the appearance of this circulating anticoagulant. Spontaneous bleeding, however, is uncommon and thrombosis is more characteristic.

The platelet count, Venereal Disease Research Laboratories (VDRL) test, and activated partial thromboplastin time are reasonable screening tests but are not totally reliable in detecting abnormalities induced by the presence of the lupus anticoagulant. Specific assays have been developed and are generally available.

Antiphospholipid antibodies are responsible for a variety of clinical and laboratory abnormalities in patients with SLE.[342] Patients with antiphospholipid antibodies have repeated episodes of venous and arterial thromboses,[343,344] coma, thrombocytopenia, livedo reticularis,[345] and labile hypertension. Spontaneous recurrent abortions and cardiovascular crises such as myocardial infarction and valvular lesions[346–348] have been observed in young adults.

Table 7-32 Anticardiolipin Antibodies

Antigenic specificity	Phospholipids (diphosphotidyl glycerol)
Mechanism of action	Inhibition of prothrombin activator complex (Xa, V, Ca^{++}, lipid), platelet aggregation, ↓ PGI_2 release
Clinical correlations	Biologic false-positive test for syphilis (VDRL), circulating anticoagulant, recurrent venous and arterial thromboses, livedo reticularis, emboli, stroke, chorea, hypertension, thrombocytopenia, spontaneous abortions, and fetal loss

Antiphospholipid antibodies are not restricted to patients with SLE. They can be detected in a wide variety of neoplastic, infectious, inflammatory, and autoimmune diseases. In one study,[349] one-half of the patients did not have SLE.

A similar antibody species directed against phospholipid is responsible for the biologic false-positive reaction for syphilis seen in this disease (positive VDRL). This abnormality is documented in approximately 15 percent of individuals who either have or will develop SLE. The more specific tests for syphilis (FTA) are not affected.

RHEUMATOID FACTORS

Rheumatoid factors (RFs) are found in approximately 10 to 30 percent of children with SLE. In comparison, RFs are uncommon in JRA, but high titers in children with lupuslike disease may suggest a diagnosis of mixed connective-tissue disease.

Complement

Determination of the serum complement level is one of the most important laboratory measures of active immune complex formation in SLE.[99,299,301,305,350] Specific components of the complement sequence such as C3 and C4 may be assayed or the total serum hemolytic complement, CH_{50}, may be titrated by red cell lysis. The CH_{50} reflects the integrity of the total complement cascade and is abnormally low in approximately 90 percent of patients with active nephritis. The C3 concentration appears to be depressed less frequently than that of CH_{50}. Depression of the C4 concentration is usually found to be a consistent and reliable indicator of nephritis in SLE.

Immune Complex Assays

Assays of circulating immune complexes are occasionally useful in managing a child with SLE, especially when there is uncertainty concerning interpretation of clinical status, anti-nDNA antibody titers, and serum complement levels.[308] The simplest assays involve measurement of cryoglobulins and anticomplementary activity of serum. Methods employing C1q binding[351] and Raji cells[352] are the most reliable in SLE. Extensive reviews of the complexity and multiplicity of these assays have been published,[353,354] and their clinical applicability to the problems of immune complex disease in SLE has been evaluated.[355–357]

Synovial Fluid

The synovial fluid in SLE is usually a group I non-inflammatory fluid (Appendix). The white cell count is low ($<2,000/mm^3$; $<2.0 \times 10^9/L$), and the protein content varies from transudative to exudative levels. Complement levels are low, in part undoubtedly reflecting hypocomplementemia.

Urine

Most children with active glomerulonephritis have urinary sediment abnormalities characteristic of their type of renal involvement or have a telescoped urine (a urinary sediment that shows, at one time, the sequential features characteristic of the evolution and progression of glomerulotubulonephritis).[358]

Proteinuria is probably the most common urinary abnormality, but hematuria and red blood cell casts are more important hallmarks of active glomerulitis. The latter are also useful clinical markers in following the course of treatment. Proteinuria is indicative of both glomerular and tubular abnormalities and, like the creatinine clearance, may not be a satisfactory short-term indicator of therapeutic response.

In severe renal disease, the sediment also contains increased numbers of cellular and fatty casts. With the onset of the nephrotic syndrome, doubly refractile bodies appear and assume the form of Maltese crosses on polarizing microscopy (oval fat bodies).

Profuse proteinuria and a fixed specific gravity (1.010) are characteristic of the chronic phases of lupus nephritis. Broad casts of renal failure are seen at that time, and there may be few cellular elements in the sediment. Other abnormalities may include renal tubular acidosis. Immunoglobulin and light chain excretion are also increased in nephritis.

TREATMENT

General Measures

The importance of general supportive care of the child who is severely ill with SLE should not be underestimated in the treatment program. Factors warranting attention include nutrition, fluid and electrolyte balance, diagnosis and treatment of infection, management of congestive heart failure, and control of hypertension.

As with other illnesses in childhood, rigorous restraints on general activity are often unnecessary and undesirable. The child with SLE should be encouraged to attend school whenever symptoms and strength permit. Physical education should be monitored with the school in order to match the program to the child's endurance. The child should be encouraged to participate in appropriate extracurricular activities as the disease allows. Finally, most children benefit from continuing contact with the same physician and pediatric rheumatology team over the long course of their disease. This continuity enables the team to provide the child and family with an understanding of SLE and its complex treatment. Anxieties and fears contributing to noncompliance are best handled by this team approach. Although SLE is a serious problem, the chronic course of the disease in children justifies a conservative approach to the patient and family and sympathetic but energetic treatment of each exacerbation. Constant surveillance is indispensable. It is our opinion that careful attention to all of the details of managing SLE has contributed as much to the improved prognosis of children with the disease as any single therapeutic program or drug.

Treatment should be tailored to the individual child and based on the extent and severity of the disease. Each child must be thoroughly examined before any treatment program is considered. The initial diagnostic program invariably includes a full evaluation of the nature and extent of renal disease.

Certain general aspects of treatment are of primary importance (Table 7-33). The dangers of exposure to

Table 7-33 Treatment of SLE in Children

Prophylaxis: adequate rest, appropriate sun screens
Management of infections
Salicylates for musculoskeletal symptoms
Hydroxychloroquine for cutaneous disease
Prednisone
    Low-dose
    High-dose
        Oral
        Intravenous
Immunosuppressive drugs
Experimental therapy

excessive sunlight and unnecessary drugs and transfusions should be stressed to each patient. The appropriate sunscreens should be prescribed, e.g., those with high PSF numbers. The physician should be aware of the development of infectious complications so that they may be diagnosed correctly and treated promptly.

A fever accompanied by elevation of a previously low white blood cell count into the normal range $(5,000-10,000/mm^3; 50-100 \times 10^9/L)$ should be considered to be of infectious origin until proved otherwise. Blood cultures should be performed at these times. Basilar pneumonitis should always be regarded as bacterial, and cultures and Gram stains of the sputum should be obtained. Unexplained changes in renal sediment or function should be considered first to represent pyelonephritis. The many complications of granulomatous disease such as tuberculosis should be included in each differential diagnosis. CNS disease should also be regarded initially as related to infection; therefore, a CSF examination and cultures and India ink preparations for *Cryptococcus* should be performed. Antibiotics should not be used prophylactically.

Aspirin and Other Nonsteroidal Anti-inflammatory Drugs

The anti-inflammatory action of aspirin is of value for certain manifestations of SLE, such as arthralgia and myalgia. Patients with SLE may be at risk to develop elevation of the serum transaminases after high-dose salicylate administration (Ch. 3).[359] Liver function must be monitored carefully; however, significant liver cell necrosis is almost never seen in this setting. Patients with thrombocytopenia or the lupus anticoagulant should not be treated with anti-inflammatory doses of aspirin. Certain of the NSAIDs may be contraindicated in SLE because of an association with specific toxicities, e.g., ibuprofen with aseptic meningitis.[360]

Antimalarial Drugs

Antimalarial drugs such as the 4-aminoquinolines (e.g., hydroxychoroloroquine sulfate) are most often used as an adjunct to a planned reduction of corticosteroid dosage or an aid in control of the dermatitis of SLE. The starting dosage is 6–7 mg/kg/day taken in one or two divided doses with meals. This dosage is maintained for approximately 2 months and then is lowered to about 5 mg/kg/day.[361,362] *It is imperative that children receiving antimalarial drugs have a complete ophthalmologic examination initially and every 4 to 6 months while receiving therapy.*

Corticosteroid Drugs

It is generally considered that optimal therapy for children with SLE includes the administration of corticosteroids in the minimum dosage necessary to control symptoms.[19,180,363] Many of the potential benefits from sustained corticosteroid regimens in children can be nullified, however, by the serious complications that develop from this form of treatment.

Prednisone is usually preferred to treat the more severe manifestations of SLE (Table 7-34 and 7-35),[364] although newer glucocorticoids may be superior when approved for use.[365] A tuberculin skin test and controls should be performed before therapy is begun if at all practical (i.e., seriousness of the illness, prior BCG vaccination). Isoniazid prophylaxis should be used only in children who have a positive tuberculin reaction and no evidence of current activity of tuberculosis indicated by the chest roentgenogram. Because of the danger of exacerbating SLE with isoniazid, we do not recommend routine prophylactic use

Table 7-34 Approaches to the Medical Management of Seriously Ill Children with Life-Threatening SLE

Corticosteroid program
Prednisone (oral): 0.25–2.0 mg/kg/day
Steroid-pulse therapy
IV methylprednisolone 10–30 mg/kg/day for 1–3 days
Oral pulse therapy
Immunosuppressive regimen
Azathioprine: 1–2 mg/kg/day
Cyclophosphamide
Oral: 1–2 mg/kg/day
IV pulse: 500–750 mg/M^2/month
Plasmapheresis
Total lymphoid irradiation

Table 7-35 Oral Prednisone Treatment for Patients with SLE

Initial therapy: individualize
    Average dose: 15–40 mg/day
    Nephritis: 30–60 mg/day
    Hematologic crisis: 60–100 mg/day
    CNS disease: 60–100 mg/day

Maintenance therapy
    Initial dose until clinical control: 4–6 weeks
    $60 \rightarrow 20$ mg/day: decrease by 5 mg to $2\frac{1}{2}$ mg/week
    $20 \rightarrow 10$ mg/day: decrease by $2\frac{1}{2}$ mg to 1 mg/week
    10 mg/day: decrease by $\frac{1}{2}$ mg to 1 mg/2–4 weeks

of this medication. In this regard, it seems wisest to treat each child on an individual basis.

Kornreich and Hanson recommended that systemically ill children be treated initially with prednisone in a dose equivalent to 50–75 mg/M^2/day for approximately 3 to 6 weeks and that the corticosteroid should then be cautiously tapered to a level adequate to control the clinical and serologic activity of the disease. In their studies, it was necessary to divide the initial daily dose in order to control severe symptoms, and alternate-day administration of corticosteroids was rarely successful at onset or feasible until the total daily amount had been consolidated into a single morning dose. Even so, it was found that many children had exacerbations of disease when alternate-day steroid therapy was attempted. The corticosteroid program was supplemented with hydroxychloroquine in a dose of 200 mg/M^2/day in some children, and other immunosuppressive drugs were added for severe renal or CNS involvement when those facets of the disease did not respond to high-dose corticosteroids. For the latter purpose, azathioprine in a dose of 2 mg/kg/day or cyclophosphamide in a dose of 2.0–2.5 mg/kg/day was usually chosen. Meislin and Rothfield chose an initial dose in a range of 40–60 mg/M^2/day of prednisone, combined with an antimalarial drug in a dose of 200 mg/day for a period of 3 weeks, followed by gradual tapering of the steroid to a minimum dose.[19]

LOW-DOSE THERAPY

Prednisone in as low a dose as possible should be instituted and maintained to achieve the objectives of the treatment program. Low-dose therapy, defined as <0.5 mg/kg/day given in divided doses, is adequate to treat certain aspects of the disease such as fever, dermatitis, arthritis, and pleural effusion. With low-dose prednisone therapy, these manifestations are generally controlled within hours to days. Usually weeks are required for adequate control of anemia or leukopenia and reversal of abnormalities of the sedimentation rate, hypergammaglobulinemia, DNA binding, and complement. Initial doses are almost always maintained for at least a 4-week period. Before that time, tapering usually results in exacerbations of the disease.

HIGH-DOSE THERAPY

High-dose prednisone therapy in the range of 1–2 mg/kg/day in divided doses is used for control of lupus crisis, CNS disease, acute hemolytic anemia, and the more severe types of lupus nephritis. Hypertension, azotemia or uremia, and preexisting psychosis are relative contraindications to high steroid doses. Acute hemolytic anemia is often a medical emergency and is difficult to control even with high-dose prednisone therapy. The patient may relapse during tapering of the drug; splenectomy in children who fail to achieve a remission on prednisone therapy alone seems to be less efficacious than in the idiopathic form of the disease. Blood transfusions should be avoided for these patients except when absolutely necessary.

The dose of corticosteroids and the duration of treatment in the management of the various forms of lupus nephritis remain controversial (Table 7-36).[33,279,280,285,366,367] Most experts agree that the prognosis for mesangial and focal glomerulitis is good. Relatively moderate- and low-dose corticosteroid regimens sufficient to control the clinical aspects of the disease and to reverse serologic abnormalities are often sufficient for treatment of mesangial or focal nephritis. It is hoped that such treatment may also prevent or delay progression in the severity of the nephritis.[281]

The prognosis is much more guarded in severe diffuse proliferative glomerulonephritis, and a higher corticosteroid dose is recommended for a longer pe-

Table 7-36 Prednisone and Immunosuppressive Therapy for Lupus Nephritis

Initial dose
    Mesangial: symptomatic management
    Focal: 0.5 mg/kg/day for 2–4 months
    Diffuse: 1 mg/kg/day for 3–6 months; IV
        cyclophosphamide (?)
    Membranous: moderate symptomatic dose; IV
        cyclophosphamide (?)

riod of time. Clinical response and laboratory indixes of activity of the renal disease are periodically assessed to determine the length of treatment. Alterations of dose are based upon the presence of hematuria, stability of the creatinine clearance and proteinuria, and maintenance of a normal serum complement level and anti-nDNA antibody titer. In many children with proliferative nephritis, treatment with adequate doses of corticosteroids leads to a return of the urinalysis toward normal, although proteinuria and a depressed creatinine clearance are less responsive to corticosteroid therapy.

The appropriate level of the corticosteroid dose in membranous nephritis is uncertain. This form of renal impairment may be less responsive to high-dose regimens than is diffuse disease. A conservative approach with adequate symptomatic and serologic suppression is probably the wisest course of action.

The majority of children with SLE do not develop renal insufficiency if they are treated early and maintained in serologic and clinical remission. Systemic exacerbation of the lupus or loss of control by inappropriate tapering of steroid therapy usually leads to a return of the renal abnormalities. Such exacerbations are again usually responsive to adequate therapy, and severe renal insufficiency generally does not occur. Some children appear to enter permanent remissions; late in the course of the disease, gradual deterioration of renal function may again be observed (end-stage disease).

To be maximally effective in controlling the acute inflammatory manifestations of SLE, prednisone should be given in divided dosages three to four times a day. As an anti-inflammatory drug, prednisone given twice a day is less effective than the same amount divided into three doses a day. Less frequent administration is commonly used when tapering the drug in response to clinical improvement or during maintenance therapy. Once-a-day treatment is seldom effective except in minimally active or asymptomatic patients. Every-other-day programs have little to recommend them. (There are no studies in children comparing these treatment protocols.)

TAPERING THE PREDNISONE DOSE

After initial control of the disease with prednisone, tapering the dose should not be started until anti-nDNA antibodies have decreased to acceptable levels and the serum complement level has returned to normal (Fig. 7-27). Exacerbations of disease are usually heralded by the reappearance of abnormalities in these serologic parameters, and the steroid dose can be modified accordingly. The ANA titer in a specific child decreases with control of the clinical activity of the disease.

After control of the acute manifestations of the disease, the lowest possible dose of prednisone that will maintain the well-being of the child should be used. As shown in Table 7-35, a decrease in dose from high to moderate should not be greater than 5 mg/day each week. The average decrease in the lower ranges of dosages, for example, from 20 to 10 mg/day, should be slower at approximately 2.5 mg/day every 2 weeks. Below 10 mg/day, a much slower rate of tapering is necessary: 1 mg/day every 2 weeks. Such schedules cannot be arbitrary, however, and must be individualized. Metabolically, it is preferable to keep the morning dose highest and to taper the other doses first.

During tapering of corticosteroid therapy, the clinician should guard against precipitating relapses that may be difficult to control. If the disease should flare, the dose of prednisone often needs to be increased by 25 to 50 percent and maintained at that level for a while before tapering is begun again. It is generally agreed that most children with SLE are withdrawn completely from corticosteroid drugs only with great difficulty during the initial years after diagnosis. Even very-low-dose maintenance therapy with prednisone may minimize the tendency toward exacerbations.

STEROID-PULSE THERAPY

Intravenous therapy with methylprednisolone similar to that used in renal transplant rejection has been introduced into the treatment of diffuse proliferative lupus nephritis and other acute manifestations of SLE (Ch. 3). In uncontrolled studies, patients have been noted to show an improvement in deteriorating renal function within days, and severe immunologic abnormalities have been reversed.[368-372] The general medical program, especially fluid and electrolyte balance, needs to be diligently controlled in the hospital in order to prevent toxicity (see Table 3-21). This therapeutic approach has the advantage of providing high doses of drug over a brief period and ideally

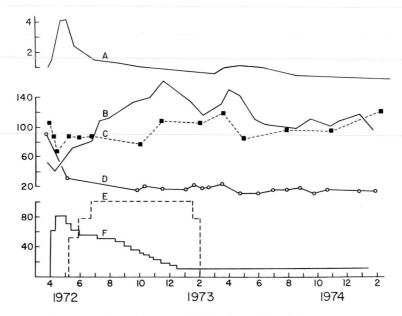

Fig. 7-27 The course of a young girl with acute SLE is charted in relation to urinary protein measured in grams per 24 hours (*A*), serum hemolytic complement units (*B*), creatinine clearance in liters per 24 hours (*C*), and anti-DNA antibody expressed as DNA binding in percent (*D*). The doses of cyclophosphamide (*E*) and prednisone (*F*) are indicated in milligrams per day. Diffuse proliferative glomerulonephritis was present on renal biopsy. Gradual resolution of her systemic disease was accompanied by a fall in the DNA binding to a normal value of less than 20 percent and a rise in the serum hemolytic complement to normal values above 110 CH_{50} units. During the second year of her disease, the hemolytic complement decreased again to subnormal levels. Resolution of the acute phase of renal disease was accompanied initially by an increase in urinary protein excretion and a decrease in the creatinine clearance, and then by a fall in daily protein excretion and a gradual rise of the creatinine clearance to relatively normal values. Initial deterioration in the creatinine clearance with corticosteroid therapy is a frequent observation, presumably related in part to rapid lysis of cells and release of DNA into the circulation.

thereby decreasing the risk of side effects consequent to long-term corticosteroid intake.

STEROID TOXICITY AND IATROGENIC CUSHING'S SYNDROME

The cumulative risks of prednisone treatment are considerable (Tables 3-16 and 3-17). Although peptic ulceration has not been common in our children, a modified four-feeding diet has been routinely prescribed. Weight gain can be minimized by reasonable caloric restriction. Limitation of sodium intake and monitoring for hypokalemia should be carried out. The blood pressure should be taken at each visit and diuretics or other antihypertensives used as indicated. For a fuller discussion of this problem, the reader is referred to Ch. 3.

Although differentiating CNS lupus from steroid-

induced psychosis may appear to be difficult, it is our impression that an acute steroid psychosis in a child with SLE is unusual (Table 7-37) (Ch. 3). Pure or-

Table 7-37 Differential Diagnosis of Lupus Encephalopathy and Steroid Psychosis

	Lupus Encephalopathy	Steroid Psychosis
Organic brain syndrome (impairment of orientation, judgment, memory)	+	−
Functional psychosis	−	+
Psychosis soon after steroid dose is started or increased	−	+
Seizures or abnormal neurologic examination	+	−
Evidence of active SLE	+	−
Cotton wool spots, peripheral vasculitis	+	−

ganic brain syndromes are sometimes best managed without psychotropic drugs. Agitated psychoses may be controlled in part by drugs of the phenothiazine (thioridazine) and butyrophenone classes (haloperidol).[373] Nonspecific sedatives in most of these children worsen the problems of encephalopathy.

CORONARY ARTERY DISEASE

Myocardial infarction may be a late effect of chronic administration of suppressive doses of prednisone to children with SLE. Accelerated atherosclerosis in patients with SLE has been observed after the long-term administration of corticosteroid drugs.[374] Abnormal lipoprotein profiles undoubtedly contribute to these developments.[375,376] In a study of 19 children with SLE, Ilowhite et al. found dyslipoproteinemia in the majority.[375] The most common findings were increases in the serum cholesterol, triglycerides, and low-density lipoproteins, with a corresponding decrease in high-density lipoproteins (dependent on whether corticosteroids had been used).

In a variety of studies, including those of adult patients, it has been estimated that approximately 5 percent of patients with SLE experience nonfatal myocardial infarctions and have an equal number of fatal infarctions.[212-214,217,219-221] However, a much larger percentage develop myocardiopathy,[214] and 45 percent have been demonstrated by angiography to have narrowing of at least one coronary artery.[223] Functional valvular disease was present in 18 percent of the patients in one series,[215] in part related to myocardial disease. (See the discussion of Libman-Sacks endocarditis.)

Immunosuppressive Agents

The disappointing results achieved with corticosteroid therapy alone in some patients with lupus nephritis and the relatively uncertain long-term outlook in this disease have led to an evaluation of the use of immunosuppressive agents for treatment of the severe manifestations of SLE.[377-380] Recent studies of the use of azathioprine or cyclophosphamide in the treatment of life-threatening SLE have been encouraging. However, long-term controlled studies have been difficult to evaluate and do not present a unified impression of the correct choices of therapeutic management. Clinically, there seems to be little question

that immunosuppressive agents aid in the control of the systemic disease when used in conjunction with prednisone. However, there are obvious and definite dangers associated with these powerful medications. They should be used only with extreme care. The long-term studies at the National Institutes of Health of immunosuppressive drug therapy have involved adult patients.[379-382] Their data and others have not consistently shown statistically impressive effectiveness of the use of azathioprine[381-385] or cyclophosphamide[381,382,386,387] in conjunction with prednisone for the treatment of severe SLE. Recent studies combining these two drugs with prednisone may give more encouraging results. Other alternative forms of treatment, such as plasmapheresis, are also being examined in controlled studies,[388-391] as are other drugs.[392,393]

It has been our clinical experience that children with SLE tolerate smaller doses of the immunosuppressive drugs than do patients with hematologic disorders. The initial dose of either azathioprine or cyclophosphamide should not exceed 1 mg/kg/day. Some children do not tolerate even this amount before developing leukopenia. Furthermore, it may not be necessary to achieve leukopenia to obtain effective levels of therapy. This is particularly worth remembering in treating patients with SLE who already have a tendency to leukopenia.

Exacerbation of systemic disease was noted in one clinical trial of long-term azathioprine therapy with the abrupt withdrawl of this drug in 7 of 9 patients.[394] These exacerbations were delayed by approximately 3 months and were often refractory to treatment. One patient died during such an exacerbation. In an analysis of treatment of children with SLE, Meislin and Rothfield stressed that immunosuppressive drugs are rarely needed.[19] Kornreich and Hanson indicated that immunosuppressive therapy was warranted in children who required frequent hospitalizations because of exacerbations of their disease or who could not be maintained in a state of clinical remission and serologic normality on small doses of steroids.[204] They treated 38 children with a combination of corticosteroid and immunosuppressive medications. Children were considered candidates for immunosuppressive therapy if they had continuing activity of diffuse lupus nephritis or severe systemic involvement of some other vital organ, especially the CNS. Nine of their patients died. One child was maintained on hemodialysis after rejection of a renal transplant. Four patients were placed on dialysis after failure to respond to the immunosuppressive and corticosteroid program. One patient on hemodialysis after rejecting a renal transplant was in remission without medication at follow-up.

Another approach to immunosuppression in patients with SLE has been treatment with total lymphoid irradiation.[395] In at least one center (Stanford) this approach has been successful in a limited number of adults and has prevented the long-term effects of cytotoxic and corticosteroid drug therapy.

Dialysis and Renal Transplantation

Dialysis and transplantation offer final approaches to maintaining life and renal function in patients with end-stage kidney disease.[396] Hemodialysis has been difficult psychologically for younger children and should be undertaken only in centers with experience in this age group. Renal transplantation has offered an alternative longer-term approach and has generally been successful.[397] Recurrences of the nephritis have been noted[398]; SLE at this stage of the disease is usually inactive serologically and permanent remissions occur.[399]

Data from 1982–1983 indicate that the 5-year survivorship rate of all patients who had end-stage renal disease was 80 percent.[400,401] In those who had undergone transplantation, 30 percent of renal allografts were functioning at 3 years, and 60 percent of related-donor kidneys were functional at the same period of time.

COURSE AND PROGNOSIS

SLE is characterized by exacerbations and remissions of varying manifestations.[19,24,402,403] The clinical course is often prolonged over many years. The disease may become acute at any time. Spontaneous remissions occur or an infection or drug hypersensitivity reaction may lead to another exacerbation. Fever and prominent constitutional symptoms are present at the onset of disease and during exacerbations. In our study,[24] there was little tendency for new organ systems to be involved after onset during exacerbations except for CNS disease. In this regard, the disease in each child with SLE tends to be mnemic.

King et al.[25] estimated that as few as 5 percent of children had mild disease with only occasional exacerbations; however, some children with severe disease went into sustained remissions. The most common course of SLE was chronic. Low-grade activity continued for many years with unpredictable exacerbations that were often severe. The most persistent problems during the course of the disease were also related to cardiac, neurologic, and renal involvement. These three organ systems were also affected somewhat more frequently during the course of the disease than at onset.

Morbidity

With the increasing life expectancy of children with SLE, a number of newly recognized factors that affect their long-term quality of life are emerging (Table 7-38). These are directly related to previously unappreciated aspects of SLE; drug therapy that has been used, especially corticosteroid drugs and immunosuppressive agents; and residual problems with physical and psychological adaptations to a chronic severe illness.

The ability to place patients with SLE on long-term peritoneal dialysis or hemodialysis or to transplant a kidney has materially changed the life expectancy of these patients. These alternative avenues of treatment have permitted the physician to focus more clearly on saving the life of a child rather than on simply preserving renal function at all costs.

Recurrent infections have emerged as a significant factor in the morbidity of surviving children with

Table 7-38 Morbidity in Children with SLE

Renal	Dialysis, transplantation
CNS	Organic brain syndrome, seizures, psychosis, neuropsychiatric dysfunction
Cardiovascular	Atherosclerosis, myocardial infarction, myocardiopathy, functional valvular disease, hypertension
Immune defense	Recurrent infections, malignancy (lymphoma), asplenia
Musculoskeletal	Osteopenia, compression fractures, osteonecrosis, stunting of linear growth (height), obesity
Ocular	Cataracts, glaucoma
Endocrine	Diabetes, infertility, fetal wastage

SLE.[404,405] It is not certain whether these infections are primarily related to the longer-term course of the disease in surviving patients or to their therapy. The development of asplenia in some children with SLE is a contributing factor.[347,348]

Important and perhaps progressive neuropsychiatric dysfunction is also emerging as a significant disability. Lipnick, White, and colleagues have summarized their data on 32 children followed for a mean duration of 4 years.[259,406] After a battery of standardized tests, 21 of 32 patients were found to have significant abnormalities. Abnormal cognitive impairment was present in 52 percent of the children, and an additional 29 percent had results considered borderline abnormal. In addition, one patient had developed a cerebral vascular accident following lupus vasculitis and an additional child had chorea.

Finally, the cardiac and atherosclerotic complications of SLE are emerging as important residual problems of the illness. The latter begin to become prominent clinically after approximately 10 years of active disease. Whether these developments are related primarily to the lupus,[214,215] to hyperlipoproteinemia,[375,376] or to long-term complications of corticosteroid therapy[374] is not clear. Undoubtedly all contribute to the final clinical observations.

Survivorship

There has been a remarkable improvement in the outcome of patients with SLE during the past three decades (Table 7-39).[19,25,34,311,404,405,407–410] Although SLE is a serious, life-threatening disease, an optimistic approach to the care of these children is now justified by current data on survivorship. Many of the factors emphasized previously in this chapter have played a role in bringing about this change for the better (Table 7-40).

The prognosis in an individual child with SLE is relatively unpredictable. Generalizations about prognosis are especially unreliable during the first 24 months after diagnosis. Estimates can be related to the degree of activity and severity of the systemic disease, the type and progression of nephritis, clinically apparent vasculitis, and the multisystemic character of the disease. The prognosis is poorest in patients with diffuse proliferative nephritis or persistent CNS disease and is best in those with minimal disease or focal nephritis.[411–413] Encephalopathy, especially

Table 7-39 Survivorship in Children with SLE

Series (yr)	No.	Percentage		
		5 yr	10 yr	15 yr
Meislin and Rothfield[19] (1968)	42	42/72[a]	—	—
Walravens and Chase[34] (1976)	50	—	60–70	—
Garin et al.[311] (1976)	49	72	—	—
King et al.[25] (1977)	108	78	—	—
Fish et al.[404] (1977)	49	—	86	—
Abeles et al.[407] (1980)	67	89/100[a]	—	—
Platt et al.[405] (1982)	70	90	85	77
Glidden et al.[409] (1983)	55	92	85	—

[a]% with renal disease/% without renal disease.

organic brain syndrome or vascular accident, has become a major factor in survivorship in recent studies.[24,250,414]

Sepsis has replaced renal failure as the most common cause of death. This fact is illustrated by the change in causes of death in children with SLE (Table 7-41).[24] Malignant hypertension, GI bleeding and perforation, acute pancreatitis, and pulmonary hemorrhage are other terminal events. Infection may involve common pathogens as well as opportunistic organisms such as fungi or protozoa. Death from lupus crisis is rare today, probably because of the efficacy of the corticosteroid drugs in managing acute exacerbations.

Table 7-40 Factors in the Observed Improvement in the Prognosis of SLE

Better appreciation of the natural course of the disease
More precise pathologic categorization of the types of lupus nephritis
Improved and more rational approach to treatment and intensive care
    Corticosteroid drugs
    Immunosuppressive agents
    Antihypertensive drugs
    Diuretics
    Antibiotics
Improved serologic evaluation of the response to treatment

Table 7-41 Causes of Death in Children with SLE[a]

Series (yr)	Died/total	Infection	Renal	CNS	Cardiac	Acute Flare	Other
Meislin and Rothfield[19] (1968)	18/42	7	6	2	—	2	1
Walravens and Chase[34] (1976)	12/50	1	4	—	5	—	3
Garin et al.[311] (1976)	6/49	2	2	2	—	—	—
King et al.[25] (1977)	28/108	8	12	—	—	—	8
Cassidy et al.[24] (1977)	11/58	8	7	1	3	—	1
Fish et al.[404] (1977)	7/49	6	—	—	—	—	—
Abeles et al.[407] (1980)	10/67	1	3	—	—	1	5
Platt et al.[405] (1982)	11/70	9	2	—	1	—	2
Glidden et al.[409] (1983)	9/55	3	3	3	—	—	1

[a] In some cases, more than one cause of death has been enumerated.

Reports on prognosis prior to 1968 were based on early experience with corticosteroids and in general were restricted to children with classic SLE and severe disease.[19,180] Meislin and Rothfield in 1968 reviewed 42 children with SLE and compared them to 200 adults followed from 1957 to 1966 (Table 7-39).[19] They found that survivorship in children with SLE was improving but was still poorer than in adult patients. Survivorship at 5 years calculated from the time of diagnosis was 42 percent for children with renal disease compared to 82 percent for adults, and 72 percent for children without renal disease, compared to 86 percent for adults. In a more recent study from the same medical center,[407] 5-year survivorship for children with renal disease improved to 89 percent compared to 83 percent for adults and was 100 percent for children without renal disease compared to 94 percent for adults. Other studies have indicated that children with diffuse proliferative nephritis have a 5-year survivorship of 61 percent[311] and 73 percent[404]

In the Los Angeles series,[25] outcome did not appear to be related to age of onset of disease. Fifteen children who had onset before 12 years of age and 13 after 12 years had died at the time of the study. There was an excess mortality in males: 9 boys (50 percent) died compared to 19 girls (17 percent), a rate perhaps related to the younger age of the boys. Platt et al. reviewed 70 children with SLE followed by 1958 to 1981.[405] Survivorship was 77 percent at 15 years (Table 7-39) (Fig. 7-28).[405] No differences were noted for younger age of onset or development of CNS disease.

Prognosis for life and renal function were poorest after 7 years of follow-up in those children with diffuse nephritis.

Estes and Christian estimated that there were no significant differences in life span between black and white patients.[402] Age of onset did not affect the prognosis in SLE; 5-year survivorship in patients younger than 20 years was

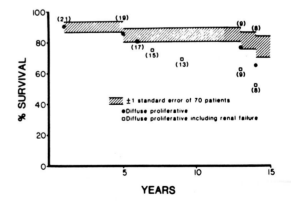

Fig. 7-28 Life table analysis of survival of 21 patients with diffuse proliferative lupus nephritis determined from time of study entry to death (solid circle) and from study entry to death or end-stage renal failure (open square). For comparison, the standard error of survival of 70 patients is indicated (shaded area). Number in parentheses is number of patients studied. (From Platt et al.,[405] with permission.)

69 percent compared to 77 percent for adults in the third decade of life. The relationship of mortality to race and sex was evaluated for a 5-year period (1968 to 1972) by the National Center for Health Statistics (Table 7-42).[415] The overall mortality rate for females of 6.3 per 10^6 person-years was 4 times that for males of 1.6 per 10^6 person-years. Furthermore, black females had a rate of 14.8, compared to 5.2 for white females. Black males and white males were much closer at 2.2 and 1.5. These epidemiologic data have been reevaluated recently and the preceding conclusions are again supported.[416]

In summary, there seems little doubt that prognosis for the child with SLE has improved considerably. Periodic assays of anti-nDNA antibodies and serum complement levels have permitted physicians to initiate and monitor therapeutic programs for maximum effectiveness and at the same time maintain corticosteroid doses at the lowest possible level commensurate with control of the disease. Until the cause or cure of SLE is discovered, we can expect that the prognosis will continue to improve modestly. This expectation is supported by current data and will be facilitated by continued development of mutual faith and support between a knowledgeable and compliant child and family and a physician expert in the care of SLE.

Overlap Syndrome

Some children with SLE have major manifestations of another connective-tissue disease. Perhaps most common are signs and symptoms of JRA involving RF seropositivity, rheumatoid nodules, and erosive synovitis of the small joints. These patients are properly referred to as having an *overlap syndrome*. *Mixed connective-tissue disease* has been reported in children and includes manifestations of SLE and other major clinical features of chronic arthritis, scleroderma, dermatomyositis, or polyarteritis (Ch. 10).[417,418] These

patients have very high serum antibody titers to an extractable nuclear antigen (ENA) that is ribonuclease- (RNAse-)sensitive (e.g., anti-U1RNP).[419–422] Anti-RNP antibodies also occur in children with SLE; however, anti-Sm antibody, detected originally in the sera of patients with mixed connective-tissue disease, is now recognized as virtually diagnostic of SLE. In our clinic, children with mixed connective-tissue disease have been uncommon. It was originally thought that adults with this type of overlap syndrome had a more favorable prognosis than those with SLE,[402] although recent reports do not substantiate that viewpoint. A few patients with mixed connective-tissue disease have developed a nephritis that is indistinguishable from lupus nephritis.

Additional experience has documented the development of SLE after a long period of disease characterized only by arthritis that was initially diagnosed as JRA (Tables 7-43 and 7-44).[205,423,424] Although children with SLE characteristically have a nondeforming arthritis and multisystemic involvement greater than that found in JRA, it may be difficult to distinguish between these two diseases when the manifestations of SLE evolve slowly, especially in the presence of a chronic erosive arthritis. A documented diagnosis of SLE may be possible only years after the onset of the inflammatory arthritis. In our study,[205] such a diagnosis only became obvious 2½ to 21 years after onset. SLE was confirmed at that time by the presence of characteristic immune complex nephritis and a positive test for antibody to nDNA. Perhaps as many as 3 percent of children in whom an initial diagnosis of JRA is made will eventually develop such a disease, indistinguishable from SLE. Sherry and Kredich also reported the development of transient thrombocytopenia (SLE) in three children with sys-

Table 7-42 Mortality in SLE of Childhood[a]

Age (Years)	White Male	White Female	Black Male	Black Female
0–4	—	—	—	—
5–9	0.1	0.4	0.2	0.6
10–14	0.3	1.5	0.8	4.4
15–19	0.9	3.8	1.8	12.9

[a] Data are expressed as mortality rates per 10^6 person-years. (Adapted from Kaslow and Masi,[415] with permission.)

Table 7-43 Evolution of JRA to SLE: Status at Diagnosis of JRA

Sex	7F:3M
Age of onset (yr)	1–14
Type of onset	9 Poly: 1 Mono
Subcutaneous nodules	4/10
Raynaud's phenomenon	3/10
ANA +	5/6
LE cell +	0/7
Anti-nDNA +	0/3
Rheumatoid factor +	3/10

Table 7-44 Evolution of JRA to SLE: Status at Diagnosis of SLE

Age at onset (yr)	5–29
Duration of JRA (yr)	2–21
Acute exacerbation of arthritis	8/10
Serositis	5/10
Seizures	3/10
Fever	5/10
Rash	5/10
ANA +	10/10
LE cell +	10/10
Anti-nDNA +	10/10
Coombs' antibody +	6/10
WBC count (mm^3)	1,800–10,700
Renal biopsy: GTN	6/6

temic-onset disease who had been initially diagnosed as JRA.[424]

Pregnancy

The pediatric rheumatologist may be called upon to deal with the subject of pregnancy in the teenage girl with active SLE.[425–428] The disease may first develop during pregnancy or may undergo an acute exacerbation during its course. There is no effect of SLE on fertility, although corticosteroid drugs may influence the conception rate.[429]

A frank discussion of contraceptive therapy is indicated in the management of these young women. Oral contraceptives per se (estrogen-containing) may exacerbate the disease. The effect of prednisone on the fetus is an area of considerable confusion.[430–432] The treatment program must be individualized, however, and not every patient responds to pregnancy in an unfavorable manner. As a generalization, the lowest possible prednisone dose tolerated by the mother is the one most acceptable during pregnancy. Prednisone per se does not cross the placenta in significant amounts.

The prior existence of hypertension or nephritis increases the possibility of an exacerbation of SLE during pregnancy, death of the mother, or premature loss of the child.[433–435] Flares of disease may occur at any time during or after pregnancy, although the 8-week period following delivery is most critical. Consideration should be given to increasing the corticosteroid dose at hospitalization to stress levels and then tapering slowly after delivery to predelivery values.

The problem of fetal loss related to anticardiolipin antibodies and neonatal disease in relation to anti-Ro antibodies should be considered.[436] The presence of anti-Ro antibody is directly related to fetal outcome in women with SLE. In one recent study,[437] 155 pregnant women were followed prospectively; 47, or 30 percent, had anti-Ro antibody and 108 did not. There were no differences in fertility or adverse fetal outcome in these two comparison groups; however, complete congenital heart block (CCHB) occurred in 6 of 96 pregnancies. All of these women had serum anti-Ro antibody. The authors calculated that the relative risk of CCHB in women with antibody was 1:20 and in those without antibody 1:60.

Anticardiolipin antibody is also related to fetal outcome. In one study,[438] pregnancies were uncomplicated in 12 of 23 women who did not have anticardiolipin antibody. In 11 women with this serum antibody activity, there were 3 instances of intrauterine fetal death and 8 cases of significant fetal distress.

THE NEONATAL LUPUS SYNDROMES

Classification

Children of mothers who have SLE may develop manifestations of lupus in the neonatal period that are mediated by the transplacental passage of maternal IgG autoantibodies.[439–442] The neonatal lupus syndromes (NLSs), especially those with predominant cutaneous manifestations, are more common in female infants than in males (Table 7-45).

The affected infant will have transiently positive ANA seropositivity, LE-cell phenomena, and depressed complement levels.[443–445] In the majority of

Table 7-45 Neonatal Lupus Syndromes

Anti-Ro/La antibodies almost invariably present

Transient (3 mo)
    Photosensitive discoid rash
    Cytopenia (white cells, red cells, platelets)
    Hepatosplenomegaly

Permanent
    Complete congenital heart block
    Endomyocardial fibroelastosis
    Structural cardiac defects (PDA, septal defects)

these babies there is no associated clinical disease, and the serologic abnormalities will regress in several weeks to months after birth in accordance with the normal half-life of maternal IgG (24–28 days).

Photosensitive Skin Rash

Erythema annulare is the characteristic cutaneous manifestation of the NLS (Fig. 7-29). It begins as an erythematosus scaly papule that expands peripherally, leaving a depressed ecchymotic central area. The rash is seldom present at birth but occurs from hours to several days after delivery. The lesions are multiple and occur anywhere on the body, including the scalp, face, palms, and soles, and may involve mucous membranes. These rashes usually heal without resi-

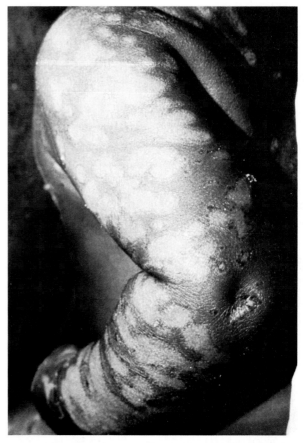

Fig. 7-30 Another child with a neonatal lupus syndrome. The rash here is more discoid in character. (Courtesy of Dr. D. Kredich.)

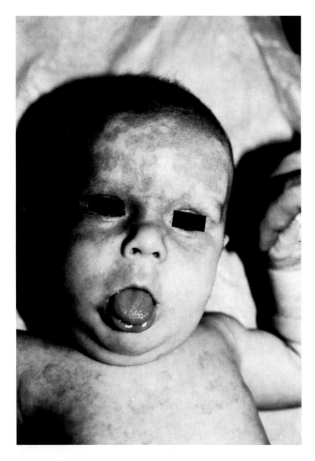

Fig. 7-29 Neonatal lupus syndrome. This erythematosus rash appeared a day after birth in this baby and was accompanied by thrombocytopenia and leukopenia. (Courtesy of Drs. D.C. Rada and T. Kestenbaum.)

dua. Other photosensitive lesions may occur in the malar area and often leave residual atrophic or pigmentary changes more suggestive of discoid lupus (Fig. 7-30).[446–449]

Complete Congenital Heart Block

Complete congenital heart block is the most serious manifestation of the NLSs.[450–459] It is signaled in utero by the sudden onset of bradycardia that results in congestive heart failure and nonimmune hydrops fetalis. It is estimated that approximately one-third of babies with CCHB have mothers with a connective-tissue disease, usually SLE. It is important that this complication be recognized and that appropriate steps be taken to safeguard the infant by emergency delivery and use of a cardiac pacemaker, if possible. This type of CCHB is permanent.

Histologically, CCHB is characterized by fibrosis of the conduction system and presence of dystrophic calcification. Endocardial fibroelastosis is frequent and other cardiac defects are sometimes present (Fig. 7-31).[450,456,460,461]

Hematocytopenia

Thrombocytopenia or neutropenia is believed to reflect maternal hematocytopenia induced by auto-antibodies to platelets or neutrophils. It is usually present at birth, persists for days to weeks, and is

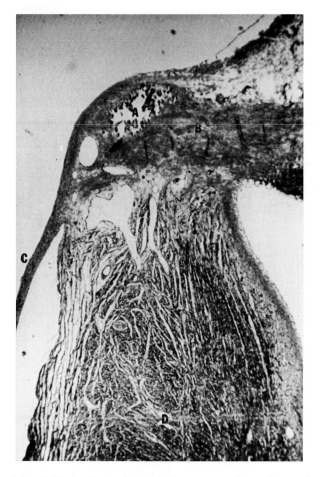

Fig. 7-31 Section of ventricular septum from fetus of mother with SLE. Baby died at birth from nonimmune hydrops secondary to CCHB. A, dystrophic calcification in region of AV; B, dense fibrosis; C, valve leaflet; D, ventricular septum.

seldom associated with clinically significant disease. The presence of petechiae may be the only indication of thrombocytopenia that may be life-threatening. GI hemorrhage occasionally occurs.

Hepatic and GI Disease

Hepatomegaly with modest elevation of the serum levels of the liver enzymes is often present. Cholestatic jaundice has been described.[462]

Pathogenesis of the Neonatal Lupus Syndromes

The pathogenesis of the NLSs is believed related to the transplacental passage of maternal IgG auto-antibodies.[436,437,439,463–466] Anti-Ro antibodies are the most characteristic of the autoimmune activities (Table 7-27). A few children with NLS and absence of CCHB who had anti-La antibodies alone but whose mothers had both anti-La (Table 7-28) and anti-Ro antibody have been reported.[319] Two cases of neonatal lupus in which anti-Ro antibody activity was absent but anti-U1RNP antibodies were present have been described (Table 7-30).[467] Maternal anti-Ro antibodies are strongly associated with CCHB even when there is no history of overt maternal lupus.[444,468–470] However, many babies whose mothers have this autoantibody are completely normal. Whether anti-Ro antibodies cause the disease or are merely associated with CCHB is not clear. The Ro antigen is widely distributed in the fetal conduction system and myocardium, as well as skin and other tissues. Antibodies to Ro are bound to the conduction system of infants dying of CCHB.[471]

Treatment and Course

Treatment of the autoimmune process (without CCHB) is seldom necessary,[445] although supportive care, and when indicated cardiac pacing, may be life-saving. Close observation of the offspring of mothers with SLE, however, may reveal more long-term problems.

An occasional mother has had successive pregnancies complicated by infants with the NLS.[469,470] One has been described with high titers of anti-Ro antibodies who subsequently had a normal infant. At least two children with NLS have had onset of idiopathic SLE later in life.[472,473]

In one family, two siblings developed CCHB with congestive heart failure. In this family, the mother had SLE and the father and paternal grandfather both had adult-onset cardiac conduction defects.[452] In a study of 24 cases of CCHB diagnosed at or before birth, 7 of 9 infants showed evidence of endomyocardial fibroelastosis at necropsy.[454] In another postmortem study of infants with CCHB born to mothers with SLE,[450] tissue sections of the conduction system suggested faulty embryonic development and early inflammatory changes of the atrioventricular node within an abnormally thick annulus fibrosis. Two additional infants had cardiomyopathy, and three had associated congenital heart disease.

OTHER HYPERSENSITIVITY DISEASES

Sjögren's Syndrome

Sjögren's syndrome can be defined as a triad of signs and symptoms consisting of the following (Table 7-46):

Table 7-46 Associated Features of Sjögren's Syndrome

Sicca complex
    Bilateral parotid enlargement
    Hashimoto's thyroiditis
    Lymphoid myositis
    Achlorhydria
    Hyposthenuria and renal tubular acidosis
    Hepatomegaly
    Pancreatitis
    Celiac syndrome

Connective-tissue disease
    Systemic lupus erythematosus
    Vasculitis
    Raynaud's phenomenon
    Nonthrombocytopenic purpura
    Chronic active hepatitis

Autoantibodies
    Rheumatoid factors
    Antinuclear antibodies
    LE-cell phenomenon
    Antibodies to SS-A, SS-B, and RAP
    Antisalivary duct antibodies
    Antitissue antibodies

Malignancy
    Pseudolymphoma
    Lymphoma
    Macroglobulinemia

1. The sicca syndrome, manifested predominantly by keratoconjunctivitis sicca and xerostomia (dry eyes and dry mouth)
2. A connective tissue disease, usually SLE
3. High titers of autoantibodies, usually ANA (anti-Ro/La) or RF

Sjögren's syndrome is a multisystemic disorder that is insidious in onset and slowly progressive.[474] It is rare in childhood and presents as recurrent parotid swelling (Table 7-47, Fig. 7-32).[475–477] In the primary syndrome, which is very rare in children, the sicca component is the dominant manifestation of the disease and is related to lymphocytic infiltration of the lacrimal and salivary glands.[474] The upper respiratory tract, larynx, stomach, and genitourinary tract are also involved. Approximately one-half of the patients have prominent manifestations of a connective-tissue disease (secondary Sjögren's syndrome).[477]

Anemia and thrombocytopenia are not usually severe, but approximately one-third of the patients have leukopenia. A striking polyclonal hypergammaglobulinemia is almost uniformly present. All pa-

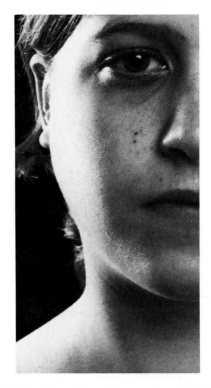

Fig. 7-32 Parotid swelling in a young girl. Two years later, she developed the clinical features of SLE.

Table 7-47 Progression of Sjögren's Syndrome to Systemic Lupus Erythematosus[a]

Age (Years)	Clinical Manifestations	Age (Years)	Clinical Manifestations
5	Persistent bilateral parotid enlargement (painless)		Compression fractures of vertebral bodies
			Grand mal convulsions
12	Xerostomia and keratoconjunctivitis sicca		Pulmonary embolism
16	Fever, pleuropericarditis	21	Acute bronchitis
	Babinski's signs		Mucocutaneous ulcerations
	Leukopenia, plus lupus erythematosus cells		Fever, arthritis
	Obtundation		Subcutaneous vasculitis
17	Pleuritis	22	Inactive disease
	Perforated duodenal ulcer	23	Grand mal convulsion
	Hematuria, lupus nephritis		Thrombophlebitis
	Lupus colitis		Subcutaneous nodules, arthritis
	Perforated gastric ulcer		Acute lupus flare
18	Laryngitis sicca		Fever, arthritis
	Perforated gastric ulcer		Mucocutaneous ulcerations
19	Thrombophlebitis		Subcutaneous vasculitis
	Grand mal convulsions		Leukopenia, plus lupus erythematosus cells
	Exfoliative dermatitis (diphenylhydantoin)	24	Acute arthritis
	Cerebral thrombosis, left hemiparesis	25	Postphlebitic syndrome, left leg
	Perforated gastric ulcer	27	Gastric ulcer
	Candida septicemia	29	Moderate esophageal stricture
	Multiple pulmonary embolisms and cardiac arrest		Arthritis
		31	Osteonecrosis, humeral heads
	Tracheitis	32	Severe hypertension
	Urticaria (penicillin)	35	Widespread vasculopathy with digital gangrene
20	Severe Cushing's syndrome and osteoporosis	36	Uremia and death

[a] Onset of disease at age 5 years; positive lupus erythematosus cell test at age 16 years; episodic, multisystemic disease since that time with prolonged survival in spite of many life-threatening exacerbations and complications of long-term treatment, first with prednisone and later with cyclophosphamide. Sjögren's syndrome and nephritis both confirmed by biopsy.

tients have high titers of other autoantibodies such as ANAs, most commonly directed to the antigens Ro (SS-A) and La (SS-B) (Tables 7-27, 7-28). A speckled or nucleolar pattern of immunofluorescence is frequently found. About 15 percent of patients have LE cells even in the absence of SLE. Other antitissue antibodies are found in two-fifths of the patients.

Anti-Ro antibodies in patients with Sjögren's syndrome have been found in association with anemia, leukopenia, lymphopenia, cryoglobulinemia, and vasculitis.[91,92,94,478] More than 95 percent of patients with Sjögren's syndrome have this type of antibody activity, and 85 percent or more have it in association with anti-La antibodies.

Pathophysiologically, Sjögren's syndrome appears to be an example of increased B-cell reactivity to a variety of antigens in association with subnormal T-cell responsiveness.[138,474] The latter can be demonstrated in the laboratory by decreased lymphocyte transformation to phytohemagglutinin. Skin tests for delayed hypersensitivity are impaired. The syndrome may be an example of defective T-cell suppressor function.

Since this is a multisystem disorder, there is widespread infiltration of lymphocytic cells and, to a lesser extent, plasma cells and reticulum cells in parenchymal organs and the salivary and lacrimal glands. In some cases, germinal follicle formation is seen. There are subsequent secondary atrophy and obliteration of secretory acini. Particularly in the salivary glands, there is a proliferation of ductal lining cells to form epimyoepithelial islands. This latter histologic finding is one of the important diagnostic features of Sjögren's syndrome (Fig. 7-33).

Therapy is nonspecific. Treatment of the systemic manifestations is with NSAIDs or corticosteroids.

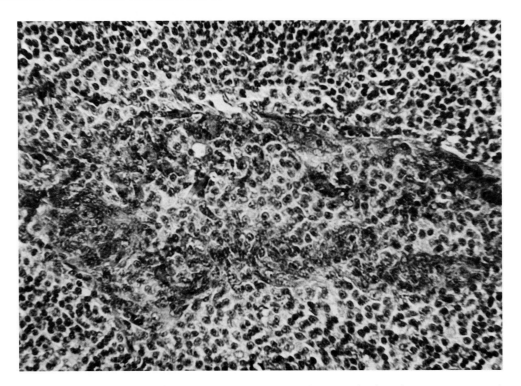

Fig. 7-33 Parotid gland. Obliteration of the normal acinar architecture by lymphocytes. Regenerative epimyoepithelial island in the center of the field.

The sicca component is managed with attention to environmental humidity, artificial tears, nasal saline douches, and sour lemon drops to stimulate production of saliva.

Autoerythrocyte Sensitization

In the syndrome of autoerythrocyte sensitization first described by Gardner and Diamond,[479] the patient reacts to minor trauma by the development of large, superficial, inflammatory lesions.[480,481] Subcutaneous injection of the patient's own red cell membranes ("ghosts") reproduces the lesions (Fig. 7-34). The syndrome has been most frequent in adolescent girls and is often associated with bizarre psychiatric disturbances. It has been described in one boy in the childhood age group.[482]

Thrombotic Thrombocytopenia Purpura

The combination of thrombocytopenia purpura and acute hemolytic anemia (Evan's syndrome) is seen in both thrombotic thrombocytopenic purpura (TTP) and SLE.[483,484] TTP may occur as a hypersensitivity reaction to drugs or recent immunization and may also complicate carcinoma, inflammatory arthritis, and pregnancy. It has been associated with a wide variety of infections; recent reports in a few patients have implicated an organism of the Bartonellaceae species.

TTP occurs primarily in young women but is similar in many ways to the *hemolytic uremic syndrome* seen in children. TTP has an acute onset and is often fatal. In addition to anemia and purpura, these patients have fever, changing central nervous system signs, and nephritis.

The primary laboratory abnormalities are seen in the peripheral blood. Leukocytosis is present. Platelets on the peripheral blood smear are absent to greatly decreased. The most striking abnormalities are microangiopathic hemolytic anemia and the presence of bizarre red blood cells, especially helmet cells. The Coombs' test is usually negative. Coagulation studies indicate that platelet consumption exceeds fibrinogen utilization; for example, primary damage to the vascular endothelium rather than intravascular coagulation occurs.

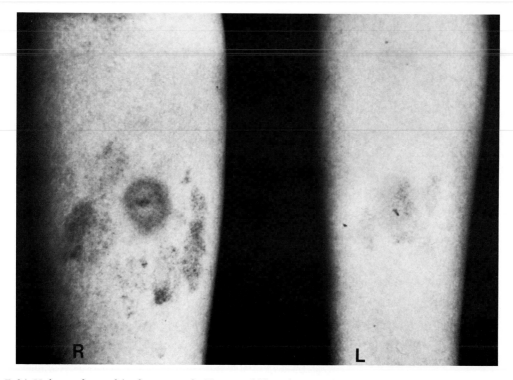

Fig. 7-34 Volar surfaces of the forearms of a 10-year-old boy diagnosed as having Gardner-Diamond syndrome. A large area of inflammatory change and ecchymosis was produced in the right forearm by the subcutaneous injection of "ghosts" prepared from his red blood cell membranes. Except for subcutaneous bleeding, no inflammatory changes were produced in the left arm by injection of a comparable amount of buffer.

Histologically, there is widespread occlusion of arterioles and capillaries by hyaline thrombi. These thrombi consist principally of fibrin products and do not contain immunoglobulins or complement. Punch biopsy of skin often reveals these changes.

Treatment is often unsuccessful, and the patient's illness pursues a short, fulminant course. Corticosteroids and anticoagulants have been used successfully in some persons, and splenectomy is occasionally done. Plasmapheresis and blood exchange have been suggested as experimental treatments.

Relapsing Polychondritis

Relapsing polychondritis is a rare, widespread inflammation of cartilage associated with marked systemic features. It has seldom been described in children.[485,486] The disease may affect the cartilage of the ear and then spreads to involve the upper respiratory and ocular tracts and hyaline cartilage of the joints.[487] Arthritis occurs in approximately 80 percent of cases.[488] The course initially is episodic but becomes progressive in the majority of patients. Etiology is unknown; however intrauterine transmission has been described. Although separate from Wegener's granulomatosis, vasculitis can occur in this syndrome along with dilatation of the aortic root. Ocular inflammation and uveitis have been reported. Corticosteroids are suppressive. Death is often due to respiratory collapse.[489]

REFERENCES

1. Maini RN, Glass DN, Scott JT: Immunology of the rheumatic diseases, no. 7. In Turk J (ed): Current Topics in Immunology. Williams & Wilkins, Baltimore, 1977, p. 146
2. Koffler D, Agnello V, Thoburn R et al: Systemic lupus erythematosus: prototype of immune complex nephritis in man. J Exp Med 134:169, 1971
3. Tan EM, Cohen AS, Fries JF et al: The 1982 revised criteria for the classification of systemic lupus erythematosus. Arthritis Rheum 25:1271, 1982

4. Cohen AS, Reynolds WE, Franklin EC et al: Preliminary criteria for the classification of systemic lupus erythematosus. Bull Rheum Dis 21:643, 1971

5. Trimble RB, Townes AS, Robinson H et al: Preliminary criteria for the classification of systemic lupus erythematosus (SLE). Evaluation in early diagnosed SLE and rheumatoid arthritis. Arthritis Rheum 17:184, 1974

6. Passas CM, Wong RL, Peterson M et al: A comparison of the specificity of the 1972 and 1982 American Rheumatism Association criteria for the classification of systemic lupus erythematosus. Arthritis Rheum 28:620, 1985

7. Gribetz D, Henley WL: Systemic lupus erythematosus in childhood. J Mt Sinai Hosp (NY) 26:289, 1959

8. Smith CD, Cyr M: The history of lupus erythematosus: from Hippocrates to Osler. Rheum Dis Clin North Am 14:1, 1988

9. Kaposi M: New reports on knowledge of lupus erythematosus. Arch Dermatol u Syph 4:36, 1872

10. Osler W: On the visceral complications of erythema exudativum multiforme. Am J Med Sci 110:629, 1895

11. Libman E, Sacks B: A hitherto undescribed form of valvular and mural endocarditis. Arch Intern Med 33:701, 1924

12. Gross L: Cardiac lesions in Libman-Sacks disease with a consideration of its relationship to acute diffuse lupus erythematosus. Am J Pathol 16:375, 1940

13. Baehr G, Klemperer P, Schifrin A: A diffuse disease of the peripheral circulation usually associated with lupus erythematosus and endocarditis. Trans Assoc Am Physicians 50:139, 1935

14. Hargraves MM, Richmond H, Morton R: Presentation of two bone marrow elements: the "Tart" cell and "L.E." cell. Mayo Clin Proc 23:25, 1948

15. Nobrega FT, Ferguson RH, Kurland LT et al: Lupus erythematosus in Rochester, Minnesota 1950–65: a preliminary study. In Bennett PH, Wood PHN (eds): Population Studies of the Rheumatic Diseases. International Congress Series, No. 148, Excepta Medica Foundation, New York, 1968

16. Fessel WJ: Systemic lupus erythematosus in the community. Incidence, prevalence, outcome, and first symptoms: the high prevalence in black women. Arch Intern Med 134:1027, 1974

17. Fessel WJ: Epidemiology of systemic lupus erythematosus. Rheum Dis Clin North Am 14:15, 1988

18. Siegel M, Lee ML: The epidemiology of systemic lupus erythematosus. Semin Arthritis Rheum 3:1, 1973

19. Meislin AG, Rothfield NF: Systemic lupus erythematosus in childhood. Analysis of 42 cases with comparative data on 200 adult cases followed concurrently. Pediatrics 42:37, 1968

20. Zetterström R, Berglund G: Systemic lupus erythematosus in childhood. A clinical study. Acta Paediatr Scand 45:189, 1956

21. Cook CD, Wedgwood RJP, Craig MJ et al: Systemic lupus erythematosus. Description of 37 cases in children and a discussion of endocrine therapy in 32 of the cases. Pediatrics 26:570, 1960

22. Peterson RDA, Vernier RL, Good RA: Lupus erythematosus. Pediatr Clin North Am 10:941, 1963

23. Robinson MJ, Williams AL: Systemic lupus erythematosus. Aust Paediatr J 3:36, 1967

24. Cassidy JT, Sullivan DB, Petty RE et al: Lupus nephritis and encephalopathy. Prognosis in 58 children. Arthritis Rheum 20:315, 1977

25. King KK, Kornreich HK, Bernstein BH et al: The clinical spectrum of systemic lupus erythematosus in childhood. Arthritis Rheum 20:287, 1977

26. Jacobs JC: Treatment of systemic lupus erythematosus in childhood. Arthritis Rheum 20:304, 1977

27. Dubois EL, Tuffanelli DL: Clinical manifestations of systemic lupus erythematosus. Computer analysis of 520 cases. JAMA 190:104, 1964

28. Harvey AM, Shulman LE, Tumulty PH et al: Systemic lupus erythematosus. A review of the literature and clinical analysis of 138 cases. Medicine 33:291, 1954

29. Kornreich H: Systemic lupus erythematosus in childhood. Clin Rheum Dis 2:429, 1976

30. Celermajer DS, Thorner PS, Baumal R et al: Sex differences in childhood lupus nephritis. Am J Dis Child 138:586, 1984

31. Norris DG, Colón AR, Stickler GB: Systemic lupus erythematosus in children: the complex problems of diagnosis and treatment encountered in 101 such patients at the Mayo Clinic. Clin Pediatr 16:774, 1977

32. Lee P, Urowitz MB, Bookman AAM et al: Systemic lupus erythematosus: a review of 110 cases with reference to nephritis, the nervous system, infections, aseptic necrosis and prognosis. Q J Med 46:1, 1977

33. Hagge WW, Burke EC, Stickler GB: Treatment of systemic lupus erythematosus complicated by nephritis in children. Pediatrics 40:822, 1967

34. Walravens PA, Chase HP: The prognosis of childhood systemic lupus erythematosus. Am J Dis Child 130:929, 1976

35. Kaslow RA: High rate of death caused by systemic lupus erythematosus among U.S. residents of Asian descent. Arthritis Rheum 25:414, 1982

36. Feng PH, Boey ML: Systemic lupus erythematosus

in Chinese: the Singapore experience. Rheumatol Int 2:151, 1982

37. Lee BW, Yap HK, Yip WC et al: A 10 year review of systemic lupus erythematosus in Singapore children. Aust Paediatr J 23:163, 1987

38. Chen JH, Lin CY, Chen WP et al: Systemic lupus erythematosus in children. Chin J Microbiol Immunol 20:23, 1987

39. Tejani A, Nicastri AD, Chen CK et al: Lupus nephritis in Black and Hispanic children. Am J Dis Child 137:481, 1983

40. Moreton RO, Gershwin MD, Brady C et al: The incidence of systemic lupus erythematosus in North American Indians. J Rheumatol 3:186, 1976

41. Delgado EA, Malleson PN, Carter J et al: Pulmonary manifestations of childhood systemic lupus erythematosus. Arthritis Rheum 30:S27, 1987

42. Fritzler M: Proceedings 1st International Conference on Systemic Lupus Erythematosus. J Rheumatol, (suppl. 13), 1987

43. Miller ML, Magilavy DB, Warren RW: The immunologic basis of lupus. Pediatr Clin North Am 33:1191, 1986

44. Michlmayr G, Pathouli C, Huber C et al: Antibodies for T lymphocytes in systemic lupus erythematosus. Clin Exp Immunol 24:18, 1976

45. Tan P, Pang G, Wilson JD: Immunoglobulin production in vitro by peripheral blood lymphocytes in systemic lupus erythematosus: helper T cell defect and B cell hyperreactivity. Clin Exp Immunol 44:548, 1981

46. Ichikawa Y, Lavastida MT, Gonzales EB et al: Defective expression of OKT4 antigen on the cell surface of helper T lymphocytes in a patient with systemic lupus erythematosus. Clin Exp Rheumatol 1:299, 1983

47. Morimoto C, Steinberg AD, Letvin NL et al: A defect of immunoregulatory T cell subsets in systemic lupus erythematosus patients demonstrated with anti-2H4 antibody. J Clin Invest. 79:762, 1987

48. Hahn BH, Ando D, Ebling FN et al: T cell upregulation of B cells via their idiotypes contributing to the development of systemic lupus erythematosus. A hypothesis. Am J Med 85:suppl., 6A, 32, 1988

49. Bluestein HG, Zvaifler NJ: Brain-reactive lymphocytotoxic antibodies in the serum of patients with systemic lupus erythematosus. J Clin Invest 57:509, 1976

50. Bresnihan B, Oliver M, Gregor R: Brain reactivity of lymphocytotoxic antibodies in systemic lupus erythematosus with and without cerebral involvement. Clin Exp Immunol 30:333, 1977

51. Bluestein HG, Williams GW, Steinberg AD: Cerebrospinal fluid antibodies to neuronal cells: association with neuropsychiatric manifestations of systemic lupus erythematosus. Am J Med 70:240, 1981

52. Bresnihan B, Jasin HE: Suppressor function of peripheral blood mononuclear cells in normal individuals and in patients with systemic lupus erythematosus. J Clin Invest 59:106, 1977

53. Horowitz S, Borcherding W, Moorthy AV et al: Induction of suppressor T cells in systemic lupus erythematosus by thymosin and cultured thymic epithelium. Science 197:999, 1977

54. Calabrese LH, Bach JF, Currie T et al: Development of systemic lupus erythematosus after thymectomy for myasthenia gravis. Studies of suppressor cell function. Arch Intern Med 141:253, 1981

55. Perl A, Gonzalez-Cabello R, Láng I et al: Depressed natural and lectin-dependent cell-mediated cytotoxicity against adherent HEp-2 cells in patients with systemic lupus erythematosus. Immunol Commun 11:431, 1982

56. Katz P, Zaytoun AM, Lee JH, Jr et al: Abnormal natural killer cell activity in systemic lupus erythematosus: an intrinsic defect in the lytic event. J Immunol 129:1966, 1982

57. Oshimi K, Sumiya M, Gonda N et al: Natural killer cell activity in untreated systemic lupus erythematosus. Ann Rheum Dis 41:417, 1982

58. Kaufman DB: Natural killer augmentation in systemic lupus erythematosus via a soluble mediator derived from human lymphocytes. Arthritis Rheum 25:562, 1982

59. Miller ML, Lantner R, Pachman LM: Natural and antibody-dependent cellular cytotoxicity in children with systemic lupus erythematosus and juvenile dermatomyositis. J Rheumatol 10:640, 1983

60. Strannegård O, Hermodsson S, Westberg G: Interferon and natural killer cells in systemic lupus erythematosus. Clin Exp Immunol 50:246, 1982

61. Hahn BH, Pletscher LS, Muniain M et al: Suppression of the normal autologous mixed leukocyte reaction by sera from patients with systemic lupus erythematosus. Arthritis Rheum 25:381, 1982

62. De Faucal P, Godard A, Peyrat MA et al: Impaired IL2 production by lymphocytes of patients with systemic lupus erythematosus. Ann Immunol 135D:161, 1984

63. Miller JJ, III, Olds LC: Interleukin-2 production by lymphocytes from blood of children with arthritis is less suppressed than in systemic lupus or cystic fibrosis. J Rheumatol 14:736, 1987

64. Schwartz RS: Viruses and systemic lupus erythematosus. N Engl J Med 293:132, 1975

65. Phillips PE: The role of infectious agents in childhood

rheumatic diseases. Models and evidence. Arthritis Rheum 20:459, 1977

66. Norton WL: Endothelial inclusions in active lesions of systemic lupus erythematosus. J Lab Clin Med 74:369, 1969

67. Hurd ER, Eigenbrodt E, Ziff M et al: Cytoplasmic tubular structures in kidney biopsies in systemic lupus erythematosus. Arthritis Rheum 12:541, 1969

68. Klippel JH, Decker JL: Epstein-Barr virus antibody and lymphocyte tuboloreticular structures in systemic lupus erythematosus. Lancet 2:1057, 1973

69. Klippel JH, Grimley PM, Decker JL: Lymphocyte inclusions in newborns of mothers with systemic lupus erythematosus. N Engl J Med 290:96, 1974

70. Mellors RC, Mellors JW: Antigen related to mammalian type-C RNA viral p30 proteins is located in renal glomeruli in human systemic lupus erythematosus. Proc Natl Acad Sci USA 73:233, 1976

71. Phillips PE, Hargrave-Granda R: Type C oncornavirus isolation studies in systemic lupus erythematosus. II: Attempted detection by viral RNA-dependent DNA polymerase assay. Ann Rheum Dis 37:225, 1978

72. Carr RI, Hoffman AA, Harbeck RJ: Comparison of DNA binding in normal population, general hospital laboratory personnel, and personnel from laboratories studying SLE. J Rheumatol 2:178, 1975

73. Beaucher WN, Garman RH, Condemi JJ: Familial lupus erythematosus. Antibodies to DNA in household dogs. N Engl J Med 296:982, 1977

74. Lewis RM: Animal model: canine systemic lupus erythematosus. Am J Pathol 69:537, 1972

75. Reinersten JL, Kaslow RA, Klippel JH et al: An epidemiologic study of households exposed to canine systemic lupus erythematosus. Arthritis Rheum 23:564, 1980

76. Hollinger FB, Sharp JT, Lidsky MD et al: Antibodies to viral antigens in systemic lupus erythematosus. Arthritis Rheum 14:1, 1971

77. Phillips PE: Raised antibody titres in systemic lupus erythematosus. Lancet 1:382, 1972

78. Phillips PE, Christian CL: Virus antibodies in systemic lupus erythematosus and other connective tissue diseases. Ann Rheum Dis 32:450, 1973

79. Hurd ER, Dowdle W, Casey H et al: Virus antibody levels in systemic lupus erythematosus. Arthritis Rheum 15:267, 1972

80. Reichlin M, Harley JB: Immune response to the RNA protein particles in systemic lupus erythematosus. Am J Med 85:suppl., 6A, 35, 1988

81. Lahita RG, Bradlow HL, Ginzler E et al: Low plasma androgens in women with systemic lupus erythematosus. Arthritis Rheum 30:241, 1987

82. Travers RL, Hughes GRV: Oral contraceptive therapy and systemic lupus erythematosus. J Rheumatol 5:448, 1978

83. Jungers P, Dougados M, Pélissier C et al: Influence of oral contraceptive therapy on the activity of systemic lupus erythematosus. Arthritis Rheum 25:618, 1982

84. Landwirth J, Berger A: Systemic lupus erythematosus and Klinefelter syndrome. Am J Dis Child 126:851, 1973

85. Schlegelberger T, Kekow J, Gross WL: Impaired T-cell-independent B-cell maturation in systemic lupus erythematosus: coculture experiments in monozygotic twins concordant for Klinefelter's syndrome but discordant for systemic lupus erythematosus. Clin Immunol Immunopathol 40:365, 1986

86. Fam AG, Izsak M, Saiphoo C: Systemic lupus erythematosus and Klinefelter's syndrome (letter). Arthritis Rheum 23:124, 1980

87. Howie JB, Helyer BJ: The immunology and pathology of NZB mice. Adv Immunol 9:215, 1968

88. Talal N: Animal models for systemic lupus erythematosus. Clin Rheum Dis 1:485, 1975

89. Klotzin BL, Palmer E: Genetic contributions to lupus-like disease in NZB/NZW mice. Am J Med 85:suppl., 6A, 29, 1988

90. McCarty GA, Valencia DW, Fritzler MJ: Antinuclear Antibodies: Contemporary Techniques and Clinical Application to Connective Tissue Diseases. Oxford University Press, New York, 1984

91. Nakamura RM, Peebles CL, Rubin RL et al: Autoantibodies to Nuclear Antigens (ANA). 2nd Ed. American Society of Clinical Pathologists Press, Chicago, 1985

92. Fritzler MJ: Antinuclear antibodies in the investigation of rheumatic diseases. Bull Rheum Dis 35:1, 1985

93. Harmon CE: Antinuclear antibodies in autoimmune disease. Med Clin North Am 69:547, 1985

94. Tan EM: Antinuclear antibodies: diagnostic markers and clues to the basis of systemic autoimmunity. Pediatr Infect Dis 7:53, 1988

95. Koffler D, Schur PH, Kunkel HG: Immunological studies concerning the nephritis of systemic lupus erythematosus. J Exp Med 126:607, 1967

96. Kunkel H: Mechanisms of renal injury in systemic lupus erythematosus (editorial). Am J Med 45:165, 1968

97. Izui S, Lambert PH, Miescher PA: In vitro demonstration of a particular affinity of glomerular basement membrane and collagen for DNA. A possible basis for a local formation of DNA-anti-DNA complexes in systemic lupus erythematosus. J Exp Med 144:428, 1976

98. Gilboa N, Durante D, McIntosh RM: Glomerular deposition of renal tubular epithelial antigen in patients with systemic lupus erythematosus: its possible role in lupus nephritis. J Rheumatol 4:358, 1977

99. Gewurz H, Pickering RJ, Mergenhagen SE et al: The complement profile in acute glomerulonephritis, systemic lupus erythematosus and hypocomplementemic chronic glomerulonephritis. Int Arch Allergy 34:556, 1968

100. Rothfield N, Ross HA, Minta JO et al: Glomerular and dermal deposition of properdin in systemic lupus erythematosus. N Engl J Med 287:681, 1972

101. Gershwin ME, Steinberg AD: Qualitative characteristics of anti-DNA antibodies in lupus nephritis. Arthritis Rheum 17:947, 1974

102. Steward MW, Katz FE, West NJ: The role of low affinity antibody in immune complex disease. The quantity of anti-DNA antibodies in NZB/W F1 hybrid mice. Clin Exp Immunol 21:121, 1975

103. Winfield JB, Faiferman I, Koffler D: Avidity of anti-DNA antibodies in serum and IgG glomerular eluates from patients with systemic lupus erythematosus. Association of high avidity antinative DNA antibody with glomerulonephritis. J Clin Invest 59:90, 1977

104. Leon SA, Green A, Ehrlich GE et al: Avidity of antibodies in SLE. Relation to severity of renal involvement. Arthritis Rheum 20:23, 1977

105. Hale GM, Highton J, Kalmakoff J et al: Changes in anti-DNA antibody affinity during exacerbations of systemic lupus erythematosus. Scand J Rheumatol 15:243, 1986

106. Sher JH, Pertschuk LP: Immunoglobulin G deposits in the choroid plexus of a child with systemic lupus erythematosus. J Pediatr 85:385, 1974

107. Buckman KJ, Moore SM, Ebbin AJ et al: Familial systemic lupus erythematosus. Arch Intern Med 138:1674, 1978

108. Miller KB, Schwartz RS: Familial abnormalities of suppressor-cell function in systemic lupus erythematosus. N Engl J Med 301:803, 1979

109. Lehman TJ, Hanson V, Zvaifler N et al: Antibodies to nonhistone nuclear antigens and antilymphocyte antibodies among children and adults with systemic lupus erythematosus and their relatives. J Rheumatol 11:644, 1984

110. Lieberman E, Heuser E, Hanson V et al: Identical 3-year-old twins with disseminated lupus erythematosus: one with nephrosis and one with nephritis. Arthritis Rheum 11:22, 1968

111. Brunner CM, Horwitz DA, Davis JS, IV: Identical twins discordant for systemic lupus erythematosus: an experiment in nature (abstract). Arthritis Rheum 14:373, 1971

112. Block SR, Winfield JB, Lockshin MD et al: Studies of twins with systemic lupus erythematosus. A review of the literature and presentation of 12 additional sets. Am J Med 59:533, 1975

113. Zaharia L, Hill JM, Loeb E et al: Systemic lupus erythematosus in twin sisters following ten years of hyperglobulinemic purpura (Waldenström). Acta Med Scand 199:429, 1976

114. Thai AC, Teoh PC, Feng PH: Systemic lupus erythematosus in a pair of male twins. Singapore Med J 21:775, 1980

115. Schroeder JL, Hahn BH, Beale MG et al: Genetic, hormonal, and immune studies in a pair of identical twin boys discordant for lupus. Arthritis Rheum 26:1399, 1983

116. Kaplan D: The onset of disease in twins and siblings with systemic lupus erythematosus. J Rheumatol 11:648, 1984

117. Shigematsu H, Irabu N, Ishii T et al: Different histological manifestations of glomerular lesions in familial systemic lupus erythematosus. Acta Pathol Jpn 29:607, 1979

118. Lahita RG, Chiorazzi N, Gibofsky A et al: Familial systemic lupus erythematosus in males. Arthritis Rheum 26:39, 1983

119. Leonhardt ETG: Family studies in systemic lupus erythematosus. Clin Exp Immunol 2:743, 1967

120. Larsen RA: Family studies in systemic lupus erythematosus. J Chronic Dis 25:187, 1972

121. DeHoratius RJ, Pillarisetty R, Messner RP et al: Antinucleic acid antibodies in systemic lupus erythematosus patients and their families. Incidence and correlation with lymphocytotoxic antibodies. J Clin Invest 56:1149, 1975

122. Mitchell AJ, Rusin LJ, Diaz LA: Circumscribed scleroderma with immunologic evidence of systemic lupus erythematosus. Arch Dermatol 116:69, 1980.

123. Lippman SM, Arnett FC, Conley CL et al: Genetic factors predisposing to autoimmune diseases. Autoimmune hemolytic anemia, chronic thrombocytopenic purpura, and systemic lupus erythematosus. Am J Med 73:827, 1982

124. Smith CK, Cassidy JT, Bole GG: Type I dysgammaglobulinemia, systemic lupus erythematosus, and lymphoma. Am J Med 48:113, 1970

125. Milligan DW, Chang JG: Systemic lupus erythematosus and lymphoma. Acta Haematol 64:109, 1980

126. Berliner S, Shoenfeld Y, Sidi Y et al: Systemic lupus erythematosus and lymphoma. A family study. Scand J Rheumatol 12:310, 1983

127. Efremidis A, Eiser AR, Grishman E et al: Hodgkin's lymphoma in an adolescent with systemic lupus erythematosus. Cancer 53:142, 1984

128. Tsunematsu Y, Koide R, Sasaki M et al: Acute myeloid leukemia with preceding systemic lupus erythematosus and autoimmune hemolytic anemia. Jpn J Clin Oncol 14:107, 1984

129. Saulsbury FT, Sabio H, Conrad D et al: Acute leukemia with features of systemic lupus erythematosus. J Pediatr 105:57, 1984

130. Thomas JR, III, Su WP: Concurrence of lupus erythematosus and dermatitis herpetiformis. A report of nine cases. Arch Dermatol 119:740, 1983

131. Rosenstein ED, Wieczorek R, Raphael BG et al: Systemic lupus erythematosus and angioimmunoblastic lymphadenopathy: case report and review of literature. Semin Arthritis Rheum 16:146, 1986

132. Cleland LG, Bell DA, Willans M et al: Familial lupus. Family studies of HLA and serologic findings. Arthritis Rheum 21:183, 1978

133. Lowenstein MB, Rothfield NF: Family study of systemic lupus erythematosus. Analysis of the clinical history, skin immunofluorescence, and serologic parameters. Arthritis Rheum 20:1293, 1977

134. Black CM, Welsh KI, Fielder A et al: HLA antigens and Bf allotypes in SLE: evidence for the association being with specific haplotypes. Tissue Antigens 19:115, 1982

135. Reinertsen JL, Klippel JH, Johnson AH et al: Family studies of B lymphocyte alloantigens in systemic lupus erythematosus. J Rheumatol 9:253, 1982

136. Fielder AH, Walport MJ, Batchelor JR et al: Family study of the major histocompatibility complex in patients with systemic lupus erythematosus: importance of null alleles of C4A and C4B in determining disease susceptibility. Br Med J 286:425, 1983

137. Arnett FC, Reveille JD, Wilson RW et al: Systemic lupus erythematosus: current state of the genetic hypothesis. Semin Arthritis Rheum 14:24, 1984

138. Arnett FC, Goldstein R, Duvic M et al: Major histocompatibility complex genes in systemic lupus erythematosus, Sjögren's syndrome, and polymyositis. Am J Med 85:suppl 6A, 38, 1988

139. Fronek Z, Timmerman LA, Alper CA et al: Major histocompatibility complex associations with systemic lupus erythematosus. Am J Med 85:suppl., 6A, 42, 1988

140. Woodrow JC: Immunogenetics of systemic lupus erythematosus (editorial). J Rheumatol 15:197, 1988

141. Agnello V: Complement deficiency states. Medicine 57:1, 1978

142. Atkinson JP: Complement deficiency. Predisposing factor to autoimmune syndromes. Am J Med 85:suppl., 6A, 45, 1988

143. Lehman TJA, Hanson V, Singsen BH et al: Serum complement abnormalities in the antinuclear anti-body-positive relatives of children with systemic lupus erythematosus. Arthritis Rheum 22:954, 1979

144. Sano Y, Nishimukai H, Kitamura H et al: Hereditary deficiency of the third component of complement in two sisters with systemic lupus erythematosus-like symptoms. Arthritis Rheum 24:1255, 1981

145. Steinsson K, McLean RH, Marrow M et al: Selective complete C1q deficiency associated with systemic lupus erythematosus. J Rheumatol 10:590, 1983

146. Iida K, Mornaghi R, Nussenzweig V: Complement receptor (CRI) deficiency in erythrocytes from patients with systemic lupus erythematosus. J Exp Med 155:1427, 1982

147. Osterland CK, Epinoza L, Parker LP et al: Inherited C2 deficiency and systemic lupus erythematosus: studies on a family. Ann Intern Med 82:323, 1975

148. Gewurz A, Lint TF, Roberts JL et al: Homozygous C2 deficiency with fulminant lupus erythematosus: severe nephritis via the alternative complement pathway. Arthritis Rheum 21:28, 1978

149. Roberts JL, Schwartz MM, Lewis EJ: Hereditary C2 deficiency and systemic lupus erythematosus associated with severe glomerulonephritis. Clin Exp Immunol 31:328, 1978

150. Ochs HD, Rosenfeld SI, Thomas ED et al: Linkage between the gene (or genes) controlling synthesis of the fourth component of complement and the major histocompatibility complex. N Engl J Med 296:470, 1977

151. Schaller JG, Gilliland BG, Ochs HD et al: Severe systemic lupus erythematosus with nephritis in a boy with deficiency of the fourth component of complement. Arthritis Rheum 20:1519, 1977

152. Berliner S, Weinberger A, Zimir R et al: Familial systemic lupus erythematosus and C4 deficiency. Scand J Rheumatol 10:280, 1981

153. Tappeiner G, Hintner H, Scholz S et al: Systemic lupus erythematosus in hereditary deficiency of the fourth component of complement. J Am Acad Dermatol 7:66, 1982

154. Kjellman M, Laurell AB, Löw B et al: Homozygous deficiency of C4 in a child with a lupus erythematosus syndrome. Clin Genet 22:331, 1982

155. Mascart-Lemone F, Hauptmann G, Goetz J et al: Genetic deficiency of C4 presenting with recurrent infections and a SLE like disease. Genetic and immunologic studies. Am J Med 75:295, 1983

156. Meyer O, Hauptmann G, Tappeiner G et al: Genetic deficiency of C4, C2 or C1q and lupus syndromes. Association with anti-Ro (SS-A) antibodies. Clin Exp Immunol 62:678, 1985

157. MacFarlane PS, Speirs AL, Sommerville RG: Fatal granulomatous disease of childhood and benign lym-

phocytic infiltration of the skin (congenital dysphag-ocytosis). Lancet 1:408, 1967

158. Schaller JG: Illness resembling lupus erythematosus in mothers of boys with chronic granulomatous disease. Ann Intern Med 76:747, 1972

159. Kohler PF, Percy J, Campion WM et al: Hereditary angioedema and "familial" lupus erythematosus in identical twin boys. Am J Med 56:406, 1974

160. Massa MC, Connolly SM: An association between C1 esterase inhibitor deficiency and lupus erythematosus: report of two cases and review of the literature. J Am Acad Dermatol 7:255, 1982

161. Raum D, Glass D, Carpenter CB et al: The chromosomal order of genes controlling the major histocompatibility complex, properdin factor B, and deficiency of the second component of complement. J Clin Invest 58:1240, 1976

162. Sussman GL, Rivera VJ, Kohler PF: Transition from systemic lupus erythematosus to common variable hypogammaglobulinemia. Ann Intern Med 99:32, 1983

163. Tsokos GC, Smith PL, Balow JE: Development of hypogammaglobulinemia in a patient with systemic lupus erythematosus. Am J Med 81:1081, 1986

164. Cleland LG, Bell DA: The occurrence of systemic lupus erythematosus in two kindreds in association with selective IgA deficiency. J Rheumatol 5:288, 1978

165. Petty RE, Palmer NR, Cassidy JT et al: The association of autoimmune diseases and anti-IgA antibodies in patients with selective IgA deficiency. Clin Exp Immunol 37:83, 1979

166. Yewdall V, Cameron JS, Nathan AW et al: Systemic lupus erythematosus and IgA deficiency. J Clin Lab Immunol 10:13, 1983

167. Miller JJ, III: Drug-induced lupus-like syndromes in children. Arthritis Rheum 20:308, 1977

168. Jacobs JC: Drug-induced lupus. JAMA 222:1557, 1972

169. Hess EV: Introduction to drug-related lupus. Arthritis Rheum 24:vi, 1981

170. Hanlon TM, Binkiewicz A, Feingold M et al: Procainamide HCl-induced lupus syndrome in a child with myotonia congenita. Am J Dis Child 113:491, 1967

171. Searles RP, Plymate SR, Troup GM: Familial thioamide-induced lupus syndrome in thyrotoxicosis. J Rheumatol 8:498, 1981

172. Vanheula BA, Carswell F: Sulphasalazine-induced systemic lupus erythematosus in a child. Eur J Pediatr 140:66, 1983

173. Walshe JM: Penicillamine and the SLE syndrome. J Rheumatol 7:155, 1981

174. Grossman L, Barland P: Histone reactivity of drug-induced antinuclear antibodies. A comparison of symptomatic and asymptomatic patients. Arthritis Rheum 24:297, 1981

175. Fritzler M, Ryan P, Kinsella TD: Clinical features of systemic lupus erythematosus patients with antihistone antibodies. J Rheumatol 9:46, 1982

176. Alarcón-Segovia D, Wakim KG, Worthington JW et al: Clinical and experimental studies on the hydralazine syndrome and its relationship to systemic lupus erythematosus. Medicine 46:1, 1967

177. Alarcón-Segovia D: Drug induced systemic lupus erythematosus and related syndromes. Clin Rheum Dis 1:573, 1975

178. Lee SL, Chase PH: Drug-induced systemic lupus erythematosus: a critical review. Semin Arthritis Rheum 5:83, 1975

179. Beernink DH, Miller JJ, III: Anticonvulsant-induced antinuclear antibodies and lupus-like disease in children. J Pediatr 82:113, 1973

180. Jacobs JC: Systemic lupus erythematosus in childhood. Report of 35 cases, with discussion of seven apparently induced by anticonvulsant medication, and of prognosis and treatment. Pediatrics 32:257, 1963

181. Singsen BH, Fishman L, Hanson V: Antinuclear antibodies and lupus-like syndromes in children receiving anticonvulsants. Pediatrics 57:529, 1976

182. Irias JJ: Hydralazine-induced lupus erythematosus-like syndrome. Am J Dis Child 129:862, 1975

183. Hahn BH, Sharp GC, Irvin WS et al: Immune responses to hydralazine and nuclear antigens in hydralazine-induced lupus erythematosus. Ann Intern Med 76:365, 1972

184. Johansson E, Mustakallio KK, Mattila MJ: Polymorphic acetylator phenotype and systemic lupus erythematosus. Acta Med Scand 210:193, 1981

185. Baer AN, Woosley RL, Pincus T: Further evidence for the lack of association between acetylator phenotype and systemic lupus erythematosus. Arthritis Rheum 29:508, 1986

186. Gardner DL: Systemic lupus erythematosus. In Gardner DL (ed): Pathology of the Connective Tissue Diseases. 2nd Ed. Williams & Wilkins, Baltimore, 1965, p. 144

187. Klemperer P, Pollack AD, Baehr G: Pathology of disseminated lupus erythematosus. Arch Pathol 32:569, 1941

188. Schrager MA, Rothfield NF: The lupus band test. Clin Rheum Dis 1:597, 1975

189. Grossman J, Schwartz RH, Callerame ML et al: Systemic lupus erythematosus in a 1-year-old child. Am J Dis Child 129:123, 1975

190. Wertheimer D, Barland P: Clinical significance of immune deposits in the skin in SLE. Arthritis Rheum 19:1249, 1976

191. Davis BM, Gilliam JN: Prognostic significance of subepidermal immune deposits in uninvolved skin of patients with systemic lupus erythematosus: a 10-year longitudinal study. J Invest Dermatol 83:242, 1984

192. James TN, Rupe CE, Monto RW: Pathology of the cardiac conduction system in systemic lupus erythematosus. Ann Intern Med 63:402, 1965

193. Bahrati S, de la Fuente DJ, Kallen RJ et al: Conduction system in systemic lupus erythematosus with atrioventricular block. Am J Cardiol 35:299, 1975

194. Libman E, Sacks B: A hitherto undescribed form of valvular and mural endocarditis. Arch Intern Med 33:701, 1924

195. Johnson RT, Richardson EP: The neurological manifestations of systemic lupus erythematosus. A clinical-pathological study of 24 cases and review of the literature. Medicine 47:337, 1968

196. Aronson AJ, Ordoñez NG, Diddie KR et al: Immune-complex deposition in the eye in systemic lupus erythematosus. Arch Intern Med 139:1312, 1979

197. Caeiro F, Michielson FM, Bernstein R et al: Systemic lupus erythematosus in childhood. Ann Rheum Dis 40:325, 1981

198. Schaller J: Lupus in childhood. Clin Rheum Dis 8:219, 1982

199. Lee LA, Weston WL: Lupus erythematosus in childhood. Dermatol Clin 4:151, 1986

200. Emery H: Clinical aspects of systemic lupus erythematosus in childhood. Pediatr Clin North Am 33:1177, 1986

201. Kaufman DB, Laxer RM, Silverman ED et al: Systemic lupus erythematosus in childhood and adolescence—the problem, epidemiology, incidence, susceptibility, genetics, and prognosis. Curr Probl Pediatr 16:545, 1986

202. Ansell BM: Perspectives in pediatric systemic lupus erythematosus. J Rheumatol 13:177, 1987

203. Reiter D, Myers AR: Asymptomatic nasal septal perforations in systemic lupus erythematosus. Ann Otol Rhinol Layngol 89:78, 1980

204. Kornreich HK, Hanson V: The rheumatic diseases of childhood. Curr Probl Pediatr 4:1, 1974

205. Ragsdale CG, Petty RE, Cassidy JT et al: The clinical progression of apparent juvenile rheumatoid arthritis to systemic lupus erythematosus. J Rheumatol 7:50, 1980

206. Foote RA, Kimbrough SM, Stevens JC: Lupus myositis. Muscle Nerve 5:65, 1982

207. Smith FE, Sweet DE, Brunner CM et al: Avascular necrosis in SLE. An apparent predilection for young patients. Ann Rheum Dis 35:227, 1976

208. Griffiths ID, Maini RN, Scott JT: Clinical and radiological features of osteonecrosis in systemic lupus erythematosus. Ann Rheum Dis 38:413, 1979

209. Abeles M, Urman JD, Rothfield NF: Aseptic necrosis of bone in systemic lupus erythematosus. Relationship to corticosteroid therapy. Arch Intern Med 138:750, 1978

210. Zizic TM, Marcoux C, Hungerford DS et al: Corticosteroid therapy associated with ischemic necrosis of bone in systemic lupus erythematosus. Am J Med 79:596, 1985

211. Ansari A, Larson PH, Bates HD: Vascular manifestations of systemic lupus erythematosus. Angiology 37:423, 1986

212. Englund JA, Lucas RV, Jr: Cardiac complications in children with systemic lupus erythematosus. Pediatrics 72:724, 1983

213. Badui E, Garcia-Rubi D, Robles E et al: Cardiovascular manifestations in systemic lupus erythematosus. Prospective study of 100 patients. Angiology 36:431, 1985

214. Doherty NE, Siegel RJ: Cardiovascular manifestations of systemic lupus erythematosus. Am Heart J 110:1257, 1985

215. Galve E, Candell-Riera J, Pigrau C et al: Prevalence, morphologic types and evolution of cardiac valvular disease in systemic lupus erythematosus. N Engl J Med 319:817, 1988

216. Stevens MB: Lupus carditis. (editorial) N Engl J Med 319:861, 1988

217. Mandell BF: Cardiovascular involvement in systemic lupus erythematosus. Semin Arthritis Rheum 17:126, 1987

218. Jacobson EJ, Reza MJ: Constrictive pericarditis in systemic lupus erythematosus. Demonstration of immunoglobulins in the pericardium. Arthritis Rheum 21:972, 1978

219. Ishikawa S, Segar WE, Gilbert EF et al: Myocardial infarct in a child with systemic lupus erythematosus. Am J Dis Child 132:696, 1978

220. Homcy CJ, Liberthson RR, Fallon JT et al: Ischemic heart disease in systemic lupus erythematosus in the young patients: report of six cases. Am J Cardiol 49:478, 1982

221. Spiera H, Rothenberg RR: Myocardial infarction in four young patients with SLE. J Rheumatol 10:464, 1983

222. Haider YS, Roberts WC: Coronary arterial disease in systemic lupus erythematosus; quantification of degrees of narrowing in 22 necropsy patients (21 women) aged 16 to 37 years. Am J Med 70:775, 1981

223. Laufer J, Frand M, Milo S: Valve replacement for severe tricuspid regurgitation caused by Libman-Sacks endocarditis. Br Heart J 48:294, 1982

224. Dajee H, Hurley EJ, Szarnicki RJ: Cardiac valve replacement in systemic lupus erythematosus. A review. J Thorac Cardiovasc Surg 85:718, 1983

225. Klinkhoff AV, Thompson CR, Reid GD et al: M-mode and two-dimensional echocardiographic abnormalities in systemic lupus erythematosus. JAMA 253:3273, 1985

226. Kahan A, Amor B, deVernejoul F et al: Endocarditis: the diagnostic importance of two-dimensional echocardiography. Br J Rheumatol 24:187, 1985

227. Doherty NE, III, Feldman G, Maurer G et al: Echocardiographic findings in systemic lupus erythematosus. Am J Cardiol 61:1144, 1988

228. Haupt HM, Moore GW, Hutchins GM: The lung in systemic lupus erythematosus. Analysis of the pathologic changes in 120 patients. Am J Med 71:791, 1981

229. De Jongste JC, Neijens HJ, Duiverman EJ et al: Respiratory tract disease in systemic lupus erythematosus. Arch Dis Child 61:478, 1986

230. Nadorra RL, Landing BH: Pulmonary lesions in childhood onset systemic lupus erythematosus: analysis of 26 cases, and summary of literature. Pediatr Pathol 7:1, 1987

231. Good JT, Jr, King TE, Antony VB et al: Lupus pleuritis. Clinical features and pleural fluid characteristics with special reference to pleural fluid antinuclear antibodies. Chest 84:714, 1983

232. Jay MS, Jerath R, Van Derzalm T et al: Pneumothorax in an adolescent with fulminant systemic lupus erythematosus. J Adolesc Health Care 5:142, 1984

233. Ramirez RE, Glasier C, Kirks D et al: Pulmonary hemorrhage associated with systemic lupus erythematosus in children. Radiology 153:409, 1984

234. Nadorra RL, Nakazato Y, Landing BH: Pathologic features of gastrointestinal tract lesions in childhood-onset systemic lupus erythematotus: study of 26 patients, with review of the literature. Pediatr Pathol 7:245, 1987

235. Hamdan JA, Ahmad MS, Saádi AR: Malacoplakia of the retroperitoneum in a girl with systemic lupus erythematosus. Pediatrics 70:296, 1982

236. Tsukahara M, Matsuo K, Kojima H: Protein-losing enteropathy in a boy with systemic lupus erythematosus. J Pediatr 97:778, 1980

237. Chase GJ, O'Shea PA, Collins E et al: Protein-losing enteropathy in systemic lupus erythematosus. Hum Pathol 13:1053, 1982

238. Weiser MM, Andres GA, Brentjens JR et al: Systemic lupus erythematosus and intestinal venulitis. Gastroenterology 81:570, 1981

239. Schousboe JT, Koch AE, Chang RW: Chronic lupus peritonitis with ascites: review of the literature with a case report. Semin Arthritis Rheum 18:121, 1988

240. Oddis C, McGlynn TJ: Abdominal computed tomography scan in acute lupus abdominal serositis. J Comput Assist Tomogr 8:337, 1984

241. Reynolds JC, Inman RD, Kimberly RP et al: Acute pancreatitis in systemic lupus erythematosus: report of twenty cases and a review of the literature. Medicine 61:25, 1982

242. Simons-Ling N, Schachner L, Penneys N et al: Childhood systemic lupus erythematosus. Association with pancreatitis, subcutaneous fat necrosis, and calcinosis cutis. Arch Dermatol 119:491, 1983

243. Zizic TM, Classen JN, Stevens MB: Acute abdominal complications of systemic lupus erythematosus and polyarteritis nodosa. Am J Med 73:525. 1982

244. Hall S, Czaja AJ, Kaufman DK et al: How lupoid is lupoid hepatitis? J Rheumatol 13:95, 1986

245. Gibson T, Myers AR: Subclinical liver disease in systemic lupus erythematosus. J Rheumatol 8:752, 1981

246. Mackay IR, Taft LI, Cowling DC: Lupoid hepatitis. Lancet 2:1323, 1956

247. Dillon AM, Stein HB, English RA: Splenic atrophy in systemic lupus erythematosus. Ann Intern Med 96:40, 1982

248. Malleson P, Petty RE, Nadel H et al: Functional asplenia in childhood onset systemic lupus erythematosus. J Rheumatol 15:1648, 1988

249. Sergent JS, Lockshin MD, Klempner MS et al: Central nervous system disease in systemic lupus erythematosus. Therapy and prognosis. Am J Med 58:644, 1975

250. Yancy CL, Doughty RA, Athreya BH: Central nervous system involvement in childhood systemic lupus erythematosus. Arthritis Rheum 24:1389, 1981

251. Herd JK, Medhi M, Uzendoski DM et al: Chorea associated with systemic lupus erythematosus: report of two cases and review of the literature. Pediatrics 61:308, 1978

252. Kukla LF, Reddy C, Silkalns G et al: Systemic lupus erythematosus presenting as chorea. Arch Dis Child 53:345, 1978

253. Arisaka O, Obinata K, Sasaki H et al: Chorea as an initial manifestation of systemic lupus erythematosus. A case report of a 10-year-old girl. Clin Pediatr 23:298, 1984

254. Bruyn GW, Padberg G: Chorea and systemic lupus erythematosus. A critical review. Eur Neurol 23:435, 1984

255. Asherson RA, Derksen RH, Harris EN et al: Chorea in systemic lupus erythematosus and "lupus-like" disease: association with antiphospholipid antibodies. Semin Arthritis Rheum 16:253, 1987

256. Groothuis JR, Groothuis DR, Mukhopadhyay D et al: Lupus-associated chorea in childhood. Am J Dis Child 131:1131, 1977

257. Feinglass EJ, Arnett FC, Dorsch CA et al: Neuro-

psychiatric manifestations of systemic lupus erythematosus: diagnosis, clinical spectrum, and relationship to other features of the disease. Medicine 55:323, 1976

258. McCune WJ, Golbus J: Neuropsychiatric lupus. Rheum Dis Clin North Am 14:149, 1988

259. Silber TJ, Chatoor I, White PH: Psychiatric manifestations of systemic lupus erythematosus in children and adolescents. A review. Clin Pediatr 23:331, 1984

260. Ostrov SG, Quencer RM, Gaylis NB et al: Cerebral atrophy in systemic lupus erythematosus: steroid- or disease-induced phenomenon? AJNR 3:21, 1982

261. DelGiudice GC, Scher CA, Athreya BH et al: Pseudotumor cerebri and childhood systemic lupus erythematosus. J Rheumatol 13:748, 1986

262. Smith CA, Pinals RS: Optic neuritis in systemic lupus erythematosus. J Rheumatol 9:963, 1982

263. Winfield JB, Brunner CM, Koffler D: Serologic studies in patients with systemic lupus erythematosus and central nervous system dysfunction. Arthritis Rheum 21:289, 1978

264. Keeffe EB, Bardana EJ, Jr, Harbeck RJ et al: Lupus meningitis: antibody to deoxyribonucleic acid (DNA) and DNA-anti-DNA complexes in cerebrospinal fluid. Ann Intern Med 80:58, 1974

265. Bonfa E, Golombek SJ, Kaufman LD et al: Association between lupus psychosis and anti-ribosomal P protein antibodies. N Engl J Med 317:265, 1987

266. Temesvari P, Denburg J, Denburg S et al: Serum lymphocytotoxic antibodies in neuropsychiatric lupus: a serial study. Clin Immunol Immunopathol 28:423, 1983

267. Carette S, Urowitz MB, Grosman H et al: Cranial computerized tomography in systemic lupus erythematosus. J Rheumatol 9:855, 1982

268. Gaylis NB, Altman RD, Ostrov S et al: The selective value of computed tomography of the brain in cerebritis due to systemic lupus erythematosus. J Rheumatol 9:850, 1982

269. Kaell AT, Shetty M, Lee BC et al: The diversity of neurologic events in systemic lupus erythematosus. Prospective clinical and computed tomographic classification of 82 events in 71 patients. Arch Neurol 43:273, 1986

270. Hiraiwa M, Nonaka C, Abe T et al: Positron emission tomography in systemic lupus erythematosus: relation of cerebral vasculitis to PET findings. AJNR 4:541, 1983

271. Pinching AJ, Travers RL, Hughes GRV et al: Oxygen-15 brain scanning for detection of cerebral involvement in systemic lupus erythematosus. Lancet 1:898, 1978

272. Muehrcke RC, Kark RM, Pirani CL et al: Lupus nephritis: a clinical and pathologic study based on renal biopsies. Medicine 36:1, 1957

273. Pollak VE, Pirani CL, Schwartz FD: The natural history of the renal manifestations of systemic lupus erythematosus. J Lab Clin Med 63:537, 1964

274. Comerford FR, Cohen AS: The nephropathy of systemic lupus erythematosus: an assessment by clinical, light and electron microscopic criteria. Medicine 46:425, 1967

275. Pollak VE, Pirani CL: Renal histologic findings in systemic lupus erythematosus. Proc Mayo Clin 44:630, 1969

276. Morris MC, Cameron JS, Chantler C et al: Systemic lupus erythematosus with nephritis. Arch Dis Child 56:779, 1981

277. Phadke K, Trachtman H, Nicastri A et al: Acute renal failure as the initial manifestation of systemic lupus erythematosus in children. J Pediatr 105:38, 1984

278. Kozeny GA, Hurley RM, Fresco R et al: Systemic lupus erythematosus presenting with hyporeninemic hypoaldosteronism in a 10-year-old girl. Am J Nephrol 6:321, 1986

279. Baldwin DS, Lowenstein J, Rothfield NF et al: The clinical course of the proliferative and membranous forms of lupus nephritis. Ann Intern Med 73:929, 1970

280. Baldwin DS, Gluck MC, Lowenstein J et al: Lupus nephritis. Clinical course as related to morphologic forms and their transitions. Am J Med 62:12, 1977

281. Donadio JV, Jr: Renal involvement in SLE: the argument for aggressive treatment. In Bacon PA, Hadler NM (eds): The Kidney and Rheumatic Disease. Butterworth Scientific, Boston, 1982, p. 45

282. Diamond H: Progression of mesangial and focal to diffuse lupus nephritis. N Engl J Med 291:693, 1974

283. Ginzler EM, Nicastri AD, Chen C-K et al: Progression of mesangial and focal to diffuse lupus nephritis. N Engl J Med 291:693, 1974

284. Magil AB, Ballon HS, Rae A: Focal proliferative lupus nephritis. A clinicopathologic study using the W.H.O. classification. Am J Med 72:620, 1982

285. Rothfield N, Baldwin D: The clinical course of the proliferative and membranous forms of lupus nephritis. Ann Intern Med 73:929, 1970

286. Morel-Maroger L: The course of lupus nephritis: contribution of serial renal biopsies. In Hamburger J (ed): Advances in Nephrology, Vol. 6. Year Book Medical Publishers, Chicago, 1976, p. 79

287. Zimmerman SW, Jenkins PG, Shelf WD et al: Progression from minimal or focal to diffuse proliferative lupus nephritis. Lab Invest 32:665, 1975

288. Libit SA, Burke B, Michael AF et al: Extramembranous glomerulonephritis in childhood: relationship to systemic lupus erythematosus. J Pediatr 88:394, 1976

289. Ty A, Fine B: Membranous nephritis in infantile sys-

temic lupus erythematosus associated with chromosomal abnormalities. Clin Nephrol 12:137, 1979

290. The Southwest Pediatric Nephrology Study Group: Comparison of idiopathic and systemic lupus erythematosus-associated membranous glomerulonephropathy in children. Am J Kidney Dis 7:115, 1986

291. Brentjens JR, Sepulveda M, Baliah T et al: Interstitial immune complex nephritis in patients with systemic lupus erythematosus. Kidney Int 7:342, 1975

292. Striker GE, Kelley MR, Quadracci LJ et al: The course of lupus nephritis: a clinical-pathological correlation of fifty patients. In Kincaid-Smith P, Mathew TH, Becker EL (eds): Glomerulonephritis: Morphology, Natural History and Treatment. Part II. John Wiley & Sons, New York, 1973, p. 1141.

293. Woolf A, Croker B, Osofsky SG et al: Nephritis in children and young adults with systemic lupus erythematosus and normal urinary sediment. Pediatrics 64:678, 1979

294. Weis LS, Pachman LM, Potter EV et al: Occult lupus nephropathy: a correlated light, electron and immunofluorescent microscopic study. Histopathology 1:401, 1977

295. Mahajan SK, Ordoñez NG, Feitelson PJ et al: Lupus nephropathy without clinical renal involvement. Medicine 56:493, 1977

296. Leehey DJ, Katz AI, Azaran AH et al: Silent diffuse lupus nephritis: long-term follow-up. Am J Kidney Dis 2:188, 1982

297. Bennett WM, Bardana EJ, Norman DJ et al: Natural history of "silent" lupus nephritis. Am J Kidney Dis 1:359, 1982

298. Magil AB, Ballon HS, Chan V et al: Diffuse proliferative lupus glomerulonephritis. Determination of prognostic significance of clinical, laboratory and pathologic factors. Medicine 63:210, 1984

299. Cassidy JT: Clinical assessment of immune-complex disease in children with systemic lupus erythematosus (editorial). J Pediatr 89:523, 1976

300. Tan EM, Schur PH, Carr RI et al: Deoxyribonucleic acid (DNA) and antibodies to DNA in the serum of patients with systemic lupus erythematosus. J Clin Invest 45:1732, 1966

301. Schur PH, Sandson J: Immunologic factors and clinical activity in systemic lupus erythematosus. N Engl J Med 278:533, 1968

302. Pincus T, Hughes GRV, Pincus D et al: Antibodies to DNA in childhood systemic lupus erythematosus. J Pediatr 78:981, 1971

303. Hughes GRV, Cohen AS, Christian CL: Anti-DNA activity in systemic lupus erythematosus. A diagnostic and therapeutic guide. Ann Rheum Dis 30:259, 1971

304. Adler MK, Baumgarten A, Hecht B et al: Prognostic significance of DNA-binding capacity patterns in patients with lupus nephritis. Ann Rheum Dis 34:444, 1975

305. Schur PH: Complement in lupus. Clin Rheum Dis 1:519, 1975

306. Garin EH, Donnelly WH, Shulman ST et al: The significance of serial measurements of serum complement C3 and C4 components and DNA binding capacity in patients with lupus nephritis. Clin Nephrol 12:148, 1979

307. Sliwinski AJ, Zvaifler NJ: Decreased synthesis of the third component of complement (C3) in hypocomplementemic systemic lupus erythematosus. Clin Exp Immunol 11:21, 1972

308. Abrass CK, Nies KM, Louie JS et al: Correlation and predictive accuracy of circulating immune complexes with disease activity in patients with systemic lupus erythematosus. Arthritis Rheum 23:273, 1980

309. Stamenkovic I, Favre H, Donath A et al: Renal biopsy in SLE irrespective of clinical findings: long-term follow-up. Clin Nephrol 26:109, 1986

310. Balow JE, Austin HA, Muenz LR et al: Effects of treatment on the evolution of renal abnormalities in lupus nephritis. N Engl J Med 311:491, 1984

311. Garin EH, Donnelly WH, Fennell RS, III et al: Nephritis in systemic lupus erythematosus in children. J Pediatr 89:366, 1976

312. Rothfield NF: Systemic lupus erythematosus. Laboratory studies. Arthritis Rheum 20:299, 1977

313. McCarty GA: Update on laboratory studies and relationship to rheumatic and allergic diseases. Ann Allergy 55:1, 1985

314. Zein N, Ganuza C, Kushner I: Significance of serum C-reactive protein elevation in patients with systemic lupus erythematosus. Arthritis Rheum 22:7, 1979

315. Maury CP, Helve T, Sjöblom C: Serum beta 2-microglobulin, sialic acid, and C-reactive protein in systemic lupus erythematosus. Rheumatol Int 2:145, 1982

316. Pepys MB, Lanham JG, DeBeer FC: C-reactive protein in SLE. Clin Rheum Dis 8:91, 1982

317. Karpatkin S, Strick BS, Karpatkin MB et al: Cumulative experience in the detection of antiplatelet antibody in 234 patients with idiopathic thrombocytopenic purpura, systemic lupus erythematosus and other clinical disorders. Am J Med 52:776, 1972

318. Hughes GRV: Autoantibodies in lupus and its variants: experience in 1,000 patients. Br Med J 285:339, 1984

319. Harley JB, Gaither KK: Autoantibodies. Rheum Dis Clin North Am 14:43, 1988

320. Tan EM: Autoantibodies to nuclear antigens: their immunobiology and medicine. Adv Immunol 33:167, 1982

321. Hardin JA, Craft JE: Patterns of autoimmunity to nucleoproteins in patients with systemic lupus erythematosus. Rheum Dis Clin North Am 13:37, 1987

322. Lehman TJ, Hanson V, Singsen BH et al: The role of antibodies directed against double-stranded DNA in the manifestations of systemic lupus erythematosus in childhood. J Pediatr 96:657, 1980

323. Morimoto C, Sano H, Abe T et al: Correlation between clinical activity of systemic lupus erythematosus and the amounts of DNA in DNA/anti-DNA antibody immune complexes. J Immunol 129:1960, 1982

324. Miller JJ, III, Hsu YP, Osborne CL et al: Comparison of three assays for anti-DNA with three assays for the measurement of the role of complement in systemic lupus erythematosus in adolescents. J Rheumatol 7:660, 1980

325. Crowe W, Kushner I: An immunofluorescent method using Crithidia luciliae to detect antibodies to double-stranded DNA. Arthritis Rheum 20:811, 1977

326. Deng JS, Rubin RL, Lipscomb MF et al: Reappraisal of the Crithidia luciliae assay for nDNA antibodies: evidence for histone antibody kinetoplast binding. Am J Clin Pathol 82:448, 1984

327. Maddison PJ, Provost TT, Reichlin M: Serological findings in patients with "ANA-negative" systemic lupus erythematosus. Medicine 60:87, 1981

328. Gillespie JP, Lindsley CB, Linshaw MA et al: Childhood systemic erythematosus with negative antinuclear antibody test. J Pediatr 98:578, 1981

329. Clark G, Reichlin M, Tomasi TB, Jr: Characterization of a soluble cytoplasmic antigen reactive with sera from patients with systemic lupus erythematosus. J Immunol 102:117, 1969

330. Wasicek CA, Reichlin M: Clinical and serological differences between systemic lupus erythematosus patients with antibodies to Ro versus patients with antibodies to Ro and La. J Clin Invest 69:835, 1982

331. Harmon CE, Deng J, Peebles CL et al: The importance of tissue substrate in the SS-A (Ro) antigen-antibody system. Arthritis Rheum 27:166, 1984

332. Arroyave CM, Giambrone MJ, Rich KC et al: The frequency of antinuclear antibody (ANA) in children by use of mouse kidney (MK) and human epithelial cells (HEp-2) as substrates. J Allergy Clin Immunol 82:741, 1988

333. Wechsler HL, Stavrides A: Systemic lupus erythematosus with anti-Ro antibodies: clinical, histologic and immunologic findings. J Am Acad Dermatol 6:73, 1982

334. Barada FA, Jr, Andrews BS, David JS, IV et al: Antibodies to Sm in patients with systemic lupus erythematosus. Correlation of Sm antibody titers with disease activity and other laboratory parameters. Arthritis Rheum 24:1236, 1981

335. Beaufils M, Kouki F, Mignon F et al: Clinical significance of anti-Sm antibodies in systemic lupus erythematosus. Am J Med 74:201, 1983

336. Fritzler MJ, Tan EM: Antibodies to histone in drug-induced and idiopathic lupus erythematosus. J Clin Invest 62:560, 1978

337. Fritzler MJ, Ryan JP, Kinsella TD: Clinical features of SLE patients with antihistone antibodies. J Rheumatol 9:46, 1982

338. Portanova JP, Arndt RE, Tan EM et al: Anti-histone-antibodies in idiopathic and drug-induced lupus recognize distinct intrahistone regions. J Immunol 138:293, 1987

339. Rubin RL, Joslin GF, Tan EM: Specificity of anti-histone antibodies in systemic lupus erythematosus. Arthritis Rheum 25:779, 1982

340. Conley CL, Hartmann RC: A hemorrhagic disorder caused by circulating anticoagulant in patients with disseminated lupus erythematosus. J Clin Invest 31:621, 1952

341. Bajaj SP, Rapaport SI, Fierer DS et al: A mechanism for the hypoprothrombinemia of the acquired hypoprothrombinemia-lupus anticoagulant syndrome. Blood 61:684, 1983

342. Harris EN, Hughes GRV, Charavi AE: Antiphospholipid antibodies: an elderly statesman dons new garments. J Rheumatol 14:suppl., 13, 208, 1987

343. St Clair W, Jones B, Rogers JS et al: Deep venous thrombosis and a circulating anticoagulant in systemic lupus erythematosus. Am J Dis Child 135:230, 1981

344. Appan S, Boey ML, Lim KW: Multiple thromboses in systemic lupus erythematosus. Arch Dis Child 62:739, 1987

345. Weinstein C, Miller MH, Axtens R et al: Livedo reticularis associated with increased titers of anticardiolipin antibodies in systemic lupus erythematosus. Arch Dermatol 123:596, 1987

346. Asherson RA, Lubbe WF: Cerebral and valve lesions in SLE: association with antiphospholipid antibodies (editorial). J Rheumatol 15:539, 1988

347. Lubbe WF, Asherson RA: Intracardiac thrombus in systemic lupus erythematosus associated with lupus anticoagulant. Arthritis Rheum 31:1453, 1988

348. Brown JH, Doherty CC, Allen DC et al: Fatal cardiac failure due to myocardial microthrombi in systemic lupus erythematosus. Br Med J 296:1505, 1988

349. Schleider MA, Nachman RL, Jaffe EA et al: A clinical study of the lupus anticoagulant. Blood 48:499, 1976

350. Singsen BH, Bernstein BH, King KK et al: Systemic lupus erythematosus in childhood: correlations be-

tween changes in disease activity and serum complement levels. J Pediatr 89:358, 1976

351. Levinsky RJ, Cameron JS, Soothill JF: Serum immune complexes and disease activity in lupus nephritis. Lancet 1:564, 1977

352. Theofilopoulos AN, Wilson CB, Bokisch VA et al: Binding of soluble immune complexes to human lymphoblastoid cells. II: Use of Raji cells to detect circulating immune complexes in animal and human sera. J Exp Med 140:1230, 1974

353. Lambert PH: A WHO collaborative study for the evaluation of 18 methods for detecting immune complexes in serum. J Clin Lab Immunol 1:1, 1978

354. Maini RN, Holborow EJ (eds): Detection and measurement of circulatory soluble antigen-antibody complexes and anti-DNA antibodies. Ann Rheum Dis 36:suppl., 1, 1976

355. Harbeck RJ, Bardana EJ, Kohler PF et al: DNA-anti-DNA complexes: their detection in systemic lupus erythematosus sera. J Clin Invest 52:789, 1973

356. Bardana EJ, Jr, Harbeck RJ, Hoffman AA et al: The prognostic and therapeutic implications of DNA: anti-DNA immune complexes in systemic lupus erythematosus (SLE). Am J Med 59:515, 1975

357. Coppo R, Bosticardo GM, Basolo B et al: Clinical significance of the detection of circulating immune complexes in lupus nephritis. Nephron 32:320, 1982

358. Krupp MA: Urinary sediment in visceral angiitis (periarteritis nodosa, lupus erythematosus, Libman-Sacks "disease"): quantitative studies. Arch Intern Med 71:54, 1943

359. Seaman WE, Ishak KG, Plotz PH: Aspirin-induced hepatotoxicity in patients with systemic lupus erythematosus. Ann Intern Med 80:1, 1974

360. Samuelson CO, Williams HJ: Ibuprofen-associated aseptic meningitis in systemic lupus erythematosus. West J Med 131:57, 1979

361. Laaksonen A-L, Koskiahde V, Juva K: Dosage of antimalarial drugs for children with juvenile rheumatoid arthritis and systemic lupus erythematosus. A clinical study with determination of serum concentrations of chloroquine and hydroxychloroquine. Scand J Rheumatol 3:103, 1974

362. Rudnicki RD, Gresham GE, Rothfield NF: The efficacy of antimalarials in systemic lupus erythematosus. J Rheumatol 2:323, 1975

363. Hanson V, Kornreich H: Systemic rheumatic disorders ("collagen disease") in childhood: lupus erythematosus, anaphylactoid purpura, dermatomyositis and scleroderma. Bull Rheum Dis 17:435, 1967

364. Axelrod L: Glucocorticoid therapy. Medicine 55:39, 1976

365. Imbimbo B, Tuzi T, Porzio F et al: Clinical equivalence of a new glucocorticoid, deflazacort and prednisone in rheumatoid arthritis and SLE patients. Adv Exp Med Biol 171:241, 1984

366. Pollak VE, Pirani CL, Kark RM: Effect of large doses of prednisone on the renal lesions and life span of patients with lupus glomerulonephritis. J Lab Clin Med 57:495, 1961

367. Urman JD, Rothfield NF: Corticosteroid treatment in systemic lupus erythematosus. Survival studies. JAMA 238:2271, 1977

368. Cathcart ES, Idelson BA, Scheinberg MA et al: Beneficial effects of methylprednisolone "pulse" therapy in diffuse proliferative lupus nephritis. Lancet 1:163, 1976

369. Kimberly RP, Lockshin MD, Sherman RL et al: High-dose intravenous methylprednisolone pulse therapy in systemic lupus erythematosus. Am J Med 70:817, 1981

370. Perez HD, Kimberly RP, Kaplan HB et al: Effect of high-dose methylprednisolone infusion on polymorphonuclear leukocyte function in patients with systemic lupus erythematosus. Arthritis Rheum 24:641, 1981

371. Barron KS, Person DA, Brewer EJ, Jr et al: Pulse methylprednisolone therapy in diffuse proliferative lupus nephritis. J Pediatr 101:137, 1982

372. Ponticelli C, Zucchelli P, Banfi G et al: Treatment of diffuse proliferative lupus nephritis by intravenous high-dose methylprednisolone. Q J Med 51:16, 1982

373. Shields WD, Bray PF: A danger of haloperidol therapy in children. J Pediatr 88:301, 1976

374. Bulkley BH, Roberts WC: The heart in systemic lupus erythematosus and the changes induced in it by corticosteroid therapy. A study of 36 necropsy patients. Am J Med 58:243, 1975

375. Ilohite NT, Samuel P, Ginzler E et al: Dyslipoproteinemia in pediatric systemic lupus erythematosus. Arthritis Rheum 31:859, 1988

376. Smith GW, Hannan SF, Scott PJ et al: Immune complex-like activity associated with abnormal serum lipoproteins in systemic erythematosus. Clin Exp Immunol 48:8, 1982

377. Steinberg AD: Efficacy of immunosuppressive drugs in rheumatic diseases. Arthritis Rheum 16:92, 1973

378. Wagner L: Immunosuppressive agents in lupus nephritis: a critical analysis. Medicine 55:239, 1976

379. Carette S, Klippel JH, Decker JL et al: Controlled studies of oral immunosuppressive drugs in lupus nephritis. A long-term follow-up. Ann Intern Med 99:1, 1983

380. Klippel JH, Austin HA, III, Balow JE et al: Studies of immunosuppressive drugs in the treatment of lupus nephritis. Rheum Dis Clin North Am 13:47, 1987

381. Steinberg AD, Decker JL: A double-blind controlled trial comparing cyclophosphamide, azathioprine and placebo in the treatment of lupus glomerulonephritis. Arthritis Rheum 17:923, 1974

382. Decker JL, Klippel JH, Plotz PH et al: Cyclophosphamide or azathioprine in lupus glomerulonephritis. A controlled trial: results at 28 months. Ann Intern Med 83:606, 1975

383. Hahn BH, Kantor OS, Osterland CK: Azathioprine plus prednisone compared with prednisone alone in the treatment of systemic lupus erythematosus. Report of a prospective controlled trial in 24 patients. Ann Intern Med 83:597, 1975

384. Barnett EV, Dornfeld L, Lee DB et al: Longterm survival of lupus nephritis patients treated with azathioprine and prednisone. J Rheumatol 5:275, 1978

385. Ginzler E, Sharon E, Diamond H et al: Long-term maintenance therapy with azathioprine in systemic lupus erythematosus. Arthritis Rheum 18:27, 1975

386. Donadio JV, Jr, Holley KE, Ferguson RH et al: Treatment of diffuse proliferative lupus nephritis with prednisone and combined prednisone and cyclophosphamide. N Engl J Med 299:1151, 1978

387. McCune WJ, Golbus J, Zeldes W et al: Clinical and immunologic effects of monthly administration of intravenous cyclophosphamide in severe systemic lupus erythematosus. N Engl J Med 318:1423, 1988

388. Lockwood CM, Pussell B, Wilson CB et al: Plasma exchange in nephritis. Adv Nephrol 8:383, 1979

389. Johannessen A, Gutteberg T, Husby G: Plasma exchange in the treatment of severe, childhood onset systemic lupus erythematosus. Acta Paediatr Scand 71:347, 1982

390. Wallace DJ, Goldfinger D, Bluestone R et al: Plasmapheresis in lupus nephritis with nephrotic syndrome: a long-term follow-up. J Clin Apheresis 1:42, 1982

391. Wei N, Klippel JH, Huston DP et al: Randomised trial of plasma exchange in mild systemic lupus erythematosus. Lancet 1:17, 1983

392. Hadidi T, Decker JL, El-Nagdy L et al: Ineffectiveness of levamisole in systemic lupus erythematosus: a controlled trial. Arthritis Rheum 24:60, 1981

393. Hall RP, Lawley TJ, Smith HR et al: Bullous eruption of systemic lupus erythematosus. Dramatic response to dapsone therapy. Ann Intern Med 97:165, 1982

394. Sharon E, Kaplan D, Diamond HS: Exacerbation of systemic lupus erythematosus after withdrawal of azathioprine therapy. N Engl J Med 288:122, 1973

395. Strober S, Fariñas MC, Field EH et al: Treatment of lupus nephritis with total lymphoid irradiation. Arthritis Rheum 31:850, 1988

396. Pollock CA, Ibels LS: Dialysis and transplantation in patients with renal failure due to systemic lupus erythematosus. The Australian and New Zealand experience. Aust NZ J Med 17:321, 1987

397. Advisory Committee to the Renal Transplant Registry: Renal transplantation in congenital and metabolic diseases: a report from the ACH/NIH Renal Transplant Registry. JAMA 232:148, 1975

398. Kumano K, Sakai T, Mashimo S et al: A case of recurrent lupus nephritis after renal transplantation. Clin Nephrol 27:94, 1987

399. Brown CD, Rao TKS, Maxey RW et al: Regression of clinical and immunological expression of SLE consequent to the development of uremia. Kidney Int 16:884, 1979

400. Jarrett MP, Santhanam S, Del Greco F: The clinical course of end-stage renal disease in systemic lupus erythematosus. Arch Intern Med 143:1353, 1983

401. Kramer P, Boyer M, Brunner FP et al: Combined report on regular dialysis and transplantation in Europe. XII, 1981. Proc Eur Dial Transplant Assoc 19:29, 1982

402. Estes D, Christian CL: The natural history of systemic lupus erythematosus by prospective analysis. Medicine 50:85, 1971

403. Wedgwood RJ: Prognostic factors in childhood systemic lupus erythematosus. Arthritis Rheum 20:295, 1977

404. Fish AJ, Blau EB, Westberg NG et al: Systemic lupus erythematosus within the first two decades of life. Am J Med 62:99, 1977

405. Platt JL, Burke BA, Fish AJ et al: Systemic lupus erythematosus in the first two decades of life. Am J Kidney Dis 2:212, 1982

406. Lipnick R, Papero P, White P: Neuropsychological deficits in SLE. Abstracts of the AAP Section on Rheumatology 1988.

407. Abeles M, Urman JD, Weinstein A et al: SLE in the younger patient: survival studies. J Rheumatol 7:515, 1980

408. Wallace DJ, Podell T, Weiner J et al: Systemic lupus erythematosus—survival patterns. Experience with 609 patients. JAMA 245:934, 1981

409. Glidden RS, Mantzouranis EC, Borel Y: Systemic lupus erythematosus in childhood: clinical manifestations and improved survival in fifty-five patients. Clin Immunol Immunpathol 29:196, 1983

410. Dumas R: Lupus nephritis. Collaboratory study by the French Society of Paediatric Nephrology. Arch Dis Child 60:126, 1985

411. Rush PJ, Baumal R, Shore A et al: Correlation of renal histology with outcome in children with lupus nephritis. Kidney Int 29:1066, 1986

412. Harisdangkul V, Nilganuwonge S, Rockhold L:

Cause of death in systemic lupus erythematosus: a pattern based on age at onset. South Med J 80:1249, 1987

413. Austin HA, III, Muenz LR, Joyce KM et al: Prognostic factors in lupus nephritis. Contribution of renal histologic data. Am J Med 75:382, 1983

414. Bennahum DA, Messner RP: Recent observations on central nervous system lupus erythematosus. Semin Arthritis Rheum 4:253, 1975

415. Kaslow RA, Masi AT: Age, sex, and race effects on mortality from systemic lupus erythematosus in the United States. Arthritis Rheum 21:473, 1978

416. Gordon MF, Stolley PD, Schinnar R: Trends in recent systemic lupus erythematosus mortality rates. Arthritis Rheum 24:762, 1981

417. Singsen BH, Kornreich HK, Koster-King K et al: Mixed connective tissue disease in children. Arthritis Rheum 20:355, 1977

418. Fraga A, Gudiño J, Ramos-Niembro F et al: Mixed connective tissue disease in childhood. Relationship to Sjögren's syndrome. Am J Dis Child 132:263, 1978

419. Sharp GC, Irvin WS, May CM et al: Association of antibodies to ribonucleoprotein and Sm antigens with mixed connective-tissue disease, systemic lupus erythematosus and other rheumatic diseases. N Engl J Med 295:1149, 1976

420. Grennan DM, Bunn C, Hughes GRV et al: Frequency and clinical significance of antibodies to ribonucleoprotein in SLE and other connective tissue disease subgroups. Ann Rheum Dis 36:442, 1977

421. Sharp GC: Subsets of SLE and mixed connective tissue disease. Am J Kidney Dis 2:201, 1982

422. Kusukawa R, Sharp GC (eds): Mixed Connective Tissue Disease and Anti-Nuclear Antibodies: Proceedings of the International Symposium on Mixed Connective Tissue Disease and Anti-Nuclear Antibodies. Excerpta Medica, New York, 1987

423. Saulsbury FT, Kesler RW, Kennaugh JM et al: Overlap syndrome of juvenile rheumatoid arthritis and systemic lupus erythematosus. J Rheumatol 9:610, 1982

424. Sherry DD, Kredich DW: Transient thrombocytopenia in systemic onset juvenile rheumatoid arthritis. Pediatrics 76:600, 1985

425. Estes D, Larson DL: Systemic lupus erythematosus and pregnancy. Clin Obstet Gynecol 8:307, 1965

426. Cecere FA, Persellin RH: The interaction of pregnancy and the rheumatic diseases. Clin Rheum Dis 7:747, 1981

427. Varner MW, Meehan RT, Syrop CH et al: Pregnancy in patients with systemic lupus erythematosus. Am J Obstet Gynecol 145:1025, 1983

428. Mintz G, Miz J, Gutierrez G et al: Prospective study of pregnancy in systemic lupus erythematosus. Results of a multidisciplinary approach. J Rheumatol 13:732, 1986

429. Fraga A, Mintz G, Orozco J et al: Sterility and fertility rates, fetal wastage and maternal morbidity in systemic lupus erythematosus. J Rheumatol 1:293, 1974

430. Zurier R: SLE and motherhood (editorial). J Rheumatol 7:591, 1980

431. Bear R: Pregnancy and lupus nephritis. A detailed report of six cases with a review of the literature. Obstet Gynecol 47:715, 1976

432. Tozman ECS, Urowitz MB, Gladman DD: Systemic lupus erythematosus and pregnancy. J Rheumatol 7:624, 1980

433. Zulman JI, Talal N, Hoffman GS et al: Problems associated with the management of pregnancies in patients with systemic lupus erythematosus. J Rheumatol 7:37, 1980

434. Gimovsky ML, Montoro M, Paul RH: Pregnancy outcome in women with systemic lupus erythematosus. Obstet Gynecol 63:686, 1984

435. Imbasciati E, Surian M, Bottino S et al: Lupus nephropathy and pregnancy. A study of 26 pregnancies in patients with systemic lupus erythematosus and nephritis. Nephron 36:46, 1984

436. Singsen BH, Akhter JE, Weinstein MM et al: Congenital complete heart block and SSA antibodies: obstetric implications. Am J Obstet Gynecol 512:655, 1985

437. Ramsey-Goldman R, Hom D, Deng JS et al: Anti-SS-A antibodies and fetal outcome in maternal systemic lupus erythematosus. Arthritis Rheum 29:1269, 1986

438. Lockshin MD, Druzin ML, Goei S et al: Antibody to cardiolipin as a predictor of fetal distress or death in pregnant patients with systemic lupus erythematosus. N Engl J Med 313:152, 1985

439. Bridge RG, Foley FE: Placental transfer of the lupus erythematosus factor. Am J Med Sci 227:1, 1954

440. Vonderheid EC, Koblenzer PJ, Ming PM et al: Neonatal lupus erythematosus. Report of four cases with review of the literature. Arch Dermatol 112:698, 1976

441. Schaller JG: Lupus phenomena in the newborn. Arthritis Rheum 20:312, 1977

442. Lane AT, Watson RM: Neonatal lupus erythematosus. Am J Dis Child 138:663, 1984

443. Kephart DC, Hood AF, Provost TT: Neonatal lupus erythematosus: new serologic findings. J Invest Dermatol 77:331, 1981

444. Watson RM, Lane AT, Barnett NK et al: Neonatal lupus erythematosus. A clinical, serological and immunogenetic study with review of the literature. Medicine 63:362, 1984

445. Gross KR, Lum VK, Petty RE et al: Maternal auto-

antibodies and fetal disease. Arthritis Rheum 30:S105, 1987

446. McCuistion CH, Schoch EP: Possible discoid lupus erythematosus in a newborn infant. Arch Dermatol Syphil 70:782, 1954

447. Epstein HC, Litt JZ: Discoid lupus erythematosus in a newborn infant. N Engl J Med 265:1106, 1961

448. Jackson R: Discoid lupus in a newborn infant of a mother with lupus erythematosus. Pediatrics 33:425, 1964

449. Reed WB, May SB, Tuffanelli DL: Discoid lupus erythematosus in a newborn. Arch Dermatol 96:64, 1967

450. Chameides L, Truex RC, Vetter V et al: Association of maternal systemic lupus erythematosus with congenital complete heart block. N Engl J Med 297:1204, 1977

451. McCue CM, Mantakos ME, Tinglestad JB et al: Congenital heart block in newborns of mothers with connective tissue disease. Circulation 56:82, 1977

452. Winkler RB, Nora AH, Nora JJ: Familial congenital complete heart block and maternal systemic lupus erythematosus. Circulation 56:1103, 1977

453. Hardy JD, Solomon S, Banwell GS et al: Congenital complete heart block in the newborn associated with maternal systemic lupus erythematosus and other connective tissue disorders. Arch Dis Child 54:7, 1979

454. Esscher E, Scott JS: Congenital heart block and maternal systemic lupus erythematosus. Br Med J 1:1235, 1979

455. Waterworth RF: Systemic lupus erythematosus occurring with congenital complete heart block. NZ Med J 92:311, 1980

456. Stephensen O, Cleland WP, Hallidie-Smith K: Congenital complete heart block and persistent ductus arteriosus associated with maternal systemic lupus erythematosus. Br Heart J 46:104, 1981

457. Lanham JG, Walport MJ, Hughes GRV: Congenital heart block and familial connective tissue disease. J Rheumatol 10:823, 1983

458. Litsey SE, Noonan JA, O'Connor WN et al: Maternal connective tissue disease and congenital heart block. Demonstration of immunoglobulin in cardiac tissue. N Engl J Med 312:98, 1985

459. Houssiau FA, Lebacq EG: Neonatal lupus erythematosus with congenital heart block associated with maternal systemic lupus erythematosus. Clin Rheumatol 5:505, 1986

460. Hogg GR: Congenital, acute lupus erythematosus associated with subendocardial fibroelastosis: report of a case. Am J Clin Pathol 28:648, 1957

461. Hull D, Binns BAO, Joyce D: Congenital heart block and widespread fibrosis due to maternal lupus erythematosus. Arch Dis Child 41:688, 1966

462. Laxer RM, Roberts EA, Cutz E et al: Cholestatic jaundice and hepatitis in neonatal lupus erythematosus. Arthritis Rheum 30:S81, 1987

463. Franco HL, Weston WL, Peebles C: Autoantibodies directed against sicca syndrome antigens in the neonatal lupus syndrome. J Am Acad Dermatol 4:67, 1981

464. Reed BR, Lee LA, Harmon C et al: Autoantibodies to SS-A/Ro in infants with congenital heart block. J Pediatr 103:889, 1983

465. Lin RY, Cohen-Addad N, Krey PR et al: Neonatal lupus erythematosus, multiple thromboses, and monoarthritis in a family with Ro antibody. J Am Acad Dermatol 12:1022, 1985

466. Jordan SC, Lemire JM, Border W et al: False-negative anti-DNA antibody activity in infantile systemic lupus erythematosus (SLE). J Clin Immunol 4:156, 1984

467. Provost TT, Watson R, Gammon WR et al: The neonatal lupus syndrome associated with U1RNP (nRNP) antibodies. N Engl J Med 316:1135, 1987

468. Scott JS, Maddison RJ, Taylor PV et al: Connective tissue disease, antibodies to ribonucleoprotein and congenital heart block. N Engl J Med 309:209, 1983

469. Lee LA, Lillis PJ, Fritz KA et al: Neonatal lupus syndrome in successive pregnancies. J Am Acad Dermatol 9:401, 1983

470. Buyon J, Roubey R, Swersky S et al: Complete congenital heart block: risk of occurrence and therapeutic approach to prevention. J Rheumatol 15:1104, 1988

471. Taylor PV, Scott JS, Gerlis LM et al: Maternal autoantibodies against fetal cardiac antigens in congenital complete heart block. N Engl J Med 315:667, 1986

472. Fox RJ, Jr, McCuistion CH, Schoch EP, Jr: Systemic lupus erythematosus. Association with previous neonatal lupus erythematosus. Arch Dermatol 115:340, 1979

473. Callen JP, Fowler JF, Kulick KB et al: Neonatal lupus erythematosus occurring in one fraternal twin. Serologic and immunogenetic studies. Arthritis Rheum 28:271, 1985

474. Moutsopoulos HM, Klippel JH, Pavlidis N et al: Correlative histologic and serologic findings of sicca syndrome in patients with systemic lupus erythematosus. Arthritis Rheum 23:36, 1980

475. Bernstein B, Koster-King K, Singsen B et al: Sjögren's syndrome in childhood. Arthritis Rheum 20:361, 1977

476. Krause A, Alarcón-Segovia D: Primary juvenile Sjögren's syndrome. J Rheumatol 15:803, 1988

477. Palcoux JB, Janin-Mercier A, Campagne D et al: Sjögren syndrome and lupus erythematosus nephritis. Arch Dis Child 59:175, 1984

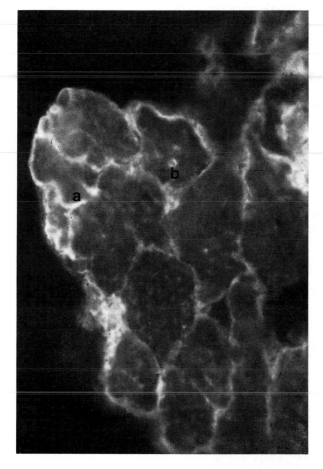

Fig. 8-32 Immunoglobulin deposition around the peri-mysium of myofibers, *a*, and the wall of a small blood vessel, *b*. Cryostat section of muscle reacted with fluorescein conjugated anti-IgG (225×).

in the lesions.[26] Diffuse linear and occasionally granular vascular wall deposits of IgM, C3d, and fibrin were also observed in the areas of noninflammatory vasculopathy. Electron microscopy, however, has revealed no evidence of subendothelial deposition of immunoglobulins within the vessel walls as might have been expected in classic immune complex disease, although circulating complexes and anti-complementary activity are often present in the blood.[75,161]

Veins

In the veins intramural and perivascular mono-nuclear cell inflammatory infiltrates are seen frequently and may or may not be associated with immunoglobulin deposition.[26,71] The endothelial cells frequently contain inclusions.

CONNECTIVE TISSUES

It is not known whether the connective tissues or collagen are directly involved in the pathogenesis of JDM. In human muscle, types I and III collagens are found in the endomysium and perimysium, although the endomysium predominantly contains type I collagen.[162,163] Basement membranes contain type IV collagen, and type V collagen is found in the small blood vessels and endomysium. The synthesis of collagen appears to be excessive in myositis.

Skin

A capillary endothelial change similar to that seen in muscle is almost always present in involved skin.[26] Biopsy specimens from the skin of patients with dermatomyositis may show epidermal atrophy, liquefaction degeneration of the basal cells, vascular dilatation, and lymphocytic infiltration of the dermis.[164] An increase in acid mucopolysaccharides has been found in both involved and uninvolved skin in approximately one-third of the patients.[165] Tubular inclusions may be seen also in epidermal cells. In a study of the histopathology of Gottron papules,[166] basal layer vasculopathy, periodic acid-schiff-(PAS) positive basement membrane thickening, upper dermal mucin deposition, and a diffuse upper dermal mononuclear infiltrate were frequent. Epidermal hyperplasia consisting of acanthosis or papillomatosis was often present. Epidermal atrophy was rare.

In the healing phase of the disease, calcium salts, hydroxyapatite or fluorapatite,[167,168] may be found in the skin and subcutaneous tissues as well as in the interfascial planes of the muscle (Figs. 8-16 to 8-23). With calcinosis, there may be persistence of fibrosis as well as some degree of round cell and giant cell infiltration. Mechanisms for the excessive accumulation of hydroxyapatite are unknown.[75]

Gastrointestinal Tract

Ulceration or perforation resulting from vasculopathy can occur in any part of the GI tract including the esophagus.[26,106] Serious disease of this type develops in approximately 10 percent of patients.[75] Pneumatosis intestinalis has been described in JDM.[125,126] Except for the vascular disease, smooth muscle is not generally a site of involvement.[169]

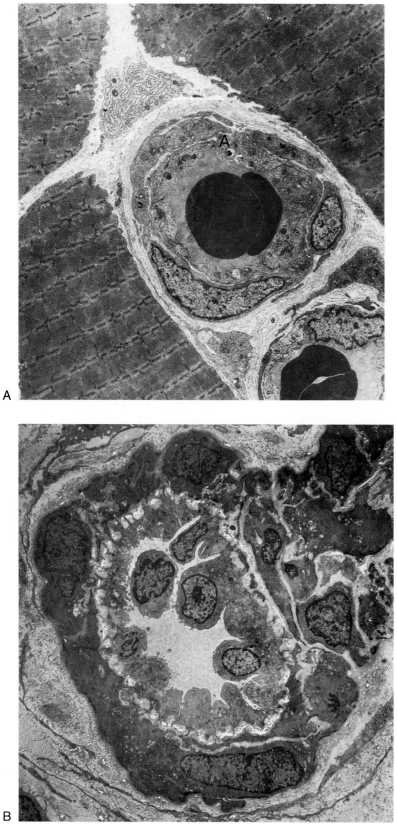

Fig. 8-33 Electron microscopic section of muscle from case in Figure 8-31. (**A**) Slight degree of endothelial cell swelling, *A*, in an arteriole (63,337×). (**B**) More marked endarteropathy (5,200×). *Figure Continues.*

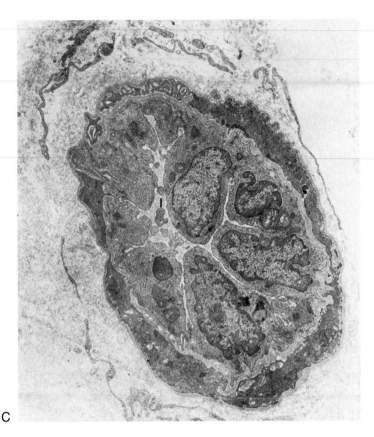

Fig. 8-33 (*Continued*). (**C**) Virtual occlusion of the lumen, *l*, of a small arteriole by extreme swelling of the endothelial cells (10,968×). Thrombosis and inflammation are not present. (Courtesy of Dr. George McClellan.)

C

Heart

Cardiac muscle is seldom clinically affected by the primary pathologic process.[169,170] A few cases of carditis have been described with areas of focal myocardial fibrosis and contraction-band necrosis. Interstitial myocarditis and narrowing of the coronary arteries have been reported.[26]

Kidneys

Although renal abnormalities have been occasionally noted in JDM, they appear to be rare.[11,106] However, in one report, histopathologic findings in five of six renal biopsies were abnormal.[11] The changes that were described included cellular hyperplasia, capillary thickening, capsular adhesions, and hyperplasia involving the small blood vessels. Renal abnormalities have not been common in postmortem reports.[17,26,130]

DIFFERENTIAL DIAGNOSIS

The differential diagnosis of JDM includes postviral myositis, primary myopathies, and inflammatory myositis accompanying another connective-tissue disease. In the presence of the characteristic skin rash and weak, painful, or tender proximal muscles, the correct diagnosis is quite straightforward. Early in the disease course, especially in the absence of the characteristic rash, the differential diagnosis becomes more difficult.

Postinfectious Myositis

Acute transient myositis follows certain viral infections, especially influenza A and B,[31,46,47] and coxsackievirus B.[43,55] Although myalgia is a characteristic complaint of acute influenza, myositis per se is rare (Table 8-10). In the 1957 series of Lund-

Table 8-10 Acute Myositis Associated with Influenza B Infection

Onset during recovery phase of the viral illness
Predominant severe bilateral pain and tenderness of the gastrocnemius and soleus muscles
Elevated serum muscle enzyme concentrations (CK, AST)
Recovery in 3 to 5 days

berg,[45] a contagious illness characterized by fever, headache, rhinitis, cough, nausea, and vomiting that lasted 2 to 3 days was followed by severe proximal calf pain (myalgia cruris epidemica). This was accompanied by circumscribed muscle tenderness that was exacerbated by movement. Complete recovery occurred after approximately 3 days. Laboratory studies revealed a slightly elevated erythrocyte sedimentation rate (ESR) and moderate leukopenia with relative lymphocytosis. Onset was most common in preadolescent boys. Although no specific infectious agent was identified in this classic study, subsequent reports have pointed to influenza B as the most common causative agent.[46] These studies have shown concomitant elevation of the serum levels of creatine kinase (CK) and aspartate aminotransferase (AST). Recognition of the correct diagnosis of these cases during influenza epidemics is important as treatment is supportive and not specific.

Coxsackievirus B can cause epidemic pleurodynia (Bornholm disease) characterized by fever and sharp pain in the muscles of the chest and abdominal wall.[171] This syndrome is sometimes preceded by a moderate to severe headache, nausea, vomiting, and pharyngitis. The illness is most common in children and adolescents and usually lasts for 3 to 5 days. Treatment is supportive.

Other infectious causes of myositis, including trichinosis, schistosomiasis, trypanosomiasis, toxoplasmosis, and staphylococcal bacteremia, should be sought.[172,173] Toxoplasmosis may be associated with a syndrome that looks very much like dermatomyositis.[36,38,173]

Trichinosis is caused by ingestion of the larval cyst of the nematoid *Trichinella spiralis* in inadequately cooked meat.[171] Initially fever, diarrhea, and abdominal pain are present; after 1 week swelling and tenderness of muscles and periorbital edema follow. The muscles of the face, neck, and chest are most frequently affected. Peripheral blood eosinophilia is often striking, and biopsy of the affected muscles shows the larvae, and later, calcified cysts. Treatment includes use of the corticosteroid drugs to diminish inflammation and agents such as thiabendazole.

Pyomyositis is an abscess of skeletal muscle most frequently caused by staphylococci after local muscle injury.[174] It occurs at all ages but is more common in boys than girls. Lesions may be solitary or multiple and are usually located in the thigh, calf, buttock, arm, scapular areas, or chest wall. The abscess is tender and, if not too deep, warm. Low-grade fever is usually present. The symptoms last for a few days to a week and, if associated with the lower extremity, may cause a limp. Ultrasonography or gallium 67 citrate scanning helps in localizing the lesion. Severe pustular acne may occasionally be associated with inflammatory disease of muscle (as well as arthritis).[175]

Neuromuscular Diseases and the Myopathies

In the absence of characteristic skin changes, the differential diagnosis of JDM includes a wide variety of neuromuscular disorders in children (Table 8-11)[111,176] (see Appendix). The clinician should consider the type of onset of the disease, the site of muscle involvement (proximal, distal, or combined), and the age of the patient at onset of the illness (Tables 8-12 to 8-14).

The possibility of muscular dystrophy is suggested by a positive family history, along with an insidious onset and a selective, slowly progressive pattern of muscle weakness. Constitutional signs, muscle tenderness, and cutaneous abnormalities are absent. In Duchenne type muscular dystrophy, there is characteristic hypertrophy of the calves along with markedly elevated CK levels in both the child and the mother. Enlargement of muscle groups may be seen in JDM, although this change is not common.[27] Familial inflammatory myopathy has been commented upon and is very rare. The other congenital myopathies, myotonias, and hypotonic syndromes and the metabolic and endocrine myopathies must also be considered. Paroxysmal myoglobinuria may occasionally be encountered. Certain drugs or toxins, including alcohol, clofibrate, penicillamine, corticosteroids, and hydroxychloroquine, can cause a myopathy.[177,178]

Metabolic myopathies such as phosphorylase deficiency can be confused with inflammatory myositis. The metabolic myopathies, including glycogen-storage disease and familial periodic (hypo- or hyperkalemic) paralysis, are distinguishable by appropriate biochemical testing and tissue analysis. McArdle syndrome is a chronic, inherited disease of muscle characterized by weakness and stiffness exacerbated by exercise. In this condition there is a phosphorylase block restricted to muscle; patients are unable to degrade glycogen to lactic acid during exercise.

Table 8-11 Classification of the Major Neuromuscular Disorders of Infancy and Childhood

I. Primary myopathies
  A. The muscular dystrophies
    1. Sex-linked recessive
      a. Duchenne's type muscular dystrophy
      b. Becker's muscular dystrophy
      c. Variants (Mabry, Emery types)
    2. Autosomal dominant
      a. Fascioscapulohumeral (Dejerine-Landouzy)
      b. Distal myopathy (Welander's)
      c. Ocular myopathy
      d. Oculopharyngeal muscular dystrophy
    3. Autosomal recessive
      a. Limb-girdle (Erb's)
  B. Congenital myopathies
    1. Congenital muscular dystrophy
      a. Arthrogryposis multiplex congenita (myopathic form)
    2. Benign congenital myopathy
    3. Central core disease
    4. Nemaline myopathy
    5. Myotubular myopathy
  C. Myotonic disorders
    1. Myotonia congenita (Thomsen's disease)
    2. Dystrophia myotonia (Steinert's disease)
  D. Metabolic disorders
    1. Glycogen storage disease
      a. Type II: acid maltase deficiency (Pompe's disease)
      b. Type III: amylo-1,6-glucosidase deficiency (debrancher enzyme)
      c. Type IV: amylo-(1,4 → 1,6)transglucosidase deficiency (brancher enzyme) (Anderson)
      d. Type V: phosphorylase deficiency (McArdle syndrome)
      e. Type VII: phosphofructokinase deficiency (Tarui)
    2. Familial periodic paralysis
      a. Hyperkalemic
      b. Hypokalemic
      c. Normokalemic (Poskanzer and Karr)
    3. Carnitine deficiency
    4. Carnitine palmityl-transferase deficiency
    5. Secondary to endocrinopathies
      a. Addison's disease
      b. Cushing's syndrome
      c. Hypopituitarism
      d. Hypothyroidism
    6. Myoadenylate deaminase deficiency
    7. Chronic hemodialysis
  E. Inflammatory disease
    1. Postinfectious
      a. Viral syndromes
          Influenza B
          Coxsackievirus B
          Echovirus
          Poliomyelitis
      b. Toxoplasmosis, sarcosporidiosis
      c. Trichinosis, cysticercosis
      d. Septic (staphylococci and other pyogenic organisms)
      e. Tetanus
      f. Gas gangrene
    2. Connective-tissue disease
      a. Juvenile rheumatoid arthritis
      b. Dermatomyositis
      c. Systemic lupus erythematosus
      d. Scleroderma
      e. Polyarteritis
  F. Genetic abnormalities
    1. Osteogenesis imperfecta
    2. Ehlers-Danlos syndrome
    3. Mucopolysaccharidoses
  G. Trauma
    1. Physical
      a. Crush syndrome
      b. Exhaustive physical exertion (rhabdomyolysis)
    2. Toxic
      a. Snakebite
    3. Drugs
      a. Corticosteroids
      b. Hydroxychloroquine
      c. Diuretics, licorice
      d. Amphotericin B
      e. Alcohol
      f. Vincristine
      g. D-Penicillamine
      i. Cimetidine
II. Neurogenic atrophies
  A. Spinal muscular and anterior horn-cell dysfunction
    1. Infantile and juvenile muscle atrophy
      a. Type I: Acute infantile (Werdnig-Hoffman atrophy)
      b. Type II: Infantile spinal muscular atrophy, chronic variant
      c. Type III: Juvenile spinal muscular atrophy (Kugelberg-Welander disease)
    2. Arthrogryposis multiplex congenita
    3. Amyotrophic lateral sclerosis
  B. Peripheral nerve dysfunction
    1. Peroneal muscular atrophy (Charcot-Marie-Tooth disease)
    2. Neurofibromatosis
    3. Acute infectious polyneuritis (Guillain-Barré syndrome)
  C. Disorders of neuromuscular transmission
    1. Congenital myasthenia gravis
    2. Botulism
    3. Tick paralysis
    4. Organophosphate poisoning

(Adapted from The Research Group On Neuromuscular Diseases,[176] with permission.)

Table 8-12 Classification of Neuromuscular Disorders by Disease Course

Acute course
  Muscular dystrophy (Duchenne's type)
  Alcoholic polymyopathy
  Paroxysmal myoglobinuria

Chronic course
  Dermatomyositis
  Muscular dystrophy (Dejerine-Landouzy dystrophy)
  Congenital hypotonia
  Central core disease and nemaline myopathy
  Glycogen storage disease
  Myoadenylate deaminase deficiency
  Endocrine myopathy
  Nutritional myopathy
  Amyloidosis

Episodic course
  Paramyotonia congenita
  Familial periodic paralysis
  Hypokalemia
  Myasthenia gravis
  Myasthenia of malignancy

(Adapted from Cassidy,[249] with permission.)

Table 8-13 Classification of Neuromuscular Disorders by Site of Muscle Involvement

Proximal muscles
  Dermatomyositis
  Muscular dystrophy
  Thyrotoxic myopathy
  Sarcoid myopathy
  Proximal familial neuromuscular diseases
  Steroid myopathy

Distal muscles
  Myotonic dystrophy
  Distal muscular dystrophy
  Peroneal muscular atrophy
  Motor system diseases

Proximal or distal distribution
  Floppy infant syndrome
  Myotonia congenita
  Dystrophic ophthalmoplegia
  Periodic paralysis
  Myasthenia gravis

(Adapted from Cassidy,[249] with permission.)

Muscular underdevelopment and hypotonia are frequent in Marfan's syndrome.[179] These features may be so prominent as to suggest a primary disorder of muscle. The muscle cell is normal, however, and the presentation is probably secondary to abnormalities of bones, joints, or perimysial connective tissue.

Myoadenylate deaminase deficiency (MDD) was first described in 1978 by Fishbein (Table 8-15).[180] This disorder presents in a primary form that is presumably autosomal recessive and as an acquired disease associated with rheumatic and neuromuscular disorders. Current data suggest that MDD is relatively common in that 2 percent of muscle biopsies have been found to be deficient in enzyme activity (<2 percent in primary, <15 percent in secondary). The male-to-female ratio is approximately 2 to 1. Muscle fatigue, stiffness, and cramping after exercise are noted, beginning in childhood (23 percent) or adolescence (26 percent). Patients with MDD have a decreased muscle mass, hypotonia, and weakness. There may be a mild elevation of the serum CK concentration. With forearm exercise there is a failure of plasma ammonia to rise along with inosine monophosphate. Electromyography (EMG) findings are nonspecific. The muscle biopsy specimen in the primary cases is normal except for absence of adenosine monophosphate (AMP) deaminase (EC3.5.4.6). Enzyme activity is normal in other tissues.

Endocrinopathies, especially hyper- and hypothyroidism, hyper- and hypoparathyroidism, diabetes mellitus, and the myopathy associated with Cushing's syndrome, should be carefully considered and eliminated.[181] Myasthenia gravis can occur in children but is rare. The diagnosis of this disease is suggested by a decremental response to repetitive nerve stimulation or activity, involvement of ocular and distal muscles, and improvement of the weakness after administration of cholinergic drugs.

Any evidence of neurologic disease should be sought and appropriate studies performed to document signs of involvement of the central or peripheral system. The neurogenic atrophies include infantile and juvenile spinal muscular atrophy, benign congenital hypotonia, and peroneal atrophy. Proximal muscle weakness is seen in all of these entities. The age at onset, course and progression of the disease, and lack of association with either cutaneous abnormalities or constitutional symptoms suggest the correct diagnosis. Sensory changes or the presence of long-tract signs on the physical examination, de-

Table 8-14 Classification of Neuromuscular Disorders by Age of Patients at Onset

Congenital
    Congenital muscular dystrophy
    Central core disease
    Nemaline myopathy
    Congenital hypoplasia
    Benign hypotonia

Childhood
    Muscular dystrophy (Duchenne)
    Glycogen storage diseases
    Myoadenylate deaminase deficiency

Late childhood and adolescence
    Muscular dystrophy (Dejerine-Landouzy)
    Myotonia congenita
    Periodic paralysis

Onset at any age
    Dermatomyositis
    Trichinosis
    Myasthenia gravis
    Steroid and hydroxchloroquine myopathies

(Adapted from Cassidy,[249] with permission.)

Table 8-15 Myoadenylate Deaminase Deficiency

Male:female ratio   2:1
Muscle fatigue, stiffness, or cramping after exercise
Decreased muscle mass, hypotonia, and weakness, often since childhood
Mild elevation of serum creatine kinase concentration
Failure of plasma ammonia to rise with forearm exercise
Nonspecific electromyographic abnormalities
Frequently normal muscle biopsy histopathology except absent adenylate deaminase
Autosomal recessive (?); acquired (associated with rheumatic and neuromuscular disorders)

creased nerve conduction times or fasciculation on EMG, or fiber-type grouping and atrophy on the muscle biopsy would be confirmatory of neurogenic atrophy. The serum levels of muscle enzymes, including the CK, can be elevated in these diseases.[182,183] The acute phase reactants are usually normal.

Myositis with Other Connective-Tissue Diseases

It is not likely that JRA or one of the seronegative spondyloarthropathies will be a source of diagnostic confusion, but children with SLE may have similar constitutional symptoms and signs to those with early JDM (Ch. 7). The child with JDM may have a malar flush similar in distribution to the butterfly rash of SLE, but often lacking the relatively well defined borders and extension to the forehead. Furthermore, one does not expect to encounter in children with SLE the degree of upper eyelid suffusion and periorbital edema of JDM. Although isolated cutaneous lesions may occur, children with SLE do not have the fully developed erythematous rash over the extensor surfaces of the elbows and knees and the dorsal surfaces of the small joints of the hands. Systemic features of

SLE such as pericarditis and pleural effusions are rare in JDM. The arthritis of JDM is both uncommon and mild; that of SLE is much more frequent and, although nonerosive, may be quite florid at onset and extremely painful. Laboratory evaluation shows normal or slightly elevated serum levels of the muscle enzymes in SLE (presumably on the basis of vasculitic involvement of the muscle), compared to marked elevations in JDM. This difference alone is usually sufficient to differentiate these two diseases.

Occasionally an overlap syndrome[184] between JDM and JRA occurs. Although rare, it was present in two children whom we have seen. One girl appeared to have the simultaneous onset of both diseases accompanied by subcutaneous rheumatoid nodules. Eosinophilic fasciitis and mixed connective-tissue diseases are distinctive syndromes within this category (Ch. 10).[185,186] A steroid-responsive myositis, differentiated from dermatomyositis by absence of vasculopathy on muscle biopsy, is seen in infancy.[187]

Scleroderma, on the other hand, poses unique diagnostic problems in that approximately 20 percent of children with this disorder may present with a primary myositis not unlike that seen in JDM. Although early cutaneous abnormalities of scleroderma and JDM are quite different, during the courses of these diseases the skin changes tend to merge in character.

Muscle abnormalities in uncomplicated JRA, rheumatic fever, SLE, or scleroderma include focal accumulations of lymphocytes, patchy fiber atrophy, and increased interstitial connective tissue.[188-190] Perifascicular atrophy has been described in SLE.[191] In Sjögren's syndrome, muscle fiber degeneration and atrophy, sarcoplasmic degeneration, and microcyst formation have been noted.[192] In polyarteritis, a necrotizing vasculitis with muscle-fiber degeneration may be seen along with areas of neurogenic atrophy.

Miscellaneous Disorders

A number of rare forms of myositis have been described in adults, including inclusion body myositis,[193] eosinophilic myositis,[194] and disease restricted to one muscle group or extremity such as localized nodular myositis[195,196] and proliferative myositis.[197] Reducing body myopathy has been reported, however, in a number of children.[198,199] It begins in early childhood; pursues a relentless, severe course; and results in death in months to a few years after onset.

The exclusions should also include the myositis occasionally observed in multicentric reticulohistiocytosis[200] and giant cell myositis.[201] In sarcoidosis, there should be biopsy evidence of a granulomatous myositis.[202] Poliomyelitis and the Guillain-Barré syndrome are other diagnostic possibilities.

Rhabdomyolysis may follow an upper respiratory infection, trauma, or extreme muscular exertion.[203] Onset is generally acute and characterized by profound weakness, myoglobinuria, and occasionally oliguria and renal failure. It may also be seen after a snakebite, in heatstroke, and in the familial malignant hyperpyrexia syndrome.

Myositis ossificans progressiva, a rare, sporadic disorder sometimes referred to as fibrodysplasia ossificans progressiva, results in inflammatory, painful swelling of muscle and fascia, followed by fibrosis and calcification.[204,205] The child may present with a spontaneous joint contracture. The clinical diagnosis is often elusive until calcification (and, later, ossification) appears on the radiograph. Biopsy findings of affected sites at an early stage may be misleading and may be interpreted as a malignant sarcoma.

Boys are affected more often than girls, with onset usually within the childhood period. The back of the neck and posterior trunk are often involved initially, followed by the muscles of the limbs. Palmar and plantar fascia may be affected as well. The great toes are often congenitally short, and the thumbs are sometimes involved. The disease appears as exacerbations and remissions and is slowly progressive to severe debilitation and immobility. All attempts at treatment have failed (Fig. 8-34).

LABORATORY EXAMINATION AND DIAGNOSTIC STUDIES

Routine laboratory studies are of little diagnostic help in the child with JDM. Nonspecific tests of inflammation such as the ESR and C-reactive protein (CRP) level tend to correlate with the degree of clinical inflammation or be of no clinical usefulness (except in helping to differentiate JDM from the non-inflammatory myopathies).[206,207] Leukocytosis and anemia are uncommon at onset except in the child with associated GI bleeding. Urinalysis is usually normal although a few children have microscopic hematuria.[11]

There are no specific abnormalities of immunoglobulin levels,[206,208] although a dermatomyositislike disease has been observed in children with agammaglobulinemia and common variable immune deficiency (Ch. 11).[209–211]

Myoglobin, a normal constituent of cardiac and skeletal muscle with a molecular weight of approximately 17,000, is increased in serum in approximately 50 percent of patients with inflammatory myositis.[212–214] This elevation does not always correlate with an increase in CK serum levels. Antibodies to myoglobin are found in 70 percent of patients and may interfere with its quantitation.[215] Studies by Dickerson and Widdowson[216] and Hallgren et al.[217] have estimated that a normal adult with 30 kg of muscle mass would release 0.3 mg of myoglobin per day. Although myoglobin is much more renotoxic than hemoglobin, myoglobinuria seldom reaches levels that are associated with renal damage.

Autoantibodies

Children with JDM are almost always rheumatoid factor (RF) seronegative. Antinuclear antibodies (ANAs) have been reported in a variable frequency of 10 to 50 percent.[13,15,28,218] Specific ANAs have been described in dermatomyositis and polymyositis (Table 8-16). Particularly important are ANAs directed against one of a number of extractable nuclear antigens that are soluble in saline at neutral or acid pH. Antibodies reactive with PM-1 antigens are found in up to 60 percent of adults with polymyositis,[219] but only a minority of children.[75] The PM-1 antibody was found in 4 of 18 patients in Pachman's series,[75,220–222] and in 3 of 21 in the series by Crowe et al.[26] Other specificities described in adults include the Jo-1 antigens,[223] Mi antigens,[244,225] and Ku antigen.[226] Antibodies to other known nuclear antigens including double-stranded deoxyribonucleic acid (DNA) and Sm are absent, and serum complement determinations are normal.[227–229]

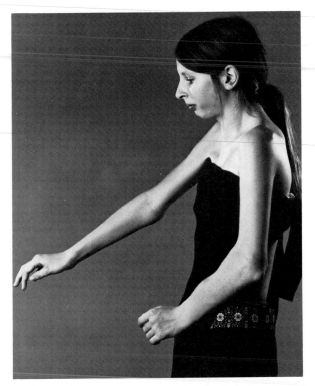

Fig. 8-34 Myositis ossificans progressiva. This young girl presented with an extension contracture of the left wrist and later developed the diagnostic features of this disorder. In this photograph the fixed deformity is visible, along with tumorous ossification of the forearm and a fixed contracture of the elbow. The movement of the left shoulder is greatly restricted, and muscle atrophy around that joint is present. A receding chin and short thumbs are present and characteristic.

Half of the children show evidence of circulating immune complexes that may be involved in the pathogenesis of the vascular injury.[67,75,228] It is possible that they also interfere with the accurate serologic detection of other antibodies and potential antigens.

The frequency of antibodies to myosin, muscle, and nuclei is the same for patients with inflammatory myopathy, the muscular dystrophies, or denervation atrophy.[227,230] Therefore these antibodies may be secondary to muscle damage rather than primary phenomena.

Specific Studies

The three most helpful laboratory abnormalities are elevated serum levels of the muscle enzymes, abnormal electromyographic changes, and specific his-

Table 8-16 Antibodies to Nuclear, Nucleolar, and Cytoplasmic Antigens in Dermatomyositis and Polymyositis in Adults

Name	Frequency	Antigenic Specificity
PM-1	PM/DM 65%, PM/scleroderma 85%	Acidic nuclear protein
Ku	PM/scleroderma (55%) and SLE overlap	Acidic nuclear protein
Mi-1	PM/DM (10%)	Nuclear nonhistone basic protein
Mi-2	PM/DM (5%)	Nuclear proteins
PM-Scl	PM/DM/scleroderma (8%)	Nucleolar proteins
Jo-1	PM (15–30%)	Histidyl-tRNA synthetase
PL-7	PM/DM (3%)	Threonyl-tRNA synthetase
PL-12	Rare	Alanyl-tRNA synthetase
tRNA	Rare	Transfer RNA

Table 8-17 Specific Diagnostic Studies at Onset of Dermatomyositis in Children

Study	Percentage
Elevation of serum levels of the muscle enzymes	90–98
Aspartate aminotransferase	87
Creatine kinase	85
Aldolase	65
Lactic dehydrogenase	64
Abnormal electromyography	93–96
Abnormal muscle biopsy (inflammation)	79

topathologic abnormalities on muscle biopsy (Table 8-17).

SERUM MUSCLE ENZYMES

The serum muscle enzymes are important for diagnosis and for monitoring the effectiveness of therapy. Some individual variation in the pattern of enzyme elevation is observed in JDM; it is recommended, therefore, at least early in the disease, that CK, AST, and aldolase be measured in order to provide a reliable base-line evaluation (Table 8-17). The height of the increase in serum concentration is variable but ranges from 20 to 40 times normal for the CK or AST. Regenerating skeletal muscle releases the MB isozyme of CK.[231] Therefore, in muscle inflammation, there may be a persistent elevation of the MB band in contrast to the transient increase observed in myocardial infarction.

Rarely, children are seen who have no increase in the serum level of CK during the acute phase of the disease, and other children are also encountered who have a persistent elevation of this enzyme late in the course of the disease without any other clinical indication of muscle inflammation. In the latter instance, evaluation of serum CK levels in family members may reveal an unrelated, but unsuspected, genetic abnormality. In addition to abnormalities of enzyme concentrations, the age-related urinary creatine/creatinine ratio is increased.[206]

Lactic dehydrogenase (LDH) and alanine aminotransferase (ALT) are elevated in many children with JDM but are relatively less specific. Serum levels of all muscle enzymes usually decrease 3 to 4 weeks before improvement in muscle strength and rise 5 to 6 weeks before clinical relapse. Occasionally they remain entirely within the normal range in spite of active myositis, especially later in the course of the disease.

It should be noted that serum levels of all of these enzymes are increased in a wide variety of other diseases. Serum CK is elevated in many cases of muscle injury, motor neuron diseases, vasculitis, metabolic disorders, endocrinopathies, toxic reactions, and infections. Extreme elevations are most commonly associated with JDM and, to a somewhat lesser extent, with muscular dystrophy.

Creatine Kinase

Creatine kinase catalyzes the transfer of a phosphoryl group from creatine phosphate to adenosine diphosphate (ADP) in order to regenerate adenosine triphosphate (ATP) in the mitochondria of muscle, brain, and heart. The ATP available to muscle is sufficient to sustain contractile activity for only a fraction of a second.

In skeletal muscle, CK constitutes up to 20 percent of the soluble sarcoplasmic protein. Total CK activity is 225 to 12,000 units/g of muscle. CK is a dimeric molecule with two subunits: M(muscle) and B(brain). Both consist of 360 aminoacids with a molecular weight of 41 kD. Three isoenzymes exist. MM (CK-3) is found in muscle and myocardium; BB (CK-1)) in brain; and MB (CK-2) in myocardium and regenerating muscle. The adult pattern of isozymes is achieved by age 4 years.

Creatine kinase is released from inflamed or injured muscle cells. Abnormalities of the junctional sites between the T tubules and the sarcoplasmic reticulum in JDM may serve as the primary sites of leakage of the enzyme. These abnormal anastomoses are far more extensive in the perifascicular than in the centrofascicular myofibers. It is also evident that the serum levels of the muscle enzymes probably could not result from destruction of muscle tissue alone. These enzymes are not released in diseases in which there is generally no loss of sarcolemmal integrity (e.g., steroid myopathy and disuse atrophy).

Creatine is synthesized in the liver from arginine and glycine by an amidotransferase to form ornithine and guanidoacetic acid. The latter is transmethylated by interaction with S-adenosylmethionine to form creatine and S-adenosylhomocysteine. Creatine circulates in the plasma in relatively low concentrations of <0.6 mg/dl in adults. It is stored in muscle as creatine phosphate and serves as the reserve energy pool for muscular activity.

In muscle, creatine is converted to the anhydride creatinine at a constant rate of approximately 2 percent per day. Creatinine diffuses passively into the plasma and is excreted by the kidney. If the body pool of creatine decreases, the creatinine excretion per unit of time is also decreased. Therefore, endogenous creatinine excretion is an important laboratory index of body creatine stores and total muscle mass. Creatinuria in dermatomyositis is not simply a matter of failure of uptake by inflamed muscle or a decreased muscle mass, but rather a failure to maintain normal membrane permeability.

It is difficult to use the urinary creatine/creatinine ratio in children, as opposed to adults, as a laboratory guide to the activity of the inflammatory disease. As stated, creatinine excreted per 24 hours is an excellent indicator of intrinsic muscle mass in children between the ages of 3 and 18 years. Urinary creatinine in males increases from approximately 0.36 g/day at age 5 years to 1.6 g/day at age 17 years. Boys begin to excrete significantly larger amounts of creatinine than girls at puberty.

Creatine excretion, however, bears an inverse relationship to age and is much higher in the younger child. A 24-hour urine collection would have to show extremely large or infinitesimally small amounts of creatine before it could be judged to be abnormal in a child. After the age of 12 years the creatine/creatinine ratio is more reliable. The changes in creatine metabolism with age are suggestive of a slowly changing metabolic adjustment associated with normal growth and development. At no age in childhood is there a significant sex difference in the excretion of creatine.

Transaminases

AST (formerly SGOT) and ALT (formerly SGPT) are cytosolic and mitochondrial enzymes with a wide tissue distribution. AST has two dimeric isoenzymes; one in the cytosol and the other in the mitochondria. The half-life in human plasma is 47 hours for ALT, 6 hours for mitochondrial AST, and 12 to 17 hours for cytosolic AST. Plasma levels fall to the range of normal adult concentrations by one year of age.

Aldolase

Adolase (1,6-diphosphofructoaldolase) is found in myocardium, liver, cerebral cortex, kidneys, and erythrocytes, but is present in much higher concentrations in skeletal muscles. There are three cytosolic isoenzymes: aldolase A, which predominants in muscle, aldolase B in liver, and aldolase C in brain. It is aldolase A that is increased in the serum of children with active JDM. Aldolase is one of the principle glycolytic enzymes that catalyse the conversion of D-fructose-1,6-diphosphate to dihydroxyacetone phosphate and D-glyceraldehyde-3-phosphate.

Lactic Dehydrogenase

Lactic dehydrogenase is abundant in myocardium and skeletal muscle. There are five isoenzymes: I (30 percent), II (40 percent), III (20 percent), IV (6 percent), and V (4 percent). In acute adult polymyositis there is relatively less I and relatively more II, III, IV, and V. In chronic disease, only I and II are disproportionately elevated. In contrast, patients with active muscular dystrophy exhibit an increase in isoenzymes I and II and a decrease in III, IV, and V, especially in the younger patient.

ELECTROMYOGRAPHY

Electromyography (EMG) is useful in confirming the diagnosis of JDM and in aiding in the selection of the best site for performing a muscle biopsy. EMG should be performed on one side of the body only so that the muscle biopsy, if necessary, can be performed on the opposite extremity without any artifact created by a needle puncture. The procedure may be troublesome in the young child and sedation is often necessary. An EMG is not mandatory and need not be done unless the diagnosis is in doubt.

The characteristic EMG changes are those of myopathy and denervation (Table 8-18). EMG findings are typical of those associated with membrane instability (increased insertional activity, fibrillations, and positive sharp waves) and random fiber destruction (decreased amplitude and duration of the action po-

tentials). The electrical changes in denervation probably result from segmental myonecrosis of the endplate, although the terminal axons may also be affected.[145] Reinnervation following the acute phase of the disease may occur.[232]

The value of EMG in identifying continuing inflammatory activity of the muscles during the course of JDM has not been adequately documented. Quantitative EMG may be more informative in this regard.[233–236] In following the course of the disease, increasing muscle strength correlates with less spontaneous activity and a decreasing proportion of high-frequency components. Early in the initial period of treatment, however, a temporary increase in high-frequency signals is expected. Nerve conduction velocities and latencies are normal in JDM unless severe muscle atrophy is present with a decrease in the number of muscle fibers in a motor unit and electrical irritability of the sarcolemmal membrane or terminal axonal fibers.

MUSCLE BIOPSY

A muscle biopsy is indicated in the initial assessment of a child if the diagnosis is in any way uncertain or if medicolegal support for instituting long-term corticosteroid therapy or immunosuppressive drugs is needed. A muscle biopsy performed for diagnostic reasons immediately documents the possibility of another disease and provides valuable prognostic information, based upon the studies of Banker et al.[106] and Crowe et al.[26]

The muscles to be biopsied, usually the deltoid or quadriceps, should be clinically involved as demonstrated by muscle testing or EMG, but not atrophied. Since muscle involvement in JDM is often spotty, a generous specimen should be obtained (for example, 2 to 3 cm). Care should be taken to prepare the specimen in accordance with the instructions of the pathologist.

Table 8-18 Electromyography in Juvenile Dermatomyositis

Myopathic motor units (decreased amplitude, short duration, polyphasic)

Denervation potentials (positive sharp waves), spontaneous fibrillations, and insertional activity

High-frequency repetitive discharges

Biopsy results are more likely to be negative if the biopsy is inadequate in size, obtained from an inappropriate muscle, or done late in the disease when the pathologic changes may no longer be specific. In an occasional child, there is no evidence of inflammatory changes on the muscle biopsy specimens even though characteristic abnormalities such as perifascicular atrophy are present.[140] Although an open biopsy is most often performed, needle biopsy may become more popular. The latter technique may be performed sequentially in selected children during the course of the disease if questions concerning appropriate therapeutic interventions arise.[139]

RADIOLOGIC CHANGES

Radionuclide scanning can detect early abnormal changes in blood flow in diseased muscles.[237–241] Plain radiographs, computed tomography, and magnetic resonance imaging may prove useful in documenting changes in muscle mass and atrophy and extent of early calcinosis.[242–245]

TREATMENT

An early study by Bitnum et al. analyzed 168 children,[11] of whom approximately one-third died, one-third totally recovered, and one-third were crippled from a moderate to a severe extent. Most of the patients in this study had been treated before the use of corticosteroids in the management of this disease.

The introduction of the corticosteroid hormones has revolutionzed the treatment and prognosis for children with JDM.[9,13–15,21,108–114,218,246–249] In addition, the team approach and general supportive care, including bed rest and positioning early in the disease and individualized physical therapy, are essential.

General Supportive Care

In acute disease, attention must be given to the adequacy of ventilatory effort and swallowing. Occasionally weakness is so profound that respiratory assistance, nasogastric feeding, and frequent oral suctioning may be required. Each patient should be monitored carefully for swallowing, adequacy of airway, and depth of breathing. Hypoxia may super-

vene in a quite insidious manner. In the older child, vital capacity measurements can be a valuable objective measure of response to therapy. Although respiratory problems occur in approximately one-third of severely affected children, tracheostomy is seldom required. Profound involvement of the thoracic and respiratory muscles is seen in a few children and leads rapidly to increasing dyspnea at rest, agitation, respiratory insufficiency, aspiration, or death.[131]

Skin care is especially important in children who develop fissures in the axillae, groin, or striae of the skin or over pressure points. Emollients and padding of pressure areas may help prevent breakdown and ulceration (Fig. 8-35). These ulcerations are open sites for secondary infections and abscesses, complications that are abetted by the administration of the corticosteroid drugs. Late in the disease the dermatitis may become markedly photosensitive and water-based sun screens with high SPF numbers are necessary. The rash may or may not respond to the use of corticosteroid creams. Their use is generally not recommended because of the secondary atrophic effects that may result from long-term application.

Frequent counseling and education of patient and parents are necessary to help allay anxiety and permit understanding of the necessarily slow pace of treatment and recovery. Systemic complications, particularly abdominal pain or GI bleeding, require urgent

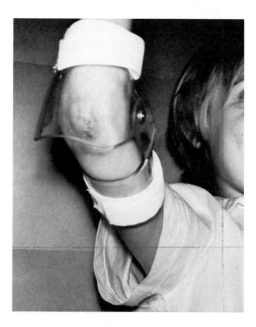

Fig. 8-35 Elbow pad.

surgical consultation and may be life-threatening, especially early in the disease. Attention to nutritional status and limitation of total caloric and sodium intake may help minimize the side effects of the corticosteroid drugs.

Physical and Occupational Therapy

Physiotherapy should be initiated at the time of diagnosis. While the skeletal muscles are actively inflamed, the focus of attention should be on preventing loss of range by twice- to thrice-daily passive range of motion to all joints with gentle stretching to regain lost range if present. Splinting of knees, elbows, or wrists at night or during rest periods helps to achieve these goals.

The average child with JDM pursues a progressively improving course with full functional recovery. During the healing phase the physical therapy program is increased to normalize function as nearly as possible and to minimize development of contractures secondary to muscle weakness or atrophy. Muscle strengthening should be added to the exercise program only when clinical evidence of acute inflammation has subsided.

Periodic grading of muscle strength by an experienced observer is important in following the course of the child with JDM (Table 8-19).[250,251] A quantitative musculoskeletal examination using a standard scale should be sequentially recorded by the same individual. The importance of this examination becomes even more critical during the course of the disease when serum muscle enzyme concentrations may be less dependable indicators of activity. Selected muscles that should always be evaluated are the neck flexors and extensors; shoulder abductors; elbow flexors and extensors; hip flexors, extensors, and abductors; and knee flexors and extensors.

Additional observations should include those related to function such as gait, head control, getting up off the floor, bending over, and performing the activities of daily living. New mechanical techniques to grade selected large muscles by more objective procedures are perhaps more applicable to the distal muscles than to the proximal groups.

Corticosteroid Drugs

Acute disease is treated with suppressive doses of the synthetic corticosteroid drugs (Table 8-20).[13,15] Prednisone is preferred to other synthetic steroids

Table 8-19 Scale for Grading Muscle Strength

Grade	Percentage of Function	Activity Level
0—None	0	No evidence of muscle contractility
1—Trace	15	Evidence of slight contractility; no effective joint motion
2—Poor	25	Full range of motion without gravity
3—Fair	50	Full range of motion against gravity
4—Good	75	Complete range of motion against gravity with some resistance
5—Normal	100	Complete range of motion against gravity with full resistance

(Modified from the National Foundation,[251] with permission.)

Table 8-20 Medical Treatment of Juvenile Dermatomyositis

Basic medical program
  Corticosteroid program
    Initial: prednisone 2 mg/kg/day for 1 month
    Course: prednisone 1 mg/kg/day followed by a gradual taper over approximately 2 years
  Hydroxychloroquine
    Initial: 7 mg/kg/day for 6 weeks
    Maintenance: 5 mg/kg/day

Experimental therapy
  Steroid-pulse therapy
    IV methylprednisolone 10–30 mg/kg for 1 to 3 days
    High-dose oral pulse therapy
  Immunosuppressive regimen
    Methotrexate 0.35–0.65 mg/kg/week
    Cyclophosphamide
      Oral: 1 mg/kg/day
      IV pulse: 500 mg/M^2/month
    Azathioprine 1–3 mg/kg/day
  Plasmapheresis

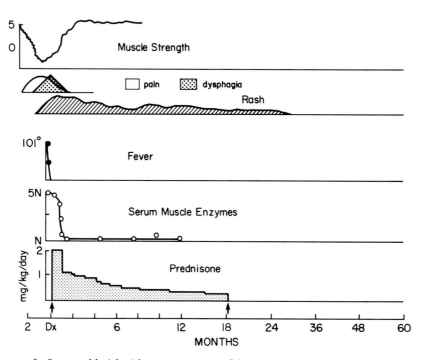

Fig. 8-36 Course of a 5-year-old girl with an acute onset of dermatomyositis and eventual complete recovery. Dysphagia resolved within the first month, muscle strength returned to normal during the first year, and the rash ultimately subsided by 3 years, as did all other signs of the disease. (Courtesy of Dr. D. B. Sullivan.)

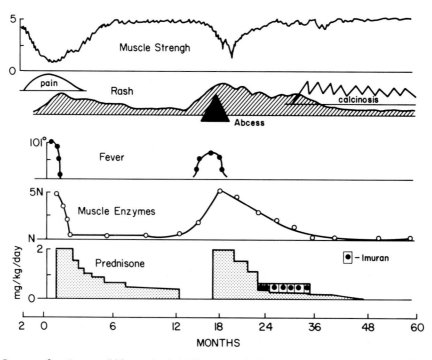

Fig. 8-37 Course of an 8-year-old boy who initially responded to steroid treatment that was discontinued after 12 months. At 18 months, a gluteal abscess developed and an acute relapse that required combined immunosuppressive therapy because of the development of clinically significant steroid toxicity occurred. (Courtesy of Dr. D. B. Sullivan.)

such as dexamethasone or triamcinolone because these steroids may have more potent myopathic effects (Ch. 3). The dosage of prednisone is in the range of 2 mg/kg/day in four divided doses for the first month of the disease and then, if indicated by the clinical response and a fall in the serum levels of the muscle enzymes, by a reduction in dosage to 1 mg/kg/day, also given in divided doses. Thereafter, the steroid is gradually tapered by careful monitoring of improvement in muscle weakness and symptoms, and by assay of serum levels of the muscle enzymes.

In our experience alternate-day steroid therapy is useful only late during the recovery phase of the disease. It is axiomatic that satisfactory clinical control is not attained until the serum enzymes have returned to normal or nearly normal levels and have remained there during tapering of the steroids and a planned increase in the level of physical activity of the child.

The clinical response of the child to steroid management is not entirely predictable. The fever should abate within a few days of instituting steroids, and the serum enzymes should show an appreciable decrease in concentration in the first 1 to 2 weeks of therapy (Figs. 8-36 and 8-37). Muscle strength may not show any significant change for 1 to 2 months after instituting corticosteroid drugs.

Improvement in the dermatitis is unpredictable. The status of the skin rash at any point is generally not an indication for a change in steroid therapy as its course does not parallel that of the inflammatory myopathy. An extensive rash at onset or a generalized progression of the dermatitis is, however, a poor prognostic sign.[15]

It is difficult to be certain when corticosteroids can be totally discontinued without risking an exacerbation of the disease. It is apparently necessary to maintain many children on low-dose corticosteroids even many years after "control" of the myositis.

Children who require high-dose steroids for long periods of time also develop osteopenia, and some cases progress to vertebral compression fractures (Fig. 8-38). It is unsettled whether supplementation with dietary calcium and vitamin D can prevent this osteopenia. Cushing's syndrome and growth retardation result in any child placed on suppressive doses for a period of months. The dosage of the drug and duration of its use should, therefore, be kept as low as possible commensurate with the clinical and laboratory responses to therapy.

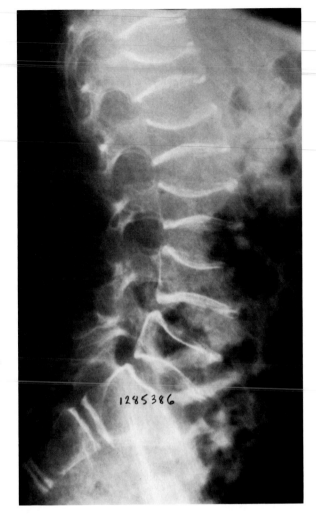

Fig. 8-38 Extreme osteopenia of the lumbar spine with multiple vertebral compression fractures in a 15-year-old girl with a long history of chronic polycyclic dermatomyositis and steroid treatment.

The physician must be wary of the possible development of steroid myopathy, which might be misinterpreted as an exacerbation of the basic disease process (Ch. 3). The manifestations are insidious onset of hip flexor weakness and atrophy, with normal serum muscle enzyme assays and minimal myopathic changes on EMG (Table 8-21). The presence of steroid myopathy can only be confirmed by a marked improvement in the child's weakness that follows a drastic reduction in the steroid dose or change to an

Table 8-21 Characteristics of Steroid-Induced Myopathy

Insidious onset
Hip-flexor weakness and atrophy
Normal serum muscle enzyme concentrations
Minimal myopathic changes on electromyography
Type II fiber atrophy on muscle biopsy

alternate-day schedule. A muscle biopsy may be warranted because of diagnostic confusion and shows type II fiber atrophy.

Hydroxychloroquine

Recently hydroxychloroquine has been used as a steroid-sparing agent and as a drug that is effective on the dermatitis (in a dose similar to that employed in SLE).[252] Although the evidence is only anecdotal, our observations support the efficacy of this regimen.

Calcinosis and Its Management

The development of calcinosis occurs late in the course of JDM and is of unknown cause. Rarely, it is accompanied by hypercalcemia.[253] In one study, patients with calcinosis had abnormal excretion of gamma carboxyglutamate.[254] Trauma has been thought to play a role as calcific deposits tend to occur in surgical incision sites.

None of the many approaches to the treatment of calcinosis has been consistently effective.[167,168,253–265] Medications that have been used include colchicine, aluminum hydroxide, probenecid, diphosphonate, intravenous (IV) EDTA, and warfarin. Colchicine may suppress local and systemic signs associated with calcinosis. Surgical excision of calcifications that mechanically interfere with function or are associated with breakdown of skin may be indicated.[266] It should be noted that the natural history of most calcific deposits associated with JDM is that they spontaneously begin to disappear after months or years. The one-fourth of children who have calcinosis in interfascial places tend to have persistent lesions, however.[122]

Experimental Therapy

Various forms of experimental therapy have been suggested for the child who fails to respond to corticosteroid in reasonable dose, who is steroid-toxic, or who develops problems later in the disease that are steroid-unresponsive (Table 8-20). Steroid-pulse IV therapy has been tried in order to regain control without subjecting the child to long-term, high-dose daily steroids (Ch. 3).[267–270]

An initial publication by Laxer et al.[270] indicated a satisfactory response in six children with JDM to steroid-pulse therapy. Subsequently, two additional patients were treated. Both were boys who had fairly mild early disease; a single pulse of IV methylprednisolone, 30 mg/kg, led to a fall in the enzyme levels and improved muscle strength over 2 months. There may be a subgroup of children with JDM in whom an initial approach such as this to management of the disease will be successful and will abrogate the need for long-term corticosteroid treatment on a daily basis. This approach to therapy in JDM must be evaluated further. If chosen, treatment would be initiated with IV corticosteroid-pulse therapy that could be repeated up to three times if necessary as indicated by the clinical state and enzyme concentrations in the child under treatment. If control by this process is not complete, then oral steroids should be started according to the more traditional regimen. It is estimated by these authors[270] that perhaps 30 percent of children with JDM may respond to this treatment protocol and need no oral corticosteroid therapy.

Immunosuppressive regimens[271–273] have used methotrexate,[274–277] azathioprine,[278,279] cyclophosphamide,[26] or more recently cyclosporin A (Ch. 3). Of the immunosuppressive regimens, methotrexate is used most frequently. No controlled study has been published on the consistency of response to this drug; however, a report of 22 adult patients suggested a favorable improvement of greater than 75 percent without major toxicity or hepatic disease.[276] Immunosuppressive drugs also appear to have a steroid-sparing effect.

Plasmapheresis has recently been advanced as a form of therapy.[140,280–284] It may have to be accompanied by immunosuppression, and the effects of plasmapheresis cannot usually be dissociated from those of the administered immunosuppressive drugs. It, however, may play an important adjunctive role in the treatment of those children demonstrated to have high circulating levels of soluble immune complexes. Certainly all of these forms of experimental

therapy should be reserved for the 10 percent or fewer children who have the most severe and progressive forms of the disorder.

The immense long-term implications of these various forms of therapy in children are well publicized. Informed consent must be obtained, and the facilities to monitor such therapy must be present before experimental therapy can be undertaken (Ch. 3).

Steroid resistance of the disease in a specific child should be carefully defined and differentiated from *steroid-dependent disease*: Either type may be justification for the introduction of an immunosuppressive program. In steroid resistance there should have been an inadequate improvement in muscle strength and a failure to lower the serum muscle enzyme concentrations in response to a closely monitored corticosteroid program. It can also be defined in terms of the amount of prednisone that is required, for example, ≥ 1 to 2 mg/kg/day, and the duration of time that has elapsed since initiation of therapy, for example, ≥ 3 to 4 months. Later during the course of the disease, steroid dependence may become evident and be characterized by a failure of the disease to respond favorably to a gradual reduction of the corticosteroid program to an acceptable level, recurrence of progressive muscle weakness in spite of continuing therapy, or unacceptable steroid toxicity.

COURSE OF THE DISEASE AND PROGNOSIS

At present, the long-term survival in JDM is approximately 90 percent, but in the presteroid era, dermatomyositis was associated with a high mortality rate that approached 40 percent.[15,26,285–287] Children who survived often had devastating residual problems of contractures and muscular atrophy. Adverse factors that influence the outcome of JDM at this time are shown in Table 8-22. The single factor with greatest impact upon a favorable outcome that can be controlled is early adequate steroid treatment.[12,15] Functional outcome appears best in children who have been seen early and treated vigorously. The majority of survivors should be able to function independently as adults, although some will have residual atrophy of skin or muscle.

The course of JDM in children can be divided into four clinical phases, as outlined in Table 8-23.[288] The early prodromal phase is supplanted by a period of progressive muscle weakness and rash that then stabilizes for 1 to 2 years before recovery. In our experience approximately 80 percent of children pursue

Table 8-22 Dermatomyositis in Children: Factors That Adversely Influence Outcome

Disease-related
    Rapid onset and extensive involvement
    Extensive cutaneous vasculitis
    Severe endarteropathy and infarction in muscle biopsy specimens

Therapy-related
    Delay in diagnosis and institution of therapy
    Inadequate dose or duration of corticosteroid therapy
    Minimal response to initial corticosteroid therapy

Table 8-23 Clinical Phases of Dermatomyositis in Childhood

1. Prodromal period with nonspecific symptoms (weeks to months)
2. Progressive muscle weakness and rash (days to weeks)
3. Persistent weakness, rash, and active myositis (up to 2 years)
4. Recovery with or without residual muscle atrophy, contractures, and calcinosis

(Modified from Hanson,[17] with permission.)

this type of course.[13,15] The entire disease duration may be as brief as 8 months with complete recovery, or may last 2 or more years with a continuing requirement for treatment with corticosteroids during that time. Twenty percent of children in our experience have had repeated acute exacerbations and remissions without any stabilization of the initial course of the disease.

The studies of Crowe et al. have identified a group of children with noninflammatory vasculopathy who have extensive and chronic ulcerative cutaneous disease (Table 8-24).[26] These children and a similar group reported earlier by Banker and Victor may develop significant systemic complications, including fatal GI hemorrhage.[106] At a minimum, children with severe generalized erythroderma and cutaneous ulcerations often behave poorly in terms of outcome relative to the development of extensive calcinosis and overall functional impairment.

Late progression of JDM has been reported with a recurrence of active disease after a prolonged remission[288,289] or smoldering persistence of activity many years after onset.[290] Of interest in this regard

Table 8-24 Course of Dermatomyositis in Children

Type of Course	Extent of Involvement	Steroid Response	Residual Disease	Number	(%)	Death
Monocyclic	Limited disease	Responsive	None	9/33	(27)	0
Chronic ulcerative	Cutaneous and GI ulcerations Active disease present for years	Unresponsive	Long-term severe calcinosis and residual disability	11/33	(33)	3 (1 respiratory failure; 2 GI ulcerations)
Chronic nonulcerative	Progressive weakness Limitation of motion	Good initial response Relapses	Permanent disability, calcinosis, severe weakness	13/33	(40)	1

(Modified from Crowe et al.,[26] with permission.)

is the risk from pregnancy in women who have had or have dermatomyositis.[291,292] Dependent upon the activity of the disease, residual muscle weakness, calcinosis, and general debility, pregnancy should be considered high-risk for both mother and baby.

OUTCOME

Function

In children with the typical uniphasic course, the functional outcome is usually excellent, although minor flexion contractures and residual skin changes may persist (Table 8-25). In children in whom the disease remains active beyond 3 years, there may be smoldering myositis and dermatitis with the deposition of calcium salts and progressive functional loss.

Table 8-25 Overall Prognosis of Dermatomyositis in Childhood

Outcome	Percentage
Normal to good functional outcome	64–78
Minimal atrophy or contractures	24
Calcinosis[a]	20–40
Wheelchair dependence	5
Death	7–10

[a] Children with calcinosis were also included in the other categories.

This outcome occurs in approximately 20 to 30 percent of children.

Development of Other Diseases

Approximately 5 percent of children with JDM eventually develop a clinical disease that is more typical of systemic vasculitis[26,106] or scleroderma with sclerodactyly and cutaneous atrophy.[15]

Psychosocial Outcome

A study by Miller et al. suggested that a number of children who enter adulthood continue to have psychological problems and learning disabilities based upon unrecognized cerebral abnormalities at onset of disease.[287] A major study of late outcome in JDM by Chalmers et al. indicated that educational achievement and employment status in the 18 patients who were studied were better than those of a comparable group who had had JRA or of the general adult population.[293] Significant disability related to calcinosis or contractures was present in three patients, six had persistent muscle weakness, and seven had recurrent rash. Raynaud's phenomenon (33 percent), arthritis (22 percent), and subcutaneous nodules were present in others, and minor increases in the serum concentration of CK that did not correlate with the presence of muscle weakness or rash were noted in seven patients.

Death

Death occurs most often within 2 years after onset and is often associated with progressive involvement of skin or muscle that is steroid-unresponsive. This observation suggests that the basic nature of the inflammatory disease, its early treatment and response, presence of vasculitis, and involvement of other organ systems such as the GI or pulmonary tracts are major factors that should be assessed in estimating prognosis. Deaths most frequently result from respiratory insufficiency or pneumonitis, or from acute GI ulceration and bleeding. Surgical intervention in the latter group of children has generally not been of benefit.

There have been 6 deaths in the Ann Arbor series of 71 children with JDM. One death in a young girl 5 years after onset was related to cardiorespiratory collapse. Necropsy examination showed no active myositis. Three patients died 2 months, 6 months, and 4 years after onset from multiple sites of GI hemorrhage. Another girl died from a subdural hematoma caused by a fall from a wheelchair. A boy died shortly after onset of disease from respiratory insufficiency and hypoxia. In the series of Spencer et al.,[294] 7 of 66 patients died. Five deaths were early during the course of the disease (1 to 11 months from diagnosis) and were related to sepsis (1), GI perforation (2), and unresponsive muscle weakness and pneumonitis (2). Two late deaths occurred at 9 and 16 years from pulmonary fibrosis with cor pulmonale and suicide.

In the recent report of 39 patients with JDM by Miller et al.,[287] there were 10 deaths (26 percent); 8 of these occurred in children seen prior to 1972. No child who had received intensive corticosteroid treatment (and, in some cases, azathioprine) died. All deaths were associated with bowel perforation and aspiration pneumonitis and occurred an average of $2\frac{1}{2}$ years after onset. The improved outcome since 1972 (92 percent survival rate) was judged to be related to early and appropriate steroid regimens, better clinical assessment and follow-up with sequential serum muscle enzyme determinations, and management of complications. Five of the 24 surviving patients were still on corticosteroids at follow-up.

REFERENCES

1. Pearson CM: Polymyositis. Annu Rev Med 17:63, 1966
2. Bohan A, Peter JB: Polymyositis and dermatomyositis. N Engl J Med 292:344, 1975
3. Hanissian AS, Masi AT, Pitner SE et al: Polymyositis and dermatomyositis in children: an epidemiologic and clinical comparative analysis. J Rheumatol 9:390, 1982
4. Hepp P: Ueber einen Fall von acuter parenchymatöser Myositis, welche Geschwülste bildete und Fluctuation vortäuschte. Klin Wochenschr 24:389, 1887
5. Jackson H: Myositis universalis acuta infectiosa, with a case. Boston Med Surg J 116:498, 1887
6. Wagner E: Ein Fall con acuter Polymyositis. Dtsch Arch Klin Med 40:241, 1887
7. Unverricht H: Ueber eine eigenthümliche Form von acuter Muskelentzündung mit einem der Trichinose ähnlenden Kraukheitsbilde. Munch Med Wochenschr 34:488, 1887
8. Karelitz S, Welt SK: Dermatomyositis. Am J Dis Child 43:1134, 1932
9. Wedgwood RJP, Cook CD, Cohen J: Dermatomyositis: report of 26 cases in children with a discussion of endocrine therapy in 13. Pediatrics 12:447, 1953
10. Carlisle JW, Good RA: Dermatomyositis in childhood: report of studies on 7 cases and a review of literature. Lancet 79:266, 1959
11. Bitnum S, Daeschner CW, Jr, Travis LB et al: Dermatomyositis. J Pediatr 64:101, 1964
12. Hanson V, Kornreich H: Systemic rheumatoid disorders of childhood: lupus erythematosus, anaphylactoid purpura, dermatomyositis and scleroderma. Parts I and II. Bull Rheum Dis 17:435, 1967
13. Sullivan DB, Cassidy JT, Petty RE: Prognosis in childhood dermatomyositis. J Pediatr 80:555, 1972
14. Rose AL: Childhood polymyositis: a follow-up study with special reference to treatment with corticosteroids. Am J Dis Child 127:518, 1974
15. Sullivan DB, Cassidy JT, Petty RE: Dermatomyositis in the pediatric patient. Arthritis Rheum 20:327, 1977
16. Batten FE: Case of dermatomyositis in a child, with pathological report. Br J Child Dis 9:247, 1912
17. Hanson V: Dermatomyositis, scleroderma, and polyarteritis nodosa. Clin Rheum Dis 2:445, 1976
18. Scheuermann H: Zur Klinik und Pathogenese der Dermatomyositis (Polymyositis). Arch Dermatol U Syph 178:414, 1939
19. Hecht MS: Dermatomyositis in childhood. J Pediatr 17:791, 1940
20. Selander P: Dermatomyositis in early childhood. Acta Med Scand [Suppl] 246:187, 1950
21. Rose AL, Walton JN: Polymyositis: a survey of 89 cases with particular reference to treatment and prognosis. Brain 89:747, 1966
22. Medsger TA, Dawson WN, Masi AT: The epidemiology of polymyositis. Am J Med 48:715, 1970

23. Benbassat J, Geffel D, Zlotnick A: Epidemiology of polymyositis-dermatomyositis in Israel 1960–1976. Isr J Med Sci 16:197, 1980

24. Barwick DD, Walton JN: Polymyositis. Am J Med 35:646, 1963

25. Cook CD, Rosen FS, Banker BQ: Dermatomyositis and focal scleroderma. Pediatr Clin North Am 10:979, 1963

26. Crowe WE, Bove KE, Levinson JE et al: Clinical and pathogenetic implications of histopathology in childhood polydermatomyositis. Arthritis Rheum 25:126, 1982

27. Thompson CE: Polymyositis in children. Clin Pediatr 7:24, 1968

28. Whitaker JN: Inflammatory myopathy: a review of etiologic and pathogenetic factors. Muscle Nerve 5:573, 1982

29. Denman AN: Aetiology. Inflammatory disorders of muscle. Clin Rheum Dis 10:9, 1984

30. Landry M, Winkelman RK: Tubular cytoplasmic inclusion in dermatomyositis. Mayo Clin Proc 47:479, 1972

31. Middleton PJ, Alexander RM, Szymanski MT: Severe myositis during recovery from influenza. Lancet 2:533, 1970

32. Cotterill JA, Shapiro H: Dermatomyositis after immunization. Lancet 2:1158, 1978

33. Ehrengut W: Dermatomyositis and vaccination. Lancet 1:1040, 1978

34. Hanissian AS, Martinez J, Jabbour JT et al: Vasculitis and myositis secondary to rubella vaccination. Arch Neurol 28:202, 1973

35. Kass E, Straume S, Munthe E: Dermatomyositis after B.C.G. vaccination. Lancet 1:772, 1978

36. Hendrickx GF, Verhage J, Jennekens FG et al: Dermatomyositis and toxoplasmosis. Ann Neurol 5:393, 1979

37. Phillips PE, Kassan SS, Kagen LJ: Increased toxoplasma antibodies in idiopathic inflammatory muscle disease. A case-controlled study. Arthritis Rheum 22:209, 1979

38. Pollock JL: Toxoplasmosis appearing to be dermatomyositis. Arch Dermatol 115:736, 1979

39. Kagen LJ, Kimball AC, Christian CL: Serological evidence of toxoplasmosis among patients with polymyositis. Am J Med 56:186, 1974

40. Schröter HM, Sarnat HB, Matheson DS et al: Juvenile dermatomyositis induced by toxoplasmosis. J Child Neurol 2:101, 1987

41. Ruff RL, Secrist D: Viral studies in benign acute childhood myositis. Arch Neurol 39:261, 1982

42. Bowles NE, Dubowitz V, Sewry CA et al: Dermatomyositis, polymositis, and Coxsackie-B-virus infection. Lancet 1:1004, 1987

43. Christensen ML, Pachman LM, Maryjowski MC et al: Antibody to coxsackie B virus: increased incidence in sera from children with recently diagnosed juvenile dermatomyositis. (abstract) Arthritis Rheum 26:S24, 1983

44. Christensen ML, Pachman LM, Schneiderman R et al: Prevalence of Coxsackie B virus antibodies in patients with juvenile dermatomyositis. Arthritis Rheum 29:1365, 1986

45. Lundberg A: Myalgia crures epidemica. Acta Paediatr 46:18, 1957

46. Dietzman DE, Schaller JG, Ray CG et al: Acute myositis associated with influenza B infection. Pediatrics 57:255, 1976

47. Chou SM, Miike T: Ultrastructural abnormalities and perifascicular atrophy in childhood dermatomyositis with special reference to transverse tubular system sarcoplasmic reticulum junctions. Arch Pathol Lab Med 105:76, 1981

48. Chou SM: Myxovirus-like structures in a case of human chronic polymyositis. Science 158:1453, 1967

49. Burch GE, Sohal RS, Colcolough HL, III et al: Virus-like particles in skeletal muscle after heat stroke. Arch Environ Health 17:984, 1968

50. Baringer JR, Swoveland T: Tubular aggregates in endoplasmic reticulum: evidence against their viral nature. J Ultrastruct Res 41:270, 1972

51. Katsuragi S, Miyayama H, Takeuchi T: Picornavirus-like inclusions in polymyositis—aggregation of glycogen particles of the same size. Neurology 31:1476, 1981

52. Ben-Bassat M, Machtev I: Picornavirus-like structures in acute dermatomyositis. Am J Clin Pathol 58:245, 1972

53. Chou SM, Gutmann L: Picornavirus-like crystals in subacute polymyositis. Neurology 20:205, 1970

54. Fukuyama Y, Ando T, Yokota I: Acute fulminant myoglobinuric polymyositis with picornavirus-like crystals. J Neurol Neurosurg Psychiatry 40:775, 1977

55. Gyorkey F, Cabral GA, Gyorkey PK: Coxsackievirus aggregates in muscle cells of a polymyositis patient. Intervirology 10:69, 1978

56. Mastaglia FL, Watson JM: Coxsackie virus-like particles in skeletal muscle from a case of polymyositis. J Neurol Sci 11:593, 1970

57. Hashimoto K, Robinson I, Velayos F et al: Dermatomyositis: electron microscopic, immunologic and tissue culture studies of paramyxovirus-like inclusions. Arch Dermatol 103:120, 1971

58. Norton WL: Comparison of the microangiopathy of systemic lupus erythematosus, dermatomyositis, scleroderma, and diabetes mellitus. Lab Invest 22:301, 1970

59. Saunders M, Knowles M, Currie S: Lymphocyte

stimulation with muscle homogenate in polymyositis and other muscle-wasting disorders. J Neurol Neurosurg Psychiatry 32:569, 1969

60. Currie S, Sander M, Knowles M et al: Immunological aspects of polymyositis. The in vitro activity of lymphocytes on incubation with muscle antigen and with muscle cultures. Q J Med 40:63, 1971

61. Esiri MM, Maclennan ICM, Hazleman BL: Lymphocyte sensitivity to skeletal muscle in patients with polymyositis and other disorders. Clin Exp Immunol 14:25, 1973

62. Mastaglia FL, Currie S: Immunological and ultrastructural observations on the role of lymphoid cells in the pathogenesis of polymyositis. Acta Neuropathol 18:1, 1971

63. Lisak RP, Zweiman B: Mitogen and muscle extract induced in vitro proliferative responses in myasthenia gravis, dermatomyositis and polymyositis. J Neurol Neurosurg Psychiatry 38:521, 1975

64. Currie S: Destruction of muscle cultures by lymphocytes from cases of polymyositis. Acta Neuropathol 15:11, 1970

65. Dawkins R, Mastaglia FL: Cell-mediated cytotoxicity to muscle in polymyositis. Effect of immunosuppression. N Engl J Med 288:434, 1973

66. Johnson RL, Fink CW, Ziff M: Lymphotoxin formation by lymphocytes and muscle in polymyositis. J Clin Invest 51:2435, 1972

67. Haas DC, Arnason BGW: Cell-mediated immunity in polymyositis. Creatine phosphokinase release from muscle cultures. Arch Neurol 31:192, 1974

68. Iannaccone ST, Bowen DE, Samaha FJ: Cell-mediated cytotoxicity and childhood dermatomyositis. Arch Neurol 39:400, 1982

69. Miller ML, Lantner R, Pachman LM: Natural and antibody-dependent cellular cytotoxicity in children with systemic lupus erythematosus and juvenile dermatomyositis. J Rheumatol 10:640, 1983

70. Haas DC: Absence of cell-mediated cytoxicity to muscle cultures in polymyositis. J Rheumatol 7:671, 1980

71. Whitaker JN, Engel WK: Vascular deposits of immunoglobulin and complement in idiopathic inflammatory myopathy. N Engl J Med 286:333, 1972

72. Spencer CH, Jordon SC, Hanson V: Circulating immune complexes in juvenile dermatomyositis. Arthritis Rheum 23:750, 1980

73. Iannaccone ST, Bowen D, Yarcom A et al: In vitro study of cytotoxic factors against endothelium in childhood dermatomyositis. Arch Neurol 41:862, 1984

74. Kissel JT, Mendell JR, Rammohan KW: Microvascular deposition of complement membrane attack complex in dermatomyositis. N Engl J Med 314:329, 1986

75. Pachman LM, Cooke N: Juvenile dermatomyositis: a clinical and immunologic study. J Pediatr 96:226, 1980

76. Webster AD: Inflammatory disorders of muscle. Echovirus disease in hypogammaglobulinaemic patients. Clin Rheum Dis 10:189, 1984

77. Carroll JE, Silverman A, Isobe Y et al: Inflammatory myopathy, IgA deficiency and intestinal malabsorption. J Pediatr 89:216, 1976

78. Leddy JP, Griggs RC, Klemperer MR et al: Hereditary complement (C2) deficiency with dermatomyositis. Am J Med 58:83, 1975

79. Solomon SD, Maurer KH: Association of dermatomyositis and dysgerminoma in a 16-year-old patient (letter). Arthritis Rheum 26:572, 1983

80. Page AR, Hansen AE, Good RA: Occurrence of leukemia and lymphoma in patients with agammaglobulinemia. Blood 21:197, 1963

81. Takayanagi T: Immunohistological studies of experimental myositis in relation to human polymyositis. Folia Psychiatr Neurol Jpn 21:117, 1967

82. Webb JN: Experimental immune myositis in guinea pigs. J Reticuloendothel Soc 7:305, 1970

83. Suenaga Y: Experimental pathological studies on homologous immunization with the skeletal muscle tissue of the rabbit. J Tokyo Med Coll 25:975, 1967

84. Morgan G, Peter JB, Newbould BB: Experimental allergic myositis in rats. Arthritis Rheum 14:599, 1971

85. Smith PD, Butler RC, Partridge TS et al: Current progress in the study of allergic polymyositis in the guinea-pig and man. In Rose FC (ed): Clinical Neuroimmunology. Blackwell Scientific Publications, Oxford, 1979, p. 146

86. Kakulas BA: In vitro destruction of skeletal muscle by sensitized cells. Nature 210:1115, 1966

87. Kakulas BA: Destruction of differentiated muscle cultures by sensitized lymphoid cells. J Pathol Bacteriol 91:495, 1966

88. Currie S: Experimental myositis. The in vivo and in vitro activity of lymph node cells. J Pathol 105:169, 1971

89. Hathaway PW, Engel WK, Zellweger K: Experimental myopathy after microarterial embolization. Comparison with childhood X-linked pseudohypertrophic muscular dystrophy. Arch Neurol 22:365, 1970

90. Mendell JR, Engel WK, Derrer EC: Duchenne muscular dystrophy: functional ischemia reproduces its characteristic lesions. Science 172:1143, 1971

91. Grimley PM, Friedman RM: An arboviral infection of voluntary striated muscle. J Infect Dis 122:45, 1970

92. Melnick JL, Godman GC: Pathogenesis of coxsackie

virus infections: multiplication of virus and evolution of the muscle lesion in mice. J Exp Med 93:247, 1951

93. Ytterberg SR, Mahowald ML, Messner RP: T cells are required for coxsackievirus B1 induced murine PM. J Rheumatol 15:475, 1988.

94. Craighead JE: Pathogenicity of the M and E variants of the encephalomyocarditis (EMG) virus. I: Myocardiotropic and neurotropic properties. Am J Pathol 48:333, 1966

95. Seay AR, Griffin DR, Johnson RT: Experimental viral polymyositis: age dependency and immune responses to Ross River virus infection in mice. Neurology 31:656, 1981

96. Lambie JA, Duff IF: Familial occurrence of dermatomyositis. Ann Intern Med 59:839, 1963

97. Lewkonia RM, Buxton PH: Myositis in father and daughter. J Neurol Neurosurg Psychiatry 36:820, 1973

98. Christianson HB, Brunsting LA, Perry HO: Dermatomyositis: unusual features, complications and treatment. AMA Arch Dermatol 74:581, 1956

99. Harati Y, Niakan E, Bergman EW: Childhood dermatomyositis in monozygotic twins. Neurology 36:721, 1986

100. Rose T, Nothjunge J, Schlote W: Familial occurrence of dermatomyositis and progressive scleroderma after injection of a local anesthetic for dental treatment. Eur J Pediatr 143:225, 1985

101. Pachman LM, Jonasson O, Cannon RA et al: Increased frequency of HLA-B8 in juvenile dermatomyositis. Lancet 2:1238, 1977

102. Friedman J, Pachman LM, Maryjowski ML et al: Immunogenetic studies of juvenile dermatomyositis. HLA antigens in patients and their families. Tissue Antigens 21:45, 1983

103. Friedman JM, Pachman LM, Maryjowski ML et al: Immunogenetic studies of juvenile dermatomyositis: HLA-DR antigen frequencies. Arthritis Rheum 26:214, 1983

104. Hirsch TJ, Enlow RW, Bias WB et al: HLA-D related (DR) antigens in various kinds of myositis. Hum Immunol 3:181, 1981

105. Roberts HM, Brunsting LA: Dermatomyositis in childhood. A summary of 40 cases. Postgrad Med 16:396, 1954

106. Banker BQ, Victor M: Dermatomyositis (systemic angiopathy) of childhood. Medicine 45:261, 1966

107. Hill RH, Wood WS: Juvenile dermatomyositis. Can Med Assoc J 103:1152, 1970

108. Schaller JG: Dermatomyositis. J Pediatr 83:699, 1973

109. Kornreich HK, Hanson V: The rheumatic diseases of childhood. Curr Probl Pediatr 4:3, 1974

110. Goel KM, Shanks RA: Dermatomyositis in childhood. Review of eight cases. Arch Dis Child 51:501, 1976

111. Dubowitz V: Muscle Disorders in Childhood. WB Saunders, Philadelphia, 1978

112. Winkelman RK: Dermatomyositis in childhood. J Dermatol 18:13, 1979

113. Malleson P: Juvenile dermatomyositis: a review. J R Soc Med 75:33, 1982

114. Goel KM, King M: Dermatomyositis-polymyositis in children. Scott Med J 31:15, 1986

115. Donoghue FD, Winklemann RK, Moersch J, II: Esophageal defects in dermatomyositis. Ann Otol Rhinol Laryngol 69:1139, 1960

116. Woo TR, Rasmussen J, Callen JP: Recurrent photosensitive dermatitis preceeding juvenile dermatomyositis. Pediatr Dermatol 2:207, 1985

117. Spencer-Green G, Crowe WE, Levinson JE: Nailfold capillary abnormalities and clinical outcome in childhood dermatomyositis. Arthritis Rheum 25:954, 1982

118. Maricq HR, Spencer-Green G, LeRoy EC: Skin capillary abnormalities as indicators of organ involvement in scleroderma (systemic sclerosis), Raynaud's syndrome and dermatomyositis. Am J Med 61:862, 1976

119. Spencer-Green G, Schlesinger M, Bove KE et al: Nailfold capillary abnormalities in childhood rheumatic diseases. J Pediatr 102:341, 1983

120. Nussbaum AI, Silver RM, Maricq HR: Serial changes in nailfold capillary morphology in childhood dermatomyositis. Arthritis Rheum 26:1169, 1983

121. Hamlin C, Shelton JE: Management of oral findings in a child with an advanced case of dermatomyositis: clinical report. Pediatr Dent 6:46, 1984

122. Bowyer SL, Blane CE, Sullivan DB et al: Childhood dermatomyositis: factors predicting functional outcome and development of dystrophic calcification. J Pediatr 103:882, 1983

123. Blane CE, White SJ, Braunstein EM et al: Patterns of calcification in childhood dermatomyositis. AJR 142:397, 1984

124. Thompson JW: Spontaneous perforation of the esophagus as a manifestation of dermatomyositis. Ann Otol Rhinol Laryngol 93:464, 1984

125. Fischer TJ, Cipel L, Stiehm ER: Pneumatosis intestinalis associated with fatal childhood dermatomyositis. Pediatrics 61:127, 1978

126. Braunstein EM, White SJ: Pneumatosis intestinalis in dermatomyositis. Br J Radiol 53:1011, 1980

127. Schullinger JN, Jacobs JC, Berdon WE: Diagnosis and management of gastrointestinal perforations in childhood dermatomyositis with particular reference to perforations of the duodenum. J Pediatr Surg 20:521, 1985

128. Magil HL, Hixson SD, Whitington G et al: Duodenal perforation in childhood dermatomyositis. Pediatr Radiol 14:28, 1984

129. Farber S, Vawter GF: Clinical pathological conference. J Pediatr 57:784, 1960

130. Boylan RC, Sokoloff L: Vascular lesions in dermatomyositis. Arthritis Rheum 3:379, 1960

131. Dubowitz LM, Dubowitz V: Acute dermatomyositis presenting with pulmonary manifestations. Arch Dis Child 39:293, 1964

132. Dickey BF, Myers AR: Pulmonary disease in polymyositis/dermatomyositis. Semin Arthritis Rheum 14:60, 1984

133. Duncan PE, Griffin JP, Garcia A et al: Fibrosing alveolitis in polymyositis. A review of histologically confimed cases. Am J Med 57:621, 1974

134. Singsen BH, Tedford JC, Platzker ACG et al: Spontaneous penumothorax: a complication of juvenile dermatomyositis. J Pediatr 92:771, 1978

135. Schwartz MI, Matthay RA: Sahn SA et al: Interstitial lung disease in polymyositis and dermatomyositis. Analysis of six cases and review of the literature. Medicine 55:89, 1976

136. Shaumburg HH, Nielson SL, Yurchar PM: Heart block in polymyositis. N Engl J Med 284:480, 1971

137. Lynch PE: Cardiac involvement in chronic polymyositis. Br Heart J 33:416, 1971

138. Fernandez-Herlihy L: Heart block in polymyositis. N Engl J Med 284:1101, 1971

139. Walton J: The inflammatory myopathies. J R Soc Med 76:998, 1983

140. Bennington JL, Dau PC: Patients with polymyositis and dermatomyositis who undergo plasmapheresis therapy. Pathologic findings. Arch Neurol 38:553, 1981

141. Carpenter S, Karpati G, Rothman S et al: The childhood type of dermatomyositis. Neurology 26:952, 1976

142. Munsat T, Cancilla P: Polymyositis without inflammation. Bull Los Angeles Neurol Soc 39:113, 1974

143. Giorno R, Barden MT, Kohler PF et al: Immunohistochemical characterization of the mononuclear cells infiltrating muscle of patients with inflammatory and noninflammatory myopathies. Clin Immunol Immunopath 30:405, 1984

144. Hughes JT, Esiri MM: Ultrastructural studies in human polymyositis. J Neurol 25:347, 1975

145. Matsubara S, Mair WGP: Ultrastructural changes in polymyositis. Brain 102:701, 1979

146. Rose AL, Walton JN, Pearce GW: Polymyositis: an ultramicroscopic study of muscle biopsy material. J Neurol Sci 5:457, 1967

147. Shafiq SA, Milhorat AT, Gorycki MA: An electron microscope study of muscle degeneration and vascular changes in polymyositis. J Pathol Bacteriol 94:139, 1967

148. Whitaker JN, Bertorini TE, Mendell JR: Immunocytochemical studies of cathepsin D in human skeletal muscle. Ann Neurol 10:91, 1981

149. Mastaglia FL, Kakulas BA: A histological and histochemical study of skeletal muscle regeneration in polymyositis. J Neurol Sci 10:471, 1970

150. Cros D, Pearson C, Verity MA: Polymyositis-dermatomyositis. Diagnostic and prognostic significance of muscle alkaline phosphatase. Am J Pathol 101:159, 1980

151. Engel WK, Cunningham GG: Alkaline phosphatase-positive abnormal muscle fibers of humans. J Histochem Cytochem 18:55, 1970

152. Oxenhandler R, Adelstein EH, Hatt MN: Immunopathology of skeletal muscle. The value of direct immunofluorescence in the diagnosis of connective tissue disease. Hum Pathol 8:321, 1977

153. Bodensteiner JB, Engel AG: Intracellular calcium accumulation in Duchenne dystrophy and other myopathies: a study of 567,000 muscle fibers in 114 biopsies. Neurology 28:439, 1978

154. Obere MA, Engel WK: Ultrastructural localization of calcium in normal and abnormal skeletal muscle. Lab Invest 36:566, 1977

155. Banker BQ: Dermatomyositis of childhood. Ultrastructural alternations of muscle and intramuscular blood vessels. J Neuropathol Exp Neurol 34:46, 1975

156. Eady RAJ, Odland GF: Intraendothelial tubular aggregates in experimental wounds. Br J Dermatol 93:165, 1975

157. Oshima Y, Becker LE, Armstrong DL: An electron microscopic study of childhood dermatomyositis. Acta Neuropathol 47:189, 1979

158. Mastalgia FL, Walton JN: An ultrastructural study of skeletal muscle in polymyositis. J Neurol Sci 12:473, 1971

159. Chou SM, Nonaka I, Voice GF: Anastomoses of transverse tubules with terminal cisternae in polymyositis. Arch Neurol 37:256, 1980

160. Yunis EJ, Samaha FJ: Inclusion body myositis. Lab Invest 25:240, 1971

161. Jerusalem F, Rukusa M, Engel AG et al: Morphometric analysis of skeletal muscle capillary ultrastructure in inflammatory myopathies. J Neurol Sci 23:391, 1974

162. Duance VC, Black CM, Dubowitz V et al: Polymyositis—an immunofluorescence study on the distribution of collagen types. Muscle Nerve 3:487, 1980

163. Foidart M, Foidart J-M, Engel WK: Collagen local-

ization in normal and fibrotic human skeletal muscle. Arch Neurol 38:152, 1981

164. Bowyer SL, Clark RA, Ragsdale CG et al: Juvenile dermatomyositis: histological findings and pathogenic hypothesis for the associated skin changes. J Rheumatol 13:753, 1986

165. Janis JF, Winkelmann RK: Histopathology of the skin in dermatomyositis: a histopathologic study of 55 cases. Arch Dermatol 97:640, 1968

166. Hanno R, Callen JP: Histopathology of Gottron's papules. J Cutan Pathol 12:389, 1985

167. Loewi G, Dorling J: Calcinosis, histological and chemical analysis. Ann Rheum Dis 23:272, 1964

168. Sewell JR, Liyanage B, Ansell BM: Calcinosis in juvenile dermatomyositis. Skeletal Radiol 3:137, 1978

169. Denbow CE, Lie JT, Tancredi RG et al: Cardiac involvement in polymyositis. A clinicopathologic study of 20 autopsied patients. Arthritis Rheum 22:1088, 1979

170. Haupt HM, Hutchins GM: The heart and cardiac conduction system in polymyositis-dermatomyositis: a clinico-pathologic study of 16 autopsied patients. Am J Cardiol 50:998, 1982

171. Baker JP, Goldstein M: Myositis (postinfluenza, coxsackievirus, Trichinella spiralis). In Feigin RD, Cherry JD (eds): Textbook of Pediatric Infectious Diseases. 2nd Ed. WB Saunders, Philadelphia, 1987, p. 783

172. Levin MJ, Gardner P, Waldvogel FA: "Tropical" polymyositis: an unusual infection due to Staphylococcus aureus. N Engl J Med 284:196, 1971

173. Topi GC, d'Alessandro L, Catricala C et al: Dermatomyositis like syndrome due to toxoplasma. Br J Dermatol 101:589, 1979

174. Grose C: Bacterial myositis and pyomyositis. In Feigin RD, Cherry JD (eds): Textbook of Pediatric Infectious Diseases. 2nd Ed. WB Saunders, Philadelphia, 1987, p. 780

175. Noseworthy JH, Heffernan LP, Ross JB et al: Acne fulminans with inflammatory myopathy. Ann Neurol 8:67, 1980

176. The Research Group on Neuromuscular Diseases: Classification of the neuromuscular disorders. J Neurol Sci 6:165, 1968

177. Hicklin JA: Choroquine neuromyopathy. Ann Phys Med 9:189, 1968

178. Schraeder PL, Peters HA, Dahl DS: Polymyositis and penicillamine. Arch Neurol 27:456, 1972

179. McKusick VA: Heritable Disorders of Connective Tissue. 4th Ed. CV Mosby, St. Louis, 1972

180. Sabina RL, Sevain JL, Holmes EW: Myoadenylate deaminase deficiency. In Sevian CR, Beaudet AL, Sly WS et al (eds): The Metabolic Basis of Inherited Disease. 6th Ed. McGraw-Hill, New York, 1989

181. Newman AJ, Lee C: Hypothyroidism simulating dermatomyositis. J Pediatr 97:772, 1980

182. Panitch HS, Franklin GM: Elevation of serum creatine phosphate in amyotrophic lateral sclerosis. Neurology 22:964, 1972

183. Mastaglia FL, Walton JN: Histological and histochemical changes in skeletal muscle from cases of chronic juvenile and early adult spinal muscular atrophy (the Kugelberg-Welander syndrome). J Neurol Sci 12:15, 1971

184. Allen RC, St-Cyr C, Maddison PJ et al: Overlap connective tissue syndromes. Arch Dis Child 61:284, 1986

185. Sills EM: Diffuse fasciitis with eosinophilia in childhood. Johns Hopkins Med J 151:203, 1982

186. Everhardt K, Svantesson H, Svensson B: Follow-up study of 6 children presenting with a MCTD-like syndrome. Scand J Rheumatol 10:62, 1981

187. Thompson CE: Infantile myositis. Dev Med Child Neurol 24:307, 1982

188. Brooke MH, Kaplan H: Muscle pathology in rheumatoid arthritis, polymyalgia rheumatica, and polymyositis. Arch Pathol 94:101, 1972

189. Medsger TA, Jr, Rodnan GP, Moossey J et al: Skeletal muscle involvement in progressive systemic sclerosis. Arthritis Rheum 11:554, 1968

190. Graudal H: Myopathy in rheumatoid arthritis. Rheumatism 17:81, 1961

191. Adams RD: The pathologic substratum of polymyositis. In Pearson CM, Mastofi EF (eds): The Striated Muscle. Williams & Wilkins, Baltimore, 1973, p. 292

192. Denko CW, Old JW: Myopathy in the sicca syndrome (Sjögren's syndrome). Am J Clin Pathol 51:631, 1969

193. Carpenter S, Karpati G, Heller I et al: Inclusion body myositis. A distinct variety of idiopathic inflammatory myopathy. Neurology 28:8, 1978

194. Layzer RB, Shearn MA, Satya-Murti S: Eosinophilic polymyositis. Ann Neurol 1:65, 1977

195. Cumming WJK, Weiser R, Teoh R et al: Localized nodular myositis: A clinical and pathological variant of polymyositis. Q J Med 66:531, 1977

196. Heffner RR, Barron SA: Polymyositis beginning as a focal process. Arch Neurol 38:439, 1981

197. Enzinger FM, Dulcey F: Proliferative myositis. Report of thirty-three cases. Cancer 20:2213, 1967

198. Brooke MH, Neville HE: Reducing body myopathy. Neurology 22:829, 1972

199. Neville HE: Ultrastructural changes in muscle disease. In Dubowitz V, Brooke MH (eds): Muscle Biopsy-A Modern Approach. WB Saunders, London, 1973, p. 438

200. Anderson TE, Carr AJ, Chapman RS et al: Myositis

and myotonia in a case of multicentric reticulohistiocytosis. Br J Dermatol 80:39, 1968

201. Burke JS, Medline NM, Katz A: Giant cell myocarditis and myositis associated with thymoma and myasthenia gravis. Arch Pathol 88:359, 1969

202. Silverstein A, Siltzbach LE: Muscle involvement in sarcoidosis. Arch Neurol 21:235, 1969

203. Savage DCL, Forbes M, Pearce GW: Idiopathic rhabdomyolysis. Arch Dis Child 46:594, 1971

204. Smith R, Russell RGG, Woods CG: Myositis ossificans progressiva: clinical features of eight patients and their response to treatment. J Bone Joint Surg 52B:4B, 1976

205. Hentzer B, Jacobsen HH, Asboe-Hansen G: Fibrous dysplasia ossificans progressiva. Scand J Rheumatol 6:161, 1977

206. Vignos PJ, Goldwyn J: Evaluation of laboratory tests in the diagnosis and management of polymyositis. Am J Med Sci 263:291, 1972

207. Haas RH, Dyck RF, Dubowitz V et al: C-reactive protein in childhood dermatomyositis. Ann Rheum Dis 41:483, 1982

208. Lisak RP, Zweiman B: Serum immunoglobulin levels in myasthenia gravis, polymyositis and dermatomyositis. J Neurol Neurosurg Psychiatry 39:34, 1976

209. Gotoff SP, Smith RD, Sugar O: Dermatomyositis with cerebral vasculitis in a patient with agammaglobulinemia. Am J Dis Child 123:53, 1972

210. Giuliano VJ: Polymyositis in a patient with acquired hypogammaglobulinemia. Am J Med Sci 268:53, 1974

211. Bardelas JA, Winkelstein JA, Seto DSY et al: Fatal ECHO 24 infection in a patient with hypogammaglobulinemia. Relationship to dermatomyositis-like syndrome. J Pediatr 90:396, 1977

212. Askmark H, Osterman PO, Roxin LE et al: Radioimmunoassay of serum myoglobulin in neuromuscular diseases. J Neurol Neurosurg Psychiatry 44:68, 1981

213. Kagen IJ: Myoglobulinemia in inflammatory myopathies. JAMA 237:1448, 1977

214. Nishikai M, Reichlin M: Radioimmunoassay of serum myoglobulin in polymyositis and other conditions. Arthritis Rheum 20:1514, 1977

215. Nishikai M, Homma M: Circulating autoantibody against human myoglobulin in polymyositis. JAMA 237:1842, 1977

216. Dickerson JW, Widdowson EM: Chemical changes in skeletal muscle during development. Biochem J 74:247, 1960

217. Hallgren R, Karlsson FA, Roxin L-E et al: Myoglobulin turnover—influence of renal and extrarenal factors. J Lab Clin Med 91:246, 1978

218. Ansell BM, Hamilton E, Bywaters EG: Course and prognosis in juvenile dermatomyositis. In Kakulas BA (ed): Second International Congress on Muscle Disease, Part 2. Publication 295. International Congress Series. Excerpta Medica, Amsterdam, 1973

219. Wolfe JF, Adelstein E, Sharp GC: Antinuclear antibody with distinct specificity for polymyositis. J Clin Invest 59:176, 1977

220. Pachman LM, Maryjowski, MC: Juvenile dermatomyositis and polymyositis. Clin Rheum Dis 10:95, 1984

221. Pachman LM, Friedman JM, Maryjowski-Sweeney ML et al: Immunogenetic studies of juvenile dermatomyositis. III: Study of antibody to organ-specific and nuclear antigens. Arthritis Rheum 28:151, 1985

222. Pachman LM: Juvenile dermatomyositis. Pediatr Clin North Am 33:1097, 1986

223. Nishikai M, Reichlin M: Heterogeneity of precipitating antibodies in polymyositis and dermatomyositis. Characterization of the Jo-1 antibody system. Arthritis Rheum 23:881, 1980

224. Nishikai M, Reichlin M: Purification and characterization of a nuclear non-histone basic protein (Mi-1) which reacts with anti-immunoglobulin sera and the sera of patients with dermatomyositis. Mol Immunol 17:1129, 1980

225. Reichlin M, Mattioli M: Description of a serological reaction characteristic of polymyositis. Clin Immunol Immunopathol 5:12, 1976

226. Mimori T, Akizuki M, Yamagata H et al: Characterization of a high molecular weight acidic nuclear protein recognized by autoantibodies in sera from patients with polymyositis-scleroderma overlap. J Clin Invest 68:611, 1981

227. Stern GM, Rose AL, Jacobs K: Circulating antibodies in polymyositis. J Neurol Sci 5:181, 1967

228. Behan WMH, Behan PO: Complement abnormalities in polymyositis. J Neurol Sci 34:241, 1977

229. Scott JP, Arroyave C: Activation of complement and coagulation in juvenile dermatomyositis. Arthritis Rheum 30:572, 1987

230. Caspary EA, Gubbay SS, Stern GM: Circulating antibodies in polymyositis and other muscle-wasting disorders. Lancet 2:941, 1964

231. Zweig MH, Adornato B, Van Steirteghem AC et al: Serum creatine kinase BB and MM concentrations determined by radioimmunoassay in neuromuscular disorders. Ann Neurol 7:324, 1980

232. Mechler F: Changing electromyographic findings during the chronic course of polymyositis. J Neurol Sci 23:237, 1974

233. Haridasan G, Sanghvi SH, Jindal GD et al: Quantitative electromyography using automatic analysis. A comparative study with a fixed fraction of a subject's

maximum effort and two levels of thresholds for analysis. J Neurol Sci 42:53, 1979

234. Sandstedt PE, Henriksson KG, Larrsson LE: Quantitative electromyography in polymyositis and dermatomyositis. Acta Neurol Scand 65:110, 1982

235. Partanen J, Lang H: EMG dynamics in polymyositis. A quantitative single motor unit potential study. J Neurol Sci 57:221, 1982

236. Smyth DP: Quantitative electromyography in babies and young children with primary muscle disease and neurogenic lesions. J Neurol Sci 56:199, 1982

237. Brown M, Swift TR, Spies SM: Radioisotope scanning in inflammatory muscle disease. Neurology 26:517, 1976

238. Guillet GY, Guillet J, Blanquet P et al: A new non-invasive evaluation of muscular lesions in dermatomyositis: thallium 201 muscle scans. J Am Acad Dermatol 5:670, 1981

239. Guillet J, Blanquet P, Guillet G et al: The use of technetium Tc 99m medronate scintigraphy as a prognostic guide in childhood dermatomyositis (letter). Arch Dermatol 117:451, 1981

240. Yonker RA, Webster EM, Edwards NL et al: Technetium pyrophosphate muscle scans in inflammatory muscle disease. Br J Rheumatol 26:267, 1987

241. Smith WP, Robinson RG, Gobuty AH: Positive whole-body ^{67}Ga scintigraphy in dermatomyositis. Am J Roentgenol 133:126, 1979

242. Steiner RM, Glassman L, Schwartz MW et al: The radiological findings in dermatomyositis of childhood. Radiology 111:385, 1974

243. Ozonoff MB, Flynn FJ: Roentgenologic features of dermatomyositis of childhood. Am J Roentgenol 118:206, 1973

244. Fishel B, Diamant S, Papo I et al: CT assessment of calcinosis in a patient with dermatomyositis. Clin Rheumatol 5:242, 1986

245. Kaufman LD, Gruber BL, Gerstman DP et al: Preliminary observations on the role of magnetic resonance imaging for polymyositis and dermatomyositis. Ann Rheum Dis 46:569, 1987

246. Dubowitz V: Treatment of dermatomyositis in childhood. Arch Dis Child 51:494, 1976

247. Winkelmann RK: Dermatomyositis in childhood. Clin Rheum Dis 8:353, 1982

248. Ansell BM: Management of polymyositis and dermatomyositis. Clin Rheum Dis 10:205, 1984

249. Cassidy JT: Dermatomyositis in children. In Hicks RV (ed): Vasculopathies of Childhood. PSG Publishing Co, Littleton, 1988, p. 205.

250. Resnick JS, Mammel M, Mundale MO et al: Muscular strength as an index response to therapy in childhood dermatomyositis. Arch Phys Med Rehabil 62:12, 1981

251. National Foundation: Publication No. 60, 1946

252. Woo TY, Callen JP, Voorhees JJ et al: Cutaneous lesions of dermatomyositis are improved by hydroxychloroquine. J Am Acad Dermatol 10:592, 1984

253. Wilsher ML, Holdaway IM, North JD: Hypercalcaemia during resolution of calcinosis in juvenile dermatomyositis. Br Med J 288:1345, 1984

254. Lian JB, Pachman LM, Gundberg CM et al: Gamma-carboxyglutamate excretion and calcinosis in juvenile dermatomyostitis. Arthritis Rheum 25:1094, 1982

255. Ames EL, Posch JL: Calcinosis of the flexor and extensor tendons in dermatomyositis—case report. J Hand Surg 9:876, 1984

256. Nassin JR, Connolly CK: Treatment of calcinosis universalis with aluminum hydroxide. Arch Dis Child 45:118, 1970

257. Taborn J, Bole GG, Thompson GR: Colchicine suppression of local and systemic inflammation due to calcinosis universalis in chronic dermatomyositis. Ann Intern Med 89:648, 1978

258. Fuchs D, Fruchter L, Fishel B et al: Colchicine suppression of local inflammation due to calcinosis in dermatomyositis and progressive systemic sclerosis. Clin Rheumatol 5:527, 1986

259. Skuterud E, Sydnes OA, Haavik TK: Calcinosis in dermatomyositis treated with probenecid. Scand J Rheumatol 10:92, 1981

260. Dent CE, Stamp TCB: Treatment of calcinosis circumscripta with probenecid. Br Med J 1:216, 1972

261. Uttley WS, Belton NR, Syme J et al: Calcium balance in children treated with diphosphonates. Arch Dis Child 50:187, 1975

262. Herd JK, Vaughan JH: Calcinosis universalis complicating dermatomyositis—its treatment with Na_2EDTA. Report of two cases in children. Arthritis Rheum 7:259, 1964

263. Weinstein RS: Focal mineralization defect during disodium etidronate treatment of calcinosis. Calcif Tissue Int 34:224, 1982

264. Metzger AL, Singer FR, Bluestone R et al: Failure of disodium etidronate in calcinosis due to dermatomyositis and scleroderma. N Engl J Med 291:1294, 1974

265. Miller G, Heckmatt JZ, Dubowitz V: Drug treatment of juvenile dermatomyositis. Arch Dis Child 58:445, 1983

266. Shearin JC, Pickrell K: Surgical treatment of subcutaneous calcifications of polymyositis or dermatomyositis. Ann Plast Surg 5:381, 1980

267. Miller JJ, III: Prolonged use of large intravenous steroid pulses in the rheumatic diseases of children. Pediatrics 65:989, 1980

268. Yanagisawa T, Sueishi M, Nawata Y et al: Methyl-

prednisolone pulse therapy in dermatomyositis. Dermatologica 167:47, 1983

269. Wollina U, Schreiber G: Prednisolone pulse therapy for childhood systemic lupus erythematosus with prominent dermatomyositis. A case report. Dermatologica 171:45, 1985

270. Laxer RM, Stein LD, Petty RE: Intravenous pulse methylprednisolone treatment of juvenile dermatomyositis. Arthritis Rheum 30:328, 1987

271. Haas DC: Treatment of polymyositis with immunosuppressive drugs. Neurol 23:55, 1973

272. Niakan E, Pitner SE, Whitaker JN et al: Immunosuppressive agents in corticosteroid-refractory childhood dermatomyositis. Neurology 30:286, 1980

273. Hollingworth P, de Vere Tyndall A, Ansell BM et al: Intensive immunosuppression versus prednisolone in the treatment of connective tissue diseases. Ann Rheum Dis 41:557, 1982

274. Malyaviya AN, Many A, Schwartz RS: Treatment of dermatomyositis with methotrexate. Lancet 2:485, 1968

275. Sokoloff M, Goldberg LS, Pearson CM: Treatment of corticosteroid-resistant polymyositis with methotrexate. Lancet 1:14, 1971

276. Metzger AL, Bohan A, Goldberg LS et al: Polymyositis and dermatomyositis: combined methotrexate and corticosteroid therapy. Ann Intern Med 81:182, 1974

277. Fischer TJ, Rachelelfsky GS, Klein RB et al: Childhood dermatomyositis and polymyositis. Treatment with methotrexate and prednisone. Am J Dis Child 133:386, 1979

278. Benson MD, Aldo MA: Azathioprine therapy in polymyositis. Arch Intern Med 132:547, 1973

279. Jacobs JC: Methotrexate and azathioprine treatment of childhood dermatomyositis. Pediatrics 59:212, 1977

280. Brewer EJ, Jr, Giannini EH, Rossen RD et al: Plasma exchange therapy of a childhood onset dermatomyositis patient. Arthritis Rheum 23:509, 1980

281. Singsen BH: Plasmapheresis: a pediatric perspective. J Pediatr 98:232, 1981

282. Anderson L, Ziter FA: Plasmapheresis via central catheter in dermatomyositis: a new method for selected pediatric patients. J Pediatr 98:240, 1981

283. Dau PC, Bennington JL: Plasmapheresis in childhood dermatomyositis. J Pediatr 98:237, 1981

284. Dau PC: Plasmapheresis in idiopathic inflammatory myopathy. Experience with 35 patients. Arch Neurol 38:544, 1981

285. Hochberg MC, Lopez-Acuna D, Gittelsohn AM: Mortality from polymyositis and dermatomyositis in the United States, 1968–1978. Arthritis Rheum 26:1465, 1983

286. Taieb A, Guichard C, Salamon R et al: Prognosis in juvenile dermatopolymyositis: a cooperative retrospective study of 70 cases. Pediatr Dermatol 2:275, 1985

287. Miller LC, Michael AF, Kim Y: Childhood dermatomyositis. Clinical course and long-term follow-up. Clin Pediatr 26:561, 1987

288. Miller JJ, III: Late progression in dermatomyositis in childhood. J Pediatr 83:543, 1973

289. Lovell HB, Lindsley CB: Late recurrence of childhood dermatomyositis. J Rheumatol 13:821, 1986

290. Miller JJ, III, Koehler JP: Persistance of activity in dermatomyositis of childhood. Arthritis Rheum 20:332, 1977

291. Barnes AB, Link DA: Childhood dermatomyositis and pregnancy. Am J Obstet Gynecol 146:335, 1983

292. Gutierrez G, Dagnino R, Mintz G: Polymyositis/dermatomyositis and pregnancy. Arthritis Rheum 27:291, 1984

293. Chalmers SA, Sayson R, Walters K: Juvenile dermatomyositis: medical, social and economic status in adulthood. Can Med Assoc J 126:31, 1982

294. Spencer CH, Hanson V, Singsen BH et al: Course of treated juvenile dermatomyositis. J Pediatr 105:399, 1984

9

Vasculitis

CLASSIFICATION AND DEFINITIONS

There have been many attempts to provide a consistent and comprehensive classification of the inflammatory vasculitides that takes into account both the clinical and the histopathologic features of the disease. Unfortunately, no classification is completely satisfactory. The term *polyangiitis overlap syndrome* has been suggested in recognition of the high frequency (40 percent) of patients who exhibit features of more than one distinct vasculitis syndrome.[1] Nonetheless, an attempt to classify vasculitis serves to emphasize the complexity of the subject and the heterogeneity of the clinical spectrum of these diseases.

Table 9-1 presents a classification that accommodates the most significant histopathologic and clinical findings. This schema is based in part upon the early study by Zeek[2] and later reports that have suggested certain unique clinical findings that justify further subdivision of these disorders.[2,3] A summary of the pathologic characteristics of the clinical syndromes is provided in Table 9-2. The type of pathologic change, site of involvement, size of vessel, and systemic extent of the vascular injury determine the clinical expression of the disease and its severity.

POLYARTERITIS

A number of clinical syndromes that are characterized pathologically by the presence of fibrinoid necrosis of small- and medium-sized muscular arteries are grouped together as polyarteritis.

Polyarteritis Nodosa

The classic form of polyarteritis was initially described over 100 years ago as periarteritis nodosa by Kussmaul and Maier.[4] They identified the pathologic features of necrotizing arteritis with the formation of nodules along the walls of small- and medium-sized muscular arteries.

EPIDEMIOLOGY

The disease is rare in childhood, and the diagnosis in reported cases is sometimes uncertain. In addition, infantile polyarteritis nodosa (IPN), which we now view as a severe manifestation of Kawasaki disease (KD), was usually included in early reviews of the subject. For these reasons, the discussion in this chapter will focus on more recent studies,[5-10] but the interested reader is referred to the early reviews of Fager et al.[11] and Frohnert and Sheps.[12] Reimold et al.[5] estimate that fewer than 150 cases of polyarteritis nodosa (PAN) in infants and children had been reported up to 1976. Since that time there have been several small series.[6-10] This disease occurs with equal frequency in boys and girls and has a peak age at onset between 9 and 11 years of age (Fig. 9-1).

Table 9-1 A Classification of Primary Systemic Vasculitis in Children

Polyarteritis
    Classical polyarteritis nodosa (Kussmaul-Maier disease)
    Cutaneous polyarteritis
    Cogan's syndrome
    Kawasaki disease, including infantile polyarteritis nodosa

Leukocytoclastic vasculitis
    Anaphylactoid purpura (Henoch-Schönlein)
    Hypersensitivity vasculitis (Zeek)
    Hypocomplementemic urticarial vasculitis
    Cryoglobulinemic vasculitis

Granulomatous vasculitis
    Allergic granulomatosis (Churg-Strauss syndrome)
    Wegener's granulomatosis
    Lymphomatoid granulomatosis
    Primary angiitis of the central nervous system

Giant cell arteritis
    Takayasu's arteritis
    Temporal arteritis

Other vasculitides
    Behçet disease
    Mucha-Habermann disease
    Kohlmeir-Degos syndrome
    Soter syndrome

CLINICAL MANIFESTATIONS

The insidious onset of unexplained fever and weight loss in the presence of an elevated erythrocyte sedimentation rate (ESR) should suggest the diag-

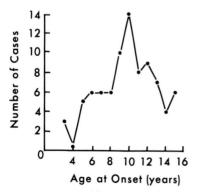

Fig. 9-1 Age at onset of polyarteritis nodosa. (Data obtained from review of published series.)

nosis of polyarteritis, in addition to diseases such as inflammatory bowel disease and malignancy. No single pattern of clinical presentation characterizes this disease, but abdominal pain, central or peripheral nervous system disease, arthritis, myalgia, and skin lesions occur in most children at some time during the course of the illness (Table 9-3). Abdominal pain may simulate that of a surgical abdomen, and biopsy specimens removed at exploratory celiotomy or appendectomy may yield the correct diagnosis. Central nervous system involvement ultimately develops in 50 to 70 percent of children. Clinical findings include organic psychosis, focal neurologic defects, unilateral blindness, seizures, and hemiparesis. A severe sensorimotor peripheral neuropathy (mononeuritis multiplex) may occur. Disabling arthralgias and myalgias may suggest another rheumatic or musculoskeletal disorder. Secondary hypertrophic osteoarthropathy is a rare cause of musculoskeletal pain in polyarteritis nodosa.[13] Cutaneous involvement includes purpura, edema, peripheral gangrene, and nodular vasculitis (Figs. 9-2, 9-3, and 9-4). A multiplicity of other signs, including testicular or epididymal swelling, pain or tenderness, or serous otitis media, rarely occur. As might be anticipated, children often have signs of primary renal disease or renovascular hypertension.

LABORATORY STUDIES

Anemia, leukocytosis, marked elevation of the erythrocyte sedimentation rate (ESR), C-reactive protein (CRP), and serum immunoglobulins, together with urinary sediment changes are frequent (Table 9-4). Rheumatoid factor (RF) and antinuclear antibody (ANA) are seldom detected. Hepatitis B antigen or a history of intravenous drug use may be present in a few persons with the onset of classic polyarteritis,[14] but this association is rare in children. Levels of factor VIII–related antigen[15] and beta thromboglobulin[16] reflect the activity of the vascular inflammation and may be useful in following the effects of treatment. Electrocardiography may reveal the ischemic effects of coronary arteritis. Demonstration by angiography of small aneurysms involving the renal, celiac, or coronary arteries is highly suggestive of this type of vasculitis[17,18] (Fig. 9-5).

The histopathologic diagnosis depends on identification of fibrinoid necrosis of the entire thickness of the walls of the medium and small muscular ar-

Table 9-2 Clinical and Pathologic Characteristics of Some of the Vasculitides in Childhood

Syndrome	Frequency	Vessels Affected	Characteristic Pathology
Polyarteritis			
PAN	Rare	Small- and medium-sized muscular arteries	Segmental (often near bifurcations), fibrinoid necrosis, GI, renal, muscular artery aneurysms; lesions at various stages
KD	Common	Coronary and other muscular arteries	Thrombosis, fibrosis, aneurysms
IPN	Rare	Coronary and other muscular arteries	Thrombosis, fibrosis, aneurysms
Leukocytoclastic vasculitis			
HSP	Common	Venules, arterioles, capillaries	Skin, kidney, GI tract
Serum sickness	Rare	Venules, arterioles, capillaries	Widespread; necrosis at same stage
Granulomatous vasculitis			
Churg-Strauss	Very rare	Medium and small muscular arteries	Granulomata, lung involvement; allergic history, eosinophilia
Wegener	Rare	Small veins, small and medium arterioles	Upper and lower respiratory tract, glomerulonephritis
Giant cell arteritis			
Takayasu's	Uncommon	Medium and large arteries	Giant cell arteritis aortic arch, branches
Temporal	Very rare	Medium and large arteries	Giant cell arteritis carotid, branches

Table 9-3 Polyarteritis Nodosa in Childhood: Clinical Characteristics

	Blau[6] $n = 11$	Fink[7] $n = 7$	Reimold[5] $n = 3$	Ettlinger[10] $n = 7^a$	Magilavy[9] $n = 8^b$	Total $n = 36$
Fever	10	6	3	7	8	94%
Hypertension	11	7	3	4	5	83%
Abdominal pain	10	4	2	6	2	67%
Arthritis	8	3	3	3	6	64%
Myalgia	7	4	1	0	7	53%
Skin						
Petechiae	6	5	3	0	0	39%
Rashes	0	7	3	6	5	58%
Edema	0	7	3	6	0	44%
Mucous membranes	0	0	0	7	0	19%
CNS						
Seizures	1	7	3	3	0	39%
Other	2	0	1	1	3	19%
Cardiac	0	4	1	6	5	44%
Respiratory	0	0	1	4	0	14%
Cervical nodes	0	0	0	3	0	8%
Splenomegaly	0	0	0	2	0	6%

[a] Excludes two infants.
[b] Excludes one patient with Churg-Strauss granulomatous arteritis.

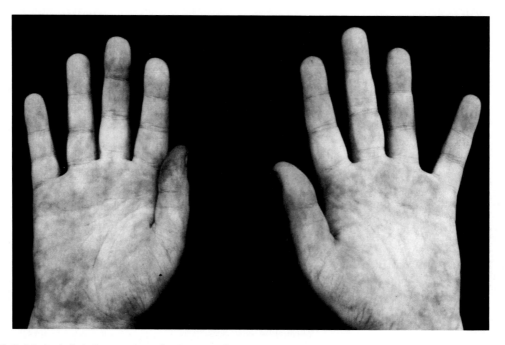

Fig. 9-2 Marked digital cyanosis and pain were characteristics of acute polyarteritis nodosa in this 9-year-old boy. Although muscle and kidney involvement were present, he made a complete recovery over a 5-year period of follow-up.

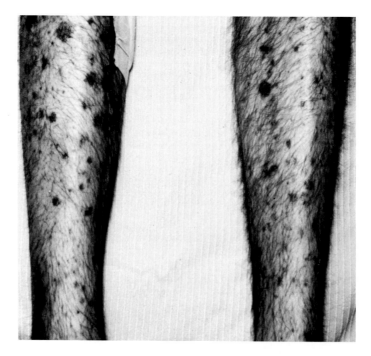

Fig. 9-3 Vascular purpura in a teenage boy with polyarteritis nodosa. Each lesion was nearly round, raised, and tender.

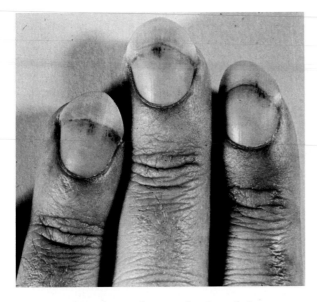

Fig. 9-4 Splinter hemorrhages under the nails in a teenage girl with polyarteritis nodosa.

teries (necrotizing vasculitis) (Figs. 9-6 to 9-8). The lesions tend to be segmental with a predilection for bifurcations of the vessels. Biopsy specimens show vasculitis in all stages of development, from acute to chronic, interspersed with areas of normal vessel wall.

TREATMENT

Corticosteroid therapy is indicated in most cases. Initial reports of the effectiveness of these agents were discouraging. More recent clinical studies have sug-

gested that suppressive doses of prednisone (1 to 2 mg/kg/day) or its equivalent can improve the life expectancy and decrease the frequency of hypertension and renal involvement.[19] Confusion regarding the effectiveness of corticosteroid therapy has resulted in part from failure to distinguish among the several forms of polyarteritis when reporting therapeutic responsiveness. There has been concern that corticosteroids could suppress the inflammatory vasculitis without allowing coincident wound healing with the resultant formation of aneurysms, or that rapid healing of the vascular lesion could lead to occlusion and peripheral anoxia or necrosis of tissue. Direct evidence that these potential effects of corticosteroids actually affect outcome in PAN is lacking, although the apparently deleterious effect of corticosteroids in patients with Kawasaki disease suggests continued caution. (See later discussion.) Cytotoxic drugs, especially cyclophosphamide (2 mg/kg/day) or azathioprine (2 mg/kg/day) by mouth, may be useful if corticosteroids fail.[20] Intravenous cyclophosphamide may be indicated in the more severe forms of the disease with involvement of the celiac and mesenteric vessels.

PROGNOSIS

The reported outcome of children with polyarteritis nodosa varies a great deal. This reflects not only improvement in prognosis with improved treatment but also, apparently, differences in the severity of the disease recognized in different series. It is difficult to rationalize these differences, but important to bear them in mind when considering any individual child.

Table 9-4 Polyarteritis in Childhood: Laboratory Abnormalities

Abnormality	Blau[6] $n = 11$	Fink[7] $n = 7$	Reimold[5] $n = 3$	Ettlinger[10] $n = 7$	Magilavy[9] $n = 8$	Total
Elevated ESR	—[a]	—	2	3	8	72%
Elevated CRP	—	—	—	—	7	88%
Leukocytosis	11	6	3	6	7	92%
Anemia	9	6	2	—	1	62%
Proteinuria	7	6	2	7	0	61%
Hematuria	8	6	2	5	2	64%
↑ BUN, Cr	6	6	2	4	1	53%
ANA present	—	—	—	—	2	25%
RF present	—	—	—	—	0	0

[a] Information not provided.

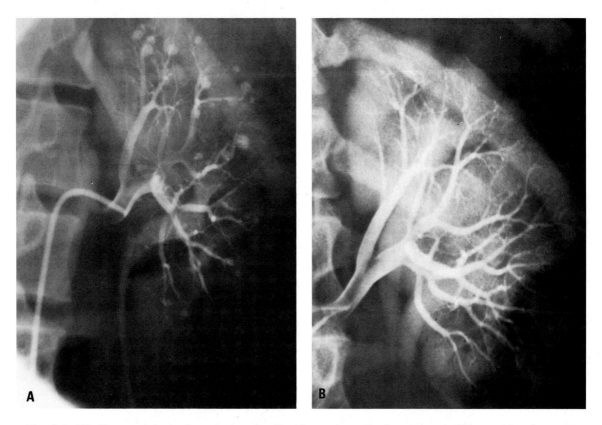

Fig. 9-5 (**A**) Characteristic renal aneurysms visualized by angiography in a 15-year-old boy with polyarteritis nodosa who presented with hypertension, myocardial infarction, and hematuria. (**B**) These lesions eventually disappeared as shown on this repeat angiogram some years after a successful course of prednisone therapy.

In one study,[9] nine children with polyarteritis had a syndrome characterized by fever, calf pain, subcutaneous nodules, elevated acute phase reactants, and multisystem vasculitis demonstrated by biopsy or arteriography. These children, most of whom had polyarteritis nodosa, were followed for a mean of 4 years and were all treated with high-dose prednisone (approximately 2 mg/kg/day orally); although serious complications (myocardial infarction, systemic hypertension, impaired renal function) had occurred, the course was a chronic one with no mortality. In contrast, the report of Fink described eight children with polyarteritis seen between 1959 and 1974, with severe hypertension, seizures, renal failure, and, in three, death.[7]

Cutaneous Polyarteritis

Although the cutaneous polyarteritis syndrome is usually primarily restricted to the skin,[21–23] evidence of systemic vasculitis should be sought. Painful, violaceous, palpable nodules or ridges of variable size develop along the course of the arterioles. Some lesions may ulcerate. The patient is usually otherwise well, although mild constitutional symptoms and acute arthritis of weight-bearing joints may occur (Fig. 9-9). The clinical course is variable and characterized by remissions and exacerbations that make evaluation of the efficacy of treatment difficult. Each crop of lesions may respond to corticosteroid drugs, or even to acetysalicylic acid, and then recur as the dose is lowered. The outcome is usually satisfactory, and the prognosis benign, although recurrences are frequent. The differential diagnosis includes livedo reticularis, panniculitis, lupus profundus, erythema nodosum, and multicentric histiocytosis. Isolated rheumatoid nodules are not tender and are usually more restricted in size and location.

Cogan's Syndrome

Nonsyphilitic interstitial keratitis with vestibuloauditory dysfunction (Cogan's syndrome)[24] is a rare syndrome that most frequently affects young adults of either sex and has been reported in only three children.[25,26] In addition to pho-

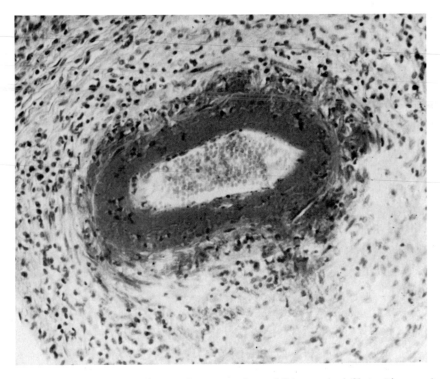

Fig. 9-6 This biopsy shows a medium-sized muscular artery that exhibits marked fibrinoid necrosis of the vessel wall. This lesion is characteristic of polyarteritis nodosa.

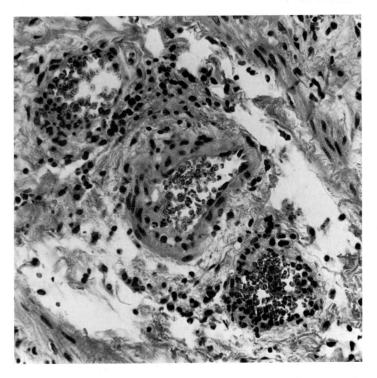

Fig. 9-7 Muscle biopsy specimen from a 6-year-old boy with polyarteritis nodosa. Vasculitis with marked mixed cellular infiltration is seen in and around the walls of arterioles and venules. Fibrinoid necrosis of the arterioles is seen.

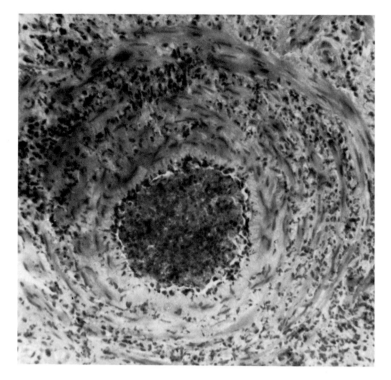

Fig. 9-8 Infiltration of mononuclear cells around the central arteriole which is surrounded by a dense fibrous scar. The lumen is occluded by a dense thrombus.

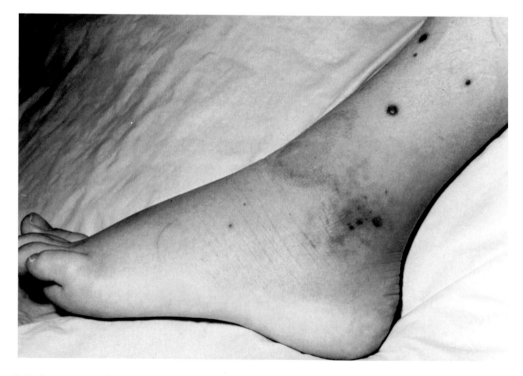

Fig. 9-9 Cutaneous polyarteritis. Acute arthritis involving the ankle and tarsometatarsal joints and vascular necrotic purpura in a 5-year-old girl.

tophobia, vertigo, and hearing loss, patients with Cogan's syndrome have evidence of widespread vasculitis,[25] including aortitis and aortic valve insufficiency. Treatment with corticosteroids is beneficial, although the hearing loss may be persistent.

Kawasaki Disease and Infantile Polyarteritis Nodosa

It now appears certain that what was formerly identified as infantile polyarteritis nodosa is a severe manifestation of a much more common disorder, Kawasaki disease. In a review of published cases of infantile polyarteritis in 1959, Monro-Faure identified a systemic clinical syndrome that characterized infants who died with infantile polyarteritis: fleeting macular skin eruption, fever, conjunctivitis, pharyngitis, cervical adenitis, and occasionally other signs or symptoms.[27] The importance of this observation was largely unrecognized until the publication by Kawasaki et al.[28,29] of a large series of children with a similar syndrome that was initially called *mucocutaneous lymph node syndrome* and is now known as Kawasaki disease.

DEFINITIONS AND CLASSIFICATION

Kawasaki disease (including the most severe manifestation, IPN) is a necrotizing arteritis of small- and medium-sized arteries that has the clinical characteristics listed in Table 9-5.[30]

EPIDEMIOLOGY

Kawasaki disease is the most common vasculitis of childhood and may well be the most common vasculitis at any age. There have been in excess of 50,000 documented cases in Japan alone.[31] A minimum annual incidence of 5.95 per 100,000 children less than 5 years old has been estimated for the metropolitan Chicago area in the United States.[32] Higher frequencies were found in younger children, boys, and children of Asian racial origin.

The mean age at onset is approximately 1.5 years, and the male:female ratio is 1.5:1. Although the disease is much more common in children of Japanese descent, it has now been recognized worldwide. The mean age at onset is somewhat higher in North America, and disease ascribed to acute KD has been reported in a few adults.[30]

A tentative association with the human leukocyte antigen (HLA) complex Bw22J2 has been made in Japan, but not in the United States.[33–35] Harada et al. have documented concordance for KD of 14.1 percent in monozygous twins and 13.3 percent in dizygotic twins in Japan.[36] They also examined HLA-A, -B, -C and -DR haplotypes in 63 members of 23 families in which 2 siblings had KD. No HLA associations were noted. Therefore, the role played by a genetic predisposition to KD is not certain but does not appear to be significant, at least in the Japanese population.

An infectious etiology is suspected, largely on the basis of the clinical presentation and the occurrence

Table 9-5 Kawasaki Disease: Frequency and Characteristics of Diagnostic Criteria[a]

1. Fever (100%)	Duration of 5 days or more
2. Conjunctivitis (85%)	Bilateral, bulbar, nonsuppurative
3. Lymph node enlargement (70%)	Cervical, nonpurulent, >1.5 cm
4. Rash (80%)	Polymorphous, no vesicles or crusts
5. Changes of lips or mucosa (90%)	Dry, red, vertically fissured lips "Strawberry" tongue Diffuse erythema of oropharynx
6. Changes of extremities (70%)	Erythema of palms or soles Indurative edema of hands or feet Desquamation of tips of fingers

[a] Diagnosis: Five of the six criteria are required for diagnosis. One of the three findings listed under (5) and (6) is sufficient to establish these criteria.
(Recommendations of the Japan Mucocutaneous Lymph Node Syndrome Research Committee 1984. From Sekiguchi et al.,[30] with permission.)

of clusters of cases grouped in time and geographical location.[37-39] There have been considerable differences in reports of seasonal variation in the occurrence of KD, but in North America most epidemics have occurred between February and May.[37] Cases occurring in Hawaii have shown some clustering in time and geographic area, suggesting an unrecognized vector, although cases among siblings or other children sharing the same home are uncommon.[38] Possible associations with mercury poisoning,[40] exposure to rug shampoo,[41] and rotavirus infection[42] have not been substantiated.

CLINICAL MANIFESTATIONS

The criteria for the diagnosis of KD are shown in Table 9-5. Other clinical characteristics are listed in Table 9-6. The disease usually begins acutely and may be divided into three phases (Fig. 9-10): (1) an acute febrile period of approximately 10 days; (2) a subacute period of approximately 2 to 4 weeks, ending with a return to normal of the platelet count; and (3) a recovery period lasting months, during which coronary artery disease may first be noted. A remittent

Table 9-6 Other Clinical Findings in Kawasaki Disease

Relatively common abnormalities
  Arthralgia/arthritis
  Meningitis
  Pneumonitis
  Anterior uveitis with photophobia
  Gastroenteritis
  Meatitis and dysuria
  Otitis

Relatively uncommon abnormalities
  Hydrops of the gallbladder
  Gastrointestinal ischemia
  Jaundice
  Central nervous system disease
    Febrile convulsions
    Encephalopathy or ataxia
  Cardiac disease
    Coronary thrombosis or aneurysms
    Cardiac tamponade
    Cardiac failure
    Myocarditis
    Pericarditis
  Petechial rash

fever, often up to 40°C or even higher, is characteristic. The fever is unresponsive to antibiotics but responds partially to antipyretics. This phase lasts from 5 to 25 days, usually approximately 10 days. Febrile seizures in such children must be distinguished from other evidence of central nervous system (CNS) involvement.

The rash is characteristically on the trunk and is polymorphous and variable over time. Scarlatinaform, macular, papular, multiform, and purpuric lesions have all been described. It is neither vesicular nor bullous, however, and crusting of the lesions does not occur. It does not appear to be pruritic. The rash usually accompanies the fever throughout the entire acute period of the disease and disappears thereafter (Fig. 9-11).

Changes in the peripheral extremities include reddish purple erythema of the palms and soles that is often accompanied by brawny edema of the dorsa of the hands and feet. A characteristic desquamation of the skin beginning at the nail margins of the fingers and toes follows and extends proximally to the PIP joints and sometimes involves the skin of the entire palm or sole (Fig. 9-12). Fine desquamation also occurs in the perineum. These cutaneous reactions are most commonly seen during the third week of the illness and may last for several weeks.

Mucous membrane changes include erythema of the lips and oropharynx, sometimes with a "strawberry" tongue. The most suggestive change is the bright red swollen lip with vertical cracking and bleeding (Fig. 9-13). Injection of the bulbar conjunctivae without purulent exudate or prominent involvement of the palpebral conjunctivae is also highly characteristic. The oral changes last throughout the febrile period, although the conjunctivitis may persist somewhat longer.

Lymphadenopathy, characteristically of the anterior cervical chain, is usually unilateral and may only involve a single node. The enlargement, which develops in the initial febrile period of the disease, may be quite marked, but of brief duration.

In addition to the classic diagnostic features described, a number of other clinical signs and symptoms frequently contribute to the overall manifestations of the disease (Table 9-6). Cough, coryza, or hoarseness early in the course of the disease suggests a viral upper respiratory tract infection. Such symptoms are usually mild and transient and are only oc-

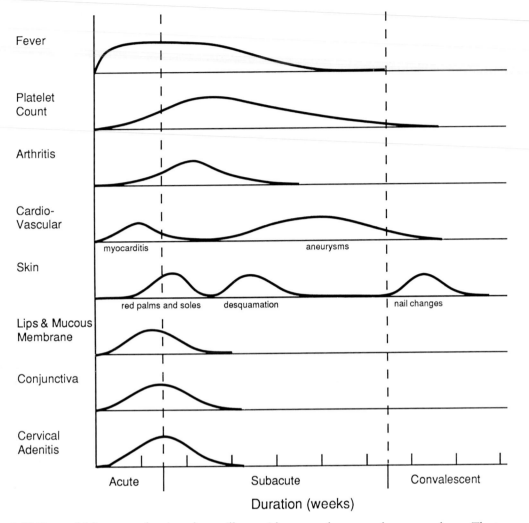

Fever

Platelet Count

Arthritis

Cardio-Vascular

myocarditis   aneurysms

Skin

red palms and soles   desquamation   nail changes

Lips & Mucous Membrane

Conjunctiva

Cervical Adenitis

Acute   Subacute   Convalescent

Duration (weeks)

Fig. 9-10 Kawasaki disease can be viewed as an illness with acute, subacute, and recovery phases. The temporal characteristics outlined in this figure are characteristic of the course of this disease.

casionally accompanied by pulmonary infiltrate or otitis media. Profuse, watery diarrhea occurs in up to one-quarter of children during the acute febrile phase and may be associated with severe abdominal pain that may represent mesenteric vasculitis or intussusception similar to that observed in children with anaphylactoid purpura. Hydrops of the gallbladder presenting as a painless abdominal mass has been described in a number of children and can be diagnosed by ultrasonography.[43] Central nervous system involvement is common, and extreme irritability is almost universally observed in children with KD. Rarely, CNS vasculitis causes focal neurologic lesions.[44,45]

Arthritis generally appears in the child during the recovery period and most commonly affects the large weight-bearing joints. It was described in approximately one-quarter of the children from Hawaii as an oligoarthritis involving the knees, ankles, or hips. Involvement of the PIP joints was much less common and was often difficult to differentiate from edema of the digits. The synovial fluid has been described as inflammatory.[46]

Cardiac disease is the most serious manifestation of KD.[47–52] Almost all of the early deaths and most of the long-term disability are related to involvement of the heart. Clinically, congestive heart failure may occur as a result of myocarditis or myocardial in-

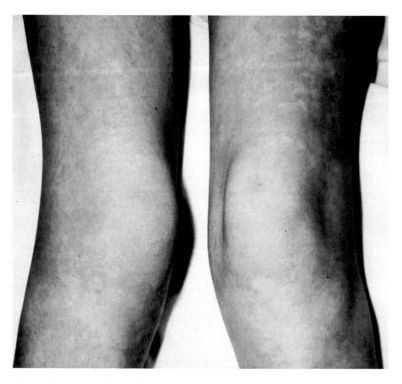

Fig. 9-11 The polymorphous exanthem of KD is shown in this photograph taken during the acute phase of the disease. It is not diagnostic in its appearance and may evolve in character as the disease progresses, although it is rarely purpuric and never has vesicles or crusts.

farction. Symptoms or signs of pericarditis (midsternal pain, muffled heart sounds, systolic murmurs or rubs) may occur, and there may be arrhythmias. Although coronary artery aneurysms require two-dimensional echocardiography or angiography for their detection (Fig. 9-14), aneurysms of other vessels, such as the brachial and femoral arteries, may be palpable clinically or demonstrated by angiography (Fig. 9-15). Left ventricular dysfunction may also be detected by echocardiography along with echodensity abnormalities that suggest vasculitis of the proximal segment of the coronary arteries.

The evolution of the cardiac lesions is documented in the study of Fujiwara et al.[49] In the coronary arteries, vasculitis predominated early but was absent in children who died after 28 days of illness. Aneurysms, thrombosis, and stenosis did not appear until 12 days of disease or later. Pericarditis, myocarditis, and endocarditis were universal early in disease, but diminished as fibrosis of the myocardium became the predominant lesion in children whose death occurred 40 or more days after the onset of the disease

(Table 9-9). The large study of Suzuki et al.[52] documents the location of the antiographic findings in 262 children. Aneurysms, dilatations, and local stenoses (that is, those associated with aneurysms) occurred with equal frequency in left and right coronary arteries; the right coronary artery was more frequently the site of segmental stenoses (89 percent) and occlusions (69 percent).

There have been several attempts to predict the degree of risk of the development of coronary artery disease in children with KD. This is increasingly important clinically because of the apparent benefit of intravenous gamma globulin in the prevention of aneurysm development and the high cost and potential risk of such treatment. The Asai score,[53] and modifications thereof (Table 9-7),[54,55] have been useful in retrospectively evaluating the efficacy of treatment, but their application to the treatment of any individual child has been extremely limited since optimal treatment should be implemented before many of the indicators of severe disease have become evident. Factors that may be of assistance in identifying the high-risk child include age under 1 year and male sex,[32,53] although these associations have not been confirmed in other studies.[54,55] White children were reported to have a higher risk of cor-

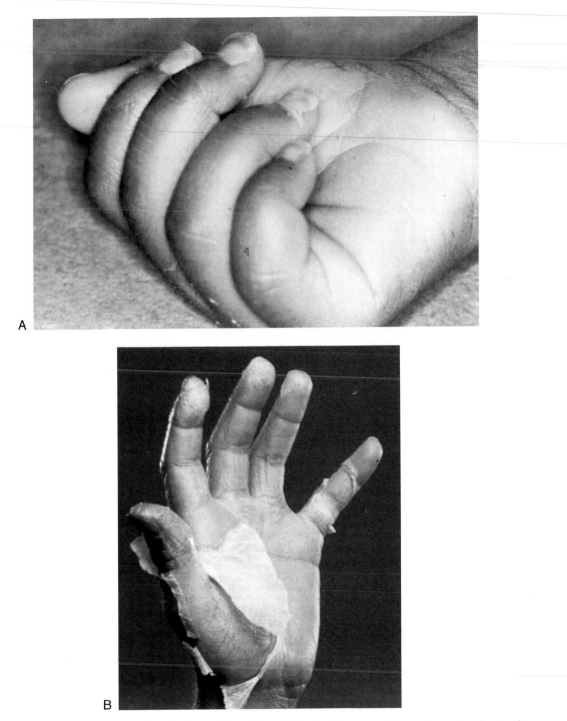

Fig. 9-12 (**A**) Edema of the hand and early pealing of the skin beginning around the nail margins during the subacute phase of KD. (**B**) Desquamation of the skin of the hand later in the subacute and early recovery phase of KD. In many children the degree of desquamation is much less than is depicted here.

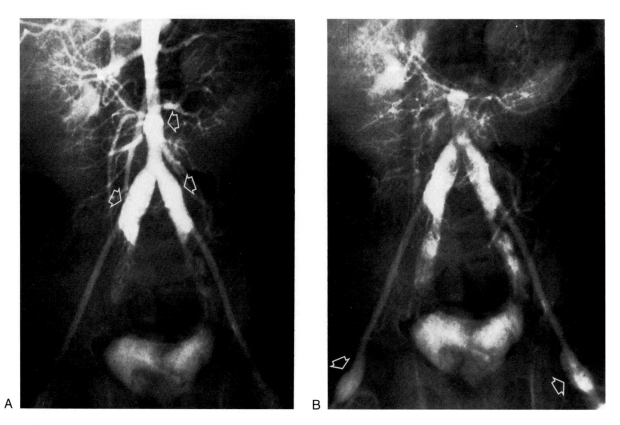

Fig. 9-15 Angiographic study of a 2-year-old boy with severe KD resulting in multiple aneurysms of the coronary, axillary, iliac, and femoral arteries. In this photograph large aneurysms of the (**A**) iliac and (**B**) femoral arteries are clearly seen. Aneurysms that were palpable in the axilla and groin in this patient later resolved. (Courtesy of Dr. G. Culham.)

other neurologic signs suggest the need for evaluation of the cerebrospinal fluid to rule out bacterial meningitis, although such symptoms are part of the picture of the acute disease. There may be early congestive heart failure secondary to myocarditis.

Table 9-8 Kawasaki Disease: Natural History of Coronary Artery Disease

	Percentage
All children with Kawasaki disease	100.0
Those with aneurysms	15.0
Aneurysms disappear	7.5
Abnormalities persist	7.5
Aneurysm	3.6
Stenosis	2.4
Irregularity	1.5

(Modified from Kato et al.,[56] with permission.)

Arrhythmias and evidence of myocardial ischemia should be repeatedly evaluated by electrocardiography. Follow-up two-dimensional echocardiography should be performed at 1 week, 6 weeks, and 3 months at a minimum, in order to detect aneurysm formation.

The treatment of KD is continuing to change as information regarding the effect of therapy on outcome accumulates. Current recommendations are outlined in Table 9-10. In contrast to other types of vasculitis, in which the mainstay of treatment is corticosteroids, these drugs should not be used to treat KD. Kato et al.[63] showed that children treated with prednisolone had the highest frequency of aneurysms (65 percent) and those treated only with aspirin had the lowest incidence (11 percent). Although this study can be criticized on many grounds, more recent studies have reached the same conclusion,[64] and, as a gen-

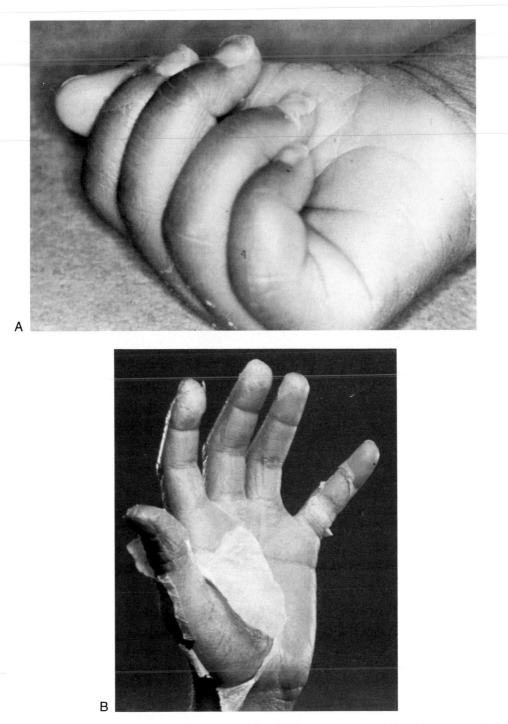

Fig. 9-12 (**A**) Edema of the hand and early peeling of the skin beginning around the nail margins during the subacute phase of KD. (**B**) Desquamation of the skin of the hand later in the subacute and early recovery phase of KD. In many children the degree of desquamation is much less than is depicted here.

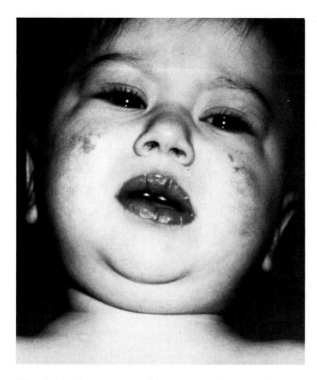

Fig. 9-13 The intense reddening, swelling, and vertical cracking of the lips is characteristic of KD. Bilateral bulbar conjunctivitis and a nonspecific facial rash are also seen in this 2-year-old boy with acute KD.

onary arteritis in one study.[32] Elevation of beta thromboglobulin[16] and early elevation of CRP and depression of platelet count[55] may also be of value in predicting the child at risk for coronary aneurysms.

It is important to consider the natural history of the coronary artery lesions when evaluating the effect of treatment or discussing prognosis with parents. An outline of the natural history of KD is provided in Tables 9-8 and 9-9.[56] Kato et al. showed that only 7.5 percent of children with KD who were treated with acetylsalicyclic acid and supportive care had a persisting coronary artery abnormality, most commonly an aneurysm. A less optimistic report found that only a minority of children with proven aneurysms had normal vessels 2 to 3 years later.[57] A recent report from the United States suggests that regression of aneurysms is more likely in girls and in infants under 1 year of age.[58] At the present time, as precise information on the course of the disease is still being

accumulated, caution should be exercised in declaring a child with KD to be entirely free of risk of late sequelae of this disease. Reports of myocardial infarction or death occurring years after KD have begun to emerge.[59,60] One lesson from these cases is the importance of recognizing a prior history of KD in an older child who is seen for a presport physical examination and obtaining the indicated cardiac evaluation (electrocardiogram [ECG], echocardiogram, and stress tests). KD is the most common cause of myocardial infarction in children.[61] Kato et al.[62] described post-KD myocardial infarction in 195 children, 141 of whom were boys. Myocardial infarction occurred within 3 months of the onset of KD in 39 percent, within 1 year in 72.8 percent, and between 1 and 7 years in 30 percent. Mortality rate after the first attack was 22 percent, after the second attack was 63 percent, and after the third attack was 83 percent. Overall mortality rate was 32 percent.

LABORATORY ABNORMALITIES

Indexes of inflammation (ESR, platelet count, white blood cell [WBC] count) are characteristically elevated early in the disease course. Although the platelet count may be low during the early acute phase of the illness, it almost always rises markedly during the second phase and may exceed 1 million per cubic millimeter (100×10^9 per liter). There may be moderate elevations of serum levels of muscle enzymes and mild anemia.

The ECG is useful in the initial workup to delineate

Table 9-7 Kawasaki Disease: Severity Score

	Score[a]		
	0	1	2
Age < 1 year	–	+	–
Sex	–	Male	–
Fever (days)	<14	14–15	>15
ESR (mm/h)	<60	60–100	>100
Elevated ESR (days)	–	–	>30
Hemoglobin < 100 g/L	–	+	–
Leukocyte count ($\times 10^9$/L)	<26	26–30	>30
Arrhythmia	–	–	+
Cardiothoracic ratio > 50%	–	+	–
Abnormal ECG findings	–	–	+

[a] Score of 6 or greater suggests increased risk of coronary aneurysms. (Adapted from Koren et al.,[54] with permission.)

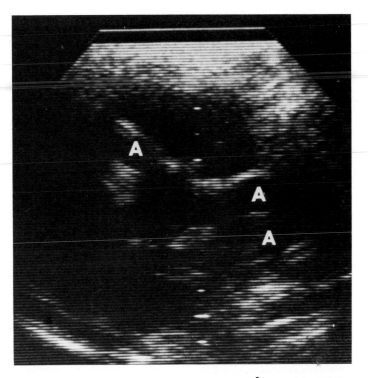

A = aneurysm

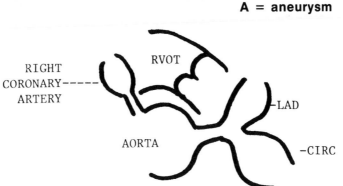

Fig. 9-14 Echocardiographic demonstration of aneurysms of the coronary arteries in a child with KD. *A,* aneurysm. (Courtesy of Dr. Dennis Crowley.)

gross abnormalities that indicate ventricular dysfunction, anoxia, or arrhythmia. Demonstration of aneurysms depends on two-dimensional echocardiography, which is effective in detecting aneurysms of >2 to 4 mm in the proximal coronary arteries (Fig. 9-14). Arteriography may be necessary to confirm the presence of aneurysms in other locations if this is clinically indicated (Fig. 9-15) or to demonstrate peripheral narrowing or occlusion of the coronary vessels.

TREATMENT OF KAWASAKI DISEASE

It is advisable to admit the child with KD to the hospital for observation, monitoring of cardiac status, and management of the multisystem manifestations of this disease. High fever (sometimes with febrile seizures), dehydration, electrolyte imbalance, and inappropriate antidiuretic hormone secretion may be associated problems. Extreme irritability or

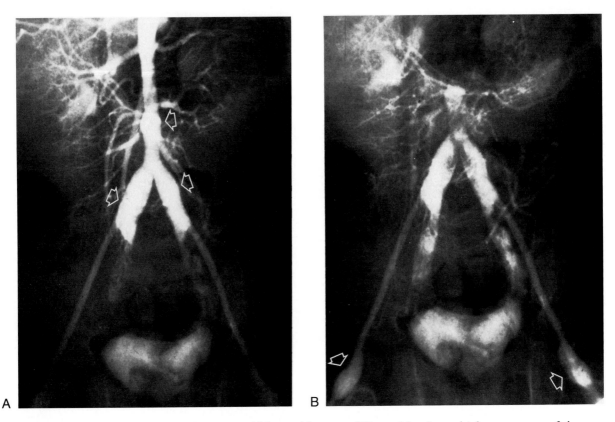

Fig. 9-15 Angiographic study of a 2-year-old boy with severe KD resulting in multiple aneurysms of the coronary, axillary, iliac, and femoral arteries. In this photograph large aneurysms of the (**A**) iliac and (**B**) femoral arteries are clearly seen. Aneurysms that were palpable in the axilla and groin in this patient later resolved. (Courtesy of Dr. G. Culham.)

other neurologic signs suggest the need for evaluation of the cerebrospinal fluid to rule out bacterial meningitis, although such symptoms are part of the picture of the acute disease. There may be early congestive heart failure secondary to myocarditis.

Table 9-8 Kawasaki Disease: Natural History of Coronary Artery Disease

	Percentage
All children with Kawasaki disease	100.0
Those with aneurysms	15.0
Aneurysms disappear	7.5
Abnormalities persist	7.5
Aneurysm	3.6
Stenosis	2.4
Irregularity	1.5

(Modified from Kato et al.,[56] with permission.)

Arrhythmias and evidence of myocardial ischemia should be repeatedly evaluated by electrocardiography. Follow-up two-dimensional echocardiography should be performed at 1 week, 6 weeks, and 3 months at a minimum, in order to detect aneurysm formation.

The treatment of KD is continuing to change as information regarding the effect of therapy on outcome accumulates. Current recommendations are outlined in Table 9-10. In contrast to other types of vasculitis, in which the mainstay of treatment is corticosteroids, these drugs should not be used to treat KD. Kato et al.[63] showed that children treated with prednisolone had the highest frequency of aneurysms (65 percent) and those treated only with aspirin had the lowest incidence (11 percent). Although this study can be criticized on many grounds, more recent studies have reached the same conclusion,[64] and, as a gen-

Table 9-9 Kawasaki Disease: Cardiac Pathology

Lesion (%)	Interval from onset to death (days)			
	0–9	12–25	28–31	40–49
Coronary artery				
Vasculitis	100	75	0	0
Aneurysms	0	85	100	85
Thrombosis	0	85	100	70
Myocardium				
Pericarditis	100	100	100	70
Myocarditis	100	85	25	0
Endocarditis	100	50	50	15
Myocardial fibrosis	0	0	0	70
Endocardial elastosis	0	0	25	40

(Modified from Fujiwara and Hamashima,[51] with permission.)

Table 9-10 Kawasaki Disease: Therapeutic Recommendations

Admit to hospital	Monitor for evidence of cardiac decompensation, other systemic complications in acute phase
Aspirin	Anti-inflammatory doses in acute phase (100 mg/kg/day); then antiplatelet doses (5–10 mg/kg/day)
Intravenous gamma globulin	400 mg/kg/day for 4 consecutive days during the first 10–12 days of the illness

eral rule, corticosteroids are contraindicated in the treatment of this disease. Exceptionally, corticosteroids may be employed in children with severe myocarditis. It is currently recommended that anti-inflammatory doses of acetylsalicylic acid (100 mg/kg/day in divided doses) be instituted during the early acute phase of the disease. When the platelet count begins to rise, usually at the onset of the subacute phase, the drug is used as an antiplatelet agent and the dose is reduced to 5 to 10 mg/kg/day. Aspirin therapy should be instituted early[65] and should be continued at the low dose until the ESR and platelet count are normal or, if aneurysms are present, indefinitely. In the event of aspirin sensitivity, another antiplatelet agent such as dipyridamole should be used to inhibit thrombus formation. Several reports have noted difficulty in achieving therapeutic salicylate levels in children with early KD, resulting from impaired absorption.[66] Care should be exercised in exceeding a dose of 100 mg/kg/day, however, since as the disease comes under control, the salicylate level may suddenly increase to toxic levels. Although aspirin has a definite effect on the fever,[67] its benefit with respect to preventing cardiac or other serious complications is not certain.[67] Theoretically, the high dose should reduce the inflammatory component of the vasculitis, and the low dose should inhibit thromboxane A_2 formation by the platelet, thus preventing thrombus formation,[68] without suppressing prostacyclin formation by the endothelium.

Table 9-11 Kawasaki Disease: Trials of Intravenous Gamma Globulin

Reference	Trial	Results
Furusho et al.[69]	Randomized, controlled, prospective multicenter trial of aspirin (30–50 mg/kg/day) vs. aspirin (as above), plus intravenous sulphonated intact gamma globulin (400 mg/kg/day × 5 days)	Aneurysm development in 42% of the aspirin treated group and in 15% of those treated with aspirin and gamma globulin ($P < .01$)
Newburger et al.[70]	Randomized, controlled, prospective multicenter trial of aspirin, 100 mg/kg/day (84 patients) vs. aspirin (as above) plus intact unmodified gamma globulin (400 mg/kg/day) 84 patients) for 4 consecutive days	Aneurysm development in 18% of the aspirin treated group and 4% of the gamma globulin treated group by 7 wk ($P = .005$)
Nagashima et al.[71]	Randomized, controlled, prospective multicenter study of aspirin, 30 mg/kg/day (67 patients) vs. aspirin (as above) plus polyethyleneglycol treated intact gamma globulin, 400 mg/kg/day × 3 days (69 patients)	Significantly reduced duration of fever and incidence of aneurysms at all intervals up to 30 days in gamma globulin treated group (16%) compared to the aspirin treated group (37%) ($P < .01$)

Administration of intravenous (IV) gamma globulin has an established role in the treatment of KD. There have been several studies demonstrating its efficacy in suppressing the clinical manifestations of the disease in general and in influencing the severity and occurrence of coronary aneurysms.[69-71] These studies are summarized in Table 9-11. It is recommended that IV gamma globulin be given within the first 10 to 12 days of the illness in a dose of 400 mg/kg/day for 4 consecutive days. The minimal effective dose has not yet been established, and there is some evidence that the earlier the initiation of treatment the smaller the total minimal effective dose. The clinician is urged to ascertain current recommendations with respect to this expensive but apparently highly effective treatment. The rationale for the use of gamma globulin is unclear. The marked T-cell activation that characterizes KD is suppressed by gamma globulin treatment.[72]

LEUKOCYTOCLASTIC VASCULITIS

Henoch-Schönlein Purpura

Anaphylactoid purpura, or Henoch-Schönlein purpura (HSP), is one of the most common vasculitides of childhood. It is characterized by a nonthrombocytopenic purpura, arthritis and arthralgia, abdominal pain and gastrointestinal hemorrhage, and nephritis.[130] This syndrome has a long and distinguished medical literary history with references to it by Heberden[73] and Willan.[74] The triad of purpuric rash, arthritis, and abnormalities of the urinary sediment was identified by Schönlein in 1837,[75] and Henoch noted the association of purpuric rash, abdominal pain with bloody diarrhea, and proteinuria.[76] The term *anaphylactoid* was applied to the syndrome by Gairdner in 1948.[77]

EPIDEMIOLOGY

Henoch-Schönlein purpura is predominantly a disease of childhood, although some adults with this disorder have been reported.[78] It occurs most frequently between the ages of 5 and 15 years and is more common in males than in females (1.5:1.0).[78] Striking seasonal variations have been noted, with most cases occurring in the winter months, often preceded by an upper respiratory tract infection.[79-81] Many reports have called attention to the preceding upper respiratory tract infection, particularly streptococcal disease.[77,82] Other investigators have doubted this association.[81,83,84] Other coincidences have been described, including those related to virus diseases such as varicella,[85,86] rubella,[86] rubeola,[86] hepatitis B infection,[87] and infection with *Mycoplasma pneumoniae*.[88] As the term *anaphylactoid purpura* suggests, allergy has also been thought by some to be the basis of the development of this disease. Reactions to insect bites[89] and drug and dietary allergens[90] have all been described.

Familial occurrence of the disease may occur either simultaneously or sequentially. No definite HLA association has been determined. HSP has been described in a number of patients with a heterozygous C2 deficiency (Ch. 11).

CLINICAL CHARACTERISTICS

The onset of the disease is often acute, with the principal manifestations appearing over a period of several days to weeks. Nonspecific constitutional signs, such as a low-grade fever or malaise, are often present. The clinical characteristics of HSP are shown in Table 9-12.

The presence of palpable purpura is essential to the diagnosis. This rash is most prominent on dependent or pressure-bearing areas, most commonly the lower extremities and buttocks, but may occur in other areas as well. The lesions range from small petechiae to large ecchymoses, but the most characteristic lesion is palpable purpura of approximately 5 mm in diameter[91] (Fig. 9-16). Lesions tend to occur in crops and progress in coloration from red to purple to brown. Ulceration may occur. The purpuric rash is often preceded by a maculopapular or urticarial lesion. Subcutaneous edema over the dorsa of the hands and feet and around the eyes, forehead, scalp, and scrotum may occur early in the disease, particularly in the child under the age of 2 years. Recurrences of the rash occur in up to half of the children, particularly the older patients, each episode usually being similar, but briefer and milder, than the preceding one.

Gastrointestinal manifestations usually occur within a week of the onset of the rash and almost

Table 9-12 Clinical Characteristics of Henoch-Schönlein Purpura

Clinical Characteristic (%)	Saulsbury[91] n = 25	Winter[92] n = 43	Emery et al.[94] n = 43
Purpura	100[a]	97	100
Arthralgia/arthritis	84	65	79
Abdominal pain	76	100[a]	63
Gastrointestinal bleeding	40	26	—[b]
Nephritis	44	—	37
Subcutaneous edema	—	—	63
Encephalopathy	8	—	—
Orchitis	4	—	—

[a] Criterion used for inclusion in the series.
[b] Information not available.

always within 30 days after the onset of the illness.[92] In the study of Winter,[92] abdominal pain was usually intermittent, colicky, and periumbilical in location. Rebound tenderness was uncommon. Vomiting occurred in 60 percent of patients and hematemesis in 7 percent. Melena occurred in 19 percent, although occult blood was present in the stools of half of the patients. Massive gastrointestinal hemorrhage and intussusception occur in less than 5 percent of children and may develop suddenly without preceding abdominal symptoms. Occasionally abdominal pain precedes the rash or other symptoms. Less common gastrointestinal disease includes intestinal gangrene and perforation, acute hemorrhagic pancreatitis,[93] ulcerative colitis, other forms of enteropathy, and steatorrhea.

Nephritis develops in approximately one-half of the children, and in 10 percent of these it is a serious and potentially life-threatening complication.[78–80, 84,86,89] The spectrum of renal manifestations is broad, ranging from microscopic hematuria and mild proteinuria to the less common nephrotic syndrome, acute nephritis, hypertension, and renal failure. Most cases of serious renal disease develop within 1 month of onset of the purpura, and the initial 3 months of the disease are the most critical in determining the eventual prognosis. In a few children, however, nephritis may not occur until much later in the disease, sometimes after a number of episodes of recurrent purpura. Thus, end-stage renal disease characteristically develops early but may not appear for a number of years. In only a small number of children do renal abnormalities antedate the rash or other features of

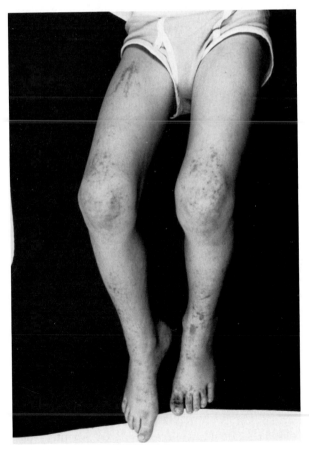

Fig. 9-16 Henoch-Schönlein purpura. These purpuric lesions appeared on the lower extremities of a 10-year-old boy who had an acute, self-limited illness characterized by fever, arthritis, melena, and transient hematuria. Note the periarticular swelling around the ankle and knee.

HSP or occur alone. Berger's nephropathy in adults may represent the latter type of case.

Arthralgia or arthritis involving a few joints occurs in the majority of children. The large joints, such as the knees and ankles, are most commonly affected, but other areas, including wrists, elbows, and small joints of the fingers, may also be involved. Characteristic findings include periarticular swelling and tenderness usually without erythema or warmth or effusions, but with considerable pain and limitation of motion. The joint disease is transient, although usually not migratory, and resolves within a few days. No residual abnormalities are found. Occasionally arthritis may precede the appearance of the rash by a day or two.[84,94]

Unusual manifestations of HSP include coma; subarachnoid hemorrhage; optic neuritis and Guillain-Barré syndrome[95,96]; ocular involvement[84,92]; intramuscular, subconjunctival, or pulmonary hemorrhage; recurrent epistaxis; parotitis[79,80]; carditis[89,97]; and orchitis.[91,98–100]

Clinical Course

In two-thirds of the children affected, the disease runs its entire course within 4 weeks of onset. Younger children generally have a shorter course and fewer recurrences than older patients. Approximately half have at least one recurrence that most commonly consists of rash and abdominal pain. The majority of these exacerbations take place within an initial 6-week period but may occur as late as 2 years after onset. They may be spontaneous or coincide with repeated respiratory tract infections.

LABORATORY INVESTIGATIONS

There are no specific diagnostic laboratory tests. It is important to ascertain that the platelet count is normal or increased, thus differentiating this form of purpura from that caused by thrombocytopenia. Similarly, studies of the coagulation pathway show normal results. A moderate leukocytosis of up to 20,000 per cubic millimeter (20×10^9 per liter) with a left shift is seen in some patients. Normochromic anemia is often related to gastrointestinal tract blood loss, which is noted in 80% of the children who have gastrointestinal complaints. Levels of complement components C1q, C3, and C4 are usually normal.[81,101] Involvement of the alternative pathway of complement activation is demonstrated by the presence of activated C3 (C3d),[102] decreased total hemolytic complement,[101] and decreased concentration of properdin in half of the children during the acute illness.[101,103] Circulating IgA-containing immune complexes[102,104,105] and cryoglobulins[106] may be present. Serum immunoglobulin A (IgA) and IgM concentrations are increased in one-half of the patients during the acute phase of the disease.[79,107] Antinuclear antibodies and rheumatoid factor are not present. Microscopic hematuria is common, and decreased concentrating ability and diminished creatinine clearance are occasionally present. Proteinuria, sometimes severe enough to cause a fall in serum albumin, may occur.[78,94]

Abdominal ultrasound is very useful in delineating the nature of the abnormalities in children with GI complaints. It shows the characteristics of decreased bowel motility with dilated loops of bowel, which are also demonstrable by barium studies. Occasionally, intussusception is demonstrated.

Skin biopsy may assist in the diagnosis of difficult cases by demonstrating a leukocytoclastic vasculitis characterized by deposition of IgA and C3. A renal biopsy is indicated only in children with persistent or major renal manifestations.

PATHOLOGY

The essential pathologic lesion in all affected organs is a leukocytoclastic vasculitis[80,108] (Fig. 9-17). In the kidney, light microscopy reveals a proliferative glomerulitis that ranges in severity from focal and segmental lesions to severe crescentic disease. The clinical renal manifestations of HSP show a direct correlation with the severity of the proliferative changes. However, renal disease may be present in the absence of urinary findings, and minimal abnormalities such as hematuria alone are not necessarily associated with a severe glomerular lesion. Levy et al. have provided a comprehensive review of the renal pathology in HSP.[80] The principal lesion is an endocapillary proliferative glomerulonephritis with an increase in endothelial and mesangial cells. All gradations of severity, from segmental to focal to diffuse, may be seen in the same biopsy specimen. There may be marked interstitial inflammatory disease as well. Arteritis is generally not seen. Fluorescence microscopy

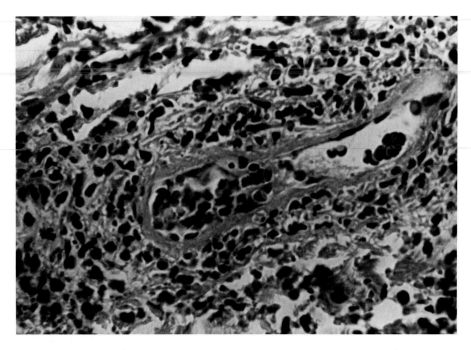

Fig. 9-17 Histopathologic demonstration of leukocytoclastic vasculitis (stained with hematoxylin and eosin). The characteristic "nuclear dust" is seen as granular dark-stained material in the vessel wall.

reveals immunoglobulin deposits, principally IgA,[109–112] but often accompanied by immunoglobulin G (IgG), fibrin, C3, and properdin, in the majority of involved glomeruli. These deposits are invariably mesangial in location, but in more severe cases, the peripheral capillary loops are involved as well. Electron microscopy confirms the presence of deposits in the mesangium and occasionally in the subendothelial regions. Thickening and splitting of the basement membrane, caused by the interposition of mesangial cell cytoplasmic material, are present.

In the gastrointestinal tract there may be edema and submucosal and intramural hemorrhage. These changes occasionally lead to intussusception or overt perforation.

DIFFERENTIAL DIAGNOSIS

HSP must be carefully distinguished from acute poststreptococcal glomerulonephritis, SLE, septicemia, disseminated intravascular coagulation, and hemolytic-uremic syndrome. Other types of polyarteritis or the vasculitis of rheumatic fever may cause diagnostic difficulty. The usual causes of an acute surgical abdomen in children with abdominal pain and

GI tract bleeding must be considered. Palpation of a tender abdominal mass indicative of intussusception or a suspicion of pancreatitis associated with a raised serum amylase level may be an important finding in some children.

TREATMENT

Treatment is supportive, with attention to maintenance of good hydration, nutrition and electrolyte balance, and control of pain with simple analgesics such as acetaminophen. Although corticosteroid drugs may dramatically decrease joint and skin symptoms, they are not usually required for the management of these manifestations of the disease. It has been customary to use prednisone or an equivalent drug in the management of severe GI disease or hemorrhage.[82] However, recent studies do not demonstrate an advantage of prednisone over supportive therapy (nasogastric suction, parenteral nutrition, antibiotics).[92] If the severity of disease prompts the clinician to use corticosteroid drugs, a dose of 1 to 2 mg/kg/day for 7 days, followed by a gradual reduction in the dose over 2 to 3 weeks, is suggested.

Corticosteroids probably have no role in the treatment of the renal disease,[79,86] although adequate trials have not been reported. There have been no trials of cytotoxic drugs in the treatment of the nephritis of HSP, and there is no evidence to suggest that they are useful.[79,86] Warfarin has also been used with disputable effect.[113]

Renal transplantation has been successful in some children with renal failure secondary to HSP, and recurrence of nephritis has been rare.[78]

PROGNOSIS

The prognosis is excellent in the great majority of affected children. Significant morbidity or mortality is associated with GI tract lesions and with nephritis. The extent of renal disease is the ultimate determinant of outcome. Overall, 5 percent of children with HSP progress to end-stage renal failure. HSP accounts for approximately 10 percent of renal failure from all causes in children.[114–116]

The prognosis of children with renal disease is highly variable. The outcome with minimal lesions is excellent, with more than 75 percent recovering within 2 years. In contrast, two-thirds of the children with more than 80 percent involvement by crescentic glomerulitis progress to terminal renal failure within the first year. Children with persistent renal abnormalities should be followed closely. In one long-term follow-up study of HSP in childhood, the worst outcome was associated with the presence of nephritis and nephrotic syndrome at onset of the disease.[114] Almost half of such children had active renal disease or renal insufficiency at follow-up more than 6 years later. The development of major indications of renal disease within the first 3 months after the onset of illness or the occurrence of numerous exacerbations associated with nephropathy is an indicator of poor prognosis for renal function.

Serum Sickness

Historically, serum sickness (hypersensitivity angiitis), one of the best examples of immune complex mediated disease in man, was encountered after the administration of heterologous antiserum to treat or prevent specific infections such as diphtheria and tetanus. A recent report of the use of equine antithymocyte globulin in the treatment of bone marrow failure indicated that most patients experienced malaise, headache, fever, cutaneous eruptions, arthralgias, arthritis, myalgias, GI complaints, and lymph node enlargement, beginning 7 to 9 days after injection and lasting 10 to 14 days.[117] Although the current use of heterologous antiserum is infrequent, it has been supplanted as a cause of serum sickness by a myriad drugs, notably penicillin, some of the sulfonamides, cefaclor, iodides, antithyroid drugs, and, rarely, other medications.[118–120] A recent report of serum sickness–like arthritis in Finland estimated the frequency of the condition at 4.7/100,000 children under the age of 16 years, making it one of the most common causes of acute arthritis in childhood.[120] The syndrome begins 7 to 14 days after primary exposure to the antigen and is characterized by fever, arthralgia, sometimes with frank arthritis, myalgia, lymphadenopathy, and a rash that may be urticarial or resemble that of HSP (Fig. 9-18). Kunnamo et al. described the presence of patchy discoloration over the affected joints with urticaria predominantly on the trunk.[120] In this study, the arthritis was transient and most commonly affected the ankles, metacarpophalangeal joints, wrists, and knees. Occasionally, pulmonary, renal, and other vasculature is affected (Fig. 9-19). Hypersensitivity angiitis may occur as an isolated idiopathic syndrome, unassociated with identifiable preceding events.

Laboratory studies show a leukocytosis, sometimes with eosinophilia, elevation of the ESR, and circulating immune complexes.[120] IgG antibodies to the putative antigen may be demonstrable. Synovial fluid examination demonstrated the presence of 8,800 to 59,000 leukocytes/mm^3, of which from 38 to 80 percent were neutrophils.[120]

Biopsy of the skin shows that small venules and capillaries are the predominantly involved vessels. Inflammatory lesions are at a similar stage of development in all involved vessels, and the cellular infiltrate contains large numbers of neutrophils and eosinophils. Allergic granulomatous angiitis may present a similar clinical pattern, but in this condition, a precipitating agent such as a drug cannot usually be identified.

The clinical course usually lasts 1 to 2 weeks with complete resolution of all abnormalities. Discontinuation of the offending drug and institution of treatment with corticosteroid agents usually suppress this disorder.

Hypocomplementemic Urticarial Vasculitis

Children, usually girls, with the rare syndrome of hypocomplementemic urticarial vasculitis have recurrent episodes of urticarial eruptions on the face, upper extremities, and trunk that typically last 1 to 2 days and disappear without residua (Fig. 9-20).[121,122] Other lesions include purpura, papules, and vesicles. Fever, arthralgia, nausea and vomiting, and abdominal pain may accompany the cutaneous disease. Arthritis, especially of the small joints, is of brief duration and without long-term consequences. Although

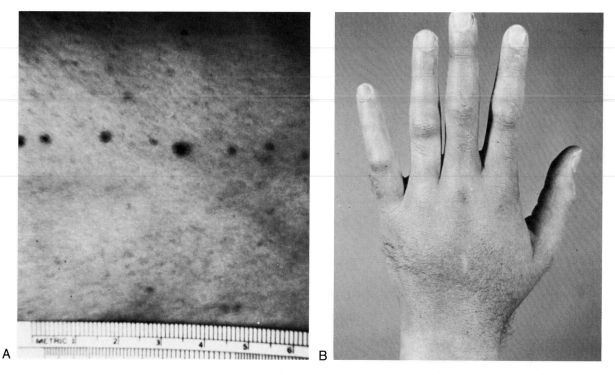

Fig. 9-18 (**A**) Hypersensitivity angiitis. Linear, palpable purpuric lesions along the course of a superficial vessel in a boy who developed vasculitis after a drug reaction. (**B**) Diffuse and periarticular swelling of the hand in a boy with acute serum sickness.

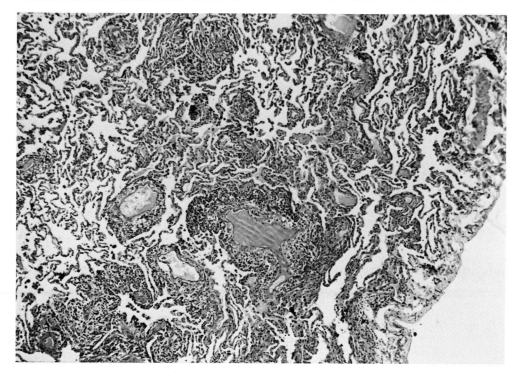

Fig. 9-19 Hypersensitivity angiitis. Lung biopsy specimen from a young drug addict with a short history of increasing dyspnea on exertion and purpura. This section shows prominent infiltration by inflammatory cells and eosinophils of the alveolar walls and around blood vessels.

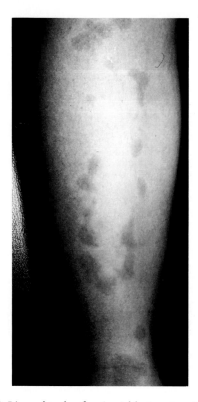

Fig. 9-20 Linear bands of urticarial lesions in a 6-year-old girl with hypocomplementemic urticarial vasculitis. These lesions were transient and recurrent.

the course is usually benign, treatment with corticosteroids may be indicated.

The pathogenesis is unknown, but an immune complex process is suggested by lesional deposits of immunoglobulins and complement and by presence of circulating immune complexes. Levels of both early and late components of the complement cascade may be depressed, the degree of hypocomplementemia paralleling the severity of the disease. ANA, RF, and cryoglobulins are usually absent. A mild membranoproliferative glomerulonephritis may accompany the predominant cutaneous disease.

Cryoglobulinemic Vasculitis

Vasculitis with mixed cryoglobulinemia clinically resembles other leukocytoclastic vasculitides such as HSP with purpura of the skin of the distal extremities, which is often precipitated by exposure to cold; arthralgia, with or without frank arthritis; and glomerulonephritis in up to half of the patients.[123] Pulmonary disease may also occur.[124] The presence of high levels of mixed cryoglobulins, containing IgG and IgM, sometimes with hepatitis B antigen[123] or

coccidioidin antigen,[125] is the serologic hallmark of the disorder. This condition has been described in at least one child.[126]

GRANULOMATOUS VASCULITIS

Allergic Granulomatosis

Allergic granulomatosis, or the Churg-Strauss syndrome, is extremely rare in childhood. It has been noted in at least five children, including a 7-year-old and a 9-year-old reported in the original description by Churg and Strauss[127] (Table 9-13). The clinical syndrome is characterized by the presence of asthma, fever, and marked eosinophilia together with variable manifestations of vasculitis. In the skin, purpura that represents leukocytoclastic venulitis and nodular lesions that represent extravascular granulomata with eosinophilic infiltrates[127] are often present. Pulmonary symptoms are almost always present, with a frequent history of asthma and the presence of infiltrates on chest radiograph. A mononeuritis multiplex, resulting in foot drop or wrist drop or other signs, occurs in the majority of adults with this disease. There is vasculitis of the coronary arteries with granulomatous pericarditis in approximately one-third of patients. GI manifestations include ulcers of stomach or colon and granulomata of the omentum.[129] Hypertension and renal involvement are somewhat less frequent.

The diagnosis is confirmed by the characteristic pathologic findings of necrotizing vasculitis with an eosinophilic infiltrate and extravascular necrotizing granulomata (Fig. 9-21).

Wegener's Granulomatosis

Wegener's granulomatosis is a necrotizing, granulomatous angiitis affecting the respiratory tract (sinuses, nasal passages, pharynx, and lungs) and kidneys (glomerulonephritis). When the lesions are limited to the upper respiratory passages and the vasculitis is minimal, the syndrome is referred to as *localized Wegener's* or *midline granuloma*. In some cases, granulomata may be more widely scattered and involve the skin, heart, CNS, GI tract, and joints (Table 9-14).[130] The disease is most commonly seen in the 25- to 50-year age group; however, the age range in

Table 9-13 Churg-Strauss Syndrome in Childhood

Reference	Sex	Age	Clinical Manifestations
Churg and Strauss[127]	F	7	Asthma, eosinophilia, pneumonia, hypertension, skin nodules and purpura, cardiac failure, renal involvement, death
	M	9	Asthma, eosinophilia, pneumonia, hypertension, skin nodules and purpura, cardiac failure, renal involvement, peripheral neuropathy
Farooki et al.[128]	M	12	Pericarditis, myocarditis, eosinophilia, history of wheezing; death
Petty et al.[8]	M	16	Fever, asthma, painful calf nodules, peripheral neuropathy, hypertension, eosinophilia
Frayha[129]	F	13	Fever, asthma, peripheral neuropathy, celiac aneurysms, eosinophilia; death

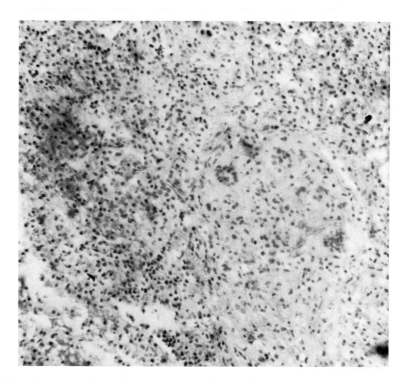

Fig. 9-21 The lung biopsy specimen from a young girl with Churg-Strauss granulomatosis. No definite vasculitis is present, but there are necrotizing granulomata with giant cells.

Table 9-14 Typical Clinicopathologic Features of Wegener's Granulomatosis

System	Frequency, Percentage	Abnormalities
Upper respiratory tract	100	Necrotizing mucosal ulceration, sinusitis, saddle nose
Lungs	100	Bilateral nodules, cavitation, fleeting infiltrates, small pleural effusions
Kidneys	80	Focal, segmental, or diffuse glomerulitis
Joints	60	Polyarthralgia, occasionally frank arthritis
Skin	50	Ulcerations
Eyes	45	Uveitis
Ears	40	Otitis media
Heart	30	Coronary arteritis, pericarditis
Nervous system	25	Peripheral and cranial neuritis

(Adapted from Wolff SM et al.,[130] with permission.)

Table 9-15 Wegener's Granulomatosis in Childhood

Reference	Age	Sex	Nose	Sinus	Ear	Lung	Kidney	Muscle	Joint	Eye
131	12	F		+	+					
132	16	F				+				
133	13	F				+				
134	16	M	+							
135	13	M	+							
136	11	M				+				
137	17	M	+							
138	14	M		+		+		+		
139	18	M				+				
140	14	M				+				
141	9	F				+	+			
142	8	M	+			+	+			
143	14	M	+			+	+			
144	18	M		+	+					
145	10	F	+							
	13	F	+	+		+				
146	11	M	+			+			+	
147	14	F	+							
	17	M				+				
	13	M	+		+				+	
	17	M	+			+				+
148	13	F					+		+	+
	7	M			+	+			+	
	12	F		+	+	+			+	+
	11	M				+			+	
149	15	M	+			+	+		+	

 Organ Involvement at Onset

published studies is from less than 1 year to 75 years.[130]

Of the 26 reported patients less than 19 years of age (Table 9-15),[130–149] 9 were girls and 17 were boys. The mean age of onset was 13 years. Epistaxis, chronic rhinorrhea, cough, and fever were the most common presenting complaints. Kidney involvement was reflected by hematuria and proteinuria in 19 percent. Sinusitis (19 percent), otitis media (19 percent), arthralgia or arthritis (27 percent), and ocular (12 percent) and muscle complaints (4 percent) were also recorded at onset (Table 9-15). Granulomatous lesions in the sinuses may extend to the orbit, producing exophthalmos and impairment of vision and potentially destructive disfigurement (Fig. 9-22). Fever, weight loss, malaise, and anorexia are common. Uremia and renal failure may develop rapidly in the absence of hypertension. The differential di-

agnosis includes other types of vasculitis, sarcoidosis, berylliosis, Löffler's syndrome, tuberculosis, disseminated fungal disease (malleomyces, blastomycosis, coccidioidomycosis, sporotrichosis), syphilis, Goodpasture's syndrome, and lymphoma.

Radiographs show pulmonary granulomata that may be discrete and solitary or multiple and bilateral and have a predilection for the lower lobes. They may be fleeting or may cavitate. Pneumothorax and pleural effusions may be present (Fig. 9-23).

Peripheral leukocytosis is frequent, but eosinophilia is uncommon. The ESR is usually markedly elevated in the early phase of the disease. RF is present in approximately half of adult patients.[151] Antinuclear antibodies are not present. Urinalysis reveals hematuria and low-grade proteinuria. Biopsy of the renal lesions shows a focal proliferative glomerulonephritis with prominent epithelial crescent formation (Fig. 9-24).[151] Electron microscopy reveals sparse subepithelial deposits.[152] Biopsy of the submucosa of the nose or sinus or of the cutaneous lesions demonstrates necrotizing granulomata. Arteritis is rare.

In the past, the prognosis was almost uniformly fatal, but great strides in the treatment of Wegener's granulomatosis have resulted in excellent long-term prognosis. Corticosteroids and cyclophosphamide provide the most effective management.[150] Using a treatment protocol consisting of cyclophosphamide, 2 mg/kg/day orally, and prednisone, 1 mg/kg/day orally, for a variable period of time, only 10 of 93 patients died, 6 with active disease and 4 from other causes. Complete remission was achieved in 93 percent of patients, with a mean duration of of approximately 4 years at the time of the report; 23 patients had been off therapy for an average of almost 3 years.[150] Intravenous cyclophosphamide given as a bolus may provide the optimal route of administration of this drug in the management of this disease, although experience to date is limited.

Lymphomatoid Granulomatosis

Lymphomatoid granulomatosis, first described by Liebow et al. in 1972,[153] is a necrotizing pulmonary vasculitis characterized by angiocentric and angiodestructive granulomatous lesions with lymphoproliferation that may progress to lymphoma. Pulmonary involvement has been described in all patients and is characterized by multiple

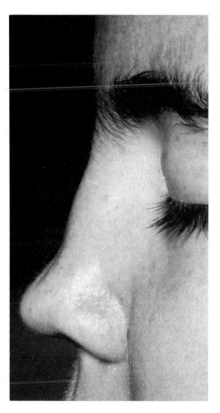

Fig. 9-22 The "saddle nose" resulting from granulomatous destruction of the nasal cartilage in this 14-year-old girl with Wegener's granulomatosus. The process was painless and occurred over several months. Later, she developed the pulmonary changes that led to the diagnosis.

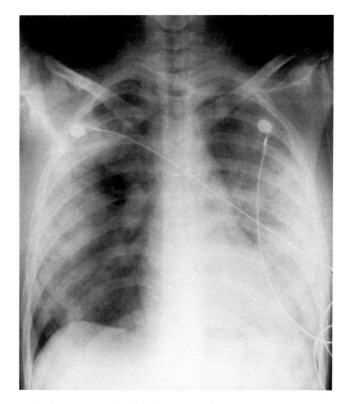

Fig. 9-23 Chest radiograph of a 14-year-old girl with Wegener's granulomatosis, showing widespread infiltrates suggestive of pulmonary hemorrhage. There were considerable day-to-day variability and eventual total resolution of these abnormalities after treatment with prednisone and cyclophosphamide. (Courtesy of Dr. G. Culham.)

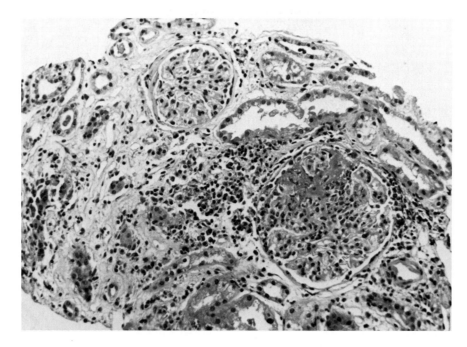

Fig. 9-24 Renal biopsy specimen from a child with Wegener's granulomatosis. The glomerulus on the right shows areas of hypercellularity and fibrinoid necrosis with interstitial inflammation.

bilateral nodular infiltrates. Skin, kidneys, and the central nervous system are affected in one-third of the patients. The renal disease consists of a nodular infiltration of the parenchyma and does not include a necrotizing arteritis. Midline sinus and upper-airway granulomata are rare. Combined treatment with prednisone (1 mg/kg on alternate days) and cyclophosphamide (2 mg/kg/day) has improved the prognosis, with remissions lasting 5 years or more in approximately half.[154] Malignant lymphoma occurred in almost all of the patients who died in one series,[154] and this disease may represent part of a continuum between diseases such as Wegener's granulomatosis, which it may resemble clinically, and malignant lymphoma.[155]

Lymphomatoid granulomatosis is extremely rare in childhood but has been reported in a 16-year-old boy,[154] a child with leukemia in remission,[155] and a child with Wiskott-Aldrich syndrome.[156] In adults the disease occurs predominantly in males in the 40- to 60-year age group.[154,157]

Primary Angiitis of the Central Nervous System

An isolated central nervous system (CNS) granulomatous angiitis was described by Cravioto and Feigin in 1959.[158] Calabrese and Mallek reviewed 40 published cases and added 8 of their own, including that of a 10-year-old girl and a 12-year-old boy who had a history or clinical findings of an unexplained acquired neurologic deficit, classic angiographic findings (multifocal areas of alternating stenosis and ectasia) or histopathologic features of angiitis within the CNS (mononuclear vasculitis of arteries and veins), but no evidence of systemic vasculitis or other systemic disease.[159] The 10-year-old girl presented with aphasia, confusion, headaches, and hemiparesis resulting from angiitis of the middle cerebral artery. She made a full recovery without treatment. The 12-year-old boy had a hemiparesis, hemianaesthesia, and nystagmus and re-

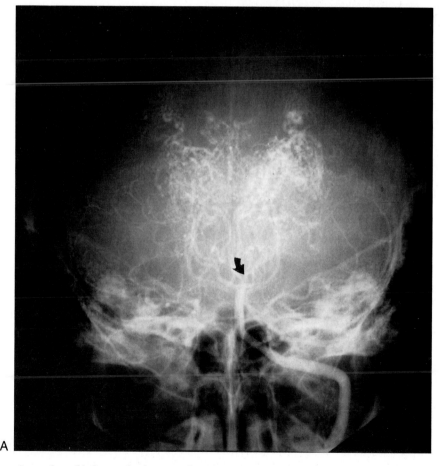

Fig. 9-25 Arteriography of left vertebral artery showing stenosis of basilar artery (arrow) just above the tentorium. The extensive collaterals are the characteristic "puff of smoke"—moyamoya. (**A**) Anteroposterior view. (*Figure continues.*)

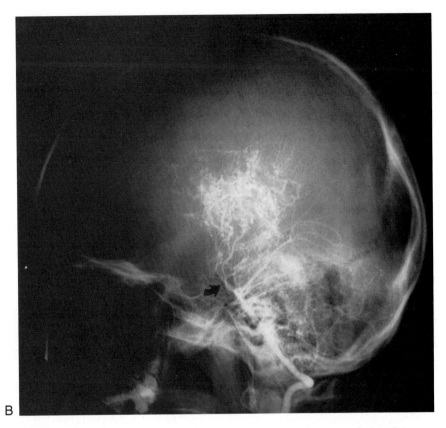

Fig. 9-25 (*Continued*) (**B**) Lateral view. (Courtesy of Dr. O. Flodmark.)

covered after treatment with prednisone. Tomography revealed cerebral infarcts in both. The cerebrospinal fluid had increased cells and protein. RF, ANA, immune complexes, and cryoglobulins were not detected and CRP was normal.

Moyamoya is a disorder that presents as vasculitis of the CNS in childhood.[160] The angiographic studies show a characteristic pattern of stenoses of the vessels around the circle of Willis (Fig. 9-25). The pathogenesis of moyamoya is unclear.

GIANT CELL ARTERITIS

Takayasu's Arteritis

DEFINITIONS

The disease Takayasu's arteritis (TA) was first described by Migito Takayasu, an ophthalmologist in Tokyo who noted the characteristic arteriovenous abnormalities of the retina in 1908.[161] Takayasu's ar-

teritis is a segmental inflammatory arteritis leading to stenosis and aneurysms of large muscular arteries, chiefly the aorta and its major branches (Table 9-16). It is known clinically by a number of names, including *pulseless disease* and *reverse coarctation*.

Table 9-16 Takayasu's Arteritis in Childhood: Patterns of Disease

Area of Inflammation	Percentage
Abdominal aorta only	20
Abdominal and descending thoracic aorta	19
Aortic arch, and descending thoracic aorta	19
Aortic arch, thoracic and abdominal aorta	16
Aortic arch and abdominal aorta	12
Descending thoracic aorta only	7
Aortic arch only	5
Aortic arch, thoracic aorta, and pulmonary arteries	2

EPIDEMIOLOGY

Takayasu's arteritis, the most common giant cell arteritis of childhood, follows Kawasaki disease and Henoch-Schönlein purpura as the most common of all vasculitides in childhood. More than 60 well-documented cases have now been reported from all over the world.[162-186] Blacks, Orientals, Latin Americans, and Sephardic Jews are at highest risk. The female:male ratio is about 8:1 in adults, closer to 2:1 in children. In Japan, 20 percent of patients are under 19 years of age, and 2 percent are under 10 years of age.

CLINICAL MANIFESTATIONS

Early systemic manifestations of the disease include fever, night sweats, weight loss, anorexia, arthralgia or arthritis, and myalgia. This type of presentation is seen in over one-half of the children and may last for a period of 3 months or many years. An erroneous diagnosis of acute rheumatic fever or juvenile rheumatoid arthritis may be made. Hypertension and disorders of the pulse supervene and lead to the diagnosis. In some children, systemic manifestations are mild or transient and the discovery of hypertension or hypertensive encephalopathy leads to the diagnosis. Takayasu's arteritis characteristically involves the aorta and its major branches and sometimes the pulmonary arteries and may be classified according to the distribution of affected vessels.[187] It is important to recognize the widespread but segmental nature of the lesions of TA. The data in Table 9-16 are collected from published cases of TA in children and indicate the frequent involvement of the abdominal aorta (sometimes with other affected areas), as well as the aortic arch and its branches. Lesions include stenosis, occlusion, dilatation, and aneurysm formation. There are curious geographic variations in the presentation of TA. Obstructive lesions are the most common in the United States, Europe, and Japan, whereas aneurysms appear to be more common in India, Thailand, and Africa. Involvement of the brachiocephalic arteries occurs in most geographic areas; the abdominal aorta is most frequently involved in Thailand,[172] and the descending thoracic aorta in India.[168,169] The significance of these differences, if they are real, is unknown.

ETIOLOGY AND PATHOGENESIS

On the basis of the racial groups at risk for TA, it has been postulated that genetic factors may play a role in its pathogenesis. Cases of TA and other rheumatic diseases have been described within families. The mother of one of our patients with systemic lupus erythematosus died of TA. It has been reported in monozygotic twin sisters, and there may be an association with the haplotype A11,B40.[183] Many reports noted the association of TA with pulmonary tuberculosis,[167,180,189] although this is by no means a constant observation, especially in North America.

PATHOLOGY

The characteristic pathologic pattern involves a focal or diffuse loss of the muscular and elastic tissues of the arterial wall. The diagnostic lesions are often segmental and spotty, and areas of the vessel directly contiguous with the disease may be entirely normal. Extensive fibrosis of the media and characteristic destruction of the elastic lamina are seen. Giant cells often surround these areas of destruction (Fig. 9-26). Stenosis is a direct result of intimal thickening, and dilatation is secondary to medial degeneration. IgG, IgM, and properdin are found in the lesions.[188,189] Dermal hyperplasia with inflammatory cells in the adventitia is characteristic. The vasa vasorum are also involved.

DIAGNOSIS

The erythrocyte sedimentation rate and other acute-phase reactants and the WBC count are usually elevated. Factor VIII–related antigen, an indicator of activated endothelium, is also elevated and may be the most specific serologic marker of inflammation of large vessels.[15] Normochromic, normocytic anemia occurs in at least half of the children. Antinuclear antibodies are rare, but rheumatoid factor is occasionally present.

Plain radiographs may reveal calcification of the aorta or widening related to prestenotic dilatation or aortic insufficiency. Pulsed Doppler and ultrasound interrogation of peripheral arteries, arteriography, and magnetic resonance imaging may dramatically

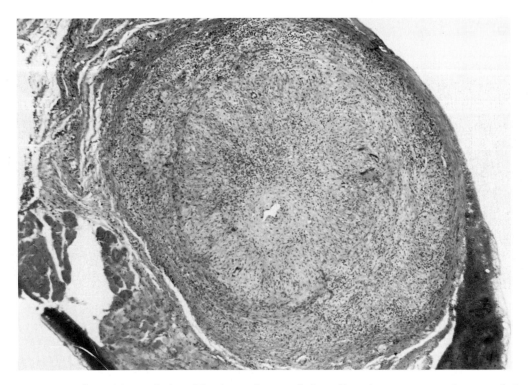

Fig. 9-26 Giant cell arteritis. Marked proliferation and accumulation of lymphocytes, macrophages, and plasma cells are present. The internal elastic lamina is fragmented and giant cells are present. Fibrinoid necrosis is not present.

demonstrate the extent of narrowing, dilatation, and diminished flow (Fig. 9-27).[171]

TREATMENT

There is some disagreement about the efficacy of any treatment in TA.[187,190] However, recent studies support the use of corticosteroid drugs, and in unresponsive patients, of cyclophosphamide.[191] Anti-inflammatory drugs are useful for alleviation of the symptoms of the disease. The use of antiplatelet agents (low-dose aspirin or dipyridimole) may be indicated in the chronic occlusive phase. Prosthetic surgery with grafting has been successful but is not advisable for patients with active disease.

Temporal (Cranial) Arteritis

Temporal arteritis is a localized variant of giant cell arteritis. Involvement of the temporal artery is often signaled by the development of a persistent headache and localized pain and tenderness over the vessel. In some patients pain may radiate to other parts of the face or there may be intermittent claudication in the jaw or tongue. Tender nodules may arise along the course of the temporal artery. Disease in the ophthalmic and central retinal arteries may lead to optic ischemia and blindness, a threat that makes early recognition of this condition and prompt institution of corticosteroid therapy imperative. The diagnosis is established by a generous temporal artery biopsy, because involvement of the arterial wall is discontinuous. This form of vasculitis is very rare in children,[192] occurring most frequently over the age of 50 years, when it is often associated with polymyalgia rheumatica.[193]

OTHER VASCULITIS SYNDROMES

Behçet's Syndrome

DEFINITIONS

In 1937, the Turkish dermatologist Behçet described the syndrome that bears his name: the triad of aphthous stomatitis, genital ulceration, and iri-

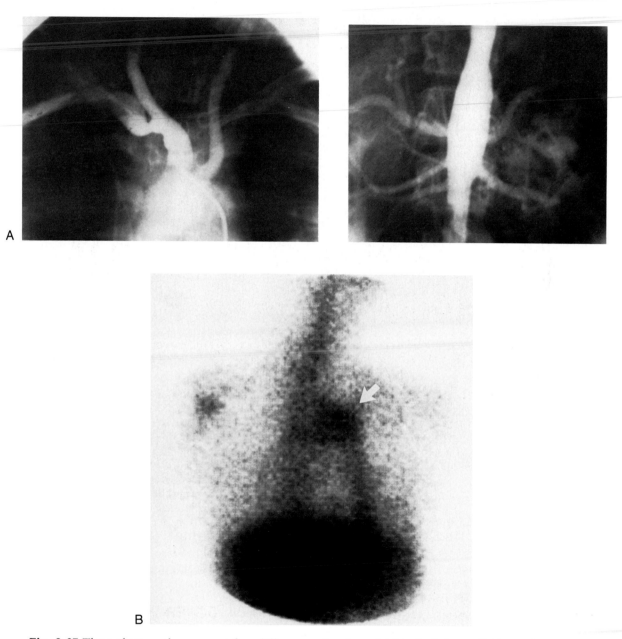

Fig. 9-27 These photographs represent four different studies documenting the lesions of Takayasu's arteritis. (**A**) There is dilatation, irregularity, and stenosis of the right innominate artery and its branches. The left subclavian artery is not visualized in this angiogram. (Courtesy of Dr. G. Culham.) (**B**) This gallium scan shows increased uptake of the isotope in the region of the aortic arch (arrow), supporting the diagnosis of inflammation of this structure. (Courtesy of Dr. H. Nadel.) (*Figure continues.*)

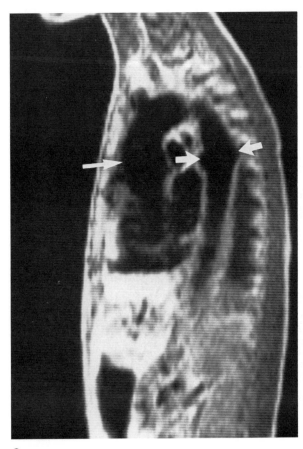

C

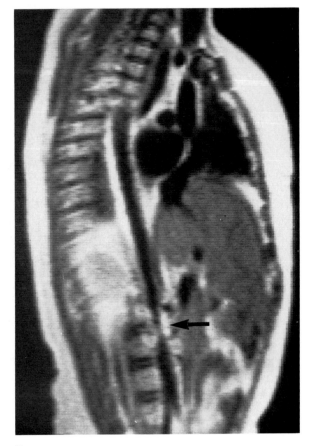

D

Fig. 9-27 (*Continued*) (**C & D**) Magnetic resonance image showing the dilated aortic arch and localized aneurysms of the thoracic portion of the decending aorta (arrows) and stenotic region in the abdominal aorta (arrow). (Courtesy of Dr. G. Culham.) (*Figure continues.*)

tis.[194] There is no general agreement about the definition of this syndrome.[195] In addition to the clinical triad that was originially described, the syndrome often includes other signs, and the criteria of Mason and Barnes may more accurately reflect the entire spectrum of the disease.[196] These authors suggested that the diagnosis of Behçet's syndrome could be made in the presence of three of four major criteria (buccal ulceration, genital ulceration, eye lesions, skin lesions) or a combination of two major criteria in addition to two minor criteria (gastrointestinal lesions, thrombophlebitis, cardiovascular lesions, arthritis, central nervous system disease, family history). Less stringent[195] and more stringent criteria[197] have also been used.

EPIDEMIOLOGY

Behçet's syndrome is rare in childhood. In the series of 32 patients seen in northern England, 8 had onset of the disease in the first decade and another 8 in the second decade.[198] In Japan, only 5.5 percent of patients were under 16 years of age.

In adults, Behçet's syndrome is almost twice as common in males as in females. The sex ratio in children may be closer to 1:1, although the small number of patients reported makes any firm conclusion impossible. Behçet's syndrome is much more common in certain geographic areas, particularly the eastern Mediterranean and Japan, where the prevalence is 1/1000,[199] than in the remainder of the world: the prevalence in Minnesota is estimated at 1/25,000.[195] Familial Behçet's syndrome, including a mother and her two adolescent daughters,[200] has been re-

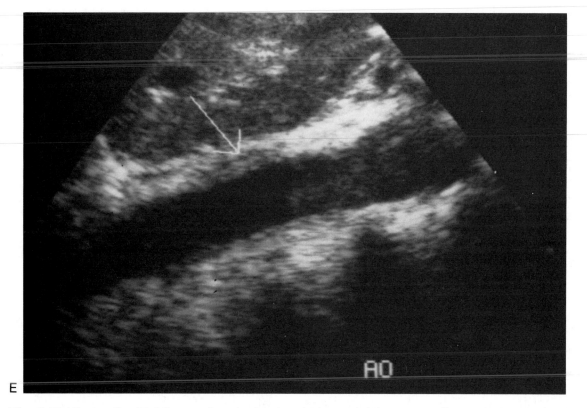

E

Fig. 9-27 *(Continued)* (**E**) Ultrasound study showing thickening of the aortic wall in a child with active Takayasu's arteritis (sagittal section). (Courtesy of Dr. J. Buckley.)

ported, but no specific mode of inheritance has been delineated. Histocompatibility antigen B5 has been associated with the syndrome in Turkish,[201] Japanese,[202] Italian,[203] and Mexican Mestizo populations,[204] but not in North American[195] or English patients.[205] No associations with HLA-DR or DQw antigens were demonstrable in North American patients.[206]

ETIOLOGY

The etiology of Behçet's syndrome is unknown, but its similarity to Reiter's syndrome and to inflammatory bowel disease has led many investigators to believe that an infectious etiology and hypersensitivity pathogenesis are likely. That an antibody-mediated process may be responsible is suggested by the observation of transient neonatal Behçet's syndrome in offspring of a mother with the disorder.[207,208]

CLINICAL CHARACTERISTICS

The frequencies of the various clinical features of Behçet's syndrome are shown in Table 9-17.

Apthous Stomatitis

Oral ulceration always occurs and may be present for much of the time. Crops of extremely painful ulcers appear on lips, tongue, palate, and elsewhere in the gastrointestinal tract (Fig. 9-28). They usually last for 3 to 10 days, sometimes longer, and usually heal without scarring. The exception to this rule is in neonatal Behçet's syndrome, in which extensive scarring may result.[207]

Genital Ulceration

In the male, recurrent painful ulceration of the glans penis, prepuce, and scrotum and in the female, of the vulva and vagina are characteristic. Ulcers may cause scarring when they heal.

Cutaneous Disease

Skin ulceration, erythema nodosum, erythema multiforme, and other rashes, including psoriasis, have been associated with Behçet's syndrome[196] (Fig.

Table 9-17 Frequency of Manifestations of Behçet's Syndrome

	Adults[a]	Children[b]
Major manifestations		
Aphthous stomatitis	100	100
Genital ulceration	75	62
Cutaneous disease	56	77
Ocular disease	70	54
Minor manifestations		
Gastrointestinal	20	69
Thrombophlebitis	20	0
Cardiovascular	<5	15
Arthritis	70	62
Central nervous system	25	38
Family history	20	—

[a] Adult data derived from Mason and Barnes,[196] and Wright and Moll.[209]
[b] Data for children calculated from data in Ammann et al.,[210] Mundy and Miller,[211] and Adorno et al.[203]

9-29). An unusual cutaneous pustular reaction to a needle puncture (pathergy) has been described.[201]

Ocular Disease

Inflammation of the anterior and posterior uvea may result in blindness. Hypopyon, corneal ulceration, and retrobulbar neuritis occur.[196] Uveitis is almost always bilateral and is more frequent in males.[212]

Gastrointestinal Lesions

GI tract lesions indistingishable from those of Crohn's disease[213] or ulcerative colitis[196] may be seen in patients with Behçet's syndrome. Aphthous stomatitis, erythema nodosum, arthritis, and uveitis may also be seen in both diseases.

Cardiovascular Lesions

Superficial or deep venous thrombosis is quite common.[196] Arteritis and arterial aneurysms may also be seen.[214–216] Pericarditis is rarely noted.[196]

Central Nervous System

Meningoencephalitis, characterized by headache, stiff neck, and cerebrospinal fluid pleocytosis, and focal neurological abnormalities may be seen.[217]

Arthritis

Polyarthritis is most common in knees, ankles, wrists, and elbows but may occur in other joints as well. It does not usually cause erosion or joint destruction. The association with sacroiliitis is not clear. Although some studies found mild sacroiliitis in the majority of patients,[218] the association has not been found in other studies.[219]

DIAGNOSIS

In general, the aphthous stomatitis is the presenting sign and other components of the syndrome may not appear for decades. The diagnosis is a clinical one, the laboratory supplying supporting evidence only. There is a generalized increase in acute-phase reactants, but ANA and RF are absent. Synovial fluid analysis shows a predominance of PMN leukocytes in relatively low numbers ($<15,000/mm^3$, $<15 \times 10^9/L$) with no distinguishing features. Synovial histology shows only nonspecific inflammation. In the skin, the basic lesion is vasculitis, which may be necrotizing but does not exhibit fibrinoid degeneration.

TREATMENT

Behçet syndrome is difficult to treat. Some patients are steroid-responsive; others may respond to colchicine,[220] levamisol,[221] chlorambucil,[222] or thalidomide.[223] The disease tends to run a very long relapsing course, and the ocular and CNS manifestations in particular are extremely incapacitating.

Mucha-Habermann Disease

Mucha-Habermann disease (pityriasis lichenoides et varioliformis acuta [PLEVA]) is a cutaneous vasculitis that has the early appearance of chronic or recurrent chickenpoxlike lesions that become atrophic and scarred. It is accompanied by fever and joint pain and swelling (Fig. 9-30). Histologically, the lesion is characterized by inflammation of the capillaries and venules of the upper dermis. It has been reported in association with a chronic arthritis resembling juvenile rheumatoid arthritis and with severe acrosclerosis and scleroderma.[224] A third patient with similar cutaneous findings has been reported by Lister and Hollingworth,[225] and we have observed a fourth patient, a young girl, who has PLEVA and recurrent bland arthritis and whose sister also has PLEVA.

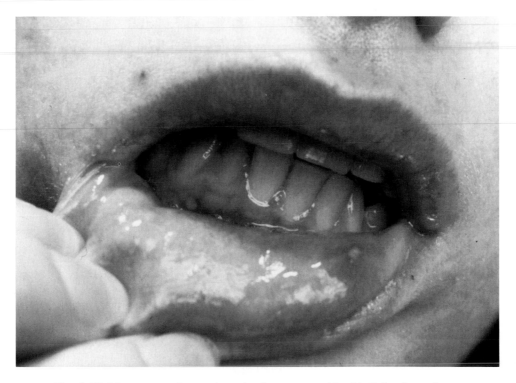

Fig. 9-28 Mucous membrane ulceration in a young girl with Behçet's syndrome.

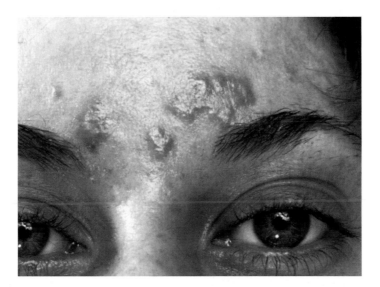

Fig. 9-29 Vesicular rash over the forehead of a young girl with Behçet's syndrome.

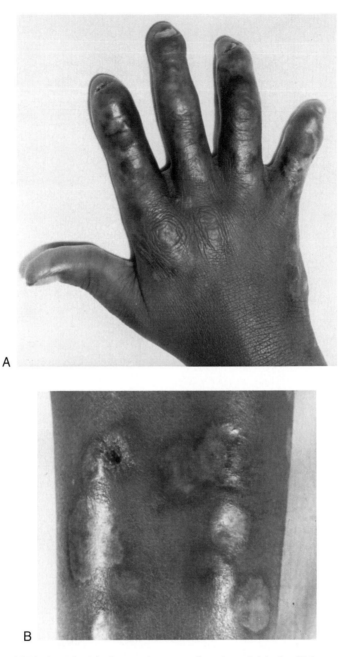

A

B

Fig. 9-30 An 11-year-old black girl with destructive acrosclerosis and Mucha-Habermann disease. (**A**) The hand. (**B**) The forearm. Characteristic cutaneous lesions of the latter disorder are seen, along with advanced ischemic digital changes.

Kohlmeir-Degos Syndrome

The Kohlmeir-Degos syndrome has a number of other names, including papulosis atrophicans maligna[226] and progressive arterial occlusive disease.[227] It is a very rare, often fatal vasculitis of cutaneous and gastointestinal small- and medium-sized arteries resulting in their occlusion by fibrosis. It has been recognized almost exclusively in young men and has been reported in three teenage boys.[227]

Cutaneous Necrotizing Venulitis in Patients with Cystic Fibrosis

Soter et al.[228] described two males with cystic fibrosis who had palpable purpura. Histologic examination demonstrated necrotizing venulitis.

SYNDROMES THAT RESEMBLE VASCULITIS

Sweet's Syndrome

Febrile neutrophilic dermatosis (Sweet's syndrome),[229] is a perivasculitis characterized by spiking fever and tender raised red plaques or nodules on face, extremities, and sometimes the trunk. Some patients have arthritis. It occurs most commonly in young women but has been described in at least six children.[230–234]

The disease is of unknown etiology, biopsy shows a prominent perivascular infiltration of neutrophils and eosinophils. There is a prompt and complete response to corticosteroid.

Goodpasture's Syndrome

In 1919, Goodpasture described a patient who developed pulmonary hemorrhage and severe proliferative glomerulonephritis with crescent formation leading to death.[235] This disease predominantly affects young men, with a male:female ratio of 9:1. It is rare in children. Levin et al.[236] described the disease in three children under the age of 10 years, and two other case reports have been published.[237,238]

The disease is mediated by antibody that cross-reacts with constituents of basement membrane in the lung and the glomerulus. These antibodies are demonstrated as linear staining by direct or indirect immunofluorescence. This disease has occurred after ingestions of D-penicillamine, in heavy metal poisoning, and in patients with other rheumatic diseases.

Pulmonary hemorrhage is often the initial manifestation and may precede renal abnormalities by a period of weeks to years. Progression may be quite rapid. Constitutional symptoms (fever, chills, increased sweating) occur in one-fourth of patients, and pulmonary complaints (dyspnea, weakness, chest pain, wheezing) are common.

In children, idiopathic pulmonary hemosiderosis, Wegener's granulomatosis, hemolytic-uremic syndrome, and systemic lupus erythematosus (SLE) are all considerations in the differential diagnosis. The presence in the serum of antibodies to glomerular basement membrane is virtually diagnostic.

Treatment includes the use of corticosteroids, plasmapheresis, and immunosuppressives with varying results.[236] The rationale for this combined approach is that circulating antibasement membrane antibodies are removed by the plasmapheresis and their synthesis is limited by the immunosuppressive agents. Nonetheless, survival rate of patients with Goodpasture's syndrome is often disappointing. Death is often related to asphyxia, pulmonary hemorrhage, or uremia.

Stevens-Johnson Syndrome

The Stevens-Johnson syndrome is a severe form of mucocutaneous erythema multiforme typified by systemic symptoms.[239] There are usually numerous bullous and papular lesions on the mucosal and cutaneous surfaces (Fig. 9-31). The anal, genital, and ocular orifices are often affected, and scarring may result. The onset is usually abrupt and is associated with fever, profound constitutional symptoms, and appearance of periarticular swelling and pain or frank arthritis. Stomatitis, conjunctivitis, and corneal ulceration may develop. A vesiculobullous hemorrhagic eruption involves the face, hands, feet, and orifices.

Histopathologic studies show a perivasculitis with no evidence of actual vasculitis. The etiology is unknown, but a preceding infectious illness with or without the ingestion of antibiotics (especially Bactrim, penicillin, or erythromycin) is commonly documented.

Supportive care is usually the only treatment needed for this self-limited disease, although in severe cases, corticosteroids are necessary.[240]

Left Atrial Myxoma

A myxoma affecting the left atrium may simulate vasculitis by embolization and should be considered in the diagnosis of an obscure vasculitislike syndrome.[241] Echocardiography demonstrates the lesion, and surgical removal is curative.

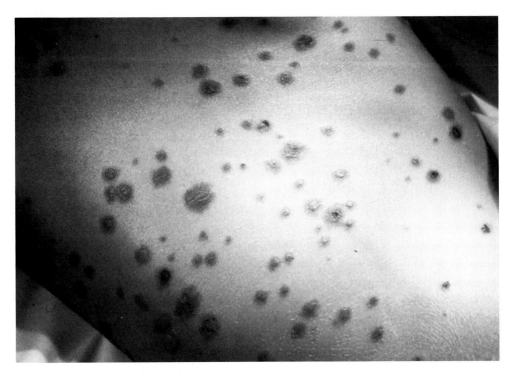

Fig. 9-31 Vesicular erythematous lesions of erythema multiforme in a young boy with Stevens-Johnson syndrome. Such children may have bullous lesions around body orifices.

REFERENCES

1. Leavitt RY, Fauci AS: Polyangiitis overlap syndrome. Am J Med 81:79, 1986
2. Zeek PM: Periarteritis nodosa and other forms of necrotizing angiitis. N Engl J Med 248:764, 1953
3. Fauci AS, Haynes BF, Katz P: The spectrum of vasculitis. Clinical, pathologic, immunologic and therapeutic considerations. Ann Int Med 89:660, 1978
4. Kussmaul A, Maier R: Ueber eine bisher nicht beschriebene eigenthümliche Arterienerkrankung (Periarteritis nodosa), die mit Morbus Brightii und rapid fortschreitender allgemeiner Muskellähmung einhergeht. Arch Klin Med 1:484, 1866
5. Reimold EW, Weinberg AG, Fink CW, Battles ND: Polyarteritis in children. Am J Dis Child 130:534, 1976
6. Blau EB, Morris RF, Yunis EJ: Polyarteritis nodosa in older children. Pediatrics 60:227, 1977
7. Fink CW: Polyarteritis and other disease with necrotizing vasculitis in childhood. Arthritis Rheum, suppl., 20:378, 1977
8. Petty RE, Magilavy DB, Cassidy JT et al: Polyarteritis in childhood. A clinical description of eight cases. Arthritis Rheum, suppl., 20:392, 1977
9. Magilavy DB, Petty RE, Cassidy JT et al: A syndrome of childhood polyarteritis. J Pediatr 91:25, 1977
10. Ettlinger RE, Nelson AM, Burke EC, Lie JT: Polyarteritis nodosa in childhood. A clinical pathologic study. Arthritis Rheum 22:820, 1979
11. Fager DB, Bigler JA, Simonds JP: Polyarteritis nodosa in infancy and childhood. J Pediatr 39:65, 1951
12. Frohnert PP, Sheps SG: Long-term followup study of periarteritis nodosa. Am J Med 43:8, 1967
13. Woodward AH, Andreini PH: Periosteal new bone formation in polyarteritis nodosa. Arthritis Rheum 17:1017, 1974
14. Gocke DJ, Hsu K, Morgan C et al: Association of polyarteritis and Australia antigen. Lancet 2:1149, 1970
15. Woolf AD, Wakerly G, Wallington TB et al: Factor VIII related antigen in the assessment of vasculitis. Ann Rheum Dis 46:441, 1987
16. Burns JC, Glode MP, Clarke SH et al: Coagulopathy and platelet activation in Kawasaki syndrome. Iden-

tification of patients at high risk for development of coronary artery aneurysms. J Pediatr 105:206, 1983

17. McLain LG, Bookstein JJ, Kelsch RC: Polyarteritis nodosa diagnosed by renal arteriography. J Pediatr 80:1032, 1972

18. Yousefzadeh DK, Chow KC, Benson CA: Polyarteritis nodosa: regression of arterial aneurysms following immunosuppressive and corticosteroid therapy. Pediatr Radiol 10:139, 1981

19. Sack M, Cassidy JT, Bole GG: Prognostic factors in polyarteritis. J Rheumatol 2:4, 1975

20. Fauci AS, Katz P, Haynes BF et al: Cyclophosphamide therapy of severe necrotizing vasculitis. N Engl J Med 301:235, 1979

21. Diaz-Perez JL, Winkelmann RK: Cutaneous periarteritis nodosa. Arch Dermatol 110:407, 1974

22. Copeman PWM: Cutaneous angiitis. J R Coll Physicians 9:103, 1975

23. Cream JJ: Clinical and immunological aspects of cutaneous vasculitis. Q J Med 45:340, 1976

24. Cogan DG: Syndrome of nonsyphilitic interstitial keratitis and vestibuloauditory symptoms. Arch Ophthalmol 33:144, 1945

25. Kundell SP, Ochs HD: Cogan syndrome in childhood. J Pediatr 97:96, 1980

26. Cheson BD, Bluming AZ, Alroy J: Cogan's syndrome: a systemic vasculitis. Am J Med 60:549, 1976

27. Munro-Faure H: Necrotizing arteritis of the coronary vessels in infancy. Pediatrics 23:914, 1959

28. Kawasaki T: Acute febrile mucocutaneous syndrome with lymphoid involvement with specific desquamation of the fingers and toes. Jpn J Allerg 16:178, 1967

29. Kawasaki T, Kosaki F, Odawa S et al: A new infantile acute febrile mucocutaneous lymph node syndrome (MCLNS) prevailing in Japan. Pediatrics 54:271, 1974

30. Sekiguchi M, Takao A, Endo M et al: On the mucocutaneous lymph nodes syndrome or Kawasaki disease. In Yu PN, Goodwin JF (eds): Progress in Cardiology 13. Lea & Febiger, Philadelphia, 1985, p. 97

31. Watanabe N: Kawasaki disease (MCLS). Jpn J Rheumatol 1:3, 1986

32. Shulman ST, McAuley JB, Pachman LM et al: Risk of coronary abnormalities due to Kawasaki disease in urban area with small Asian population. Am J Dis Child 141:420, 1987

33. Kato S, Kimura M, Tsuji K et al: HLA antigens in Kawasaki disease. Pediatrics 61:252, 1978

34. Matsuda I, Hayttori S, Nagata JL et al: HLA antigens in mucocutaneous lymph node syndrome. Am J Dis Child 131:1417, 1977

35. Krensky AM, Berenberg W, Shanley K et al: HLA antigens in mucocutaneous lymph node syndrome in New England. Pediatrics 67:741, 1981

36. Harada F, Sada M, Kamiya T et al: Genetic analysis of Kawasaki syndrome. Am J Hum Genet 39:537, 1986

37. Bell DM, Morens DM, Holman RC et al: Kawasaki syndrome in the United States 1976 to 1980. Am J Dis Child 137:211, 1983

38. Dean AG, Melish ME, Hicks R et al: An epidemic of Kawasaki disease in Hawaii. J Pediatr 100:552, 1982

39. Meade RH, Brandt L: Manifestations of Kawasaki disease in New England outbreak of 1980. J Pediatr 100:558, 1982

40. Orlowski J, Mercer RD: Urine mercury levels in Kawasaki disease. Pediatrics 66:633, 1980

41. Patriarca PA, Rogers MF, Morens DM et al: Kawasaki syndrome: association with the application of rug shampoo. Lancet 2:578, 1982

42. Matsuno S, Utagawa E, Sugiura A: Association of rotavirus infection with Kawasaki syndrome. J Infect Dis 148:177, 1983

43. Magilavy DB, Speert DP, Silver TM et al: Mucocutaneous lymph node syndrome: report of two cases complicated by gallbladder hydrops and diagnosed by ultrasound. Pediatr 61:699, 1978

44. Amano S, Hazama F: Neural involvement in Kawasaki disease. Acta Pathol Jpn 30:265, 1980

45. Laxer RM, Dunn HG, Flodmark O: Acute hemiplegia in Kawasaki disease and infantile polyarteritis nodosa. Dev Med Child Neurol 26:814, 1984

46. Melish ME, Hicks RM, Larson EJ: Mucocutaneous lymph node syndrome in the United States. Am J Dis Child 130:599, 1976

47. Amano S, Hazama F, Hamashima Y: Pathology of Kawasaki disease. I: Pathology and morphogenesis of the vascular changes. Jpn Circ J 43:633, 1979

48. Amano S, Hazama F, Hamashima Y: Pathology of Kawasaki disease. II: Distribution and incidence of the vascular lesions. Jpn Circ J 43:741, 1979

49. Fujiwara H, Kawai C, Hamashima Y: Clinicopathologic study of the conduction systems in 10 patients with Kawasaki's disease (mucocutaneous lymph node syndrome). Am Heart J 96:744, 1978

50. Honda S, Sunagawa H, Mizoguchi Y et al: Left ventricular performance and compliance following acute febrile mucocutaneous lymph node syndrome. Jpn Circ J 44:848, 1980

51. Fujiwara H, Hamashima Y: Pathology of the heart in Kawasaki disease. Pediatrics 61:100, 1978

52. Suzuki A, Kamiya T, Kuwahara N et al: Coronary arterial lesions of Kawasaki disease: cardiac catheterization findings of 1100 cases. Pediatr Cardiol 7:3, 1986

53. Asai T: Evaluation method for the degree of seriousness in Kawasaki disease. Acta Paediatr Jpn 25:170, 1983

54. Koren G, Lavi S, Rose V et al: Kawasaki disease: review of risk factors for coronary aneurysms. J Pediatr 108:388, 1986

55. Nakano H, Ueda K, Saito A et al: Scoring method for identifying patients with Kawasaki disease at high risk of coronary artery aneurysms. Am J Cardiol 158:739, 1986

56. Kato H, Ichinose E, Yoshioka Y et al: Fate of coronary aneurysms in Kawasaki disease: serial coronary angiography and long-term follow-up studies. Am J Cardiol 49:1758, 1982

57. Turner-Gomes S, Rose V, Brezina A et al: High persistence rate of established coronary artery lesions secondary to Kawasaki disease among a panethnic Canadian population. J Pediatr 108:928, 1986

58. Takahashi M, Mason W, Lewis AB: Regression of coronary aneurysms in patients with Kawasaki syndrome. Circulation 75:387, 1987

59. Nakano H, Saito A, Ueda K et al: Clinical characteristics of myocardial infarction following Kawasaki disease: report of 11 cases. J Pediatr 108:198, 1986

60. Kohr RM: Progressive asymptomatic coronary artery disease as a late fatal sequela of Kawasaki disease. J Pediatr 108:256, 1986

61. Van der Hauwaert L, Rowe RD, Takao A et al: Results from an international survey of Kawasaki disease in 1979–1982. Second World Congress of Pediatric Cardiology, New York, 1985

62. Kato H, Ichinose E, Kawasaki T: Myocardial infarction in Kawasaki disease: clinical analyses in 195 cases. J Pediatr 108:923, 1986

63. Kato H, Koike S, Yokoyama T: Kawasaki disease: effect of treatment on coronary artery involvement. Pediatr 63:175, 1979

64. Kusakawa S: Long-term administrative care of Kawasaki disease. Acta Paediatr Jpn 25:205, 1983

65. Daniels SR, Specker B, Capannari TE et al: Correlates of coronary artery aneurysm formation in patients with Kawasaki Disease. Am J Dis Child 141:205, 1987

66. Koren G, MacLeod SM: Difficulty in achieving therapeutic serum concentrations of salicylate in Kawasaki disease. J Pediatr 105:991, 1984

67. Calabro JJ, Londino AV, Weber CA: Preventing coronary involvement in Kawasaki disease. JAMA 255:200, 1986

68. Pedersen AK, FitzGerald GA: Dose-related kinetics of aspirin. N Engl J Med 311:1206, 1984

69. Furusho K, Kamiya T, Nakano H et al: High-dose intravenous gamma globulin for Kawasaki disease. Lancet 2:1055, 1984

70. Newburger JW, Takahashi M, Burns JC et al: The treatment of Kawasaki syndrome with intravenous gammaglobulin. N Engl J Med 315:341, 1986

71. Nagashima M, Matsushima M, Matsuoka H et al: High-dose gammaglobulin therapy for Kawasaki disease. J Pediatr 110:710, 1987

72. Leung DYM, Burns JC, Newburger JW et al: Reversal of lymphocyte activation in vivo in the Kawasaki Syndrome by intravenous gammaglobulin. J Clin Invest 79:468, 1987

73. Heberden W: Commentaries on the History and Cure of Diseases. London, 1896, p. 396

74. Willan R: On cutaneous diseases. J Johnson, London, 1808

75. Schonlein JL: Allgemeine und specialle pathologie und therapie. 3rd Ed. Herisana, Lit-Comp 2:48, 1837

76. Henoch EHH: About a peculiar form of purpura. Am J Dis Child 128:78, 1974 (translated from Berlin Klin Wochenschr 11:641, 1874)

77. Gairdner D: The Schönlein-Henoch syndrome (anaphylactoid purpura) Q J Med 17:95, 1948

78. Habib R, Cameron JS: Schönlein-Henoch purpura. In Bacon PA, Hadler NM (eds): The Kidney and Rheumatic Diseases. Butterworth, London 1982. p 178

79. Habib R, Broyer M, Levy M: Schönlein-Henoch purpura glomerulonephritis in children. In Pediatric Nephrology. Vol 4. Strauss J (ed): Garland Press, New York 1977, p. 155

80. Levy M, Broyer M, Assan A et al: Anaphylactoid purpura nephritis in childhood: natural history and immunopathology. Adv Nephrol 6:183, 1976

81. Atkinson SR, Barker DJ: Seasonal distribution of Henoch-Schönlein purpura. Br J Prev Soc Med 30:22, 1976

82. Allen DM, Diamond LK, Howell DA: Anaphylactoid purpura in children (Schönlein-Henoch syndrome): review with a follow-up of the renal complications. Am J Dis Child 99:833, 1960

83. Ayoub EM, Hoyer J: Anaphylactoid purpura: streptococcal antibody titers and beta 1c-globulin levels. J Pediatr 75:193, 1969

84. Ansell BM: Henoch-Schönlein purpura with particular reference to the prognosis of the renal lesion. Br J Dermatol 82:211, 1970

85. Pedersen FK, Petersen EA: Varicella followed by glomerulonephritis. Treatment with corticosteroids and azathioprine resulting in recurrence of varicella. Acta Paediatr Scand 64:886, 1975

86. Meadows SR, Glasgow EF, White RHR et al: Schönlein-Henoch nephritis. Q J Med 41:242, 1972

87. Maggiore G, Martini A, Grideo S et al: Hepatitis B virus infection and Schönlein-Henoch purpura. Am J Dis Child 138:681, 1984

88. Liew SW, Kessel I: Mycoplasmal pneumonia preceding Henoch-Schönlein purpura. Arch Dis Child 49:912, 1974

89. Kobayashi O, Wada H, Ikawa K et al: Schönlein-Henoch syndrome in children. Contrib Nephrol 4:48, 1977

90. Ackroyd JK: Allergic purpura, including purpura due to foods, drugs and infections. Am J Med 14:605, 1953

91. Saulsbury FT: Henoch-Schönlein purpura. Pediatr Dermatol 1:195, 1984

92. Winter HS: Steroid effects on the course of abdominal pain in children with Henoch-Schönlein purpura. Pediatrics 79:1018, 1987

93. Garner JAM: Acute pancreatitis as a complication of anaphylactoid (Henoch-Schönlein) purpura. Arch Dis Child 52:971, 1977

94. Emery H, Larter W, Schaller JG: Henoch-Schönlein vasculitis. Arthritis Rheum suppl., 20:385, 1977

95. Lewis ID, Philpot MG: Neurological complications of the Schönlein-Henoch syndrome. Arch Dis Child 31:369, 1956

96. Kaplan JM, Quintana P, Samson J: Facial nerve palsy with anaphylactoid purpura. Am J Dis Child 119:452, 1970

97. Imai J, Matsumoto S: Anaphylactoid purpura with cardiac involvement. Arch Dis Child 45:727, 1970

98. Sahn DJ, Schwartz AD: Schönlein-Henoch syndrome: observations on some atypical clinical presentations. Pediatrics 49:614, 1972

99. Naiman JL, Harcke T, Sebastinanelli J et al: Scrotal imaging in the Henoch-Schönlein syndrome. J Pediatr 92:1021, 1978

100. O'Regan S, Robitaille P: Orchitis mimicking testicular torsion in Henoch-Schönlein's purpura. J Urol 126:834, 1981

101. Garcia-Fuentes M, Martin A, Chantler C et al: Serum complement components in Henoch-Schönlein purpura. Arch Dis Child 53:417, 1978

102. Kauffmann RH, Hermann WA, Meyer CJLM et al: Circulating IgA immune complexes in Henoch-Schönlein purpura. Am J Med 69:859, 1980

103. Spitzer RE, Urmson JR, Farnett JL et al: Alteration of the complement system in children with Henoch-Schönlein purpura. Clin Immunol Immunopathol 11:52, 1978

104. Levinsky RJ, Barratt TM: IgA immune complexes in Henoch-Schönlein purpura. Lancet 2:1100, 1979

105. Hall RP, Lawley TJ, Heck JA et al: IgA-containing circulating immune complexes in dermatitis herpetiformis, Henoch-Schönlein purpura, systemic lupus erythematosus and other diseases. Clin Exp Immunol 40:431, 1980

106. Garcia-Fuentes M, Chantler C, Williams DG: Cryoglobulinaemia in Henoch-Schönlein purpura. Br Med J 2:163, 1977

107. Trygstad CW, Stiehm ER: Elevated serum IgA globulin in anaphylactoid purpura. Pediatrics 47:1023, 1971

108. Sinniah R, Feng PH, Chen BT: Henoch-Schönlein syndrome: a clinical and morphological study of renal biopsies. Clin Nephrol 9:219, 1978

109. Faille-Kuyper EH, Kater L, Kuijten RH et al: Occurrence of vascular IgA deposits in clinically normal skin of patients with renal disease. Kidney Int 9:424, 1976

110. Giangiacomo J, Tsai CC: Dermal and glomerular deposition of IgA in anaphylactoid purpura. Am J Dis Child 131:981, 1977

111. Nakamoto Y, Asano Y, Dohi K et al: Primary IgA glomerulonephritis and Schönlein-Henoch purpura nephritis: clinicopathological and immunohistological characteristics. Q J Med 47:495, 1978

112. Conley ME, Cooper MD, Michael AF: Selective deposition of immunoglobulin A1 in immunoglobulin A nephropathy, anaphylactoid purpura nephritis and systemic lupus erythematosus. J Clin Invest 66:1423, 1980

113. Counahan R, Cameron JS: Henoch-Schönlein purpura. In: Massry S (ed): Contributions to Nephrology. Karger, Basel, 1977

114. Counahan R, Winterborn MH, White RHR et al: Prognosis of Henoch-Schönlein nephritis in children. Br Med J 2:11, 1977

115. Meadows SR: The prognosis of Henoch-Schönlein nephritis. Clin Nephrol 9:87, 1978

116. Coakley JC, Chambers TL: Should we follow up children with Henoch-Schönlein syndrome? Arch Dis Child 64:903, 1979

117. Bielory L, Gascon P, Lawley TJ et al: Human serum sickness. A prospective analysis of 35 patients treated with equine anti-thymocyte globulin for bone marrow failure. Medicine 67:40, 1988

118. McCarthy PL, Wasserman D, Spiesel SZ et al: Evaluation of arthritis and arthralgia in the pediatric patient. Clin Pediatr 19:183, 1980

119. Murray DL, Singer DA, Singer AB et al: Cefaclor—a cluster of adverse reactions. N Engl J Med 303:1003, 1980

120. Kunnamo I, Kallio P, Pelkonen P et al: Serum-sickness-like disease is a common cause of acute arthritis in children. Acta Paediatr Scand 75:964, 1986

121. McDuffie FC, Sams WM, Jr, Maldonado JE et al: Hypocomplementemia with cutaneous vasculitis and arthritis. Possible immune complex syndrome. Mayo Clin Proc 48:340, 1973

122. Soter NA: Chronic urticaria as a manifestation of necrotizing venulitis. N Engl J Med 296:1440, 1977

123. Levo Y, Gorevic PD, Kassab HJ et al: Association between hepatitis B virus and essential mixed cryoglobulinemia. N Engl J Med 196:1501, 1977

124. Bombardieri S, Paoletti P, Ferri C et al: Lung involvement in essential mixed cryoglobulinemia. Am J Med 66:748, 1979

125. Gamble CN, Ruggles SW: The immunopathogenesis of glomerulonephritis associated with mixed cryoglobulinemia. N Engl J Med 299:81, 1978

126. Weinberger A, Berliner S, Pinkhas J: Articular manifestations of essential cryoglobulinemia. Semin Arthritis Rheum 10:224, 1981

127. Churg J, Strauss L: Allergic granulomatosis, allergic angiitis and periarteritis nodosa. Am J Pathol 277:277, 1961

128. Farooki ZQ, Brough MB, Joseph A et al: Necrotizing arteritis. Am J Dis Child 128:837, 1974

129. Frayha RA: Churg-Strauss syndrome in a child. J Rheumatol 9:807, 1982

130. Wolff SM, Fauci AS, Horn RG et al: Wegener's granulomatosis. Ann Intern Med 81:513, 1974

131. Fahey JL, Leonard E, Churg J et al: Wegener's granulomatosis. Am J Med 17:168, 1954

132. Carrington CB, Liebow AA: Limited forms of angiitis and granulomatosis of Wegener's type. Am J Med 41:497, 1966

133. Feldman F, Fink H, Gruezo Z: Wegener's granulomatosis. Report of a case in a 13-year-old girl. Am J Dis Child 112:587, 1966

134. Roback SA, Herdman RC, Hoyer J et al: Wegener's granulomatosis in a child. Am J Dis Child 118:608, 1969

135. Lane HC, Dodd K: Idiopathic lethal granuloma of the nose and face. Pediatrics 16:461, 1955

136. Cassan SM, Coles DT, Harrison EG, Jr: The concept of limited forms of Wegener's granulomatosis. Am J Med 49:366, 1970

137. Cawson RA: Gingival changes in Wegener's granulomatosis. Br Dent J 118:30, 1965

138. Brown HA, Woolner LB: Findings referable to the upper part of the respiratory tract in Wegener's granulomatosis. Ann Otol Rhinol Laryngol 69:810, 1960

139. Atkins JP, Eisman SH: Wegener's granulomatosis. Ann Otol Rhinol Laryngol 68:524, 1959

140. Thomas K: Laryngeal manifestations of Wegener's granulomatosis. J Laryngol Otol 84:101, 1970

141. Lancos F, Erdos Z, Kadar A et al: Wegenersche granulomatose in kindesalter. Acta Paediatr Acad Sci Hung 12:285, 1971

142. Isaeva LA, Fedorova AN, Lysinka GA et al: Wegener's granulomatosis in children. Pediatriia 51:67, 1972

143. Hu H, O'Loughlin S, Winkelmann RK: Cutaneous manifestations of Wegener granulomatosis. Arch Dermatol 113:175, 1977

144. Reza MJ, Dornfeld L, Goldberg LS et al: Wegener's granulomatosis. Long-term followup of patients treated with cyclophosphamide. Arthritis Rheum 18:501, 1975

145. Moorthy AV, Chesney RW, Segar WE et al: Wegener granulomatosis in childhood: Prolonged survival following cytotoxic therapy. J Pediatr 91:616, 1977

146. Baliga R, Chang CH, Bidani AK et al: A case of generalized Wegener's granulomatosis in childhood: successful therapy with cyclophosphamide. Pediatrics 61:286, 1978

147. Orlowski JP, Clough JD, Dyment PG: Wegener's granulomatosis in the pediatric age group. Pediatrics 61:83, 1978

148. Hall SL, Miller LC, Duggan E et al: Wegener granulomatosis in pediatric patients. J Pediatr 106:739, 1985

149. Case Records of the Massachusetts General Hospital. Case 12-1986. N Engl J Med 314:834, 1986

150. Fauci A, Hynes B, Katz P et al: Wegener's granulomatosis: prospective clinical and therapeutic experience with 85 patients for 21 years. Ann Intern Med 98:76, 1983

151. Mills JA, McCroskery PA: Periarteritis nodosa, hypersensitivity angiitis and related syndromes: clinical and pathological aspects. Bacon PA, and Hadler NM (eds): The Kidney and Rheumatic Disease. Butterworth, London, 1982, p. 150

152. Rubin D, Peterson P, Meltzer JI: Renal lesions in Wegener's granulomatosis. Ann Intern Med 82:849, 1975

153. Liebow AA, Carrington CB, Friedman PJ: Lymphomatoid granulomatosis. Hum Pathol 3:457, 1972

154. Fauci AS, Haynes BF, Costa J et al: Lymphomatoid granulomatosis. Prospective clinical and therapeutic experience over 10 years. N Engl J Med 306:68, 1982

155. Shen SC, Heuser ET, Landing BH et al: Lymphomatoid granulomatosis-like lesions in a child with leukemia in remission. Hum Pathol 12:276, 1981

156. Ilowite NT, Fligner CL, Ochs HD et al: Pulmonary angiitis with atypical lymphoreticular infiltrates in Wiskott-Aldrich syndrome: possible relationship of lymphomatoid granulomatosis and EBV infection. Clin Immunol Immunopathol 41:479, 1986

157. Koss MN, Hochnolzer L, Langloss JM et al: Lymphomatoid granulomatosis: a clinicopathologic study of 42 patients. Pathology 18:283, 1986

158. Cravioto H, Feigin I: Noninfectious granulomatous angiitis with a predilection for the nervous system. Neurology 9:599, 1959

159. Calabrese LH, Mallek JA: Primary angiitis of the central nervous system. Medicine 67:20, 1988

160. Goldberg HJ: Moyamoya associated with peripheral vascular occlusive disease. Arch Dis Child 49:964, 1974

161. Takayasu M: Case with unusual changes of the central retinal vessels. Acta Soc Ophthalmol Jpn 12:554, 1908

162. Hall S, Nelson AM: Takayasu's arteritis and juvenile rheumatoid arthritis. J Rheumatol 13:431, 1986

163. Haas A, Stiehm ER: Takayasu's arteritis presenting as pulmonary hypertension. Am J Dis Child 140:372, 1986

164. Taieb A, Dufillot D, Pellegrin-Carloz B et al: Postgranulomatous anetoderma associated with Takayasu's arteritis in a child. Arch Dermatol 123:796, 1987

165. Eke F, Balfe JW, Hardy BE: Three patients with arteritis. Arch Dis Child 59:877, 1984

166. Gronemeyer PS, deMello DE: Takayasu's disease with aneurysm of right common iliac artery and iliocaval fistula in a young infant: case report and review of the literature. Pediatrics 69:616, 1982

167. Pantell RH, Goodman BW, Jr: Takayasu's arteritis: the relationship with tuberculosis. Pediatrics 67:84, 1981

168. Gupta S: Surgical and haemodynamic considerations in middle aortic syndrome. Thorax 34:470, 1979

169. Gupta S, Goswami B, Ghosh DC et al: Middle aortic syndrome as a cause of heart failure in children and its management. Thorax 36:63, 1981

170. Hall S, Barr W, Lie JT et al: Takayasu arteritis. A study of 32 North American patients. Medicine 64:89, 1985

171. Southwood TR, Buckley AR, Culham JAG et al: New techniques for detection of large vessel arteritis. Arthritis Rheum 31:R18 1988

172. Vinijchaikul AJ: Primary arteritis of the aorta and its main branches (Takayasu's arteriopathy). Medicine 43:15, 1967

173. Lomas RW, Bolande RP, Gibson WM: Primary arteritis of the aorta in a child. Am J Dis Child 97:87, 1959

174. Warshaw JB, Spach MS: Takayasu's disease (primary aortitis) in childhood: Case report with a review of the literature. Pediatrics 35:620, 1965

175. Zilleruelo GE, Ferrer P, Garcia OL et al: Takayasu's arteritis associated with glomerulonephritis. Am J Dis Child 132:1009, 1978

176. Owyang C, Miller LJ, Lie JT et al: Takayasu's arteritis in Crohn's disease. Gastroenterology 76:825, 1979

177. Gilbert EF, Levy JM, Hong R et al: Takayasu's arteriopathy with involvement of aortic valve and bacterial endocarditis. J Pediatr 83:463, 1973

178. Danaraj TJ, Ong WH: Primary arteritis of abdominal aorta in children causing bilateral stenosis of renal arteries and hypertension. Circulation 20:856, 1959

179. Danaraj TJ, Wong WO, Thomas MA: Primary arteritis of the aorta causing renal artery stenosis and hypertension. Br Heart J 25:153, 1963

180. Wiggelinkhuizen J, Cremin BJ: Takayasu arteritis and renovascular hypertension in childhood. Pediatrics 62:209, 1978

181. Wagenvoort CA, Harris LE, Brown AL et al: Giant cell arteritis with aneurysm formation in children. Pediatrics 32:861, 1963

182. Rossor E: Takayasu's arteritis as a differential diagnosis of systemic juvenile chronic arthritis. Arch Dis Child 54:798, 1979

183. Numano R, Isohisa I, Kishi U et al: Takayasu's disease in twin sisters. Possible genetic factors. Circulation 58:173, 1978

184. Feld LG, Weiss RA, Weiner S et al: Takayasu's arteritis. Asymptomatic presentation in a two-year-old boy. New York State J Med 83:229, 1983

185. Rozwadowski MA, Downing JW: Anaesthetic management for nephrectomy in a child with Takayasu's arteritis and severe renovascular hypertension. S Afr Med J 67:898, 1985

186. Kubryk N, Blanluet B, Borde M: Maladie de Takayasu. A propos d'une observation chez une enfant de quatorze ans. Sem Hôp Paris 58:1189, 1982

187. Lupi-Herrera E, Sanchez-Torres G, Marcushamer J et al: Takayasu's arteritis. Clinical study of 107 cases. Am Heart J 93:94, 1977

188. Asherson RA, Asherson GL, Schrire V: Immunological studies in arteritis of the aorta and great vessels. Br Med J 3:589, 1968

189. Nakao K, Ikeda M, Kimata S et al: Takayasu's arteritis. Clinical report of eighty-four cases and immunological studies of seven cases. Circulation 35:1141, 1967

190. Fraga A, Mintz G, Valle L et al: Takayasu's arteritis: frequency of systemic manifestations (study of 22 patients) and favorable response to maintenance steroid therapy with adrenocorticosteroids (12 patients). Arthritis Rheum 15:617, 1972

191. Shelhamer JH, Volkman DJ, Parrillo JE et al: Takayasu's arteritis and its therapy. Ann Intern Med 103:121, 1985

192. Lie JT, Gordon LP, Titus JL: Juvenile temporal arteritis: biopsy study of four cases. JAMA 234:496, 1975

193. Hunder GG, Allen GL: Giant cell arteritis: a review. Bull Rheum Dis 29:980, 1978

194. Behçet H: Uber rezidivierende Aphthose, durch ein Virus verursachte Geschwure am Mund, am Auge und an den Genitalien. Dermatol Wochenschr 105:1152, 1937

195. O'Duffy JD: Summary of international symposium on Behçet's disease. J Rheumatol 5:229, 1978

196. Mason RM, Barnes CG: Behçet's syndrome with arthritis. Ann Rheum Dis 28:5, 1969
197. Sakane T, Kotani H, Takada S et al: Functional aberration of T cell subsets in patients with Behçet's disease. Arthritis Rheum 25:1343, 1982
198. Chamberlain MA: Behçet's syndrome in 32 patients in Yorkshire. Ann Rheum Dis 36:491, 1977
199. Oshima Y, Shimizu T, Hokohari R et al: Clinical studies on Behçet's syndrome. Ann Rheum Dis 28:102, 1969
200. Pitkeathly DA: Discussion on Behçet's syndrome with arthritis. Ann Rheum Dis 28:102, 1969
201. Yazici H, Tuzun Y, Pazarli H et al: The combined use of HLA-B5 and the pathergy test as diagnostic markers of Behçet's disease in Turkey. J Rheumatol 7:206, 1980
202. Ohno S, Narayama E, Sigiura S et al: Specific histocompatibility antigens associated with Behçet's disease. Am J Ophthalmol 80:636, 1975
203. Adorno D, Pezzi PP, Bonini S et al: HLA-B5 and Behçet's disease. Tissue Antigens 14:444, 1979
204. Lavalle C, Alarcon-Segovia A, Del Giudice-Knipping JA et al: Association of Behçet's syndrome with HLA-B5 in the Mexican Mestizo population. J Rheumatol 8:325, 1981
205. Lehner T, Batchelor JR, Challacombe SJ et al: An immunogenetic basis for the tissue involvement in Behçet's syndrome. Immunology 37:895, 1979
206. Moore SB, O'Duffy JD: Lack of association between Behçet's disease and major histocompatibility complex class II antigens in an ethnically diverse North American Caucasoid patient group. J Rheumatol 13:771, 1986
207. Fam AG, Siminovitch KA, Carette S et al: Neonatal Behçet's syndrome in an infant of a mother with the disease. Ann Rheum Dis 40:509, 1981
208. Lewis MA, Priestly BL: Transient neonatal Behçet's disease. Arch Dis Child 61:805, 1986
209. Wright V, Mill JMH: Seronegative Polyarthritis. New-Holland, Amsterdam, 1976, p. 353
210. Ammann AJ, Johnson A, Fyfe G et al: Behçet Syndrome. J Pediatr 107:41, 1985
211. Mundy TM, Miller JJ, III: Behçet's disease presenting as chronic aphthous stomatitis in a child. Pediatr 62:205, 1978
212. Colvard DM, Robertson DM, O'Duffy JD: The ocular manifestations of Behçet's disease. Arch Ophthalmol 95:1813, 1977
213. O'Duffy JD: Prognosis in Behçet's syndrome. Bull Rheum Dis 29:972, 1978
214. Enoch BA, Castillo-Olivares JL, Khoo TCL et al: Major vascular complications in Behçet's syndrome. Postgrad Med J 44:453, 1968
215. Davies JD: Behçet's syndrome with haemoptysis and pulmonary lesions. J Pathol 109:351, 1973
216. Grenier P, Bletry O, Cornud F et al: Pulmonary involvement in Behçet's disease. Am J Radiol 137:565, 1981
217. O'Duffy JD, Goldstein NP: Neurologic involvement in seven patients with Behçet's disease. Am J Med 61:170, 1976
218. Dilsen AN: Sacroiliitis and ankylosing spondylitis in Behçet's disease. Scand J Rheumatol, suppl. 8, abstract 20, 1975
219. Wright V, Moll JMH: Seronegative Polyarthritis. New-Holland, Amsterdam, 1976, p. 362
220. Mizushima Y, Matsumura N, Mori M: Chemotaxis of leukocytes and colchicine treatment in Behçet's disease. J Rheumatol 6:108, 1979
221. de Merieux P, Spitler LE, Paulus HE: Treatment of Behçet's syndrome with Levamisole. Arthritis Rheum 24:64, 1981
222. Tricoulis D: Treatment of Behçet's disease with Chlorambucil. Br J Ophthalmol 60:55, 1976
223. Jorizzo JL, Schmalstieg FC, Solomon AR et al: Thalidomide effects in Behçet's syndrome and pustular vasculitis. Arch Intern Med 146:878, 1986
224. Ellsworth JE, Cassidy JT, Ragsdale CG et al: Mucha-Habermann disease in children: The association with rheumatic diseases. J Rheumatol 9:319, 1982
225. Lister PD, Hollingworth P: Arthritis associated with leukocytoclastic angiitis. Ann Rheum Dis 39:526, 1980
226. Feuerman EJ: Papulosis atrophicans maligna Degos. 94:440, 1966
227. Strole WE, Clark WH, Isselbacher KJ: Progressive arterial occlusive disease (Kohlmeier-Degos). N Engl J Med 276:195, 1967
228. Soter NA, Mihm MC, Colten HR: Cutaneous necrotizing venulitis in patients with cystic fibrosis. J Pediatr 95:197, 1979
229. Sweet RD: An acute febrile neutrophilic dermatosis. Br J Dermatol 76:349, 1964
230. Saxe N, Gordon W: Acute febrile neutrophilic dermatosis (Sweet's syndrome). S Afr Med J 53:253, 1978
231. Klock JC, Oken RL: Febrile neutrophilic dermatosis in acute myelogenous leukemia. Cancer 37:922, 1976
232. Itami S, Nishioka K: Sweet's syndrome in infancy. Br J Dermatol 103:449, 1980
233. Levin DL, Burton EN, Herman JJ et al: Sweet syndrome in children. J Pediatr 99:73, 1981
234. Larsson L-G, Baum J: Acute febrile neutrophilic dermatosis (Sweet's syndrome). Successful treatment with short term corticosteroids. J Rheumatol 12:1000, 1985
235. Goodpasture EW: The significance of certain pul-

monary lesions in relation to the etiology of influenza. Am J Med Sci 158:863, 1919

236. Levin M, Rigden SPA, Pincott JR et al: Goodpasture's syndrome: treatment with plasmapheresis, immunosuppression, and anticoagulation. Arch Dis Child 58:697, 1983

237. Anand SK, Landing BH, Heuser ET et al: Changes in glomerular basement membrane antigen(s) with age. J Pediatr 92:952, 1978

238. Siegler RL, Bond DB, Morris AH: Treatment of Goodpasture's syndrome with plasma exchange and immunosuppression. Clin Pediatr 19:488, 1980

239. Kazimierowski JA, Wuepper KD: Erythema multiforme. Clin Rheum Dis 8:415, 1982

240. Rasmussen JE: Erythema multiforme in children: response to treatment with systemic corticosteroids. Br J Dermatol 95:181, 1976

241. Byrd WE, Matthews OP, Hunt RE: Left atrial myxoma presenting as a systemic vasculitis. Arthritis Rheum 23:240, 1980

10

The Sclerodermas and Related Disorders

CLASSIFICATION

The word *scleroderma* means "hard skin." The disease scleroderma means a great deal more, although hardening of the skin is a feature common to all types of scleroderma and is the most characteristic feature. A classification of the systemic and localized sclerodermas is shown in Table 10-1.

SYSTEMIC SCLERODERMA

Progressive Systemic Sclerosis (Classic Scleroderma)

Progressive systemic sclerosis (PSS) is a systemic disorder characterized by sclerodermatous skin changes and abnormalities of the viscera. Rodnan has defined PSS as a disease in which "symmetrical fibrous thickening and hardening (sclerosis) of the skin is combined with fibrous and degenerative changes in synovium, digital arteries, and certain internal organs, most notably the esophagus, intestinal tract, heart, lungs, and kidneys."[1] According to the preliminary criteria for the classification of systemic sclerosis of the American Rheumatism Association,[2] definite identification of PSS requires the presence of the major criterion or of two minor criteria (Table 10-2).

EPIDEMIOLOGY

PSS has been described worldwide and in all races.[3] It has an estimated annual incidence of from 4.5 per million[4] to 12 per million.[5] The frequency of the disease appears to increase with age and is maximal in the 30- to 50-year age group. Childhood onset is very uncommon and accounts for a small proportion of all patients with scleroderma (Table 10-3).

There are several small published series of children with PSS, and a number of case reports totaling less than 100 patients, although there are undoubtedly many more unreported patients. Those children in whom the diagnosis of PSS is clear and for whom the appropriate data are available are summarized in Table 10-4. Girls outnumber boys 3 to 1 in the group as a whole. In adults with this disease, the overall ratio of females to males is 3:1. However, from age 15 to 44 years the ratio is 15 females to 1 male, whereas after the age of 45 years, the ratio is 1.8 females to 1 male.[4] From the available data (Table 10-4),[28] it appears that the disease occurs with equal frequency in boys and girls under 8 years of age, whereas girls outnumber boys 3 to 1 when disease onset is at 8 years of age and older.

Mortality from PSS increases throughout the life span and is higher for females than for males and higher for nonwhites than for whites (Table 10-5).[28] Although no data for children are available, studies of patients of all ages demonstrate mean survivals of

renal vasculature has been reported by some investigators.[130–132]

Central Nervous System Disease

Central nervous system involvement in scleroderma is usually a reflection of renal or pulmonary abnormalities.[133] Cerebral arteritis has been described,[134] but the most frequently described abnormality in uncomplicated scleroderma is cranial nerve involvement, especially of the sensory component of the trigeminal nerve.[135–137] In contrast, peripheral neuropathies appear to be very uncommon.[138] A more subtle abnormality, diminished perception of vibration, probably reflects the damping effect of cutaneous scleroderma on the transmission of vibration.[139]

LABORATORY STUDIES

Immunologic Abnormalities

Antinuclear antibodies are frequently demonstrated in the serum of children with PSS. Indirect immunofluorescence microscopy on HEp 2 cell line substrates shows speckled and nucleolar patterns. A recent large study of adults with systemic sclerosis demonstrated that 26 percent of patients had antibody to Scl-70 (topoisomerase 1), and 22 percent had antibody to centromere.[140] No patient had antibodies to both antigens. The anticentromere antibody occurred almost exclusively in patients with the CREST syndrome, in whom it correlated with the presence of calcinosis and telangiectasis. Antibody to Scl-70 occurred most frequently in patients with diffuse scleroderma, in whom it was associated with peripheral vascular disease (digital pitting) and pulmonary interstitial fibrosis. A correlation was also demonstrated between anticentromere antibody and HLA-DR1, and between anti-Scl-70 and HLA-DR5. A second study showed similar disease-antibody correlations, although patients with antibodies to both centromere and topoisomerase 1 were occasionally seen and an association between the presence of antibody to topoisomerase 1 and malignancy was noted.[141] Antibodies that are specific for a 70-kilodalton mitochondrial antigen have been described in a small proportion of patients with systemic scleroderma or CREST syndrome.[142]

Hematologic Abnormalities

Anemia is present in approximately one-quarter of patients with PSS[143] and may be characteristic of the anemia of chronic inflammation or, less commonly, reflect vitamin B_{12} or folic acid deficiency resulting from malabsorption by the sclerodermatous gut.[144] Anemia resulting from microangiopathic hemolysis[145] or bleeding from mucosal telangiectases also occurs. Autoimmune hemolytic anemia is rare.[146,147] Leukocytosis is not prominent but correlates with advanced visceral or muscle disease.[143]

CREST Syndrome and Its Variants

DEFINITIONS

The acronym CREST stands for calcinosis, Raynaud's phenomenon, esophageal dysmotility, sclerodactyly, and telangiectases, a syndrome that was described as acrosclerosis in the older literature. Whether it is a relatively mild form of systemic scleroderma or is an entirely separate, although related disorder is undecided.[1,148] In the CREST syndrome, the sclerotic skin changes are restricted to the distal parts of the digits, and the telangiectases, Raynaud's phenomenon, and calcinosis are more prominent than in PSS. The presence of proximal scleroderma would suggest the diagnosis of PSS rather than CREST. In other ways, however, CREST syndrome closely resembles PSS, and the division of the two may be an artificial one. It was initially believed that patients with the CREST variant had a more benign disease than those with PSS, but this distinction has been disputed. For the purpose of clarity, however, PSS and CREST are discussed separately in this chapter.

EPIDEMIOLOGY

Overall, CREST syndrome accounts for approximately half of the patients with systemic scleroderma.[149] In a comparison of CREST and PSS in two large series of adults with these diseases, CREST was noted to be more frequent among women and tended to occur at an earlier age than did PSS. It was also noted that although the overall frequency of Raynaud's phenomenon was similar in PSS and CREST

Table 10-9 CREST Syndrome and Variants in Children

Reference	Sex	Age at Onset	Clinical Features
Burge et al.[16]	Male	6 yr	CREST
Larrègue et al.[14]	Female	6½ yr	CRST
	Female	6 yr	CRST
Suarez-Almazor et al.[15]	Female	10 yr	RST

syndrome, a long interval between the onset of Raynaud's phenomenon and the detection of skin changes was characteristic of CREST, and that characteristics of the capillary microscopy could be useful in differentiating the two. Mortality caused by CREST, although less than with PSS, is substantial, with a 10-year survival rate of approximately 75 percent.[149]

Very few instances of CREST in children have been reported. Those in which the classification is clear are summarized in Table 10-9.

CLINICAL CHARACTERISTICS

The individual clinical characteristics are identical to those described for PSS, although the calcinosis is usually more severe, the Raynaud's phenomenon more frequently complicated by digital ulceration and gangrene, and the telangiectases more widespread[150] (Figs. 10-17 and 10-18). It is the concurrence of these abnormalities that leads to the grouping of such patients under the diagnosis of CREST syndrome. Incomplete forms of the syndrome (CRST, CRT, etc) merge with PSS and make differentiation of the two difficult, if not impossible. The combination of scleroderma and calcinosis is sometimes referred to as the *Thibierge-Weissenbach syndrome*.[151] Winterbauer first described CRST syndrome.[150]

Although it has been alleged that CREST is associated with a lower mortality rate than is PSS, this variant is by no means a mild disease. Severe systemic involvement, especially of lungs and pulmonary vasculature, can occur, although renal disease appears to be less frequent than in PSS.

SEROLOGIC CHARACTERISTICS

Antibody to centromere was described as the serologic hallmark of the CREST syndrome, and its presence supported the rationale for the differentiation of PSS and CREST.[148,152] It appears, however, that antibody to centromere may occur in diseases other than CREST syndrome,[153] notably primary biliary cirrhosis, occasionally PSS, Sjögren's syndrome, Raynaud's phenomenon, and rarely, rheumatoid arthritis and SLE and other connective tissue diseases. Other ANAs (anti-ssDNA, anti-RNP) may occasionally occur in CREST.[154]

Mixed Connective-Tissue Disease

In 1972 Sharp et al.[155] described the clinical and serologic findings in 25 patients with a syndrome they termed *mixed connective-tissue disease* (MCTD). The syndrome included elements of PSS, SLE, and dermatomyositis occurring in conjunction with high titers of antibodies to an extractable nuclear antigen (ENA) (RNAse-sensitive nuclear antigen, RNP). It was initially believed that the patients had a paucity of renal disease, that response to corticosteroids was excellent, and that the prognosis was, in general, favorable. However, a reassessment of the original study patients showed that over time, the arthritis, serositis, fever, and myositis became less severe, while sclerodermatous findings of sclerodactyly and esophageal disease came to dominate the clinical picture, although renal disease remained infrequent.[156] The MCTD syndrome is being recognized with increasing frequency in childhood, although few cases have been reported to date (Table 10-10). As with the disease in adults, MCTD in children is a disease that evolves from a presentation indistinguishable from that of SLE or occasionally PSS or dermatomyositis. The presence of high-titer anti-RNP should alert the physician to the probable evolution of this disease into a "mixed" connective-tissue disease pattern, encompassing elements of two or more diseases.

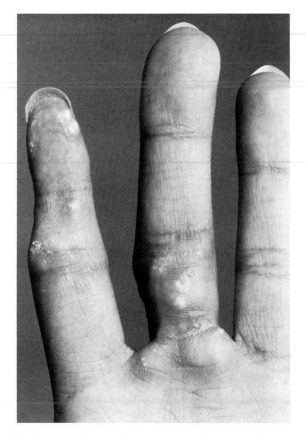

Fig. 10-17 Striking subcutaneous calcification. There may be extrusion of the material, resulting in a fistula.

CLINICAL CHARACTERISTICS

The individual disease characteristics of children with MCTD are summarized in Table 10-11. Arthritis and Raynaud's phenomenon are the most com-mon manifestations recorded. Cutaneous changes include sclerodermatous skin changes in almost one-half, with the rash of SLE in one-third, and the rash of dermatomyositis in one-third of children. Heart disease, pulmonary disease, central nervous system involvement, and esophageal dysmotility were also quite common. Although renal disease occurs, it is less common than in SLE.

IMMUNOLOGIC CHARACTERISTICS

Anti-RNP is the serologic hallmark of MCTD. This antibody may, however, be present in other diseases such as SLE, but the titer is usually low.[158] Rheumatoid factor is also commonly found, but other autoantibodies are unusual (Table 10-11). Some patients have marked elevations of immunoglobulin levels, especially of IgG,[158,160] and one patient with an isolated IgA deficiency has been reported.[157] A comparison of clinical and serologic characteristics of PSS, CREST syndrome, SLE, and MCTD is shown in Table 10-12.

PATHOLOGY

Singsen et al. described widespread vascular intimal and medial vascular wall thickening in four children with MCTD who died.[166] Renal biopsies in eight patients showed membranous change or vascular sclerosis. These authors commented that although the histopathology of MCTD resembled that of PSS, the extent of fibrosis in MCTD was less, and the intimal vascular abnormalities in larger vessels such as the coronary, pulmonary, and renal arteries and the aorta were more prominent.

Table 10-10 Mixed Connective-Tissue Disease in Childhood

Reference	N	Male	Female	Age at Onset
Sharp[155]	1		1	13 yr
Sanders[157]	1		1	8 yr
Fraga[158]	3	1	2	5 yr, 10 yr, 12 yr
Singsen[159]	14	4	10	4–16 yr (mean 10.5 yr)
Oetgen[160]	4	2	2	10 yr, 15 yr, 18 yr, 9 yr
Savouret[161]	7	2	5	(mean 10.7 yr)
Rosenberg[162]	1		1	11 yr
Peskett[163]	5	1	4	7 yr, 10 yr, 1 yr, 16 yr
Rosenthal[164]	5	2	3	7 yr, 7 yr, 10 yr, 12 yr, 16 yr
Eberhardt[165]	6	1	5	11 yr, 12 yr, 14 yr (4 patients)

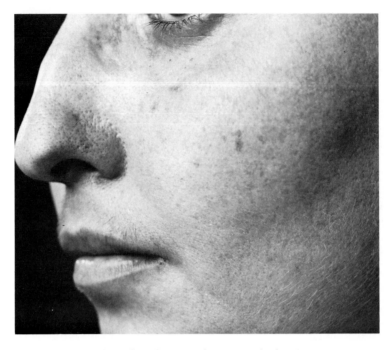

Fig. 10-18 A face showing classic round telangiectases.

Management of the Systemic Sclerodermas

The patient with systemic scleroderma presents one of the most difficult management challenges in all of pediatric rheumatology. The disease severity ranges from mild and nonprogressive to rapidly progressive and fatal. Management of the patient with PSS can be divided into three general areas: general supportive treatment, therapy directed at controlling the underlying disease process, and therapy directed at managing complications of the underlying disease.

General supportive therapy is of utmost importance in the management of any patient with a chronic unpredictable, debilitating, and potentially fatal disease. Education of the patient and parents should be undertaken early in an attempt to prevent unnecessary psychological trauma. In general, "optimistic veracity" regarding complications, outcome, and treatment is appropriate. Patient support groups may be useful, although this approach should be individualized. The therapeutic team including rheumatologist, dermatologist, nephrologist, nurse, social worker, physical and occupational therapists, and other health professionals should be involved with the patient's management from the beginning. Patients should be instructed to avoid cold and trauma. Especially in cold climates, the family should be reminded to keep the child warm both by maintaining the household temperature and by ensuring appropriate clothing, including well-insulated mitts (not gloves). On the other hand, the child should avoid excess sun exposure and heat, because of the susceptibility to hyperpigmentation of the skin and a relative inability to dissipate heat though the sclerotic skin. The child should be encouraged to be as physically active as is possible within the constraints outlined. Daily active and gentle passive range of motion exercises are essential in order to preserve maximal function. Splints may be necessary to treat or prevent contractures. General skin care should include avoidance of drying or irritating substances and application of lanolin or cream as a lubricant once or several times daily.

SPECIFIC THERAPY

The large number of different pharmacologic agents that have been used to treat generalized scleroderma is testimony to their relative inefficacy. The

Table 10-11 Disease Characteristics of Children with MCTD[a]

	No. Reported[b]	No. Present[c]	% Present
Arthritis	45	43	96
Raynaud's phenomenon	45	39	87
Sclerodermatous skin	40	19	48
Rash of SLE	40	16	36
Rash of dermatomyositis	40	16	36
Fever	34	22	65
Abnormal esophageal motility	29	14	48
Heart disease	40	12	30
Pericarditis	40	10	25
Muscle disease	45	27	60
Sjögren's syndrome	39	18	46
CNS disease	34	11	32
Lung			
Abnormal diffusion	29	5	17
Restrictive disease	29	8	27
Hypertension	29	2	7
Effusion	29	4	14
X-ray changes only	29	1	3
Splenomegaly	36	15	42
Hepatomegaly	41	16	39
Renal disease	45	13	29
LE-cell positive	8	2	25
Anti-DNA	40	5	12
Anti-Sm	32	4	12
Anti-RNP	45	45	100
Rheumatoid factor	38	25	66

[a] Data derived from 8 reports with a total of 45 children.
[b] The number of children in whom the characteristic was noted.
[c] The number in whom the abnormality was present.
(Data derived from Sanders et al.,[157] Fraga et al.,[158] Singsen et al.,[159] Oetgen et al.,[160] Savouret et al.,[161] Peskett et al.,[163] Rosenthal,[164] and Eberhardt et al.[165])

agents that are in current use are directed at suppressing the immune response (immunosuppressants), inhibiting the fibroproliferative process (colchicine), or breaking down collagen (penicillamine).

Immunosuppressants

There has been no controlled trial of the use of immunosuppressant drugs in the treatment of scleroderma in adults or in children. In spite of this, the belief that immunologic mechanisms are perpetuators, if not initiators, of the disease process has led to the use of drugs such as azathioprine[167] and chlorambucil.[168] Unfortunately, such agents have had no demonstrable benefit.

Corticosteroids, the mainstay of treatment in many of the connective-tissue disorders, are generally ineffective in the management of PSS, except for the early inflammatory stage of muscle involvement.[169] They may be contraindicated in the presence of renovascular hypertension.

Colchicine

There have been several reports that colchicine treatment (up to 0.5 mg q.i.d. in adults) results in softening of the skin in patients with PSS.[170] Sustained improvement in visceral disease is inconsistent, however.

Table 10-12 Comparison of PSS, CREST, MCTD, Dermatomyositis (DM), and SLE

Characteristic	PSS	CREST	MCTD	DM	SLE
Acrosclerosis	+ + +	+ + + +	+ +	−	−
Proximal sclerosis	+ + + +	−	+ +	−	−
Raynaud's phenomenon	+ + + +	+ + + +	+	+	+ +
Telangiectases	+ + +	+ + + +	−	+	−
Calcinosis	+ +	+ + + +	+	+ + +	−
Esophageal disease	+ +	+ + +	−	+	−
Pulmonary fibrosis	+ + + +	+ + +	+ +	+	+ +
Cardiac disease	+ + + +	−	+	+	+
Renal disease	+ + +	−	+	−	+ + + +
Muscle disease	+ + +	−	+ +	+ + + +	+
CNS disease	+	−	+ +	−	+ + +
Anti-DNA antibody	−	−	+	−	+ + +
Antinucleolar antibody	+ +	+	−	−	−
Anticentromere antibody	+	+ + + +	+	−	−
Anti-Sm antibody	−	−	−	−	+ + +
Anti-RNP					
Low titer	−	−	+	−	+
High titer	−	−	+ + + +	−	−

− rare or absent; + up to 25% of patients; + + up to 50% of patients; + + + up to 75% of patients; + + + + up to 100% of patients.

Penicillamine

Recently, D-penicillamine has been the drug most commonly used to treat PSS, in both children and adults, although results have been somewhat inconsistent.[171–173] There is, however, general agreement that if used early, penicillamine benefits the skin disease.

Penicillamine is of considerable benefit in preventing or retarding the progress of pulmonary involvement. A recent report compared D-penicillamine (n = 17 patients) with low-dose prednisone or no treatment (n = 6 patients) in the treatment of systemic sclerosis (n = 17 patients, CREST = 2 patients) or MCTD (= 4 patients). With a mean follow-up of 4½ years, DLCO/LV and DLCO remained stable in the penicillamine-treated group but decreased in the group receiving steroids or no treatment.[174] These results, together with the observation that FVC did not improve, suggested to Medsger that the drug could reverse vascular endothelial thickening but not interstitial fibrosis.[175] In vitro evidence that synthetic vitamin A analogs (retinoids) suppress synthesis of pro alpha$_1$ (I) and pro alpha$_1$ (III) collagen molecules by fibroblasts obtained from patients with scleroderma[176] suggests that these agents may be useful in the treatment of scleroderma, but to date experience is extremely limited.[177]

MANAGEMENT OF RENAL DISEASE

Until recently, the prognosis for patients with the complication of renal disease was uniformly dismal. Some success followed the use of hemodialysis with or without bilateral nephrectomy and transplantation.[178] LeRoy and Fleischmann caution that any sudden change in plasma volume should be prevented in patients with renal involvement since marked reductions in renal blood flow may precipitate the full-blown clinical problem.[179] The introduction of captopril, an inhibitor of angiotensin converting enzyme, has brought about remarkable improvement in the outlook for these patients, with effective control of blood pressure and stabilization of renal function.[180]

Management of Raynaud's Phenomenon

In addition to avoidance of precipitating circumstances such as cold or stress, specific treatment of Raynaud's phenomenon may be necessary. Useful drugs include those that affect the sympathetic nervous system, thereby indirectly causing vasodilatation, and those that act directly on the smooth muscle of the vessel wall. One drug may be effective in one patient whereas another drug is effective in others. It is, therefore, worth using several agents, one at a time, until the desired effect is obtained (Table 10-13).

Nifedipine is probably the drug of choice in the management of Raynaud's phenomenon, although the rank of this drug may change as new agents are developed. Nifedipine is a calcium channel blocker and has been shown in several controlled trials to be well tolerated and to have significant effect in reducing the frequency and severity of Raynaud's phenomenon and promoting healing of cutaneous ischemic ulcers.[189,191,192] These medications are best started in low dose, initially at bedtime. Full dosage is then achieved gradually to prevent precipitating postural hypotension. We have found phenoxybenzamine to be an effective drug in doses of 10 to 40 mg per day, divided into three or four doses, although depression may be a significant side effect. Treatment should be initiated with a small dose (10 mg) at bedtime and increased gradually because of the possibility of vasodilatation and hypotension.

Talpos et al.[199] and Winkelmann et al.[200] have used serial plasmapheresis with good effect in some patients but with no effect in others. Biofeedback has also been used as the primary mode of therapy for some patients.[201] Sympathectomy is currently used only in the treatment of gangrene or intractable pain in the digits, and then only if temporary stellate ganglion block results in good effect. Nitroglycerin paste may also be helpful.[195,202]

Eosinophilic Fasciitis

DEFINITIONS

Eosinophilic fasciitis, first described by Shulman in 1975[203] and Rodnan, et al., is an uncommon syndrome characterized by induration of the skin of the limbs, peripheral and cutaneous eosinophilia, absence of visceral involvement, and response to corticosteroid drugs.

EPIDEMIOLOGY

Eosinophilic fasciitis is rare in all age groups and has been reported in fewer than a dozen children.[204–213] In adults it is characteristically a disease of young males (male:female = 2:1). The sex ratio in children, however, is reversed, with a male:female ratio among published cases reports of 2:7 (Table 10-14). In approximately half of such patients, the symptoms begin from 2 days to several weeks after strenuous

Table 10-13 Pharmacologic Agents Used in Treatment of Raynaud's Phenomenon

Drug	Action	Reference
Drugs affecting the sympathetic nervous system		
Tolazoline	Blocks alpha-adrenergic receptors	181
Phenoxybenzamine	Blocks alpha-adrenergic receptors	182
Prazosin	Blocks alpha$_1$ receptors	182, 183
Reserpine	Depletes norepinephrine from sympathetic nerves; IV administration gives short-lived vasodilatation	181 184
Guanethidine	Interferes with norepinephrine release at sympathetic neuroeffector junctions	185
Methyldopa	Central	186
Direct-acting drugs		
Captopril	Angiotensin converting enzyme inhibitor	188
Nifedipine	Slow calcium channel blocker	189–192
PGE$_1$	Vasodilator and platelet inhibitor	193
PGI$_1$	Vasodilator	194
Glyceryl trinitrate topical	Vasodilator	195
Ketanserin	Antagonizes vasocontrictor effects of 5-HT	196
Griseofulvin	Vasodilator	197, 198

Table 10-14 Eosinophilic Fasciitis in Childhood

Reference	Sex	Age at Onset	Eosinophils (/mm³)	↑ESR	↑IgG	ANA	RF
Ansell[204]	M	14 yr	2037	+	+	–	–
Britt[205]	F	8 yr	6700	+	+	–	–
Rodnan[206]	?	11 yr	?	?	+	–	?
Caperton[207]	?	4 yr	Increased	?	+	?	?
Kaplinsky[208]	F	8 yr	Normal	–	–	–	–
Michet[209]	F	12 yr	990	+	+	–	–
Sills[210]	F	14 yr	940	+	+	1:320	+
	F	7 yr	12%	+	–	1:640	–
Frayha[211]	F	10 yr	3744	+	+	–	–
Stachow[212]	F	11 yr	?	?	?	?	?
	M	10 yr	?	?	?	?	?
Patrone[213]	M	10 yr	1030	–	?	–	–

physical exertion. This dramatic association is unique among the connective tissue diseases.

CLINICAL CHARACTERISTICS

The skin disease is characterized by the relatively abrupt onset of swelling, stiffness, and sometimes pain, but without erythema or warmth of the skin and subcutaneous tissues of the limbs (forearm, arm, thigh, or calf) or trunk. The epidermis and its appendages are not affected. The skin becomes taut and, sometimes, has the appearance of peau d'orange, secondary to fibrotic changes in the septa of the deep cutaneous tissue. The skin is not shiny, however, and sclerosis, atrophy, telangiectases, periungual vascular changes, and pigmentation changes do not occur.

Laboratory examination reveals eosinophilia, sometimes as high as 35 to 60 percent of the total white blood cell count; hypergammaglobulinemia; and elevated ESR. Biopsy of the skin, subcutaneous tissues, fascia, and muscle is required for definitive diagnosis and shows mononuclear and eosinophilic infiltrate of the subcutaneous tissue, together with fibrosis of the deep fascial layers.

The most striking differences between eosinophilic fasciitis and the other diseases related to scleroderma are the steroid responsiveness, relationship to preceding physical exertion, and absence of visceral involvement of eosinophilic fasciitis. Antinuclear antibodies (ANAs) have been reported by Sills in two patients,[201] but the experience in other series is that ANAs are absent (Table 10-14). Hematologic abnormalities, particularly hematocytopenias, have been reported in up to 10 percent of adult patients with eosinophilic fasciitis although there have been

no reports of such an association in children. The response to prednisone (0.5 to 1.0 mg/kg/day) is usually evident within the first 4 to 8 weeks of treatment, although later responses may occur. The eventual outcome appears to be good, although long-term follow-up studies of eosinophilic fasciitis in children have not been published.

LOCALIZED SCLERODERMAS

Definitions

Localized or focal sclerodermas are those disorders of connective tissue in which fibrosis is limited to the skin, subcutaneous tissue, and muscle.[214] Localized scleroderma can be further classified into morphea and linear scleroderma.

MORPHEA

Morphea is a disorder of the skin characterized by the presence of one or more oval or round circumscribed indurations that become hard and whitish. They may be located anywhere on the trunk or extremities. There is a characteristic violet border early in the disease. Lesions of morphea can become quite extensive.

LINEAR SCLERODERMA

Linear scleroderma is a disorder characterized by the presence of one or more linear streaks on the skin of the extremities, face, or scalp that involve the subcutaneous tissue, muscle, and underlying bone and that may, therefore, result in deformity or contracture of a joint. When this lesion occurs on the face or scalp it is referred to as *scleroderma en coup de sabre* (Fig. 10-19). Progressive hemifacial atrophy (Parry-Romberg syndrome) may represent an incomplete form of scleroderma en coup de sabre.[215] Lesions of morphea and linear scleroderma sometimes occur in the same child.

Epidemiology

Localized sclerodermas are much more common than the systemic sclerodermas at all ages, particularly in childhood. In one large series of localized scleroderma, morphea accounted for 434 patients, and linear scleroderma accounted for 245 patients.[214] During the same time period, the same clinic studied 365 patients with systemic sclerodermas. Children accounted for approximately half of the patients with linear scleroderma, whereas only 25 percent of those with morphea were children. The published series of localized scleroderma in children are summarized in Table 10-15.

Systemic Disease in Local Scleroderma

Underlying muscle, tendon, and bone are frequently affected in local scleroderma. Occasionally, visceral disease develops late in the disease course, suggesting an evolution of the local form of scleroderma into a systemic form. Additionally, occasional patients develop other connective tissue diseases such as systemic lupus erythematosus or mixed connective-tissue disease.[216]

Laboratory Abnormalities

The most significant laboratory abnormality is the presence of ANAs, which are present in 37 percent[209] to 67 percent.[219] Stogmann et al.[216] found ANA more frequently in children with linear scleroderma (three of six) than in those with morphea (none of five), although the reverse relationship was seen in Larrègue and associates' series,[217] and in a Japanese series ANA was found in both linear and morphea groups. Antibodies to centromere, Scl-70, nuclear RNP, Sm, and SS-B antigens were not found in this series.[218] Although antibody to centromere has been documented occasionally in patients with localized scleroderma,[220] ANA patterns are usually speckled, homogeneous, or nucleolar. Anti-DNA antibodies have been detected in up to 38 percent in one series[221] and in a much lower frequency in other studies.[218] Immunoglobulin levels are elevated, but rheumatoid factor is usually,[219] although not always,[19] absent, and immunity to all collagen types is absent.[219]

Management of Local Sclerodermas

In many instances local sclerodermatous lesions of the morphea type spontaneously regress without treatment of any kind. Linear lesions are less likely to do so, and significant local growth arrest may occur, with atrophic changes in the skin, subcutaneous tissue, and bone that may cause a significant functional and cosmetic problem. Topical and intralesional corticosteroid has been advocated by some, but the side effects of this drug on the skin itself may be prohibitive. Oral penicillamine has been advocated by Moynahan,[222] who described uniformly good results in 14 patients with linear scle-

Table 10-15 Localized Scleroderma in Childhood

Reference	Number	Male	Female	Morphea	Linear
Kornreich[19]	35	13	22	12	23[b]
Stogmann[216]	11	8	3	5	11
Larrègue[217]	27	10	17	6[a]	24
Takehara[218]	15	3	12	7	8

[a] Four patients had both linear lesions and morphea.
[b] Four patients had linear lesions on the face and scalp resulting in facial hemiatrophy in one and a skull lesion in a second patient.

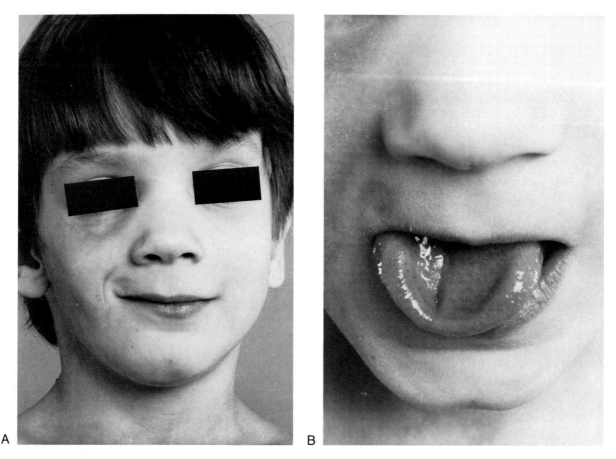

Fig. 10-19 (**A**) Scleroderma en coup de sabre showing atrophy of subcutaneous tissue and pigmentation of the skin on the right side of the face of this 6-year-old boy. (**B**) Scleroderma en coup de sabre showing an atrophic lesion on the right side of the tongue. (*Figure continues.*)

roderma and morphea, using D-penicillamine in a dose of up to 450 mg per day. The anticonvulsant diphenylhydantoin has been used in several series of patients with local (and occasionally) systemic scleroderma,[223,224] with questionable benefit. Since the skin lesions of morphea in particular may regress spontaneously, it is very difficult to assess improvement without adequately controlled studies.

Chronic Graft-Versus-Host Disease

Chronic graft-versus-host disease (GVH) is a common complication of allogeneic bone marrow transplantation for the treatment of bone marrow aplasia or malignant disease. GVH disease results from the interaction between immunocompetent T lympho-

cytes from the donor and host cells bearing different histocompatibility antigens that are therefore recognized as being foreign. Since, under the circumstances of the transplantation, the recipient is rendered immunologically incompetent, the graft attempts to "reject" the host. The resulting disease may follow acute GVH or occur de novo up to 100 days posttransplant. It is characterized by immunologically mediated disease in skin, usually beginning with erythema of the face, palms, soles, and other regions. This is followed by hyper- and hypopigmentation and scleroderma that may be distal in location or generalized. Gastrointestinal disease (severe diarrhea), hepatitis, and other visceral disease are common.[225] A comparison of chronic GVH and PSS is shown in Table 10-16.[225] Penicillamine has been claimed to be beneficial in this situation,[218] and modifications of the

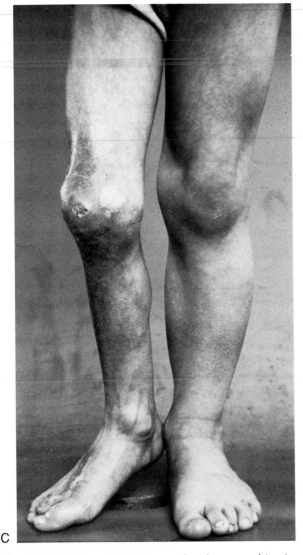

Fig. 10-19 (*Continued*). (**C**) Linear scleroderma resulting in undergrowth of the leg, taut shiny skin, and shortening of the extensor tendon to the second toe on the right foot.

Table 10-16 Comparison of Chronic GVH and PSS

System Affected	PSS% (Early) $n = 13$	PSS% (Late) $n = 36$	GVH% $n = 12$
Skin	100	100	100
Raynaud's phenomenon	100	92	42
Lungs	77	96	58
Esophagus	77	86	17
Small bowel	8	92	0
Heart	69	61	42
Kidney	15	75	8
Keratoconjunctivitis sicca	15	69	50

(Adapted from Clements et al.,[225] with permission.)

chemotherapeutic preparation of the graft recipient may offer some hope of prevention of this complication.[226]

CHEMICALLY-INDUCED SCLERODERMALIKE DISEASE

Several well-defined chemicals have been implicated in the induction of individual cases of scleroderma.

Vinyl chloride, a chemical that was initially used as an anesthetic agent,[227] is now known to cause disease, primarily among workers in the polyvinyl chloride industries. It is characterized by Raynaud's phenomenon; papular localized skin lesions, especially on fingers and hands and excluding the face and trunk; and osteolysis of the central shaft of the distal phalanges.[228]

Bleomycin, an antineoplastic agent, commonly causes skin changes resembling scleroderma[229] and pulmonary fibrosis.[230] The syndrome is not accompanied by Raynaud's phenomenon or other visceral changes and may improve with cessation of the drug.[231]

Pentazocine, a non-narcotic analgesic drug, has been reported to cause cutaneous sclerosis with or without ulceration.[232] Predisposing factors may include diabetes mellitus and alcohol abuse.

Adjuvant disease, a sclerodermalike condition that may be systemic and have visceral involvement (lung, esophagus) as well as diffuse or acrosclerotic scleroderma, has been reported to follow cosmetic surgery involving injection of paraffin or silicone.[233]

The toxic oil syndrome, caused by ingestion of cooking oil that presumably contained as yet unidentified contaminants, occurred in epidemic proportions in Spain in early 1981,[234] affecting at least 20,000 individuals and resulting in at least 350 deaths. A report of the disease in 21 children indicated that the disease may have been less severe in the young age group and that the sex ratio was closer to equal (female:male, 2.5:1) than in the adult (female:male, 6:1). The onset of the disease was characterized by fever, dyspnea secondary to pulmonary edema, pruritic rash, and malaise. There was a peripheral eosinophilia. Sclerodermatous skin lesions, alopecia, conjunctivitis sicca, Raynaud's phenomenon, myositis, neuropathy, joint contractures, dysphagia, and liver disease evolved over a period of months.[235]

PSEUDOSCLERODERMAS

The term *pseudoscleroderma* is used to describe a diverse group of disorders that are characterized by sclerodermalike fibrotic changes in the skin in association with other nonrheumatic diseases. This brief discussion is restricted to those disorders of significance in the pediatric population.

Scleroderma with Phenylketonuria

A small minority of children with phenylketonuria (phenylalanine hydroxylase deficiency) have sclerodermatous skin lesions.[236,237] The lesions, which usually appear within the first year of life, are symmetric, poorly demarcated, and may resemble those of morphea. They occur most frequently on the lower extremities and trunk. It is believed that the lesions regress with the introduction of a low-phenylalanine diet.[236] Although no difference between children with phenylketonuria with or without sclerodermatous changes was found with respect to serum phenylalanine or tryptophan levels, the urinary excretion of 5-hydroxyindoleacetic acid, indoleacetic acid, and tryptamine was much higher in children with skin changes.[236] The relationship of these biochemical abnormalities to the pathogenesis of the accompanying skin lesions or to that of the other sclerodermas is not known. The use of a low-phenylalanine diet in patients with PSS gave inconclusive results.[238]

Syndromes of Premature Aging

Two rare autosomal recessive disorders characterized by dwarfing, premature aging, and early death from atherosclerotic heart disease are associated with sclerodermatous skin changes.

Progeria is characterized by alopecia, nail dystrophy, and thickened, bound-down skin on the abdomen, flanks, proximal thighs, and upper buttocks.[239] Changes usually appear before 1 year of age.

Werner's syndrome usually presents in adolescence with generalized atrophy of muscle and subcutaneous tissue, alopecia, and sclerodermalike skin changes involving the extremities.[239] Metastatic calcifications may occur.[240]

Localized Idiopathic Fibroses

Retroperitoneal fibrosis usually occurs in the region of the promontory of the sacrum and affects vital structures in this area, notably the great vessels and ureters. It is more common in males than in females and occurs in children as well as adults. The syndrome is also associated with administration of the serotonin inhibitor methysergide. Retractile mesenteritis, mediastinal fibrosis, fibrosing pericarditis, fibrosing carditis, and peritoneal fibrosis may represent similar disorders and have been related to intake of certain drugs, notably methysergide and some antihypertensives and anticonvulsants.[241,242]

Scleredema

The disorder of scleredema usually follows streptococcal infection and is characterized by edematous induration of the face, neck, shoulders, and thorax but not of the hands. It usually lasts for 6 to 12 months and resolves spontaneously. Cardiac abnormalities have been reported.[239]

Diabetic Cheiroarthropathy

Rosenbloom et al.[243,244] have described a syndrome of juvenile-onset diabetes mellitus, short stature, and tightening of the skin and soft tissues leading to contractures of the finger joints (see Figs. 14-3, 14-4, and 14-5). In a survey of 229 diabetics aged 7 to 18 years, 28.4 percent were found to have flexion contractures of one or more joints of the fingers, most often the proximal interphalangeal joints of the fifth or fourth fingers.[245] In 7 children, stature below the third percentile was accompanied by flexion contractures of the interphalangeal and metacarpophalangeal joints in all, wrists in 6, elbows in 5, ankles in 6, toes in 3, and knees in 1. Spinal limitation was also observed. In most instances the child was unaware of any joint limitation, and pain was absent. Functional disability was uncommon. The prevalence of joint contractures increased from less than 10 percent in those with diabetes for less than 1 year to close to 50 percent in those with disease for longer than 9 years, although there did not appear to be a correlation with the severity of the diabetes or the adequacy of its control. The relationship of diabetes mellitus to contractures is unknown. Recent studies have demonstrated that the glucosylation of collagen in diabetics with this syndrome is increased, perhaps leading to connective-tissue contractures.[246] We have observed one patient in whom progressive soft tissue contractures that preceded by 3 years the onset of diabetes mellitus markedly improved after the institution of insulin therapy.[247]

Scleroderma and Porphyria

Although there have been no reports of scleroderma and porphyria in children, a recent review documented this association in 12 adult patients.[248] The skin changes were described as plaquelike and occurring predominantly on the face, neck, and upper chest and back. Some of these patients had features of other connective-tissue diseases such as discoid lupus. The basis for the association is unknown.

REFERENCES

1. Rodnan G: When is scleroderma not scleroderma? The differential diagnosis of progressive systemic sclerosis. Bull Rheum Dis 31:7, 1981
2. Masi AT, Rodnan GP, Medsger TA et al: Preliminary criteria for the classification of systemic sclerosis (scleroderma). Arthritis Rheum 23:581, 1980
3. Medsger TA, Jr: Epidemiology of progressive systemic sclerosis. In Black CM, Myers AR (eds): Systemic Sclerosis (Scleroderma). Gower Medical, New York, 1985, p. 53
4. Medsger TA, Masi AT: Epidemiology of systemic sclerosis (scleroderma). Ann Intern Med 74:714, 1971
5. Kurland LT, Hauser WA, Ferguson RH et al: Epidemiologic features of diffuse connective tissue disorders in Rochester, Minn—1951 through 1967. Mayo Clin Proc 44:649, 1969
6. Shinkai H: Epidemiology of progressive systemic sclerosis in Japan. In Black CM, Myers AR (eds): Systemic Sclerosis (Scleroderma). Gower Medical, New York, 1985, p. 79
7. Arboe-Hansen G: Epidemiology of Progressive Systemic Sclerosis in Denmark. In Black CM, Myers AR (eds): Systemic Sclerosis (Scleroderma). Gower Medical, New York, 1985, p. 78
8. Giordano M, Valentini G, Ara M et al: Epidemiology of progressive systemic sclerosis in Italy. In Black CM, Myers AR (eds): Systemic Sclerosis (Scleroderma). Gower Medical, New York, 1985, p. 72
9. Barnett AJ: Epidemiology of systemic sclerosis (scleroderma) in Australia. In Black CM, Myers AR (eds): Systemic Sclerosis (Scleroderma). Gower Medical, New York, 1985, p. 82.
10. Tuffanelli DL, LaPerriere R: Connective tissue diseases. Pediatr Clin North Am 18:925, 1971
11. Jaffe MO, Winkelmann RK: Generalized scleroderma in children. Acrosclerotic type. Arch Dermatol 83:402, 1961
12. Goel KM, Shanks RA: Scleroderma in the child. Arch Dis Child 49:861, 1974
13. Kass H, Hanson V, Patrick J: Scleroderma in childhood. J Pediatr 68:243, 1966
14. Larrègue M, Canuel C, Bazex J et al: Sclérodermie systémique de l'enfant. A propos de 5 observations. Revue de la littérature. Ann Dermatol Venereol 110:317, 1983
15. Suarez-Almazor ME, Catoggio LJ, Maldonado-Cocco JA et al: Juvenile progressive systemic sclerosis: clinical and serologic findings. Arthritis Rheum 28:699, 1985
16. Burge SM, Ryan TJ, Dawber RPR: Juvenile onset systemic sclerosis. J R Soc Med 77:793, 1984
17. Girouard M, Paré C, Camerlain M: La sclérodermie juvénile. Union Méd Can 111:546, 1982
18. Cassidy JT, Sullivan DB, Dabich L et al: Scleroderma in children. Arthritis Rheum, suppl., 20:351, 1977
19. Kornreich H, Koster King K, Bernstein N et al: Scleroderma in childhood. Arthritis Rheum, suppl., 20:343, 1977
20. Schlesinger M, Schaller JG: Progressive systemic sclerosis (PSS) of childhood. Arthritis Rheum, suppl., 24:104, 1981
21. Spencer-Green G, Schlesinger M, Bove KE et al: Nailfold capillary abnormalities in childhood rheumatic diseases. J Pediatr 102:341, 1983
22. Szymanska-Jagiello W, Rondio H, Jakubowska K: Changes in the locomotor system in progressive systemic sclerosis in children. Mater Med Pol 4:201, 1972
23. Ansell BM, Nasseh GA, Bywaters EGL: Scleroderma in childhood. Ann Rheum Dis 35:189, 1976
24. Velayos EE, Cohen BS: Progressive systemic sclerosis. Diagnosis at the age of 4 years. Am J Dis Child 123:57, 1972
25. Gray RG, Altman RD: Progressive systemic sclerosis in a family. Case report of a mother and son and review of the literature. Arthritis Rheum 20:35, 1977
26. Kennedy WP: Cardiac death from progressive systemic scleroderma in a child. Can Med Assoc J 90:33, 1964
27. Mukherjee SK, Lahiri K, Sen MK: Scleroderma in a boy of nine. J Indian Med Assoc 47:132, 1966
28. Hochberg MC, Lopez-Acuna D, Gittelsohn AM: Mortality from systemic sclerosis (scleroderma) in the United States, 1969–1977. In Black CM, Myers AR (eds): Systemic Sclerosis (Scleroderma). Gower Medical, New York, 1985, p. 61
29. Burge KM, Perry HO, Stickler GB: "Familial scleroderma." Arch Dermatol 99:681, 1969
30. Bulkley BH: Progressive systemic sclerosis: cardiac involvement. Clin Rheum Dis 5:131, 1979
31. Clements PJ, Opelz G, Terasaki PI et al: Association of HLA antigen A9 with progressive systemic sclerosis (scleroderma). Tissue Antigens 11:357, 1978

32. Van der Meulen J, van der Voort-Beelen JM, D'Amaro J et al: HLA-B8 in Raynaud's phenomenon. Tissue Antigens 15:81, 1980

33. Kallenberg CGM, Van Der Voort-Beelen JM, D'Amaro J et al: Increased frequency of B8/DR3 in scleroderma and association of the haplotype with impaired cellular immune response. Clin Exp Immunol 43:481, 1981

34. Lynch CJ, Singh G, Whiteside TL et al: Histocompatibility antigens in progressive systemic sclerosis (scleroderma). J Clin Immunol 2:314, 1982

35. Gladman DD, Keystone EC, Baron M et al: Increased frequency of HLA-DR5 in scleroderma. Arthritis Rheum 24:854, 1981

36. Black CM, Welsh KI, Maddison PJ et al: HLA antigens in scleroderma. In Black CM, Myers AR (eds): Systemic Sclerosis (Scleroderma). Gower Medical, New York, 1985, p. 84

37. Whiteside TL, Medsger TA, Jr, Rodnan GP: Studies of HLA antigens in progressive systemic sclerosis. In Black CM, Myers AR (eds): Systemic Sclerosis (Scleroderma). Gower Medical, New York, 1985, p. 89

38. Lovell CR, Nicholls AC, Duance VC et al: Characterization of dermal collagen in systemic sclerosis. Br J Dermatol 100:359, 1979

39. Brady AH: Collagenase in scleroderma. J Clin Invest 56:1175, 1975

40. Uitto J, Bauer EA, Eison AZ: Scleroderma. Increased biosynthesis of triple helical type I and type III procollagens associated with unaltered expression of collagenase by skin fibroblasts in culture. J Clin Invest 64:921, 1979

41. Peltonen L, Palotie A, Myllyla R et al: Collagen biosynthesis in systemic scleroderma: Regulation of posttranslational modifications and synthesis of procollagen in cultured fibroblasts. J Invest Dermatol 84:14, 1985

42. Blumengrantz N, Arboe-Hansen G: Subhydroxylated collagen in scleroderma. Acta Derm Venereol (Stockh) 58:359, 1978

43. Haustein UF, Herrmann K, Bohme HJ: Pathogenesis of progressive systemic sclerosis. Int J Dermatol 25:286, 1986

44. Cohen S, Johnson AR, Hurd E: Cytotoxicity of sera from patients with scleroderma. Arthritis Rheum 26:170, 1983

45. Shanahan WR, Korn JH: Cytotoxic activity of sera from scleroderma and other connective tissue diseases: lack of target cell and disease specificity (abstract). Arthritis Rheum 25:S4, 1982

46. Emerit I, Housett E, Feingold J: Chromosomal breakage and scleroderma: studies in family members. J Lab Clin Med 88:81, 1976

47. Kahaleh MB, Sherer CK, LeRoy EC: Endothelial injury in scleroderma. J Exp Med 149:1326, 1979

48. Kahaleh MB, Osborn I, LeRoy EC: Increased factor VIII/von Willebrand factor antigen and von Willebrand factor activity in scleroderma and in Raynaud's phenomenon. Ann Intern Med 94:482, 1981

49. Kalaleh MB, Osborn I, LeRoy EC: Elevated levels of circulating platelet aggregates and beta-thromboglobulin in scleroderma. Ann Intern Med 96:610, 1982

50. LeRoy EC: Scleroderma (systemic sclerosis). In Kelley WN, Harris ED, Ruddy S et al (eds): Textbook of Rheumatology. 2nd Ed. WB Saunders, Philadelphia, 1985, p. 1183

51. Wolff AD, Wakerly G, Wallington TB et al: Factor VIII related antigen in the assessment of vasculitis. Ann Rheum Dis 46:441, 1987

52. Fries JF: The microvascular pathogenesis of scleroderma: an hypothesis. Ann Intern Med 91:788, 1979

53. Sternberg EM: Pathogenesis of scleroderma: the interrelationship of immune and vascular hypotheses. Surv Immunol Res 4:69, 1985

54. Postlethwaite AE, Stuart JM, Kang AH: The cell-mediated immune system in progressive systemic sclerosis: an overview. In Black CM, Myers AR (eds): Systemic Sclerosis (Scleroderma). Gower Medical, New York, 1985, p. 319

55. Huffstutter JE, DeLustro FA, LeRoy EC: Cellular immunity to collagen and laminin in scleroderma. Arthritis Rheum 28:775, 1985

56. Braun-Falco O: Uber das verhalten der interfibrillaren grundsubstanz bei sklerodermia. Dermatol Wochenschr 136:1085, 1957 (cited by Rodnan GP: Progressive systemic sclerosis: clinical features and pathogenesis of cutaneous involvement (scleroderma). Clin Rheum Dis 5:49, 1979

57. Fleischmajer R, Perlish NS, West WP: Ultrastructure of cutaneous cellular infiltrates in scleroderma. Arch Dermatol 113:1661, 1977

58. Fleischmajer R, Perlish JS, Reeves JRT: Cellular infiltrates in scleroderma skin. Arthritis Rheum 20:975, 1977

59. Rodnan GP, Lipinski E, Luksick J: Skin thickness and collagen content in progressive systemic sclerosis and localized scleroderma. Arthritis Rheum 22:130, 1979

60. Hayes RL, Rodnan GP: The ultrastructure of skin in progressive systemic sclerosis (scleroderma). I: Dermal collagen fibers. Am J Pathol 63:433, 1971

61. Patterson JW: Pterygium inversum unguis-like changes in scleroderma. Arch Dermatol 113:1429, 1977

62. Moore CP, Wilken RF: The subcutaneous nodule. Its

significance in the diagnosis of rheumatic disease. Semin Arthritis Rheum 7:63, 1977

63. Kondo H, Rabin BS, Rodnan GP: Cutaneous antigen-stimulating lymphokine production by lymphocytes of patients with progressive systemic sclerosis (scleroderma). J Clin Invest 58:1388, 1976

64. Raynaud M: On local asphyxia and symmetrical gangrene of the extremities (1862). Arch Gen Med 1:189, 1874

65. Guntheroth WG, Morgan BL, Harbinson JA et al: Raynaud's disease in children. Circulation 36:724, 1967

66. Jung L, Dent P: Prognostic significance of Raynaud's phenomenon in children. Clin Pediatr 22:22, 1983

67. LeRoy EC, Downey JA, Cannon PJ: Skin capillary blood flow in scleroderma. J Clin Invest 50:930, 1971

68. Fries JF: Physiologic studies in systemic sclerosis (scleroderma). Arch Intern Med 123:22, 1969

69. Dabich L, Bookstein JJ, Zvaifler A et al: Digital arteries in patients with scleroderma. Arteriographic and plethysmographic study. Arch Intern Med 130:708, 1972

70. Maricq HR, Spencer-Green G, LeRoy EC: Skin capillary abnormalities as indicators of organ involvement in scleroderma (systemic sclerosis), Raynaud's syndrome and dermatomyositis. Am J Med 61:862, 1976

71. Rodnan GP, Myerowitz RL, Justh GO: Morphologic change in the digital arteries of patients with progressive systemic sclerosis (scleroderma) and Raynaud's phenomenon. Medicine 59:393, 1980

72. Winkelmann RK, Goldyne ME, Linschied RL: Influence of cold on catecholamine response of vascular smooth muscle strips from resistance vessels of scleroderma skin. Angiology 28:330, 1977

73. Winkelmann RK, Goldyne ME, Linscheid RL: Hypersensitivity of scleroderma cutaneous vascular smooth muscle to 5-hydroxytryptamine. Br J Dermatol 95:51, 1976

74. Kallenberg CGM, Vallenga E, Wouda AA et al: Platelet activation, fibrinolytic activity and circulating immune complexes in Raynaud's phenomenon. J Rheumatol 9:878, 1982

75. Majerus PW: Arachidonate metabolism in vascular disorders. J Clin Invest 72:1521, 1983

76. Rodnan GP, Medsger TA, Jr: The rheumatic manifestations of progressive systemic sclerosis (scleroderma). Clin Orthop 57:81, 1968

77. Schulman LE, Kurban AK, Harvey AM: Tendon friction rubs in progressive systemic sclerosis (scleroderma). Arthritis Rheum 4:438, 1961

78. Rodnan GP, Medsger TA, Jr: Musculoskeletal in-volvement in progressive systemic sclerosis (scleroderma). Bull Rheum Dis 17:419, 1966

79. Clark JA, Winkelmann RK, Ward LE: Serologic alterations in scleroderma and sclerodermatomyositis. Mayo Clin Proc 46:104, 1971

80. Scharer L, Smith DW: Resorption of the terminal phalanges in scleroderma. Arthritis Rheum 12:51, 1969

81. Szymanska-Jagiello W, Rondio H: Clinical picture of articular changes in progressive systemic sclerosis in children in the light of our own observations. Rheumatologia 8:1, 1970

82. Schlenker JD, Clark DD, Weckesser EC: Calcinosis circumscripta of the hand in scleroderma. J Bone Joint Surg 55A:1051, 1973

83. Rowell BR, Hopper FE: The periodontal membrane in systemic sclerosis. Br J Dermatol 93:suppl. 2, 23, 1975

84. Resnick D, Niwayama G: Diagnosis of Bone and Joint Disorders. WB Saunders, Philadelphia, 1981, p. 1212

85. Resnick D, Greenway G, Vint VC: Selective involvement of the first carpometacarpal joint in scleroderma. Am J Roentgenol 131:283, 1978

86. Clements PJ, Furst DE, Campion DS et al: Muscle disease in progressive systemic sclerosis. Arthritis Rheum 21:62, 1978

87. Medsger TA Jr, Rodnan GP, Moossy J et al: Skeletal muscle involvement in progressive systemic sclerosis (scleroderma). Arthritis Rheum 11:554, 1968

88. Norton WL, Hurd ER, Lewis DC et al: Evidence of microvascular injury in scleroderma and systemic lupus erythematosus: a quantitative study of the microvascular bed. J Lab Clin Med 71:919, 1968

89. Lindamood M, Steigerwald J: Skeletal muscle abnormalities in progressive systemic sclerosis (abstract). Arthritis Rheum 19:807, 1976

90. Alarcon-Segovia D, Ibanez G, Hernandez-Ortiz J et al: Sjögren's syndrome in progressive systemic sclerosis (scleroderma). Am J Med 57:78, 1974

91. Orringer MB, Dabich L, Zarafonetis CJD et al: Gastroesophageal reflux in esophageal scleroderma: diagnosis and implications. Ann Thoracic Surg 22:120, 1976

92. D'Angelo WA, Fries JF, Masi AT et al: Pathologic observations in systemic sclerosis (scleroderma). Am J Med 46:428, 1969

93. Meihoff WE, Hirschfield JS, Kern F: Small intestinal scleroderma with malabsorption and pneumatosis cystoides intestinalis. Report of three cases. JAMA 204:854, 1968

94. Treacy WL, Baggenstoss AJH, Slocomb CH et al: Scleroderma of the esophagus. A correlation of his-

tologic and physiologic findings. Ann Intern Med 59:351, 1963

95. Meszaroso WT:The colon in systemic sclerosis (scleroderma). Am J Roentgenol 82:1000, 1959

96. Bartholomew LG, Cain JC, Winkelmann RK et al: Chronic disease of the liver associated with systemic scleroderma. Am J Digest Dis 9:43, 1964

97. Reynolds TB, Denison EK, Frankl HD et al: Primary biliary cirrhosis with scleroderma, Raynaud's phenomenon and telangiectasia: new syndrome. Am J Med 50:302, 1971

98. Dinsmore RE, Goodman D, Dreyfus JR: The air esophagram: a sign of scleroderma involving the esophagus. Radiology 87:348, 1966

99. Martel W, Chang SF, Abell MR: Loss of colonic haustrations in progressive systemic sclerosis. Am J Roentgen 126:704, 1976

100. Meszaros WT: The colon in systemic sclerosis (scleroderma). Am J Roentgenol 82:1000, 1959

101. Smith JW, Clements PJ, Levisman J et al: Echocardiographic features of progressive systemic sclerosis (PSS). Correlation with hemodynamic and post mortem studies. Am J Med 66:28, 1979

102. Sackner MA, Heinz ER, Steinberg AJ: The heart in scleroderma. Am J Cardiol 17:542, 1966

103. Gladman DF, Gordon DA, Urowitz MB et al: Pericardial fluid analysis in scleroderma (systemic sclerosis). Am J Med 60:1064, 1976

104. Gupta MP, Zoneraich S, Zeittin W et al: Scleroderma heart disease with slow flow velocity in coronary arteries. Chest 67:116, 1975

105. Ridolfi RL, Bulkley BH, Hutchins GM: The cardiac conduction system in progressive systemic sclerosis. Am J Med 61:361, 1976

106. Clements PJ, Furst DE, Cabeen W et al: The relationship of arrhythmias and conduction disturbances to other manifestations of cardiopulmonary disease in progressive systemic sclerosis (PSS). Am J Med 71:38, 1981

107. Gottdiener JS, Moutsopoulos HM, Decker JC: Echocardiographic identification of cardiac abnormality in scleroderma and related disorders. Am J Med 66:391, 1979

108. Alexander EL, Firestein GS, Weiss JL et al: Reversible cold-induced abnormalities in myocardial perfusion and function in systemic sclerosis. Ann Intern Med 105:661, 1986

109. Trell E, Lindstrom C: Pulmonary hypertension in systemic sclerosis. Ann Rheum Dis 30:390, 1971

110. Young RH, Mark GJ: Pulmonary vascular changes in scleroderma. Am J Med 64:998, 1978

111. Bulkley BH, Ridolfi RL, Salyer WR et al: Myocardial lesions of progressive systemic sclerosis. A cause of cardiac dysfunction. Circulation 53:483, 1976

112. Steen VD, Owens GR, Fino GJ et al: Pulmonary involvement in systemic sclerosis (scleroderma). Arthritis Rheum 28:759, 1985

113. Guttadauria M, Ellman H, Kaplan D: Progressive systemic sclerosis: pulmonary involvement. Clin Rheum Dis 5:151, 1979

114. Getzowa S: Cystic and compact pulmonary sclerosis in progressive scleroderma. Arch Pathol 40:99, 1945

115. Zatuchni J, Campbell WN, Zarafonetis CJD: Pulmonary fibrosis and terminal bronchiolar ("alveolar cell") carcinoma in scleroderma. Cancer 6:1147, 1953

116. Furst DE, Davis JA, Clements PJ et al: Abnormalities of pulmonary vascular dynamics and inflammation in early progressive systemic sclerosis. Arthritis Rheum 24:1403, 1981

117. Fahey PJ, Utell MJ, Condemi JJ et al: Raynaud's phenomenon of the lung. Am J Med 76:263, 1984

118. Medsger TA, Masi AT, Rodnan BP et al: Survival with systemic sclerosis (scleroderma): a life-table analysis of clinical and demographic factors in 358 male U.S. veteran patients. J Chronic Dis 26:647, 1973

119. Cannon PJ, Hassar M, Case DB et al: The relationship of hypertension and renal failure in scleroderma (progressive systemic sclerosis) to structural and functional abnormalities of the renal cortical circulation. Medicine 53:1, 1974

120. Oliver JA, Cannon PJ: The kidney in scleroderma. Nephron 18:141, 1977

121. Tuffanelli DL, Winkelmann, RK: Systemic scleroderma. A clinical study of 727 cases. Arch Dermatol 84:359, 1961

122. LeRoy EC, Fleischmann RM: The management of renal scleroderma—experience with dialysis, nephrectomy and transplantation. Am J Med 64:974, 1978

123. Urai L, Nagy Z, Szinay G et al: Renal function in scleroderma. Br Med J 2:1264, 1958

124. Whitman HH, III, Case DB, Laragh JH et al: Variable response to oral angiotensin-converting-enzyme blockade in hypertensive scleroderma patients. Arthritis Rheum 25:241, 1982

125. Kovalchik MT, Guggenheim SJ, Silverman MH et al: The kidney in progressive systemic sclerosis: a prospective study. Ann Intern Med 89:881, 1978

126. Lester PD, Koehler PR: The renal angiographic changes in scleroderma. Radiology 99:517, 1971

127. Fisher ER, Rodnan GP: Pathologic observations concerning the kidney in progressive systemic sclerosis. Arch Pathol 65:29, 1958

128. Jarmolych JJ, Daoud AS, Landau J et al: Aortic media explants. Cell proliferation and production of mu-

copolysaccharides, collagen and elastic tissue. Exp Mol Pathol 9:171, 1968

129. Sinclair RA, Antonovych TT, Mostofi FK: Renal proliferative arteriopathies and associated glomerular changes. Hum Pathol 7:565, 1976

130. Lapenas D, Rodnan GP, Cavallo T: Immunopathology of the renal vascular lesion of progressive systemic sclerosis (scleroderma). Am J Pathol 91:243, 1968

131. Gerber MA: Immunohistochemical findings in the renal vascular lesions of progressive systemic sclerosis. Hum Pathol 6:343, 1975

132. McGivern AR, DeBoer WGR, Barnett AJ: Renal immune deposits in scleroderma. Pathology 3:145, 1972

133. Gordon RM, Silverstein A: Neurologic manifestations in progressive systemic sclerosis. Arch Neurol 22:126, 1970

134. Estey E, Lieberman A, Pinto R et al: Cerebral arteritis in scleroderma. Stroke 10:595, 1979

135. Teasdall RD, Frayha RA, Shulman LE: Cranial nerve involvement in systemic sclerosis (scleroderma): a report of 10 cases. Medicine 59:149, 1980

136. Burke MJ, Carty JE: Trigeminal neuropathy as the presenting symptom of progressive sclerosis. Postgrad Med J 55:423, 1979

137. Farrell DA, Medsger TA, Jr: Trigeminal neuropathy in progressive systemic sclerosis. Am J Med 73:57, 1982

138. Lee P, Bruni J, Sukenik S: Neurological manifestations in systemic sclerosis (Scleroderma). J Rheumatol 11:480, 1984

139. Dahlgaard T, Nielsen VK, Kristensen JK: Vibratory perception in patients with generalized scleroderma. Acta Derm Venereol 60:119, 1980

140. Steen VD, Powell DL, Medsger TA, Jr: Clinical correlations and prognosis based on serum autoantibodies in patients with systemic sclerosis. Arthritis Rheum 31:196, 1988

141. Weiner ES, Earnshaw WC, Senecal J-L et al: Clinical associations of anticentromere antibodies and antibodies to topoisomerase 1. Arthritis Rheum 31:378, 1988

142. Fregeau DR, Leung PS, Coppel RL et al: Autoantibodies to mitochondria in systemic sclerosis. Arthritis Rheum 31:386, 1988

143. Frayha RA, Shulman LE, Stevens MB: Hematological abnormalities in scleroderma. A study of 180 cases. Acta Haematol 64:25, 1980

144. Doig A, Girdwood RM: The absorption of folic acid and labeled cyanocobalamine in intestinal malabsorption with observations on the fecal excretion of fat nitrogen and the absorption of glucose and xylose. Q J Med 29:333, 1960

145. Salyer WR, Salyer DC, Heptinstall RM: Scleroderma and microangiopathic hemolytic anemia. Ann Intern Med 73:895, 1973

146. Rosenthal DS, Sack B: Autoimmune hemolytic anemia in scleroderma. JAMA 261:2011, 1971

147. Doyle JA, Connolly SM, Hoagland HC: Hematologic disease in scleroderma syndromes. Acta Derm Venerol (Stockh) 65:521, 1985

148. Fritzler MJ, Kinsella TD, Garbutt E: The CREST syndrome: a distinct serologic entity with anticentromere antibodies. Am J Med 69:520, 1980

149. Rodnan GP, Jablonska S: Classification of systemic and localized scleroderma. In Black CM, Myers AR (eds): Systemic Sclerosis (Scleroderma). Gower Medical, New York, 1985, p. 3

150. Winterbauer RH: Multiple telangiectasia, Raynaud's phenomenon, sclerodactyly and subcutaneous calcinosis: a syndrome mimicking hereditary hemorrhagic telangiectasia. Bull Johns Hopkins Hosp 114:361, 1964

151. Thibiérge G, Wiessenbach RJ: Concrétions calcaires souscutanées et sclérodermie. Ann Dermatol Syph 2:129, 1911

152. Tan EM, Rodnan GP, Garcia I et al: Diversity of antinuclear antibodies in progressive systemic sclerosis. Arthritis Rheum 23:617, 1980

153. Powell FC, Winkelmann RK, Venencie-Lemarchand F et al: The anticentromere antibody: disease specificity and clinical significance. Mayo Clin Proc 59:700, 1984

154. Furst DE, Clements PJ, Saab M et al: Clinical and serological comparison of 17 chronic progressive systemic sclerosis (PSS) and 17 CREST syndrome patients matched for sex, age and disease duration. Ann Rheum Dis 43:794, 1984

155. Sharp GG, Irvin WS, Tan EM et al: Mixed connective tissue disease—an apparently distinct rheumatic syndrome associated with a specific antibody to an extractable nuclear antigen (ENA). Am J Med 52:148, 1972

156. Nimelstein SH, Brody S, McShane D et al: Mixed connective tissue disease: a subsequent evaluation of the original 25 patients. Medicine 59:239, 1980

157. Sanders DY, Huntley CC, Sharp GC: Mixed connective tissue disease in a child. J Pediatr 83:642, 1973

158. Fraga A, Gudino J, Ramos-Niembro F et al: Mixed connective tissue disease in childhood. Am J Dis Child 132:263, 1978

159. Singsen BH, Bernstein BH, Kornreich HK et al:

Mixed connective tissue disease in childhood. J Pediatr 90:893, 1977

160. Oetgen WJ, Boice JA, Lawless OJ: Mixed connective tissue disease in children and adolescents. Pediatrics 67:333, 1981

161. Savouret J-F, Chudwin DS, Wara DW et al: Clinical and laboratory findings in presence of antibody to ribonucleoprotein containing the small nuclear ribonucleic acid U1. J Pediatr 102:841, 1983

162. Rosenberg AM, Petty RE, Cumming GR et al: Pulmonary hypertension in a child with mixed connective tissue disease. J Rheumatol 6:700, 1979

163. Peskett SA, Ansell BM, Fizzman P et al: Mixed connective tissue disease in children. Rheumatol Rehabil 17:245, 1978

164. Rosenthal M: Sharp-syndrome (mixed connective tissue disease) bei kindren. Helv Paediatr Acta 33:251, 1978

165. Eberhardt K, Svantessen H, Svennsen B: Followup studies of 6 children presenting with a MCTD-like syndrome. Scand J Rheumatol 10:62, 1981

166. Singsen BH, Swanson VL, Bernstein BH et al: A histologic evaluation of mixed connective tissue disease in childhood. Am J Med 68:710, 1980

167. Steigerwald JC: Progressive systemic sclerosis: management. III: Immunosuppressive agents. Clin Rheum Dis 5:289, 1979

168. Steigerwald JC: Chlorambucil in the treatment of progressive systemic sclerosis. In Black CM, Myers AR (eds): Systemic Sclerosis (Scleroderma). Gower Medical, New York, 1985, p. 423

169. Clements PJ, Furst DE, Campion DS et al: Muscle disease in progressive systemic sclerosis. Arthritis Rheum 21:62, 1978

170. Steigerwald JC: Colchicine vs. placebo in the treatment of progressive systemic sclerosis. In Black CM, Myers AR (eds): Systemic Sclerosis (Scleroderma). Gower Medical, New York, 1985, p. 415

171. Bluestone R, Grahame R, Holloway V et al: Treatment of systemic sclerosis with D-penicillamine. Ann Rheum Dis 29:153, 1970

172. Steen VD, Medsger TA, Jr, Rodnan GP: D-penicillamine therapy in progressive sclerosis (scleroderma) Ann Intern Med 97:652, 1982

173. Jiminez SA, Andrews RP, Myers AR: Treatment of rapidly progressive systemic sclerosis with D-penicillamine. A prospective study. In Black CM, Myers AR (eds): Systemic Sclerosis (Scleroderma). Gower Medical, New York, 1985, p. 387.

174. DeClerk LS, Dequecker J, Francx L et al: D-penicillamine therapy and interstitial lung disease in scleroderma. Arthritis Rheum 30:643, 1987

175. Medsger TA, Jr: D-penicillamine treatment of lung involvement in patients with systemic sclerosis (scleroderma). Arthritis Rheum 30:832, 1987

176. Ohta A, Uitto J: Procollagen gene expression by scleroderma fibroblasts in culture. Arthritis Rheum 30:404, 1987

177. Uhlman A, Brauningen W: Successful treatment of Sharp's syndrome and progressive systemic sclerosis with an aromatic retinoid. Z Hautkr 60:774, 1985

178. Richardson JA: Hemodialysis and kidney transplantation for renal failure from scleroderma. Arthritis Rheum 16:265, 1973

179. LeRoy EC, Fleischmann RM: The management of renal scleroderma—experience with dialysis, nephrectomy and transplantation. Am J Med 64:974, 1978

180. Beckett VL, Donadio JR, Jr, Brennan LA, Jr et al: Use of captopril as early therapy for renal scleroderma: a prospective study. Mayo Clin Proc 60:763, 1985

181. Coffman JD: Vasodilator drugs in peripheral vascular disease. N Engl J Med 300:713, 1979

182. Gifford RW, Jr: The arteriospastic diseases: clinical significance and management. Cardiovasc Clin 3:128, 1971

183. Russell IJ, Lessard JA: Prazosin treatment of Raynaud's phenomenon: a double blind single crossover study. J Rheumatol 12:94, 1985

184. McFadyen IJ, Housley E, MacPherson AIS: Intraarterial reserpine administration in Raynaud syndrome. Arch Intern Med 132:526, 1978

185. Kontos HA, Wasserman AJ: Effect of reserpine in Raynaud's phenomenon. Circulation 39:259, 1969

186. Varadi DP, Lawrence AM: Suppression of Raynaud's phenomenon by methyldopa. Arch Intern Med 124:13, 1969

187. Hansteen V, Lorentsen E: Vasodilator drugs in the treatment of peripheral arterial insufficiency. Acta Med Scand, suppl., 556:1, 1974

188. Miyazaki S, Miura K, Utaka K et al: Relief from digital vasospasm by treatment with captopril and its complete inhibition by serine proteinase inhibitors in Raynaud's phenomenon. Br Med J 284:310, 1982

189. Smith CD, McKendry RJR: Controlled trial of nifedipine in the treatment of Raynaud's phenomenon. Lancet 2:1299, 1982

190. Rodeheffer RJ, Rommer JA, Wigley F et al: Controlled double-blind trial of nifedipine in the treatment of Raynaud's phenomenon. N Engl J Med 308:880, 1983

191. Winston EL, Pariser KM, Miller KB et al: Nifedipine as a therapeutic modality for Raynaud's phenomenon. Arthritis Rheum 26:1177, 1983

192. Sauza J, Kraus A, Gonzalez-Amaro et al: Effect of the calcium channel blocker nifedipine on Raynaud's phe-

nomenon. A controlled double blind trial. J Rheumatol 11:362, 1984

193. Martin MFR, David PM, Ring EFJ et al: Prostaglandin E1 infusions for vascular insufficiency in progressive systemic sclerosis. Ann Rheum Dis 40:350, 1981

194. Belch JJF, McArdle B, Pollock JG et al: Epoprostenol (prostacyclin) and severe arterial disease. A double blind trial. Lancet 1:315, 1983

195. Coppock J, Hardman J, Bacon P et al: Objective relief of vasospasm by glyceryl trinitrate in secondary Raynaud's phenomenon. Postgrad Med J 62:15, 1986

196. Siebold JR, Jageneau AMM: Treatment of Raynaud's phenomenon with Ketanserin, a selective antagonist of the serotonin (5HT2) receptor. Arthritis Rheum 27:139, 1984

197. Giordano M, Ara M, Capelli L et al: Griseofulvin in scleroderma. In Black CM, Myers AR (eds): Systemic Sclerosis (Scleroderma). Gower Medical, New York, 1985, p. 446

198. Herxheimer A: Griseofulvin in Raynaud's phenomenon. Lancet 2:1090, 1971

199. Talpos G, Horrock M, White JM et al: Plasmapheresis in Raynaud's disease. Lancet 1:416, 1978

200. Winkelmann RK, McCune MA, Pineda AA et al: A controlled study of plasma exchange in scleroderma. In Black CM, Myers AR (eds): Systemic Sclerosis (Scleroderma). Gower Medical, New York, 1985, p. 449

201. Surwitt RS: Biofeedback: a possible treatment for Raynaud's disease. Semin Psychiatry 5:483, 1973

202. Kleckner MS, Allen EV, Wakim WG: The effect of local application of glyceryl trinitrate (nitroglycerine) on Raynaud's disease and Raynaud's phenomenon. Circulation 3:684, 1951

203. Shulman LE: Diffuse fasciitis with eosinophils: a new syndrome? Trans Assoc Am Physicians 88:70, 1975

204. Ansell BM, Nasseh GA, Bywaters EGL: Scleroderma in childhood. Ann Rheum Dis 35:198, 1976

205. Britt WJ, Duray PH, Dahl MV et al: Diffuse fasciitis with eosinophilia: a steroid responsive variant of scleroderma. J Pediatr 97:432, 1980

206. Rodnan GP, DiBartolomeo A, Medsger TA Jr: Eosinophilic fasciitis. Report of six cases of a newly recognized scleroderma-like syndrome (abstract). Arthritis Rheum 18:525, 1975

207. Caperton EM, Hathaway DE, Dehner LP: Morphea, fasciitis, and scleroderma with eosinophilia: a broad spectrum of disease (abstract). Arthritis Rheum 19:792, 1976

208. Kaplinsky N, Bubis JJ, Pras M: Localized eosinophilic fasciitis in a child. J Rheumatol 7:541, 1980

209. Michet C, Doyle J, Ginsburg W: Eosinophilic fasciitis: report of 15 cases. Mayo Clin Proc 56:27, 1981

210. Sills EM: Diffuse fasciitis with eosinophilia in childhood. Johns Hopkins Med J 151:203, 1982

211. Frayha R, Atiyah F, Karam P et al: Eosinophilic fasciitis terminating as progressive systemic sclerosis in a child. Dermatologica 171:291, 1985

212. Stachów A, Jablonska S, Kencka D: Tryptophan metabolism in scleroderma and eosinophilic fasciitis. In Black CM, Myers AR (eds): Systemic Sclerosis (Scleroderma). Gower Medical, New York, 1985, p. 130

213. Patrone NA, Kredich DW: Eosinophilic fasciitis in a child. Am J Dis Child 138:363, 1984

214. Jablonska S, Rodnan GP: Localized forms of scleroderma. Clin Rheum Dis 5:215, 1979

215. Lewkonia RM, Lowry RB: Progressive hemifacial atrophy (Parry-Romberg syndrome). Report with review of genetics and nosology. Am J Med Genetics 14:385, 1983

216. Stogmann W, Sandhofer M, Fritz J: Immunological studies in childhood scleroderma. Eur J Pediatr 124:223, 1977

217. Larrègue M, Ziegler J, Lauret P et al: Sclérodermie en bande chez l'enfant. Ann Derm Venereol 113:207, 1986

218. Takehara K, Morroi Y, Nakabayashi Y et al: Antinuclear antibodies in localized scleroderma. Arthritis Rheum 26:612, 1983

219. Bernstein RM, Pereira RS, Holden AJ et al: Autoantibodies in childhood scleroderma. Ann Rheum Dis 44:503, 1985

220. Ruffatti A, Peserico A, Glorioso S et al: Anticentromere antibody in localized scleroderma. J Am Acad Dermatol 15:637, 1986

221. Hanson V: Dermatomyositis, scleroderma and polyarteritis nodosa. Clin Rheum Dis 2:445, 1976

222. Moynahan EJ: Penicillamine in the treatment of morphoea and keloid in children. Postgrad Med J:39, 1974

223. Morgan RJ: Scleroderma: treatment with diphenylhydantoin. Cutis 8:278, 1971

224. Neldner KH: Treatment of localized linear scleroderma with phenytoin. Cutis 22:569, 1978

225. Clements PJ, Furst DE, Ho W et al: Progressive systemic sclerosis-like disease following bone marrow transplantation. In Black CM, Myers AR (eds): Systemic Sclerosis (Scleroderma). Gower Medical, New York, 1985, p. 376

226. Summerfield GP, Bellingham AJ, Bunch C et al: Successful treatment of chronic cutaneous graft-versus-host disease (GVHD) with penicillamine. Clin Lab Haematol 5:313, 1983

227. Lelbach WK, Marsteller HJ: Vinyl-chloride associated disease. Adv Intern Med Pediatr 47:1, 1981

228. Maricq HR: Vinyl chloride disease. In Black CM, Myers AR (eds): Systemic Sclerosis (Scleroderma). Gower Medical, New York, 1985, p. 105

229. Cohen I, Mosher M, O'Keefe E et al: Cutaneous toxicity of bleomycin therapy. Arch Dermatol 107:553, 1972

230. Luna MA, Bedrossian CWM, Lichtiger B et al: Interstitial pneumonitis associated with bleomycin therapy. Am J Clin Pathol 58:501, 1972

231. Finch WR, Buckingham RB, Rodnan GP et al: Scleroderma induced by bleomycin. In Black CM, Myers AR (eds): Systemic Sclerosis (Scleroderma). Gower Medical, New York, 1985, p. 114

232. Palestine RF, Millns JL, Sigel GT, et al: Skin manifestations of pentazocine abuse. J Am Acad Dermatol 2:47, 1980

233. Kondo H, Kumagai Y, Shiokawa Y: Scleroderma following cosmetic surgery ("adjuvant disease"): a review of nine cases reported in Japan. In Black CM, Myers AR (eds): Systemic Sclerosis (Scleroderma). Gower Medical, New York, 1985, p. 135

234. Alonso-Ruiz A, Zea-Mendoza AC, Salazar-Vallinas JM et al: Toxic oil syndrome: a syndrome with features overlapping those of various forms of scleroderma. Semin Arthritis Rheum 15:200, 1986

235. Izquierdo M, Mateo I, Rodrigo M et al: Chronic juvenile toxic epidemic syndrome. Ann Rheum Dis 44:98, 1985

236. Kornreich HK, Shaw KNF: Phenylketonuria and scleroderma. J Pediatr 73:571, 1968

237. Drummond KN, Michael AF, Good RA: Tryptophan metabolism in a patient with phenylketonuria and scleroderma. Can Med Assoc J 94:834, 1966

238. Nishimura N, Okamtoto M, Yasui M et al: Intermediary metabolism of phenylalanine and tyrosine in diffuse collagen diseases. II: Influences of the low phenylalanine and tyrosine diet upon patients with collagen diseases. Arch Dermatol 80:466, 1959

239. Fleishmajer R, Pollock JL: Progressive systemic sclerosis: pseudoscleroderma. Clin Rheum Dis 5:243, 1979

240. Rocco VK, Hurd ER: Scleroderma and scleroderma-like disorders. Semin Arthritis Rheum 16:22, 1986

241. Ormond JK: Idiopathic retroperitoneal fibrosis: a discussion of the etiology. J Urol 94:385, 1965

242. Marshall AJ, Baddeley M, Barrit DW: Proctolol peritonitis. A study of 16 cases and a survey of small bowel function in patients taking beta-adrenergic blockers. Q J Med 46:135, 1977

243. Rosenbloom AL, Frias JL: Diabetes, short stature and joint stiffness—a new syndrome. Clin Res 22:92A, 1974

244. Rosenbloom AL, Silverstein JH, Lezotte DC et al: Limited joint mobility in childhood diabetes mellitus indicates increased risk for microvascular disease. N Engl J Med 305:191, 1981

245. Grgic A, Rosenbloom AL, Weber FT et al: Joint contracture—common manifestation of childhood diabetes mellitus. J Pediatr 88:584, 1976

246. Buckingham BA, Uitto J, Sandborg C et al: Scleroderma-like syndrome and the non-enzymatic glucosylation of collagen in children with poorly controlled insulin dependent diabetes (abstract). Pediatr Res 15:626, 1981

247. Sherry DD, Rothstein RRL, Petty RE: Joint contractures preceding insulin-depending diabetes mellitus. Arthritis Rheum 25:1362, 1982

248. Doyle JA, Friedman SJ: Porphyria and scleroderma: a clinical and laboratory review of 12 patients. Aust J Dermatol 24:109, 1983

11

Immunodeficiencies and the Rheumatic Diseases

The frequency of the association between arthritis and immunodeficiencies suggests that insights into the pathogenesis of rheumatic diseases in general might be gained from a basic understanding of this interrelationship. It is for this reason that this association is treated separately in this textbook. Although more than 30 years has passed since the initial description of "collagen disease" in patients with agammaglobulinemia by Janeway et al. in 1956,[1] we are very little closer to understanding the pathogenic relationships that are undoubtedly represented by this association. The purpose of this chapter is to review the relationship of immunodeficiency and the rheumatic diseases in children and to comment specifically upon the most common of these associations. More comprehensive reviews of the immunodeficiencies are found in standard textbooks on the subject.

In many instances, the clinical characteristics of the rheumatic disease associated with an immunodeficiency syndrome are indistinguishable from those of rheumatic diseases occuring in immunocompetent individuals. It could be argued that most autoimmune diseases may represent the result of subtle immunodeficiencies and that the extent of the rheumatic disease–immunodeficiency association is much greater than is immediately apparent. Whether or not the identified immunodeficiency is in any direct way responsible for the development of the rheumatic disease, or whether it is associated with other, as yet unidentified, immunodeficiencies of pathogenic significance is unknown.

IMMUNODEFICIENCY DISORDERS

The extensive classification of immunodeficiency disorders suggested by a committee of the World Health Organization (Table 11-1) is somewhat unwieldly, and a simpler approach to the classification is provided in Table 11-2.

Immunodeficiency disorders may be defined as congenital or acquired defects of either the innate or the adaptive immune systems.[2] Deficiencies of the innate response include abnormalities in phagocytic cells and the complement cascade. Adaptive immunity consists of that mediated by lymphocytes and their products. A classification of deficiencies of adaptive immunity is based on the presence of abnormalities of lymphocytes of the bone marrow (B cell) or thymus (T cell) lineages or their precursors.

DISORDERS OF INNATE IMMUNITY ASSOCIATED WITH RHEUMATIC DISEASES

There is an increasing awareness of the association of rheumatic diseases with abnormalities of phago-

Table 11-1 Primary Immunodeficiency Diseases

Predominantly antibody defects
    X-linked agammaglobulinemia
    X-linked hypogammaglobulinemia with growth hormone deficiency
    Autosomal recessive agammaglobinemia
    Immunoglobulin deficiency with increased IgM
    IgA deficiency
    Selective deficiency of other immunoglobulin isotypes
    Kappa light chain deficiency
    Antibody deficiency with normal or increased immunoglobulins
    Immunodeficiency with thymoma
    Transient hypogammaglobulinemia of infancy

Common variable immunodeficiencies (CVI)
    CVI with predominant B cell defect
    CVI with predominant T cell defect
    CVI with autoantibodies to B or T cells

Predominantly cell mediated defects
    Combined immunodeficiency with predominant T cell defect
    Purine nucleoside phosphorylase deficiency
    Severe combined immunodeficiency with or without adenosine deaminase deficiency
    Immunodeficiency with unusual response to Epstein-Barr virus

Immunodeficiency associated with other defects
    Transcobalamine 2 deficiency
    Wiskott-Aldrich syndrome
    Ataxia telangiectasia
    Di George syndrome

(Modified from Rosen FS, Wedgwood RJ, Aiuti F et al. Clin Immunol Immunopathol 28: 450, 1983, with permission.)

cytic cell function or of complement pathways. These associations are listed in Table 11-3.

Disorders of Phagocytes

CHRONIC GRANULOMATOUS DISEASE

Chronic granulomatous disease (CGD), is a group of disorders in which there is an inherited inability of the polymorphonuclear leukocytes to kill bacteria, although phagocytosis is normal. As a result, viable intracellular bacteria create a granulomatous reaction.

Most children with this disease are boys, and X-linked recessive inheritance is most common. Infection, especially with *Staphylococcus aureus*, causes suppurating granulomas to develop in lymph nodes, liver and spleen, lungs, and skin and bones (especially the small bones of hands and feet).[3] Specific diagnostic studies include absence of nitroblue tetrazolium (NBT) reduction,[4] failure to generate phagocytosis-induced chemiluminescence,[5] or absence of bacterial killing as originally demonstrated.[6] Usually a marked polyclonal hypergammaglobulinemia and normal lymphocyte numbers and function are present. The carrier state can be demonstrated in female relatives by reduced, but not absent, NBT reduction or chemiluminescence.

The defect can arise from several different metabolic abnormalities of the oxygen-dependent microbicidal pathway. This pathway normally results in the generation of the superoxide ion, hydroxyl radicals, singlet oxygen, and hydrogen peroxide, all of which are microbicidal. Deficiency of enzymes in this pathway results in failure of the synthesis of these molecules during phagocytosis. As a result, the host is incapable of killing bacteria such as staphylococci that do not generate their own hydrogen peroxide although infections with pneumococci and streptococci, which synthesize hydrogen peroxide, do not cause significant difficulty.[7]

Associated Rheumatic Diseases

There have been a number of reports of discoid lupus erythematosus (DLE) in relatives, particularly mothers and maternal grandmothers, of children with CGD[8-16] (Table 11-4). Indeed, the association of the carrier state for CGD and a mucocutaneous syndrome characterized by DLE, photosensitive der-

Table 11-2 Classification of Immunodeficiency Disorders

Disorders of innate immunity
    Phagocytic abnormalities
    Complement pathway abnormalities
Disorders of adaptive immunity
    Abnormalities of both T and B lymphocytes
    Abnormalities of B lymphocytes
    Abnormalities of T lymphocytes

Table 11-3 Classification of Deficiencies of Innate Immunity Associated with Rheumatic Disease

Disorders of Innate Immunity	Rheumatic Disease Association
Phagocytic defects	
Chronic granulomatous disease	Discoid LE in mother
Lipochrome histiocytosis	Polyarthritis
Streaking leukocyte syndrome	Polyarthritis
Job's syndrome	—
Chédiak-Higashi disease	SLE-like disease in animals
Complement deficiencies	
Deficiency of C1q	SLE
Deficiency of C1r	SLE
Deficiency of C1r and C1s	SLE
Deficiency of C2	SLE, anaphylactoid purpura
Deficiency of C3	Vasculitis, arthralgias, SLE
Deficiency of C4	SLE
Deficiency of C5	SLE
Deficiency of C6	SLE, DLE
Deficiency of C7	SLE
Deficiency of C8	SLE

matitis, and recurrent aphthous stomatitis is quite common. Occasionally, other rheumatic complaints are noted and some mothers have autoantibodies to nuclear antigens, although antinuclear antibodies (ANAs) are usually absent. The frequency of defects in polymorph function in patients with DLE who lack a family history of CGD appears to be very low, however. In one study of 19 women with DLE, none was found to have abnormalities of NBT reduction or bactericidal capacity.[14]

Aside from susceptibility to septic arthritis and osteomyelitis, children with CGD have only rarely been noted to have a rheumatic disease. We have observed a bland peripheral arthritis and bursitis in two boys with CGD.

FAMILIAL LIPOCHROME HISTIOCYTOSIS

A syndrome of lipochrome histiocytosis was described in three female siblings, one of whom at age 15 developed migratory polyarthritis, rheumatoid factor, and rheumatoid nodules; a second of whom had recurrent episodes of monarthritis of brief duration; and two of whom had a photosensitive rash. All had increased susceptibility to bacterial infection, hypergammaglobulinemia, and lipo-

chrome pigment in histiocytes of lymph nodes and liver.[17] Subsequent studies revealed defects in polymorph function, which were identical to that seen in patients with CGD.[18] Unlike children with typical CGD, however, these girls did not develop granulomata and in this way resemble girls with so-called Job's syndrome.[19]

STREAKING LEUKOCYTE SYNDROME

A 14-year-old boy with severe pyoderma gangrenosum and recurrent sterile monarthritis was found to have a serum factor that enhanced random migration of leukocytes with secondary increase in chemotaxis.[20] The mechanisms of this disorder remain unknown; no further cases have been reported.

CHÉDIAK-HIGASHI SYNDROME

The rare Chédiak-Higashi syndrome is characterized by susceptibility to infection and presence of large cytoplasmic granules in polymorphs.[31] Although there have been no reports of rheumatic disease in patients with this disorder or their relatives, it is intriguing that the same leukocyte anomaly appears to occur in Aleutian mink, which have a spontaneous lupuslike disease.[22]

Table 11-4 Discoid Lupus Erythematosus and Other Abnormalities in Carrier Mothers of Children with Chronic Granulomatous Disease

Reference	Patient	Description of Maternal Disease
Schaller[8]	1	Arthralgia, DLE, photosensitivity, leukopenia, LE cells, arthritis, Raynaud's phenomenon, fever, pleuritis, oropharyngeal ulcers, recurrent upper respiratory tract infections
	2	Photosensitivity, DLE, joint stiffness, recurrent tonsillitis, stomatitis, lymphadenopathy
MacFarlane et al.[9]	1	DLE, psoriasis, rheumatic heart disease
Thompson and Soothill[10]	1	DLE; no LE cells
	2	SLE-like rash; no LE cells
	3	Polyarthritis lasting 9 months at 15 years of age; Raynaud's phenomenon
Barton and Johnson[11]	1	Photosensitive skin rash with onset at 5 years of age diagnosed as DLE; ANA and antibody to RNP present
Landing et al.[12]	1	Recurrent spontaneous abortions. Lupus (? type)
Douglas et al.[13]	1	DLE, recurrent aphthous stomatitis, photosensitive dermatitis, hypergammaglobulinemia
Humbert et al.[14]	1	DLE, ANA negative
	2	DLE, ANA negative, photosensitive dermatitis
Finlay et al.[15]	1	Photosensitive scaly facial and chest rash (sibling had same rash as mother)
Kragballe et al.[16]	1	DLE, recurrent stomatitis, photosensitivity
	2	DLE, recurrent stomatitis, photosensitivity
	3	DLE, recurrent stomatitis, photosensitivity
	4	DLE, recurrent stomatitis, photosensitivity
	5	DLE, recurrent stomatitis, photosensitivity and polyarthritis
	6	Recurrent stomatitis, photosensitivity
	7	Recurrent stomatitis, photosensitivity
	8	Recurrent stomatitis, photosensitivity
	9	Recurrent stomatitis
	10	Recurrent stomatitis

Rheumatic Disease Associated with Complement Component Deficiencies

In children with rheumatic diseases, abnormalities in the serum levels of complement components ordinarily reflect increased synthesis associated with active inflammation (increased third complement component [C3]) or consumption, as is the case in immune-complex-mediated vasculitis (decreased C3, C4, hemolytic complement). In addition, however, low levels of hemolytic complement or of individual components of the complement pathway may reflect primary deficiencies.

Genetically determined primary deficiencies of individual components of the complement pathway have been identified in association with a number of autoimmune and infectious diseases. Excellent reviews of reported cases have been published.[23–25] In general, deficiencies of the early complement components are associated with lupuslike disorders, whereas deficiencies of the later components are associated with infection, particularly with *Neisseria* species. The reported instances of patients with homozygous complement component deficiencies and rheumatic diseases are summarized in Table 11-5.[23]

Absence of C1q is the most commonly reported abnormality of the C1 complex and includes 10 children under the age of 18 years, 5 of whom had SLE usually with onset in the first 3 years of life. Deficiency of C1r, often with deficiency of C1s, was reported in 8 children, 5 of whom had SLE, and many of whom also had bacterial infections, especially meningitis.

Homozygous deficiency of C2 accounts for one-third of reported cases of complement component deficiencies associated with rheumatic diseases. Of 26 children with this abnormality,[23] 6 had SLE (1 with DLE as well), 3 had anaphylactoid purpura, 1 had acute synovitis, and 5 had idiopathic glomerulonephritis.

An example of homozygous C2 deficiency is illustrated in Figure 11-1. The patient, a 5-year-old boy with Raynaud's disease, had undetectable hemolytic complement and was C2-deficient. Both parents may have been heterozygotes for C2 deficiency, although only the mother had symptoms (Raynaud's disease). Heterozygous C2 deficiency is thought to occur in approximately 1 percent of the normal population, 1.4 percent of adults with rheumatoid arthritis, 3 percent of children with juvenile rheumatoid arthritis (JRA), and 6 percent of patients with SLE.[26] The lupuslike disease seen in these complement deficiency states, particularly in association with heterozygous C2 deficiency, tends to be a somewhat milder disease than one would expect, with less clinically significant nephritis and more florid cutaneous lesions.[23]

Almost all reported cases of homozygous C3 deficiency have been in infants or young children who have severe bacterial infection (meningitis, pneumonia, peritonitis, osteomyelitis). Other associations have included SLE (1 child), vasculitis (3 children), arthralgia (2 children), and glomerulonephritis (3 children).

Seven C4-deficient children have been recorded. Five children had SLE, one had glomerulonephritis, and three had serious infections. Deficiency of C5, although unusual, is more common in adults and older children. Both of the reported C5-deficient adolescents had *N. meningitidis* meningitis, but neither had rheumatic complaints. Absence of C6 has been reported in six children under the age of 18 years, most of whom had *N. meningitidis* meningitis. Al-

Table 11-5 Homozygous Complement Deficiencies and Rheumatic Diseases in Children

Deficient Component	No. under 18 yrs	No. (%) with associated rheumatic disease				
		SLE	GN[b]	HSP[c]	Vasculitis	Arthritis
C1q	10	5(50)	3(30)	—	—	—
C1r	8	5(62)	1(12)	—	—	—
C1s	4[a]	3(75)	—	—	—	—
C2	26	6(23)	5(19)	3(12)	—	1(4)
C3	13	1(8)	3(23)	—	3(23)	2(15)
C4	7	5(71)	1(14)	—	—	—
C5	2	—	—	—	—	—
C6	6	—	—	—	—	—
C7	11	—	—	—	—	—
C8	7	—	—	—	—	—
C9	1	—	—	—	—	—
Factor I	5	—	—	—	—	—
Factor P	2	—	—	—	—	—
Factor H	2	—	—	—	—	—

[a] These patients were also C1r-deficient.
[b] GN, glomerulonephritis.
[c] HSP, Henoch-Schönlein purpura.
(Data from Ross and Densen.[23])

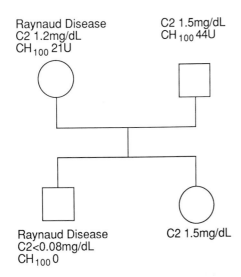

Raynaud Disease
C2 1.2mg/dL
CH$_{100}$ 21U

C2 1.5mg/dL
CH$_{100}$ 44U

Raynaud Disease
C2<0.08mg/dL
CH$_{100}$ 0

C2 1.5mg/dL

Fig. 11-1 Example of homozygous C2 deficiency. The patient is a 5-year-old boy with Raynaud's disease and undetectable hemolytic complement. C2 was below the limit of detectability. Hemolytic complement was reduced in both parents and C2 levels were half normal.

though no child with C6, C7, or C8 deficiency and a rheumatic disease has been reported, adults with these deficiencies have been noted to have DLE, Sjögren's syndrome, or SLE. Deficiencies of C9 and of the alternate pathway are very rare and have not been associated with rheumatic diseases.

The participation of the complement cascade in the inflammatory response in the rheumatic diseases might suggest that patients who are congenitally deficient in a complement component would have a much lower frequency of these diseases. The opposite appears to be the case. There are a number of possible explanations for this association. These patients have impaired host defenses to infections that may make them unable to deal effectively with rheumatogenic infectious agents. The association of C2 deficiency with SLE could be attributed to linkage with HLA genes, since genes coding for C2 and C4 are close to those coding for the HLA-DR and other loci believed to be associated with immune responses. However, hereditary angioneurotic edema, caused by a deficiency in C1 esterase inhibitor, has no known HLA association but is associated with a lupuslike disease in some families.[27,28] Patients with this disorder have poor viral neutralization lending credence to the hypothesis that deficiencies in the actual function of the

classic complement sequence may predispose patients to rheumatic diseases.

In instances of the familial occurrence of SLE, especially with very early age of onset of disease, the possibility of a complement component deficiency should be considered. In addition, in patients with normal C3 and C4 levels but deficient total hemolytic complement, in the presence of relatively inactive disease, selective deficiency of a complement component should be suspected. Measurement of total hemolytic complement in family members is also indicated in these instances.

DISORDERS OF ADAPTIVE IMMUNITY ASSOCIATED WITH RHEUMATIC DISEASES

Acquired abnormalities of adaptive immunity, as measured in the laboratory, are very common in children with rheumatic diseases. In general, it is believed that these changes (hypergammaglobulinemia, altered lymphocyte numbers or response to mitogens) reflect a response to the disease rather than a primary abnormality, although this is by no means certain. Rare but instructive examples of the association of primary immunodeficiencies and rheumatic diseases are discussed (Table 11-6).

Immunodeficiencies of T and B Lymphocytes and Rheumatic Diseases

COMBINED IMMUNODEFICIENCIES

The term *combined immunodeficiency* is applied to a group of disorders that are characterized by severe defects in both cellular and humoral immunity, whether or not they have lymphopenia or absent immunoglobulins.[29] There are two major types of this immunodeficiency: (1) severe combined immunodeficiency, characterized by lymphoid aplasia, thymic dysplasia, agammaglobulinemia, and lymphopenia and resulting in early onset of severe potentially fatal infection; and (2) Nezelof's syndrome, a cellular immunodeficiency with thymic dysplasia and normal or near normal immunoglobulin levels but defective antibody formation.

We have studied one girl with Nezelof's syndrome who had autoimmune thyroiditis, hemolytic anemia,

Table 11-6 Disorders of Adaptive Immunity Associated with Rheumatic Diseases

Disorders of Adaptive Immunity	Rheumatic Disease Association
Humoral immunodeficiencies	
IgA deficiency	JRA, SLE, RA, others
Hypogammaglobulinemia	Chronic arthritis, myositis
IgG subclass deficiencies	—
Combined immunodeficiencies	
Nezelof's syndrome	Chronic arthritis
Wiskott-Aldrich syndrome	Chronic arthritis
Immunodeficiency with thymoma	Chronic arthritis
Adenosine deaminase deficiency	—
Purine nucleoside phosphorylase deficiency	—

thrombocytopenia, and severe polyarticular arthritis, including arthritis of the knees, small joints of the hands, ankles, temporomandibular joints, and cervical spine[30] (Fig. 11-2). Needle biopsy of the knee at age 4 years showed only a mild, nonspecific synovitis. Extensive studies, including culture of the synovium, failed to detect a viral infection. Administration of transfer factor and fetal thymus transplantation failed to affect the joint disease or to reconstitute T-lymphocyte function permanently. This girl eventually died of pneumococcal sepsis. Neither of two affected siblings developed joint disease.

A third type of combined immunodeficiency, Wiskott-Aldrich syndrome, is an X-linked recessive disorder consisting of increasingly severe chronic thrombocytopenia, eczema, and recurrent bacterial and viral infection, associated with a progressive ab-

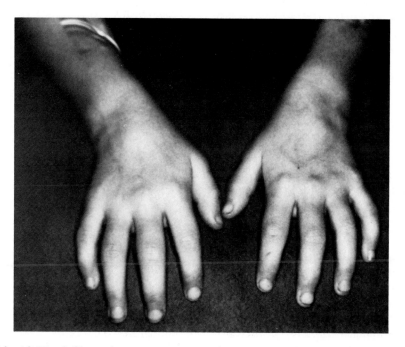

Fig. 11-2 A girl with Nezelof's syndrome at age 5 years showing swelling of the wrists, MCP and PIP joints, and dorsal tenosynovitis.

normality in both T- and B-lymphocyte function.[31] A wide variety of laboratory abnormalities is present, including a characteristic immunoglobulin pattern consisting of normal immunoglobulin G (IgG), low IgM, and very high IgA and IgE. Lymphocyte responsiveness to antigens and mitogens is diminished. The most characteristic abnormality is the failure to respond to polysaccharide antigens, including blood group antigens, so that isohemagglutinins are absent. The disease usually manifests itself in early childhood, but mild forms in adolescents or adults are occasionally seen. Overall, approximately one-quarter of the reported boys have had an associated arthritis.[32–34] Malignancy, especially sarcoma, and repeated hemorrhage are common preterminal events.

OTHER IMMUNODEFICIENCIES OF T AND B LYMPHOCYTES

The syndrome of short-limbed dwarfism with immunodeficiency is a congenital abnormality of uncertain etiology. Infants have redundant skin folds in the neck and generalized hypermobility with restriction of elbow extention. Infants with short-limbed dwarfism are highly susceptible to varicella infection. Although the presence of restricted elbow motion may raise the question of an inflammatory disorder, rheumatic diseases have not been reported.[35] Radiologic studies of these children reveal widened metaphyses, with irregular sclerosis and cystic changes, reflecting irregular chondrogenesis and osteogenesis. The costochondral junctions are flared. Progressive T-lymphocyte dysfunction occurs, sometimes with B-lymphocyte abnormalities. Cartilage-hair hypoplasia appears to be a variant of this syndrome.

A single adult with the rare syndrome of immunodeficiency with thymoma was reported to have arthritis.[36]

Deficiencies of the enzymes adenosine deaminase[37] and purine nucleoside phosphorylase[38] are associated with hypogammaglobulinemia and chondro-osseous dysplasia, although inflammatory rheumatic diseases have not been reported in these patients.

Primary Humoral Immunodeficiencies and Rheumatic Diseases

SELECTIVE IgA DEFICIENCY

Selective immunoglobulin A (IgA) deficiency, the most common of all immunoglobulin deficiencies, is defined as a serum IgA level of <10 mg/L beyond the newborn period with normal concentrations of IgG and IgM. IgA deficiency occurs in from 1 in 450 to 1 in 1,000 adult blood donors,[39] and is usually asymptomatic. Some community-based population studies estimate the frequency of IgA deficiency at closer to 1 in 1,000 individuals.[39] Both serum and secretory IgA are absent, although the secretory piece is present. In the majority of patients studied, IgA is present on lymphocyte surface membranes and in their cytoplasm, but there is excessive T-suppressor activity,[40] or a B-lymphocyte defect, accounting for failure of secretion in response to antigenic or mitogenic stimulation.[41] The variations in extent and nature of the abnormality probably contribute to the heterogeneity of the clinical and immunologic associations (Table 11-7).

The etiology is not known, but it is often familial, a pattern that may be accounted for in part by the transplacental effect of maternal anti-IgA antibodies[42] and by its association with HLA-B8.[39] For the most part, IgA deficiency is believed to be congenital and permanent, although there are several exceptions to this rule. IgA deficiency has been noted after treatment with gold[43–46] and hydroxychloroquine.[43] IgA deficiency attributed to the nonsteroidal anti-inflammatory drug fenclofenac[47] and to sulfasalazine[47–50] has also been reported. In the series reported by Cassidy et al.[51] no patient had received any of these drugs. One patient with longstanding JRA and IgA deficiency who was given plasma infusions began synthesizing her own IgA. Her rheumatic disease, which was initially diagnosed as JRA, evolved to SLE.[52] Pelkonen et al. have noted that in some children with JRA, IgA deficiency was transient.[43]

Disease Associations

The spectrum of diseases that have been associated with IgA deficiency is extremely broad, and most

Table 11-7 Selective IgA Deficiency: Immunologic Characteristics

Absent (<10 mg/L) serum and secretory IgA
B lymphocytes with normal surface IgA
± IgE deficiency
± IgG subclass deficiency
± IgG anti-IgA antibodies
± IgG antibovine protein antibodies
± T-lymphocyte defects

IgA-deficient individuals are entirely asymptomatic (Table 11-8). The rheumatic disease associations will be discussed in some detail (Table 11-9).

Chronic arthritis (JRA-like)   The most common rheumatic disease association of IgA deficiency is with chronic arthritis, which is indistinguishable from JRA. The frequency of this association appears to vary somewhat from one geographical area to another but is probably in the range of 2 to 4 percent (Table 11-9).

Of 477 patients with a diagnosis of JRA at the Uni-

versity of Michigan Pediatric Rheumatology clinic, 18 (3.8 percent) had undetectable serum IgA (<10 mg/L) and undetectable secretory IgA. An increased frequency of low but detectable levels of serum IgA (>2 standard deviations below the age-specific mean) has also been documented in children with JRA.[54]

In general, the arthritis associated with IgA deficiency is indistinguishable from JRA (Fig. 11-3 and Table 11-10).[51,53,54] The sex ratios and ages at onset of arthritis are approximately the same as those seen in the other children with JRA. In the combined series of Cassidy et al.[58] and Pelkonen et al.[43] 18 of 28 (64 percent) had oligoarticular onset (fewer than five joints), 9 (32 percent) had a polyarticular onset, and only 1 (4 percent) had systemic onset. The majority of children have not had severe disease; most are self-sufficient and active, and attend school or work. The arthritis tends to remain active for many years, often into adult life, although there may be little joint destruction discernible radiographically. Erosive arthritis did occur, however, in 28 percent of the Uni-

Table 11-8 Selective IgA Deficiency: Disease Associations

Most IgA-deficient individuals are asymptomatic

Recurrent sinusitis-otitis-pharyngitis syndrome

Rheumatic diseases
  Chronic arthritis (JRA-like)
  Systemic lupus erythematosus
  Dermatomyositis
  Ankylosing spondylitis
  Scleroderma

Autoimmune disorders
  Thyroiditis
  Chronic active hepatitis
  Pernicious anemia
  Autoimmune hemolytic anemia and thrombocyto-
    penia
  Pulmonary hemosiderosis

Gastrointestinal disease
  Nodular lymphoid hyperplasia
  Celiac disease
  Inflammatory bowel disease

CNS disease
  Ataxia-telangiectasia

Drug-induced
  Anticonvulsants
  Gold salts
  Penicillamine
  Nonsteroidal anti-inflammatory drugs

Malignancy

Chromosome 18 deletions

Other immunodeficiencies
  Chronic mucocutaneous candidiasis
  CGD
  Neutropenia

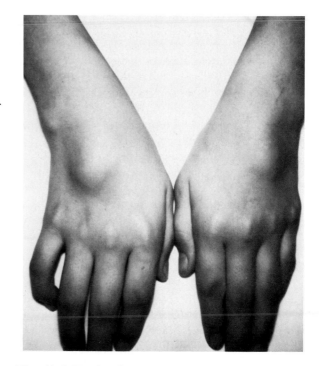

Fig. 11-3 Hands of an 11-year-old girl with chronic arthritis and selective IgA deficiency (SIgAD). Hand and wrist involvement gradually returned to normal, but a minimally symptomatic effusion of her right knee persisted.

Table 11-9 IgA Deficiency and Rheumatic Diseases

Author	Rheumatic Disease Association	No/total	%
Cassidy et al.[51,54]	Chronic arthritis (JRA-like)	18/477	4
Huntley et al.[55]	Chronic arthritis (JRA-like)	2/23	9
Panush et al.[56]	Chronic arthritis (JRA-like)	3/176	2
Pelkonen et al.[43]	Chronic arthritis (JRA-like)	11/300	4
Barkley et al.[44]	Chronic arthritis (JRA-like)	12/582	2
Amman and Hong[56]	SLE		
Bachmann et al.[57]	SLE		
Cassidy et al.[52,58,59]	SLE	10/50	5
Claman et al.[61]	SLE		
Cleland and Bell[62]	SLE	2	
Cassidy et al.[63]	Dermatomyositis	3	
Cassidy et al.[63]	Scleroderma (systemic)	1/15	6
Jay et al.[64]	Scleroderma (systemic)	1	
Spirer et al.[65]	Scleroderma (local)	1	
Cassidy et al[63]	Ankylosing spondylitis	2	
Good et al.[66]	Ankylosing spondylitis	1	
Barkley et al.[44]	Juvenile ankylosing spondylitis	1	
Siegler[67]	Sarcoidosis	7	
Thomas et al.[68]	Sarcoidosis	1	

No/total: number of IgA-deficient patients divided by number of patients with specific rheumatic disease.

versity of Michigan series (Fig. 11-4A and B), although rheumatoid nodules were seen in only 2 patients. In 1 of these children they were peripheral and located over the usual pressure areas; in the other child, nodules developed on the vocal cords and resulted in hoarseness. Chronic uveitis is also a significant risk in these children, occurring in 3 of 11 children with pauciarticular onset disease. ANAs occurred in 13 of 18 IgA-deficient children with JRA. The specificity of the ANA is largely unknown, and although antibodies to native deoxyribonucleic acid (nDNA) were reported to be associated with IgA deficiency in one study[69] levels of binding to native or denatured DNA or ribonucleic acid (RNA) were not elevated in another report.[60]

One aspect of IgA deficiency with particular relevance to patients with a rheumatic disease is the occurrence of antibodies to IgA.[59] Such antibodies are usually of the IgG class and usually react with both IgA1 and IgA2,[70] but may react with only one of the IgA subclasses or one of the allotypes of IgA2 (IgA2m1 or IgA2m2). In general, anti-IgA antibodies are more common in IgA-deficient patients with autoimmune and rheumatic diseases than they are in IgA-deficient individuals who are asymptomatic or who have allergic or infectious symptoms (Table 11-11).[59]

The role of anti-IgA antibodies is unknown, but the occurrence of IgG–anti-IgA-mediated transfusion reactions[71] suggests caution in the use of any blood product in a patient with a rheumatic disease who may be IgA-deficient. Should the need arise, any IgA-deficient patient should receive IgA-deficient blood product, if at all possible, or thoroughly washed erythrocytes.

The family of one of our patients with selective IgA deficiency is shown in Figure 11-5. The mother and three of the siblings of the patient lacked IgA. The mother had very high levels of anti-IgA antibodies detected by a hemagglutination assay. These antibodies could have crossed the placenta and induced IgA deficiency in the offspring, a possibility supported by in vitro[72] and in vivo[42] evidence.

In relation to the pathogenesis of the rheumatic disease, IgA deficiency may be only the marker of a more fundamental immunologic abnormality. In addition to anti-IgA antibodies, a variety of T-lymphocyte defects, other antibody disorders (for instance, milk precipitins), and IgG subclass deficiencies have been reported in IgA-deficient pa-

Table 11-10 Clinical Manifestations of 18 Children with Chronic Arthritis and Selective IgA Deficiency

	Percentage
Sex	
Female	78
Male	22
Age at onset of arthritis	
<4 yrs	50
5–9 yrs	45
10–12 yrs	5
Characteristics of arthritis	
Pauciarticular	61
Polyarticular	39
Systemic	0
Erosions	28
Extra-articular manifestations	
Rheumatoid nodules	11
Chronic anterior uveitis	22
Functional class at follow-up	
Class I	28
Class II	50
Class III	22
Class IV	0
Laboratory abnormalities	
ANA present	72
RF present	6
Anti-IgA antibodies present	79

tients (Table 11-7). Deficiency of ecto-5'-nucleotidase may be associated with X-linked hypogammaglobulinemia but not with selective IgA deficiency[73] and is of doubtful significance in relation to rheumatic complaints.

Other Rheumatic Diseases Associated with IgA Deficiency Selective IgA deficiency (SIgAD) has been described in patients with SLE, dermatomyositis, scleroderma, and ankylosing spondylitis. In these instances, the diseases do not appear to be different from those encountered in patients who have normal serum IgA concentrations. A lupuslike disease has occurred in 10 of our IgA-deficient patients. None of these patients has developed significant nephritis; 1 died in adulthood from a septic abortion. One patient is shown in Figure 11-6. The malar rash, oral mucocutaneous ulceration, and frontal alopecia can be seen. Over the ensuing two decades, she has had one major episode of pericarditis, ischemic necrosis of both hips, and has had two successful pregnancies.

Chronic arthritis associated with deletions of the long and short arms of chromosome 18 has been reported in two children, one of whom was also IgA-deficient.[74]

Treatment of IgA Deficiency

There is no specific treatment for the patient with SIgAD. The arthritis in these patients has responded to conventional antirheumatic therapy in a manner similar to that in other children with JRA. Treatment of connective-tissue diseases in patients with immunodeficiency is the same as that employed in the uncomplicated disease, although corticosteroid and immunosuppressive drugs should be used only with the greatest caution. Immunoglobulin replacement therapy is an essential part of the management of the child with hypogammaglobulinemia, but specific IgA replacement is not usually indicated in the child with SIgAD, since the protective effect of secretory IgA is not achieved with systemic administration, and the risk of IgG-anti-IgA transfusion reactions, especially in the child with a connective tissue disease, must be considered. Commercial intramuscular and intravenous preparations of immunoglobulin contain measurable, if low, amounts of IgA as well as IgG. Some patients with severe sinopulmonary disease have been successfully treated with IgA-free immunoglobulin preparations.

HYPOGAMMAGLOBULINEMIA AND RHEUMATIC DISEASES

The principal features of X-linked (Bruton) agammaglobulinemia and primary acquired hypogammaglobulinemia are presented in Table 11-12. Boys with X-linked agammaglobulinemia usually have onset at 6 to 9 months of age of marked susceptibility to severe bacterial infections (pneumonia, meningitis, osteomyelitis, septic arthritis). Children with non-X-linked hypogammaglobulinemia, such as the case outlined in Table 11-13, have similar complaints, although they may be later in onset and pursue a less fulminant course (Table 11-13 and Fig. 11-7).

Arthritis and Hypogammaglobulinemia

Although the association of rheumatic diseases and hypogammaglobulinemia is established, its frequency is uncertain (Table 11-14).

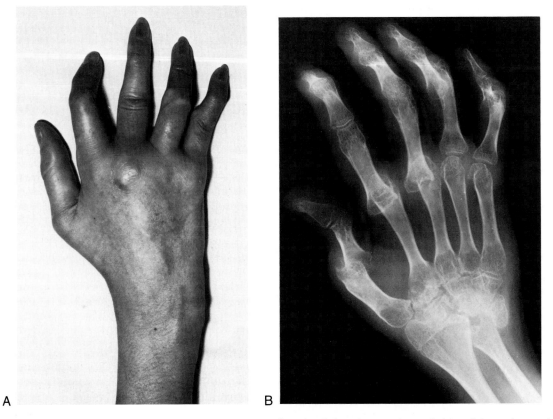

Fig. 11-4 (A) Right hand of T.P. at age 27 years. A chronic, deforming erosive arthritis of the wrists and small joints of the hands was slowly progressive from onset. These deformities and subluxation of MCP joints are evident. The second PIP joint had been fused in a functional position. **(B)** Hand of B.P., an 18-year-old girl with selective IgA deficiency and SLE, with onset of arthritis at age 7 years. Destruction of joints is already far advanced, with subluxations of ulnar side of wrist, MCP joints 1 to 3, and PIP joints 4 and 5. Erosions, destruction of articulating surfaces, microfractures and bony collapse, and extreme juxta-articular osteoporosis are present.

Table 11-11 Frequency of Anti-IgA Antibodies in Persons with Selective IgA Deficiency

		Anti-IgA Antibodies	
Diagnosis	Number	Number	Percentage
Asymptomatic blood donors	27	5	19
Miscellaneous diseases	8	2	25
Recurrent infections	10	3	30
RA-like arthritis	4	2	50
JRA-like arthritis	13	10	77
SLE-like disease	10	10	100

(Modified from Petty et al.,[59] with permission.)

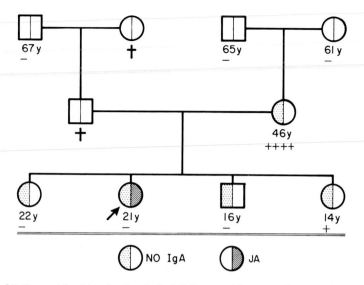

Fig. 11-5 Family of T.P., a girl with selective IgA deficiency with onset of a juvenile arthritis at age 7 years. The symbol underneath that of the sex is the anti-IgA antibody titer (− absent; + positive; + + + + strongly positive.).

Clinically the joint disease that occurs in these patients resembles that of pauciarticular JRA: onset between 3 and 15 years of age of arthritis in one to four large peripheral joints characterized by small to moderate effusions, soft tissue thickening, and limitation of motion. However, the arthritis is often minimally symptomatic. Synovial fluid from one patient contained 18,500 cells per cubic millimeter (18.5 × 10^9 per liter) that were 98 percent mononuclear. Synovial histologic examination revealed moderate hyperplasia and hypertrophy of the lining cells and villi, vascular endothelial proliferation, and subsynovial pro-

Table 11-12 Characteristics of Hypogammaglobulinemia

	X-Linked	Common Variable
Sex	Boys	Boys or girls
Genetics	X-linked recessive	Variable
Age at onset of symptoms	6 mos–2 yrs	2 yrs–adulthood
B-lymphocyte abnormalities		
Plasma cells in nodes	No	Decreased or none
Surface immunoglobulin	No	Yes
Serum IgG	<1 g/L	<5 g/L
Serum IgA, IgM	Very low	Variable
T-lymphocyte abnormalities	No	Variable
Clinical characteristics		
Recurrent severe bacterial infections	Yes	Sometimes
Malabsorption	Sometimes	Frequent
JRA-like arthritis	30%	Unknown
Control with Ig replacement	Partial	Partial

Table 11-13 Hypogammaglobulinemia and Arthritis: A Case History

History

6 months	Recurrent skin infections, otitis media, poor wound healing
5 years	Tonsillectomy
6 years	Painful, stiff shoulders
7 years	Chronic swelling of the left knee
	Rhinorrhea, wheezing, pneumonitis
14 years	Left mastoidectomy
	Frequent, bulky stools

Immunizations
    Received all routine immunizations, including live virus vaccines

Physical examination at age 15 years
    Draining left otitis media
    Axillary lymphadenopathy
    Moderate effusion and increased warmth of the left knee

Investigations at age 15 years
    Radiographs
        Sinus wall thickening and clouding
        Abnormal left mastoid
        Left knee: epiphyseal overgrowth and joint effusion
              : thermography abnormal
    Laboratory studies
        IgG 1.4 g/L; IgA 0, IgM 0.6 g/L, IgE 0.
        No antibodies to polio, diphtheria, tetanus
        No isohemagglutinins
        Schick test result positive
        Negative delayed skin tests to PPD, mumps, *Candida*, SKSD
        Impaired in vitro lymphocyte response to PHA
        Circulating lymphocytes: T cells 52%, B cells 40%
        Hemolytic complement: normal

Table 11-14 Prevalence of Chronic Arthritis with Hypogammaglobulinemia

Reference	Patient Group Studied	Arthritis	
Janeway et al.[1]	Agammaglobulinemia	5/12	42%
Good and Rotstein[75]	Agammaglobulinemia	8/27	30%
Lawrence and Bremner[76]	Hypogammaglobulinemia		
	Male	7/60	12%
	Female	0/18	
Webster et al.[77]	Variable adult-onset hypogam	5/70	7%
Schaller[78]	X-linked hypogammaglobulinemia	2/9	22%
	Variable hypogammaglobulinemia	0/20	
Cassidy et al.[79,80]	X-linked hypogammaglobulinemia	4/11	36%
	Variable hypogammaglobulinemia	5/19	26%

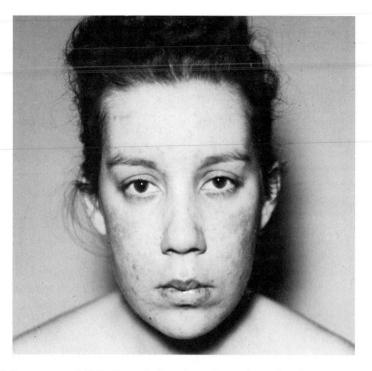

Fig. 11-6 Face of J.B. at onset of SLE. Frontal alopecia, malar rash, and oral mucocutaneous ulcerations are present. The rash was photosensitive.

liferation of fibrous tissue, but without infiltration by lymphocytes or plasma cells[79] (Fig. 11-8). Except for the lack of lymphoid cells the biopsy specimen was very similar to that seen in JRA. In one series of 30 children with hypogammalobulinemia, no patient had rheumatoid factors, ANA, nodules, or bony erosions. In spite of treatment with therapeutic amounts of intramuscular gamma globulin or with plasma or plasmin-treated intravenous gamma globulin in addition to therapeutic amounts of aspirin, the arthritis has persisted in all. In five of the patients, the arthritis began 6 months to 11 years after gamma globulin replacement therapy was initiated.[79,80] The relationship between the hypogammaglobulinemia and inflammatory joint disease illustrated by these patients seems real, although whether a pathogenic relationship exists is less clear. It is tempting to speculate that organisms such as viruses or ureaplasmal agents may be pathogenic in these immunocompromised individuals.

In a review of 96 patients with X-linked agammaglobulinemia, septic arthritis had occurred in 20 percent prior to or at the time of diagnosis.[81] In half of these cases, a bacterial cause was identified; in the remainder no pathogen was found.[81] A further 20 percent of patients developed oligoarthritis while receiving gamma globulin replacement therapy. In these cases, enteroviruses were most frequently identified in association with a dermatomyositislike syndrome. Septic bacterial arthritis appears to be prevented by gamma globulin replacement therapy. *Ureaplasma urealyticum* was identified in the joints of several patients in a number of reports.[82-84]

Table 11-15 Characteristics of the Juvenile Arthritis–Hypogammaglobulinemia Syndrome

Arthritis occurs in 20–25% of patients with hypogammaglobulinemia
Arthritis occurs after the onset of other symptoms
Arthritis is limited in extent
    Predominant involvement of the knee
    Often subtle; may be asymptomatic
    Often chronic, but nondestructive
    May cause premature osteoarthritis
    May progress to polyarticular disease
Arthritis probably not affected by gamma globulin replacement
Arthritis may occur during the course of treatment

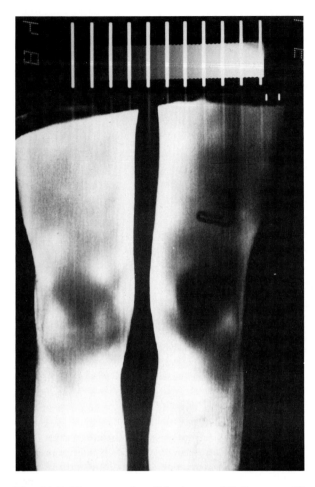

Fig. 11-7 Thermographs of the knees of R.B. at age 20 years, showing increased heat production on the left knee, the site of the inflammatory disease.

Rheumatic complaints of insufficient duration to designate as JRA or other musculoskeletal complaints are also frequent in hypogammaglobulinemia. Schaller[78] has noted transient arthritis or arthralgia in 5 of 9 patients with X-linked hypogammaglobulinemia. Of our 30 patients, in addition to 9 with chronic oligoarthritis, 2 have had septic arthritis, 6 complained of arthralgias of varying duration, and 1 developed Legg-Calvé-Perthes disease. Table 11-15 summarizes our clinical impressions concerning the appearance and course of the chronic arthritis that has been described in patients with hypogammaglobulinemia. Of particular note is its subtlety. It is asymptomatic, has a delayed onset, and can often be missed on the physical examination unless particular care is taken to document small effusions, soft tissue swelling, or decreased range of joint motion.

Hypogammaglobulinemia and a Dermatomyositislike Syndrome

There is considerable doubt that the dermatomyositislike syndrome that sometimes complicates hypogammaglobulinemia is the same disease as idiopathic dermatomyositis of childhood. Clinical characteristics of the reported cases of this syndrome are summarized in Table 11-16. This disease is characterized by edema, myalgia, muscle wasting, and, sometimes, polyarthritis followed by contractures of large joints. It is not clear from the reported cases whether the myopathy is proximal, distal, or diffuse in most instances. Cutaneous manifestations include heliotrope discoloration of the eyelids in one child,[88] rash on the extensor surfaces of the metacarpophalangeal (MCP) and proximal interphalangeal (PIP) joints in two patients,[88,89] and nonspecific rashes in two other patients. Electromyographic evidence of a myopathy was documented in one patient, and muscle biopsy abnormalities consistent with a diagnosis of dermatomyositis were present in seven. Focal calcification was present in one. Central nervous system disease and deafness frequently accompany the myositis, and a fatal outcome is common. Viral isolations (echovirus, adenovirus) from the cerebrospinal fluid and sometimes from muscle and other sites raise the question of a viral etiology of this syndrome and support a role for persistent latent viral infection in its pathogenesis.[87,89,90] A direct relationship to idiopathic dermatomyositis remains unproved, however. One patient was successfully treated with intravenous gamma globulin.[94]

IgG SUBCLASS DEFICIENCIES AND RHEUMATIC DISEASES

The availability of specific antisera for the IgG subclasses has allowed the detection of subclass deficiencies in a wide variety of normal and abnormal conditions. A 10-year-old boy with JRA and Hodgkin's disease was shown to have low IgA (0.19 g/L) and IgG2 (0.02 g/L). Another 10-year-old boy had SLE, undetectable IgA, and IgG2 of 0.02 g/L.[95] Oxelius

Table 11-16 Dermatomyositislike Disease and Hypogammaglobulinemia

Reference	n	Sex	Age	Description
Janeway et al.[1]	1	M	2 yr	Brawny edema of distal extremities; leg stiffness, contractures; gastrocnemius biopsy specimen consistent with dermatomyositis
Good et al.[85]	1	?	?	Patient with classic dermatomyositis and hypogammaglobulinemia; no other details
Page et al.[86]	1	?	?	Dermatomyositis, lymphoma
Rosen et al.[87]	2	?	?	Adenovirus 12, echovirus 9 isolated
Gotoff et al.[88]	1	M	2	Intermittent arthritis (knees) since 2 yr; at 17 yr, heliotrope rash on eyelids, MCP and PIP rash, muscle weakness, contractures, ↑LDH. Biopsy: perivascular, endomysial, perimysial lymphocytic infiltrate; normal immunofluorescence; cerebral vasculitis; death
Bardelas et al.[89]	1	M	5	Brawny edema of extremities; violaceous, telangiectatic rash over extensor aspects of legs, muscle wasting, contractures of elbows, wrists, knees. ALT↑, AST↑, CK normal; echovirus 24 in CSF; muscle biopsy: perivascular lymphocytic infiltrate; death
Wilfert et al.[90]	1	M	24	Muscle weakness, edema, rash on extensor surface of joints; contractures elbows, knees; CSF: echovirus 9; muscle biopsy: perivascular round cell infiltration; death
	1	M	12	Joint stiffness, contractures; weakness and atrophy of muscles; deafness; muscle biopsy: perivascular lymphocytic infiltration
	1	M	3	Arthritis in knees and ankles, myalgia; ↑AST ↑aldolase; EMG: myopathy; echocardiography: RBBB. CSF: echovirus 33
Webster et al.[91]	1	M	11	Polyarthritis, edema, encephalitis; muscle biopsy: mononuclear infiltration; leukocyte migration inhibited by echo 11 vaccine
Maguire et al.[92]	1	F	3 mo	Fever, muscle weakness, cellulitis, violaceous edematous eyelids, musosal ulceration; ↑CK, ↑aldolase; skin biopsy: leukocytoclastic vasculitis
Crennan et al.[93]	1	M	29	Chronic arthritis at 19 mos; in adulthood, myalgia, proximal muscle weakness, ↑CK. Gastrocnemius biopsy: active inflammatory myopathy; echovirus 11 from blood, urine, CSF, muscle

RBBB = right bundle branch block; ↑ = increased.

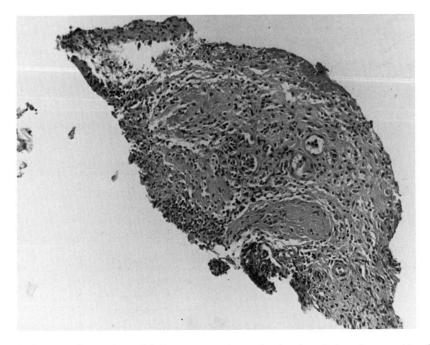

Fig. 11-8 Needle biopsy of synovium of R.B., a teenage boy who developed chronic synovitis of the left knee and was found to have common variable immunodeficiency. There is marked hypertrophy of the subsynovial layers with hyperplasia of vascular endothelium and compaction of collagen. A nonspecific infiltrate of mononuclear cells is seen, but there are no aggregations of round cells. Plasma cells are absent. Fibrin is present on the synovial surface. (From Petty et al.,[79] with permission.)

also reported IgG2 subclass deficiency in SLE.[96] Heiner et al. mention that they found low IgG4 levels (<30 mg/L) in 12 of 112 patients with "disseminated collagen vascular disease" but provide no further details.[97]

REFERENCES

1. Janeway CA, Gitlin D, Craig JM et al: "Collagen disease" in patients with congenital agammaglobulinemia. Trans Assoc Am Physicians 69:93, 1956
2. Roitt I, Brostoff J, Male D: Immunology. CV Mosby, St Louis, 1985, p. 1.1
3. Wolfson JJ, Kane WJ, Laxdal SD et al: Bone findings in chronic granulomatous disease of childhood. A genetic abnormality of leukocyte function. J Bone Joint Surg 51A:1573, 1969
4. Baehner RL, Nathan DG: Quantitative nitroblue tetrazolium test in chronic granulomatous disease. N Engl J Med 278:971, 1968
5. Johnston RB, Keele BB, Misra HP et al: The role of superoxide anion generation in phagocytic bactericidal activity. Studies with normal and chronic granulomatous disease leukocytes. J Clin Invest 55:1357, 1975
6. Holmes B, Quie PG, Windhorst DB et al: Fatal granulomatous disease of childhood. An inborn abnormality of phagocytic function. Lancet 1:1225, 1966
7. Kaplan EL, Laxdal T, Quie PG: Studies of polymorphonuclear leukocytes from patients with chronic granulomatous disease of childhood. Bactericidal capacity for streptococci. Pediatrics 41:591, 1968
8. Schaller J: Illness resembling lupus erythematosus in mothers of boys with chronic granulomatous disease. Ann Intern Med 76:747, 1972
9. MacFarlane PS, Speirs AL, Sommerville RG: Fatal granulomatous disease in childhood and benign lymphocytic infiltration of the skin (congenital dysphagocytosis). Lancet 1:408, 1967
10. Thompson EN, Soothill JF: Chronic granulomatous disease: quantitative clinicopathological relationships. Arch Dis Child 45:24, 1970
11. Barton LL, Johnson CR: Discoid lupus erythematosus and X-linked chronic granulomatous disease. Pediatr Dermatol 3:376, 1986
12. Landing BH, Shirkey HS: A syndrome of recurrent

infection and infiltration of viscera by pigmented lipid histiocytes. Pediatrics 20:431, 1957

13. Douglas SD, Davis WC, Fudenberg HH: Granulocytopathies: pleomorphism of neutrophil dysfunction. Am J Med 46:901, 1969
14. Humbert JR, Fishman CB, Weston WL et al: Frequency of the carrier state for X-linked chronic granulomatous disease among females with lupus erythematosus. Clin Genet 10:16, 1976
15. Finlay AY, Kingston HM, Holt PJA: Chronic granulomatous disease carrier geno-dermatosis (CGDCGD). Clin Genet 23:276, 1983
16. Kragballe K, Borregaard N, Brandrup F et al: Relation of monocyte and neutrophil oxidative metabolism to skin and oral lesions in carriers of chronic granulomatous disease. Clin Exp Immunol 43:390, 1981
17. Ford DK, Price GE, Culling CFA et al: Familial lipochrome pigmentation of histiocytes with hyperglobulinemia, pulmonary infiltration, splenomegaly, arthritis and susceptibility to infection. Am J Med 33:478, 1962
18. Rodey GE, Park BH, Ford DK et al: Defective bactericidal activity of peripheral blood leukocytes in lipochrome histiocytosis. Am J Med 49:322, 1970
19. Davis SD, Schaller JG, Wedgwood RJ: Job's syndrome. Recurrent "cold" staphylococcal abscesses. Lancet 1:1013, 1966
20. Jacobs JC, Goetzl EJ: "Streaking Leukocyte Factor," arthritis, and pyoderma gangrenosum. Pediatrics 56:570, 1975
21. Windhorst DB, Zellickson AS, Good RA: Chédiak-Higashi syndrome—hereditary gigantism of cytoplasmic organelles. Science 151:81, 1966
22. Windhorst DB, White JG, Dent PB et al: The Chédiak-Higashi anomaly and the aleutian trait in mink. Ann NY Acad Sci 155:818, 1968
23. Ross SC, Densen P: Complement deficiency states and infection. Epidemiology, pathogenesis and consequences of neisserial and other infections in an immune deficiency. Medicine 63:243, 1984
24. Agnello V: Lupus diseases associated with hereditary and acquired deficiencies of complement. Springer Semin Immunopathol 9:161, 1986
25. Fries LF, O'Shea JJ, Frank MM: Inherited deficiencies of complement and complement-related proteins. Clin Immunol Immunopathol 40:37, 1986
26. Glass D, Raum D, Gibson D et al: Inherited deficiency of the second component of complement. Rheumatic disease associations. J Clin Invest 58:853, 1976
27. Rosenfield GB, Partridge REH, Bartholomew W et al: Hereditary angioneurotic edema (HANE) and systemic lupus erythematosus (SLE) in one of identical twin girls. J Allergy Clin Immunol 53:68, 1974
28. Donaldson VH, Hess EV, McAdams AJ: Lupus erythematosus-like disease in three unrelated women with hereditary angioneurotic edema. Ann Intern Med 86:312, 1977
29. Amman AJ, Hong R: Disorders of the T-cell system. In Stiehm ER, Fulginiti VA (eds): Immunologic Disorders in Infants and Children. WB Saunders, Philadelphia, 1980, p. 291
30. Tubergen DG: Thymus transplant in lymphopenic immune deficiency (Nezelof's syndrome). J Pediatr 85:915, 1974
31. Perry GS, Spector BD, Schuman LM et al: The Wiskott-Aldrich syndrome in the United States and Canada (1892–1979). J Pediatr 7:72, 1980
32. Schaller JG: Immunodeficiency and autoimmunity. In Bergsma D (ed): Immunodeficiency in man and animals. Birth Defects 11:1975, 173
33. Cooper MD, Chase HP, Lowman JT et al: Wiskott-Aldrich syndrome: an immunologic deficiency disease involving the afferent limb of immunity. Am J Med 44:499, 1968
34. Wolff JA: Wiskott-Aldrich syndrome: clinical, immunologic, and pathologic observations. J Pediatr 70:221, 1967
35. Gatti RA, Platt N, Pomerance HH et al: Hereditary lymphopenic agammaglobulinemia associated with a distinctive form of short-limbed dwarfism and ectodermal dysplasia. J Pediatr 75:675, 1969
36. Adler E, Gehrmann G: Blutkrankheiten nach thymus-tumor-extirpation. Dtsch Med Wochenschr 92:423, 1907
37. Giblett ER, Anderson JE, Cohen F et al: Adenosine-deaminase deficiency in two patients with severely impaired cellular immunity. Lancet 2:1067, 1972
38. Giblett ER, Ammann AJ, Wara DW et al: Nucleoside phosphorylase deficiency in a child with severely defective T cell immunity and normal B cell immunity. Lancet 1:1010, 1975
39. Oen K, Petty RE, Schroeder ML: Immunoglobulin A deficiency: genetic studies. Tissue Antigens 19:174, 1982
40. Waldman TA, Broder S, Krakauer R et al: Defect in IgA secretion and in IgA specific suppressor cells in patients with selective IgA deficiency. Trans Assoc Am Physicians 88:215, 1976
41. Cassidy JT, Oldham G, Platts-Mills TAE: Functional assessment of a B-cell defect in patients with selective IgA deficiency. Clin Exp Immunol 35:296, 1979
42. Petty RE, Sherry DD, Johannson J: Anti-IgA antibodies in pregnancy. N Engl J Med 313:1620, 1985
43. Pelkonen P, Savilahti E, Westeren L et al: IgA deficiency in juvenile rheumatoid arthritis. Scand J Rheumatol, suppl., 8:4, 1975

44. Barkely DO, Hohermuth HJ, Howard A et al: IgA deficiency in juvenile chronic polyarthritis. J Rheumatol 6:219, 1979

45. van Riel PLCM, van de Putte LBA, Gribnau FWJ et al: IgA deficiency during aurothioglucose treatment. Scand J Rheumatol 13:334, 1984

46. Stanworth DR, Johns P, Williamson N et al: Drug-induced IgA deficiency in rheumatoid arthritis. Lancet 1:1001, 1977

47. Farr M, Struthers GR, Scott DGI et al: Fenclofenac-induced selective IgA deficiency in rheumatoid arthritis. Br J Rheumatol 24:367, 1985

48. Delamere JP, Farr M, Grindulis KA: Sulphasalazine induced selective IgA deficiency in rheumatoid arthritis. Br Med J 286:1547, 1983

49. Sarilahti E: Sulphasalazine induced immunodeficiency. Br Med J 287:759, 1983

50. Leickly FE, Buckley RH: Development of IgA and IgG2 subclass deficiency after sulfasalazine therapy. J Pediatr 108:481, 1986

51. Cassidy JT, Petty RE, Sullivan DB: Occurrence of selective IgA deficiency in children with juvenile rheumatoid arthritis. Arthritis Rheum, suppl., 20:224, 1977

52. Petty RE, Cassidy JT, Sullivan DB: Reversal of selective IgA deficiency following plasma transfusions in juvenile rheumatoid arthritis. Pediatrics 51:44, 1973

53. Panush RS, Bianco NE, Schur PH et al: Juvenile rheumatoid arthritis. Cellular hypersensitivity and selective IgA deficiency. Clin Exp Immunol 10:103, 1972

54. Cassidy JT, Petty RE, Sullivan DB: Abnormalities in the distribution of serum immunoglobulin concentrations in juvenile rheumatoid arthritis. J Clin Invest 52:1931, 1973

55. Huntley CC, Thorpe DP, Lyerly AD et al: Rheumatoid arthritis with IgA deficiency. Am J Dis Child 113:411, 1967

56. Ammann AJ, Hong R: Selective IgA deficiency: presentation of 30 cases and a review of the literature. Medicine (Baltimore) 50:223, 1971

57. Bachmann R, Laurell C-B, Svenonuis E: Studies on the serum gamma 1A-globulin level. II: Gamma 1A-deficiency in a case of systemic lupus erythematosus. Scand J Clin Lab Invest 17:46, 1965

58. Cassidy JT, Burt A, Petty RE et al: Prevalence of selective IgA deficiency in patients with connective tissue disease. N Engl J Med 280:275, 1969

59. Petty RE, Palmer NR, Cassidy JT et al: The association of autoimmune diseases and anti-IgA antibodies in patients with selective IgA deficiency. Clin Exp Immunol 37:83, 1979

60. Petty RE, Haddow M, Oen K et al: Antibodies to nucleic acid antigens in selective IgA deficiency. Clin Immunol Immunopathol 13:182, 1979

61. Claman HN, Merrill DA, Peakman D et al: Isolated severe gamma A deficiency: immunoglobulin levels, clinical disorders and chromosome studies. J Lab Clin Med 75:307, 1970

62. Cleland LG, Bell DA: The occurrence of systemic lupus erythematosus in two kindreds in association with selective IgA deficiency. J Rheumatol 5:3, 1978

63. Cassidy JT: Selective IgA deficiency and chronic arthritis in children. In Moore TD (ed): Arthritis in Childhood. Report of the Eightieth Ross Conference in Pediatric Research, 1981, p. 82

64. Jay S, Helm S, Wray BB: Progressive systemic scleroderma with IgA deficiency in a child. Am J Dis Child 135:965, 1981

65. Spirer Z, Ilie I, Pick A et al: Localized scleroderma following varicella in a 3-year-old girl with IgA deficiency. Acta Paediatr Scand 68:783, 1979

66. Good AE, Cassidy JT, Mutchnick MG et al: Ankylosing spondylitis with selective IgA deficiency and a circulating anticoagulant. J Rheumatol 4:297, 1977

67. Siegler D: Sarcoidosis and selective IgA deficiency. Br J Dis Chest 72:143, 1978

68. Thomas LLM, Alberts C, Pegels JG et al: Sarcoidosis associated with autoimmune thrombocytopenia and selective IgA deficiency. Scand J Haematol 28:357, 1982

69. Gershwin ME, Blaese RM, Steinberg AD et al: Antibodies to nucleic acids in congenital immune deficiency states. J Pediatr 89:377, 1976

70. Petty RE, Sherry DD, Johannson J: IgG anti-IgA1 and anti-IgA2 antibodies: their measurement by an enzyme-linked immunosorbent assay and their relationship to disease. Int Arch Allergy Appl Immunol 80:337, 1986

71. Rivat L, Rivat C, Daveau M et al: Comparative frequencies of anti-IgA antibodies among patients with anaphylactic transfusion reactions and among normal blood donors. Clin Immunol Immunopathol 7:340, 1977

72. Warrington RJ, Rutherford WJ, Sauder PJ et al: Homologous antibody to human immunoglobulin IgA suppresses in vitro mitogen-induced IgA synthesis. Clin Immunol Immunopathol 23:698, 1982

73. Edwards NL, Magilavy DB, Cassidy JT et al: Lymphocyte ecto-5'-nucleotidase deficiency in agammaglobulinemia. Science 201:628, 1978

74. Petty RE, Malleson P, Kalousek DK: Chronic arthritis in two children with partial deletion of chromosome 18. J Rheumatol 14:586, 1987

75. Good RA, Rotstein J: Rheumatoid arthritis and agammaglobulinemia Bull Rheum Dis 10:203, 1960

76. Lawrence JS, Bremner JM: Arthritis and hypogammaglobulinaemia. Scand J Rheumatol 5:17, 1976

77. Webster ADB, Loewi G, Dourmashkin RD et al: Polyarthritis in adults with hypogammaglobulinaemia and its rapid response to immunoglobulin treatment. Br Med J 1:1314, 1976

78. Schaller JG: Arthritis and immunodeficiency. Arthritis Rheum, suppl., 20:443, 1977

79. Petty RE, Cassidy JT, Tubergen DG: Association of arthritis with hypogammaglobulinemia. Arthritis Rheum, suppl., 20:441, 1977

80. Cassidy JT, Magilavy DB, Petty RE et al: The frequency of chronic arthritis in patients with hypogammaglobulinemia. In Munthe E (ed): The Care of Rheumatic Children. EULAR, Basel, 1977, p. 149

81. Lederman HM, Winkelstein A: X-linked agammaglobulinemia: an analysis of 96 patients. Medicine 64:145, 1985

82. Stuckey M, Quinn PA, Gelfand EW: Identification of *Ureaplasma urealyticum* (T-strain mycoplasma) in a patient with polyarthritis. Lancet 2:917, 1978

83. Webster ADB, Taylor-Robinson D, Furr PM et al: Mycoplasmal (ureaplasma) septic arthritis in hypogammaglobulinaemia. Br Med J 1:478, 1978

84. Vogler LB, Waites KB, Wright PF et al: *Ureaplasma urealyticum* polyarthritis in agammaglobulinemia. Pediatr Infect Dis 4:687, 1985

85. Good RA, Rotstein J, Mazzitello WF: The simultaneous occurrence of rheumatoid arthritis and agammaglobulinemia. J Lab Clin Med 49:343, 1957

86. Page AR, Hansen AE, Good RA: Occurrence of leukemia and lymphoma in patients with agammaglobulinemia. Blood 21:197, 1963

87. Rosen FS, Kevy SV, Janeway CA: The antibody deficiency syndromes. In Janeway CA, Rosen FS, Merler E et al (eds): The Gamma Globulins. Little Brown, Boston, 1967, p. 75

88. Gotoff SP, Smith RD, Sugar O: Dermatomyositis with cerebral vasculitis in a patient with agammaglobulinemia. Am J Dis Child 123:53, 1972

89. Bardelas JA, Winkelstein JA, Seto DS et al: Fatal ECHO 24 infection in a patient with hypogammaglobulinemia. Relationship to dermatomyositis-like syndrome. J Pediatr 90:396, 1977

90. Wilfert CM, Buckley RH, Mahanakumar T et al: Persistent and fatal central-nervous-system ECHO-virus infections in patients with agammaglobulinemia. N Engl J Med 296:1485, 1977

91. Webster AD, Tripp JH, Hayward AR et al: Echovirus encephalitis and myositis in primary immunoglobulin deficiency. Arch Dis Child 53:33, 1978

92. Maguire JF, Perez-Atayde AR, Geha RS: Vasculitis presenting in an infant with agammaglobulinemia. Ann Allergy 57:14, 1986

93. Crennan JM, Van Scoy RE, McKenna CH et al: Echovirus polymyositis in patients with hypogammaglobulinemia. Am J Med 81:35, 1986

94. Mease PJ, Ochs HD, Wedgwood RJ: Successful treatment of echovirus meningoencephalitis and myositis-fasciitis with intravenous immune globulin therapy in a patient with X-linked agammaglobulinemia. N Engl J Med 304:1278, 1984

95. Cunningham-Rundles C: Antibodies to phosphorylcholine in sera of patients with humoral immunodeficiency disease. Monogr Allergy 20:42, 1985

96. Oxelius VA: IgG subclasses and human disease. Am J Med 76:7, 1984

97. Heiner DC, Lee SI, Short JA: IgG4 subclass deficiency syndromes. Monogr Allergy 20:149, 1986

12

Arthritis Related to Infection

The relationship of infectious agents to the etiology of arthritis is an area of intense investigation. Important discoveries have led to the understanding of the etiology, pathogenesis, treatment, and cure of at least one infection-related arthritis (Lyme disease) and have given impetus to investigations of other possible arthritogenic infectious agents in childhood rheumatic diseases. Recovery of viruses such as rubella and parvovirus from synovial fluid of patients with chronic arthritis has strengthened the argument that such agents may have an etiologic role in diseases such as JRA.

CLASSIFICATION AND DEFINITIONS

Arthritis related to infection can be regarded as either septic, postinfectious, or reactive (Table 12-1). *Septic arthritis* occurs when a viable infectious agent is present or has been present in the joint space. Although direct bacterial infection of the joint space constitutes the most widely recognized form of septic arthritis, direct infection with viruses, *Borrelia*, or fungi also constitute forms of septic arthritis. *Postinfectious arthritis* may be considered to be a special type of reactive arthritis in which immune complexes containing nonviable components of the initiating infectious agent may be present in the inflamed joint. *Reactive arthritis* is a response to an infectious agent that is or has been present in some other part of the body, usually the upper airway, the gastrointestinal tract, or the genitourinary tract. By definition, infectious agents are not recoverable from the joint space in patients with reactive arthritis, which may be regarded as an autoimmune disorder resulting from immunologic cross-reactivity between articular and infectious antigens. The reactive arthritis group merges with diseases such as the seronegative spondyloarthropathies (Reiter's syndrome and possibly ankylosing spondylitis).

The relationship of infection to arthritis is complex and by no means completely understood. As techniques for the demonstration of infectious organisms improve, the frequency with which they are detected in the synovial fluid or membrane is increasing, thus lending authority to the suspicion that many of the arthritides of children are related to infectious diseases. It is, for the same reasons, difficult to categorize a disease as being postinfectious as opposed to reactive; perhaps many of the so-called reactive arthritides will be found to represent disease in which the pathogens are actually present in the joint and are, by definition, septic. In some of the viral arthritides that fit the concept of "reactive" arthritis, in that the joint disease follows the onset of the acute illness by days or weeks, virus antigen or living virus can be isolated from joint fluid, joint fluid lymphocytes, or synovial membrane when appropriate techniques are used. The same has been true for Lyme disease, in which

489

Table 12-1 Classification of Infection-Related Arthritis

Septic arthritis
    Bacterial septic arthritis, with or without
        osteomyelitis
    Viral septic arthritis
    Fungal septic arthritis
    Spirochetal septic arthritis

Postinfectious arthritis
    Arthritis associated with intestinal bypass surgery
    Musculoskeletal manifestations of systemic
        bacterial infections

Reactive arthritis
    Acute rheumatic fever
    Postdysenteric arthropathies
    Mycoplasma and arthritis

early attempts to demonstrate *Borrelia* were unsuccessful, although the organisms have now been demonstrated by silver stain in several different laboratories. The lesson implicit in all of these observations is that in chronic arthritides that we currently consider to be aseptic, concerted investigation for infectious agents, using the most powerful tools of molecular biology, may yet demonstrate the causative agent in the joint space.

Although the study of infectious agents such as viruses as possible initiators of some forms of arthritis in children has attracted much of the attention, it is important to remember that bacterial infections, both intra-articular and systemic, remain the most important curable cause of arthritis in childhood.

SEPTIC ARTHRITIS

Epidemiology

Septic arthritis of bacterial origin accounts for approximately 6.5 percent of all childhood arthritis.[1] It has been suggested that the frequency of septic arthritis may actually be increasing.[2]

SEX RATIO AND AGE AT ONSET

Septic arthritis is slightly less common in girls than in boys, who account for 55 to 62 percent of patients in reported series.[3-5] Septic arthritis is most common in the very young and the very old. The disease may

occur in the neonate, is most common in children under the age of 2 years, and diminishes in frequency throughout childhood (Table 12-2).

FAMILIALITY AND GEOGRAPHIC CLUSTERING OF CASES

There does not appear to be a genetic predisposition to bacterial septic arthritis. Cases in which no pathogen is identified tend to occur in the summer and fall months,[2] but geographic clustering has not been reported. In spirochetal septic arthritis, such as Lyme disease, there are marked geographic and seasonal outbreaks (discussed later).

PREDISPOSING FACTORS

Although preceding events are frequently noted, their significance is unknown. In one series,[2] upper respiratory tract infections preceded arthritis in approximately 50 percent of patients, and approximately one-third had received antibiotics within a week of onset of septic arthritis. A history of a mild nonpenetrating injury to the affected extremity was elicited in approximately one-third of patients. Intravenous drug users are at particular risk of septic arthritis of the sacroiliac and sternoclavicular joints, usually caused by gram-negative organisms (*Pseudomonas aeruginosa, Klebsiella, Enterobacter,* and *Serratia* species).[6] Chronic inflammatory arthritis such as juvenile rheumatoid arthritis may predispose to joint infection.[7]

Clinical Characteristics

Septic arthritis is usually accompanied by systemic signs (fever, vomiting, and headache) and may be a component of a more generalized infection including meningitis, cellulitis, osteomyelitis, or pharyngitis. Joint pain is usually severe, and the infected joint and periarticular tissues are swollen, hot, and sometimes

Table 12-2 Age of Occurrence of Bacterial Septic Arthritis

Age	2 yr	2–5 yr	6–10 yr	11–15 yr
N	341	167	109	60
% of total	50.3	24.7	16.1	8.9

(Data from Speiser et al.[5] and Fink and Nelson.[8])

Table 12-3 Extra-Articular Sites of Infection in Children with Septic Arthritis (%)

	Speiser[5] (n = 86)	Welkon[2] (n = 95)	Nelson and Koontz[3] (n = 117)
Osteomyelitis	26	12	12
Meningitis	11	4	4
Cellulitis, abscess	9		
Respiratory tract	9		19
Middle ear	3	20	
Urine	1		
Genital tract	1		4
Pericardium	1		
Pleura	1		

red. Passive and active motion of the joint is severely, often completely, restricted. Osteomyelitis frequently accompanies septic arthritis, and the presence of bone pain (as opposed to joint pain) should alert the examiner to this possibility. Other sites of infection, although less frequent, are nonetheless important (Table 12-3).

AFFECTED JOINTS

The joints of the lower extremity are most commonly infected. The knees, hips, ankles, and elbows account for 90 percent of infected joints. Septic arthritis affecting small joints of the hands or feet is rare (Table 12-4).

MULTIPLE INFECTED JOINTS

Although septic arthritis is most frequently a monarthritis, two or more joints may be infected simultaneously or during the course of the same illness. In

the large experience reported by Fink and Nelson,[8] septic arthritis was monarticular in 93.4 percent, it affected two joints in 4.4 percent, three joints in 1.7 percent, and four joints in 0.5 percent. Certain immune deficiencies such as chronic granulomatous disease may predispose to multiple joint septic arthritis.

Etiology and Pathogenesis

ORGANISMS INVOLVED

The organisms most commonly isolated from children with septic arthritis are *Hemophilus influenzae* and *Staphylococcus aureus*. There are, however, considerable interinstitutional variations in the relative frequencies with which certain pathogens are identified and, more importantly, a strong relationship to the age of the patient. *H. influenzae* type B is the most common organism identified in children under the age of 2 years; after 2 years of age, *S. aureus* becomes the most common organism. Over the age of 10

Table 12-4 Frequencies (%) of Infected Joints in Septic Arthritis

	Speiser[5] (n = 86)	Welkon[2] (n = 95)	Fink and Nelson[8] (n = 646)	Wilson and Di Paola[4] (n = 65)	Overall (n = 892)
Knee	30	46	40	29	39
Hip	29	25	23	40	25
Ankle	17	15	13	21	14
Elbow	11	5	14	3	12
Shoulder	2	4	4	3	4
Wrist	1		4	1	3
PIP, MCP, MTP	10		1		2
Other		5	1	1	1

PIP, proximal interphalangeal; MCP, metacarpophalangeal; MTP, metatarsophalangeal.

years, *H. influenzae* is rarely a cause of septic arthritis. Streptococci (groups A and B and *Streptococcus viridans*) account for a small proportion of all cases of septic arthritis in childhood and are most prevalent in the 6- to 10-year age group. *Neisseria gonorrheae* is rare in infancy but accounts for 10 percent of septic arthritis in patients in the over-10-year age group. The neonate presents a somewhat different bacteriologic picture with the majority of infants less than 1 month of age having *S. aureus* (40 to 50 percent) or *Streptococcus* (20 to 25 percent) as the causative organisms.[5,8,9] There appears to be a discrepancy between neonates with hospital-acquired infection, among whom *S. aureus* predominates, and those with community-acquired infection, among whom streptococci are most common.[9] Gram-negative organisms and *Candida* species are also significant pathogens in the neonate.

PATHOGENESIS

Septic arthritis usually arises from hematogenous spread from a focus of infection elsewhere. Direct extension of an infection from overlying soft tissue (cellulitis, abscess), bone (osteomyelitis), or traumatic invasion of the joint accounts for 15 to 20 percent of cases. The proliferation of bacteria in the synovial membrane results in accumulation of polymorphonuclear leukocytes with the inflammatory effects outlined in Ch. 2. The resulting damage to the cartilaginous surfaces of the bone and the supporting structures of the joint may be severe and permanent if treatment is not urgently initiated.

Diagnostic Procedures

It is essential that every child with an acute monarthritis have the affected joint aspirated immediately, if necessary with fluoroscopic guidance. The fluid should be examined by Gram stain, have a total white blood cell (WBC) count and differential performed, and be cultured. Synovial fluid should be aspirated under sterile conditions and immediately cultured on sheep's blood chocolate agar (for *H. influenzae* and *N. gonorrhoeae*) and MacConkey's agar (for gram-negative organisms). If an anaerobic organism is suspected, enriched medium and special anaerobic conditions are necessary. Culture for *Mycobacterium* formerly required guinea pig inoculation but is now

performed in vitro. Children in whom septic arthritis is considered should also have cultures of blood and of any potential source of infection (cellulitis, abscess, cerebrospinal fluid). In a group of children with septic arthritis in whom the bacterial agent was identified, Fink and Nelson[8] reported that the joint fluid was culture-positive in 307 of 389 patients (79 percent). The remaining 21 percent had positive culture findings from sites other than the joint: blood only (10 percent), CSF only (3.8 percent), blood and CSF (2.3 percent), vaginal culture (1.3 percent). Thus one in five children with culture-positive septic arthritis has negative synovial fluid culture results but a positive culture result elsewhere, most frequently from the blood. Although by culturing all appropriate sites, an organism can be identified in two-thirds or more of patients, there remain approximately one-third of children with septic arthritis in whom no causative organisms are ever identified. In these patients, the diagnosis of septic arthritis is made on the basis of a typical history and the demonstration of frank pus by arthrocentesis.

SYNOVIAL FLUID ANALYSIS

The characteristics of the synovial fluid depend to some extent on the duration and severity of the disease and the previous administration of antibiotics. Synovial fluid may appear normal, turbid, or grayish green with bloody streaks. The synovial fluid WBC count is frequently markedly elevated with 90 percent polymorphs. Speiser et al.[5] reported that synovial WBC count in septic arthritis was $<50,000/mm^3$ in 15 percent, between 50,000 and $100,000/mm^3$ in 34 percent, and in excess of $100,000/mm^3$ in 51 percent of children. Fink and Nelson noted a relatively low WBC count ($<25,000/mm^3$) in one-third of their patients.[8] The protein content is high (>1 g/dl) and the glucose concentration is usually low, although it may be normal. A Gram stain has a positive result in half of the untreated patients, but in only one-fifth of those who have received antibiotics. The advantage of the Gram stain is that if the findings are positive, it provides rapid confirmation of infection and tentative identification of the organism, thus permitting rational antibiotic therapy. Procedures such as counterimmunoelectrophoresis or latex agglutination may identify antigen in an occasional culture-negative fluid. These techniques have the advantage of pro-

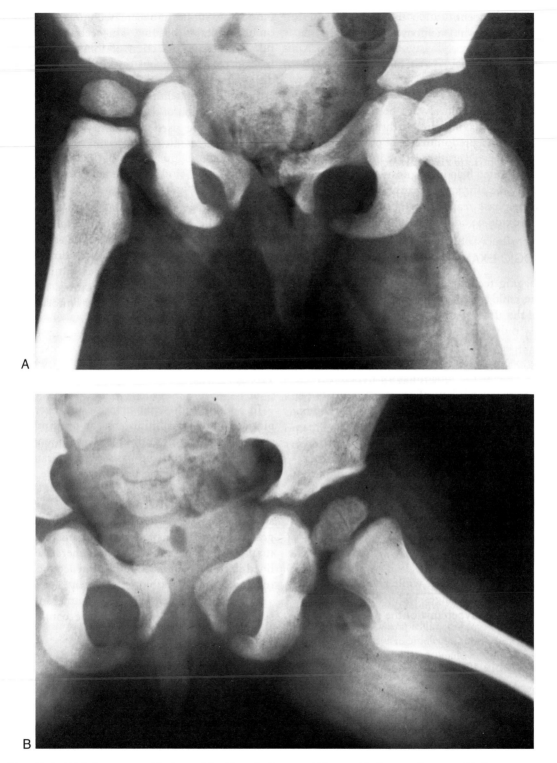

Fig. 12-1 (**A**) Joint space widening of the hip of a 2-year-old boy with fever and an irritable hip. (**B**) Repeat film taken after a delay shows subluxation and epiphyseal demineralization and irregularity.

readily leads to septic arthritis of the hip joint in the infant, since blood vessels pass between the metaphysis, through the intracapsular growth plate, and into the epiphysis. Septic arthritis of the hip joint occurs most commonly in infants and very young children, 70 percent of children being 4 years of age or younger.[15] The typical clinical picture is that of an infant or young child who has a fever, is irritable, and refuses to bear weight or walk (pseudoparalysis). Any movement of the hip is extremely painful, and the affected hip is held in a position of flexion, abduction, and external rotation. Occasionally the child has abdominal pain or tenderness in the lower abdomen, sometimes with paralytic ileus. There are often predisposing factors, particularly in very young or premature infants.[16] In a recent study of 16 children under 4 weeks of age, 11 were premature, 7 had an umbilical catheter, and 12 had septicemia. In the group aged 1 month to 3 years (13 patients), none was premature or had an umbilical catheter and only 5 had septicemia.[16] The association of septic arthritis of the hip with femoral venipuncture has been recorded[17] and may account in part for the high incidence of arthritis of this site in the premature and neonate. A high frequency of preceding or accompanying osteomyelitis of femur or pelvis has also been noted.[15]

Management of septic arthritis of the hip requires open drainage in order to minimize intra-articular pressure. Traction and immobilization for the first 2 to 3 days of treatment provide pain relief but should be followed by active and passive physiotherapy to prevent loss of range of motion. The prognosis is guarded even with the best treatment.

The anatomy of the shoulder joint is not unlike that of the hip joint with respect to vascular supply, and septic arthritis of this joint, although rare, should be treated in a similar manner.

GONOCOCCAL ARTHRITIS

Arthritis caused by *Neisseria gonorrheae* occurs most commonly in the adolescent age group, although it is occasionally seen in the neonate in association with disseminated infection.[18] It is more common in girls than in boys and is particularly likely to occur just after menstruation or with pregnancy.[19] Gonococcal arthritis usually develops in patients with primary asymptomatic genitourinary gonorrhea or with a gonococcal infection of the throat or rectum. The patient usually has a systemic illness characterized by fever and chills. A vesiculopustular rash, sparsely distributed on the extremities, commonly yields organisms on culture or Gram stain of the smear. In contrast to most patients with septic arthritis, those with gonococcal arthritis may have a purulent arthritis of several joints. In the patient with suspected gonococcal arthritis, it is important to culture the genital tract, throat, and rectum, and any vesicles, as well as the affected joint. The possibility of sexual abuse should be considered and appropriately investigated.

TUBERCULOUS ARTHRITIS

Tuberculous arthritis is seldom encountered in North America or Europe, although it is by no means a rare disease in other parts of the world. Typically, tuberculous arthritis presents as an indolent monarthritis, often of the knee or wrist, accompanying pulmonary tuberculosis and resulting in destruction of joint and surrounding bones. Tuberculous dactylitis (Fig. 12-2) with cystic expansion and destruction of bone (spina ventosa) may occur. A family or environmental history of pulmonary tuberculosis, together with a positive Mantoux skin test should suggest the possibility of tuberculous arthritis. Although synovial fluid cultures are positive in approximately three-quarters of cases, synovial membrane biopsy and culture will reveal the diagnosis in almost all patients. Synovial fluid analysis shows a WBC count of $<50,000/mm^3$ with a high proportion of mononuclear cells. Rarely, polyarthritis accompanies tuberculosis (Poncet's disease),[20] and probably represents a reactive arthritis since culture of the inflamed joints fails to demonstrate tubercle bacilli.

ARTHRITIS ASSOCIATED WITH BRUCELLOSIS

Human *Brucella* infections are uncommon in North America, but there are reports of substantial numbers of patients with this infection complicated by arthritis from Europe[21] and South America.[22,23] The species most frequently implicated are *B. melitensis*[21-23] and rarely *B. canis*.[24]

The systemic illness is often mild in children but is usually characterized by undulant fever, gastrointestinal complaints, lymphadenopathy, and some-

minimum of 21 days.[11] Providing the child's clinical state is improving (temperature returning to normal, pain diminishing, and range restriction returning to normal), and the WBC count and erythrocyte sedimentation rate are falling, the initial antibiotics should be maintained. If the patient does not appear to be responding, however, additional antibiotic coverage should be instituted intravenously.

When an organism is identified, the treatment outlined in Table 12-6 is currently suggested. Recommendations regarding antibiotic choice and duration of treatment are constantly changing, and the physician is urged to review the most current recommendations.

ASPIRATION AND DRAINAGE

The usefulness of repeated aspiration and drainage of infected joints has been hotly debated. There is no dispute that a diagnostic arthrocentesis must be performed. Indeed, any joint that appears to be under a great deal of pressure would probably benefit from aspiration, even if only from the point of view of pain relief. Studies of the importance of repeated aspirations under other circumstances, however, have failed to show a benefit. Similarly, open drainage is not better than closed needle aspiration and is attended by significantly increased morbidity. Irriga-

tion of the joint has no demonstrated benefit. Intra-articular administration of antibiotic is unnecessary since therapeutic synovial fluid antibiotic levels are readily achieved[12] and may actually induce a chemical synovitis in the infected joint.[13,14]

Prognosis

The prognosis in septic arthritis is somewhat guarded, since even with early appropriate antibiotic treatment, permanent damage to the joint is common. The child almost always recovers from the acute illness, but with the passage of time, reduction of range of motion, pain, and, eventually, degeneration of the surfaces of the affected joint may necessitate surgical intervention.

Special Cases

THE HIP

Septic arthritis of the hip is such an important problem that it merits special attention. The femoral head is intracapsular, and the arterial supply passes via the ligamentum teres through the intracapsular space. Increased intracapsular pressure, therefore, can interrupt the blood supply to the femoral head with disastrous consequences. Metaphyseal osteomyelitis

Table 12-6 Antibiotic Recommendations for Treatment of Septic Arthritis in Children

Organism	Management
None	IV antibiotic selected on the basis of the age of the patient (Table 12-5) for 7 days, oral antibiotic can be used for a further 21–28 days under closely monitored conditions with bactericidal blood titer determinations at frequent intervals to confirm compliance.
Staphylococcus aureus	IV nafcillin, 100 mg/kg/day, in divided doses until clinical response, then cloxacillin, 100 mg/kg/day, in divided doses for 21 days by mouth; bactericidal titer should be 1:8 or greater.
Hemophilus influenzae	IV cefuroxime, 100 mg/kg/day, in divided doses, or IV ampicillin, 150 mg/kg/day, or chloramphenicol, 75 mg/kg/day, if the organism is resistant to ampicillin, until clinical response, then appropriate drug for 14 days by mouth; bactericidal level should be 1:8 or greater.
Streptococcus	IV penicillin, 150,000 U/kg/day, every 4–6 h until clinical response, followed by penicillin V, 100 mg/kg/day, by mouth, for 14 days; bactericidal level should be 1:32 or greater.
Coliforms	IV gentamicin, 6 mg/kg/day, in divided doses in children; 7.5 mg/kg/day in divided doses in infants; ampicillin, 150 mg/kg/day, in divided doses in children; 75 mg/kg/day in divided doses in infants.
Gonococcus	IV penicillin, 150,000 U/kg/day, for a minimum of 7 days.

For a more comprehensive guide to antibiotic therapy the reader is referred to Nelson JD: Pocketbook of Pediatric Antimicrobial Therapy. 7th Ed. Williams & Wilkins, Baltimore, 1987.

readily leads to septic arthritis of the hip joint in the infant, since blood vessels pass between the metaphysis, through the intracapsular growth plate, and into the epiphysis. Septic arthritis of the hip joint occurs most commonly in infants and very young children, 70 percent of children being 4 years of age or younger.[15] The typical clinical picture is that of an infant or young child who has a fever, is irritable, and refuses to bear weight or walk (pseudoparalysis). Any movement of the hip is extremely painful, and the affected hip is held in a position of flexion, abduction, and external rotation. Occasionally the child has abdominal pain or tenderness in the lower abdomen, sometimes with paralytic ileus. There are often predisposing factors, particularly in very young or premature infants.[16] In a recent study of 16 children under 4 weeks of age, 11 were premature, 7 had an umbilical catheter, and 12 had septicemia. In the group aged 1 month to 3 years (13 patients), none was premature or had an umbilical catheter and only 5 had septicemia.[16] The association of septic arthritis of the hip with femoral venipuncture has been recorded[17] and may account in part for the high incidence of arthritis of this site in the premature and neonate. A high frequency of preceding or accompanying osteomyelitis of femur or pelvis has also been noted.[15]

Management of septic arthritis of the hip requires open drainage in order to minimize intra-articular pressure. Traction and immobilization for the first 2 to 3 days of treatment provide pain relief but should be followed by active and passive physiotherapy to prevent loss of range of motion. The prognosis is guarded even with the best treatment.

The anatomy of the shoulder joint is not unlike that of the hip joint with respect to vascular supply, and septic arthritis of this joint, although rare, should be treated in a similar manner.

GONOCOCCAL ARTHRITIS

Arthritis caused by *Neisseria gonorrheae* occurs most commonly in the adolescent age group, although it is occasionally seen in the neonate in association with disseminated infection.[18] It is more common in girls than in boys and is particularly likely to occur just after menstruation or with pregnancy.[19] Gonococcal arthritis usually develops in patients with primary asymptomatic genitourinary gonorrhea or with a gonococcal infection of the throat or rectum. The patient usually has a systemic illness characterized by fever and chills. A vesiculopustular rash, sparsely distributed on the extremities, commonly yields organisms on culture or Gram stain of the smear. In contrast to most patients with septic arthritis, those with gonococcal arthritis may have a purulent arthritis of several joints. In the patient with suspected gonococcal arthritis, it is important to culture the genital tract, throat, and rectum, and any vesicles, as well as the affected joint. The possibility of sexual abuse should be considered and appropriately investigated.

TUBERCULOUS ARTHRITIS

Tuberculous arthritis is seldom encountered in North America or Europe, although it is by no means a rare disease in other parts of the world. Typically, tuberculous arthritis presents as an indolent monarthritis, often of the knee or wrist, accompanying pulmonary tuberculosis and resulting in destruction of joint and surrounding bones. Tuberculous dactylitis (Fig. 12-2) with cystic expansion and destruction of bone (spina ventosa) may occur. A family or environmental history of pulmonary tuberculosis, together with a positive Mantoux skin test should suggest the possibility of tuberculous arthritis. Although synovial fluid cultures are positive in approximately three-quarters of cases, synovial membrane biopsy and culture will reveal the diagnosis in almost all patients. Synovial fluid analysis shows a WBC count of $<50,000/mm^3$ with a high proportion of mononuclear cells. Rarely, polyarthritis accompanies tuberculosis (Poncet's disease),[20] and probably represents a reactive arthritis since culture of the inflamed joints fails to demonstrate tubercle bacilli.

ARTHRITIS ASSOCIATED WITH BRUCELLOSIS

Human *Brucella* infections are uncommon in North America, but there are reports of substantial numbers of patients with this infection complicated by arthritis from Europe[21] and South America.[22,23] The species most frequently implicated are *B. melitensis*[21-23] and rarely *B. canis*.[24]

The systemic illness is often mild in children but is usually characterized by undulant fever, gastrointestinal complaints, lymphadenopathy, and some-

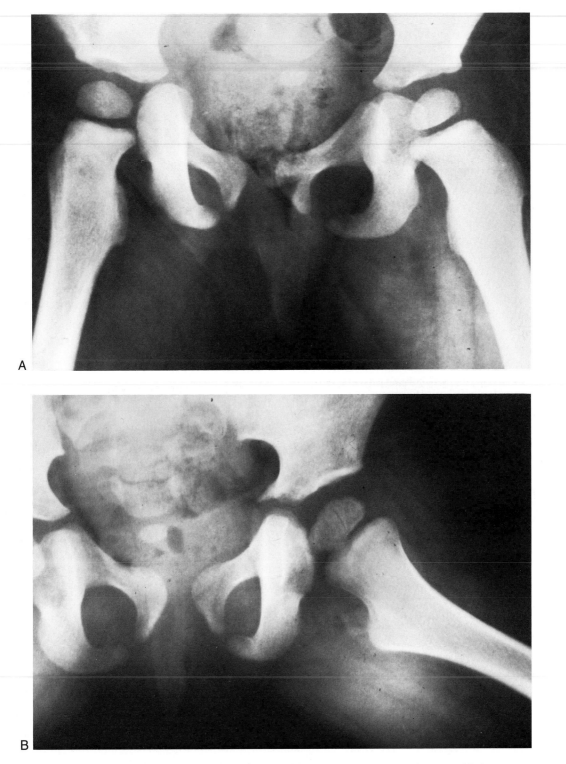

Fig. 12-1 (**A**) Joint space widening of the hip of a 2-year-old boy with fever and an irritable hip. (**B**) Repeat film taken after a delay shows subluxation and epiphyseal demineralization and irregularity.

viding antigenic identification much more rapidly than culture but do not demonstrate antibiotic sensitivities.

BLOOD STUDIES

Blood cultures should always be performed in a child suspected of having septic arthritis. An elevated WBC count with a predominance of polymorphs and bands and an elevated erythrocyte sedimentation rate, although of limited help in diagnosis, provide a baseline whereby the efficacy of treatment can be judged. Other acute phase reactants are usually elevated as well but provide no additional information.

RADIOLOGIC EXAMINATION

Three imaging techniques may be of value in evaluating the child with septic arthritis. A plain radiograph of the affected area early in the disease course may show only increased soft tissue swelling but is occasionally useful in excluding the presence of a foreign body or unsuspected trauma. Juxta-articular osteoporosis reflects the inflammatory hyperemia and occurs within several days of onset of infection. As the disease progresses, cartilage loss and narrowing of the joint space occur. They are followed by marginal erosions and eventually by ankylosis (Fig. 12-1). In the hip joint, traction applied during the radiographic procedure normally induces a radiolucent outline of the femoral head, the vacuum phenomenon. In the presence of increased intra-articular fluid this lucency is not observed.[10]

RADIONUCLIDE SCANS

During the first few days, while plain radiographs show only soft tissue changes, technetium-99m phosphate scans reflect hyperemia of the infected area on blood flow studies and increased uptake of the isotope on both sides of the joint. This technique is very useful in the early detection of joint or bone inflammation or infection but does not provide a certain differentiation between inflammatory and infectious arthritis. Radionuclide scans using isotopes of gallium or administration of the patient's indium-labeled leukocytes can be used to identify accumulations of PMNs in infected sites, including septic arthritis.

ULTRASOUND

The detection by ultrasound of an effusion in the hip of a child being treated for osteomyelitis of the femur indicates the presence of septic arthritis of that joint. Even though the antibiotics administered for osteomyelitis and septic arthritis are similar, the presence of an effusion in the hip joint is of sufficient hazard to the blood supply of the femoral head that open drainage is indicated.

Treatment

ANTIBIOTICS

In a child with septic arthritis, intravenous antibiotics should be administered as promptly as possible. The choice of antibiotic depends on the organisms suspected on the basis of the Gram stain or rapid antigen detection test, the presence of predisposing factors, and the age of the child. If Gram stain and rapid antigen detection tests are negative or not available, an approach outlined in Table 12-5 is suggested. The demonstration of organism or antigen may support or contradict the generalizations outlined in this table and should influence the physician to modify initial antibiotic treatment.

If the culture is negative, intravenous antibiotics as suggested in Table 12-5 should be continued for a

Table 12-5 Initial Therapy of Septic Arthritis Before the Etiologic Agent is Known

Age of the child	Neonate	2–10 years	>10 years
Presumed organisms	*Staphylococcus* *Streptococcus* Coliform	*Hemophilus influenzae* *Staphylococcus*	*Staphylococcus*
Antibiotics	Methicillin (or nafcillin) plus aminoglycoside	Cefuroxime or ampicillin plus methicillin (or nafcillin)	Methicillin (or nafcillin)

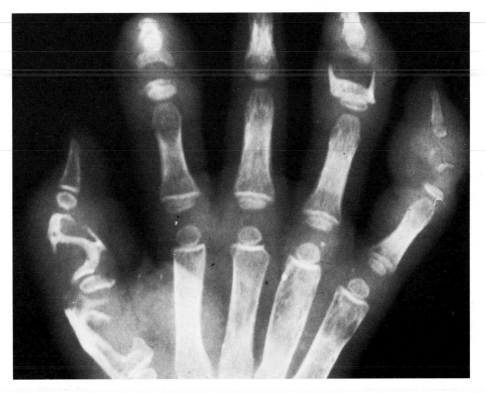

Fig. 12-2 Advanced osseous destruction in a child with tuberculous dactylitis.

times skin rash. In the large series of brucellosis patients from Peru, almost one-third were children and one-third had arthritis. In the under-15-year age group, peripheral arthritis (hip, knee) was most common, with spondylitis and sacroiliitis becoming predominant after 15 years of age. Synovial fluid analysis revealed modest white blood cell counts with a slight predominance of mononuclear cells. Culture results were positive in some patients.[22] Gomez-Reino noted that a periarthritis without effusions was most common, and that small joints and spine were not affected.[21] Whether this reflects differences in the infecting organism or in ascertainment is not known. Trimethoprim-sulfamethoxazole provides effective treatment of the acute infection, although permanent sequelae may result.[21,23]

ARTHRITIS IN IMMUNOINCOMPETENT PATIENTS

The occurrence of chronic inflammatory arthritis in immunodeficient patients is discussed elsewhere. Typical septic arthritis has been rarely reported in immunodeficient children, although there are a number of reports of recovery of *Mycoplasma* species from the synovial fluid of patients with a variety of congenital immunodeficiency syndromes (Ch. 11). *Candida albicans* is occasionally responsible for arthritis in immunosuppressed patients.[25] Patients with SLE are susceptible to septic arthritis; whether that is secondary to their disease or to the treatment is not clear.

Acquired immunodeficiency disease (AIDS) secondary to infection with human immunodeficiency virus I (HIV I) may be complicated by septic arthritis, usually of fungal origin.[26,27]

Related Disorders

DISCITIS

There is considerable dispute as to whether or not discitis is an infectious process. Intervertebral disc space infection secondary to osteomyelitis of the vertebral body is rare.[28] However, acute discitis, unassociated with vertebral osteomyelitis, is a self-limited inflammation of the intervertebral disc that may be caused by pathogens of low virulence although bacteria or viruses are seldom recovered by aspiration of the disc. Discitis occurs throughout childhood, but half of the cases occur before 4 years of age, with the peak age being in the 1- to 3-year group.[29-32] The sex ratios are approximately equal, although one review noted its occurrence more frequently in girls.[33] It is characterized by back pain and stiffness, often resulting in a characteristic tripod position during sitting or other unusual posturing. The child, who almost always has a low-grade fever, usually refuses to walk and may also complain of abdominal pain. Palpation of the spine reveals well localized tenderness, almost always in the lower lumbar region. The L4–5 interspace is most frequently affected (44 percent), followed by L3–4 (37 percent), L2–3 (7 percent), and L5–S1 (6 percent).[29-32]

Aspiration of the disc space or disc biopsy should not be necessary, although plain radiographs of the affected area and a technetium-99m phosphate bone scan are valuable diagnostic tools (Fig. 12-3). The erythrocyte sedimentation rate is usually moderately elevated. Treatment is supportive although if bacterial infection is suspected, intravenous antibiotics can be used until blood culture results are available.

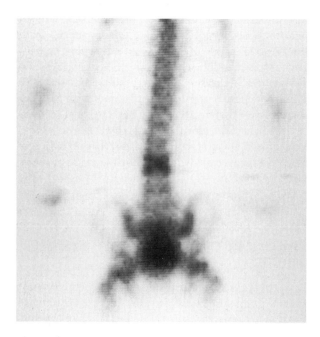

Fig. 12-3 Discitis scan. Technetium-99m bone scan of 2½-year-old girl with back pain showing increased uptake of isotope in inferior end-plate of L2 and superior end-plate of L3, characteristic of discitis. (Courtesy of Dr. H. Nadel.)

Calcification of intervertebral discs follows pyogenic or mycobacterial infection and occurs in diseases such as ochronosis. Transient calcification of a cervical or thoracic disc may occur in childhood and is associated with pain and fever lasting for up to 2 or 3 months. The etiology is unknown but is assumed to be infectious. Rarely, compression of the cord may necessitate a laminectomy.

OSTEOMYELITIS

Although osteomyelitis is most often encountered and treated by specialists in orthopedics and infectious diseases, its frequent occurrence in association with septic arthritis and the diagnostic problems that it presents require that it be included in this discussion.

Classification and Definitions

Osteomyelitis may be defined as intraosseous infection with bacteria (rarely fungi). It is classified as acute, subacute, or chronic. Acute osteomyelitis is of recent onset and short duration. It is most often hematogenous in origin but may result from trauma such as an open fracture or puncture wound. It may be metaphyseal, epiphyseal, or axial in location. Subacute osteomyelitis is of longer duration and usually caused by less virulent organisms. Chronic osteomyelitis results from ineffective treatment of acute osteomyelitis and is characterized by necrosis and sequestration of bone.

Epidemiology

Acute osteomyelitis is considerably less common than acute septic arthritis, an incidence of 16.7 cases per year being reported from the same institution where acute septic arthritis occurred at a rate of 28.4 cases per year.[8] Nade pointed out, however, that osteomyelitis is more common in the developing countries of the world.[34] Osteomyelitis occurs twice as often in boys as in girls[8,35] and is more common in younger children, although this correlation is less striking than the correlation with septic arthritis.

Clinical Characteristics

Fever, severe bone pain, and tenderness with or without local swelling should suggest the possibility of acute osteomyelitis. Although a history of prior trauma is elicited in approximately one-third of children with osteomyelitis, its significance is uncertain.

In the young infant, fever may be minimal and localization of the pain may be very difficult, except for the presence of pseudoparalysis. Evidence of systemic infection may be present. The site of infection is usually metaphyseal, and bony tenderness is elicited by pressure near or over the infected area. There may be overlying cellulitis, especially in the infant, in whom the cortex of the bone is thin and pus can break through into the periosteal structures. The presence of a joint effusion adjacent to the site of bone infection may reflect septic arthritis or a sterile noninflammatory "sympathetic" effusion. The bones of the lower extremity are the site of infection in two-thirds of patients; those of the upper extremity account for approximately 25 percent, whereas those of the skull, face, spine, and pelvis account for less than 10 percent[8,35] (Table 12-7). A small proportion (<10 percent) of children have two or more infected bones, in some cases five or more, as part of a severe septicemic illness, usually caused by staphylococci. This is to be distinguished from chronic aseptic multifocal osteomyelitis (discussed later).

Diagnostic Procedures

As in septic arthritis, it is essential that every reasonable attempt be made to identify the organism and determine its pattern of antibiotic susceptibility.[36]

Table 12-7 Comparison of Affected Sites in Chronic Recurrent Multifocal Osteomyelitis (CRMO) and Septic Osteomyelitis

Bone	CRMO (%)[47]	Osteomyelitis (%)[8,35]
Tibia	28	25
Clavicle	13	<1
Fibula	10	6
Spine	10	1
Femur	9	27
Metatarsal, metacarpal, phalangeal	9	4
Radius	6	4
Pelvis	4	6
Humerus	3	11
Ulna	3	2
Sternum	3	<1
Mandible	1	<1
Scapula	1	<1
Ribs	1	<1
Talus	1	1
Calcaneus	0	6

The aspiration of subperiosteal pus is the diagnostic procedure of choice, and together with culture of the blood, joint fluid, or infected wound should yield an organism in approximately 80 percent of patients. A bone biopsy may be necessary if other culture results are negative. *S. aureus* followed by group A streptococcus are the predominant organisms at all ages.[8] Although *H. influenzae* is a common cause of septic arthritis, it seldom causes osteomyelitis. In certain circumstances, specific organisms are likely to be found. For example, infection of the calcaneus associated with puncture wounds through athletic footwear is likely to be due to *Pseudomonas aeruginosa*.[37] Osteomyelitis caused by *Streptococcus pneumoniae* usually occurs in children with associated diseases such as sickle cell anemia,[38] asplenia,[39] or hypogammaglobulinemia,[40] although it has been noted in young infants without underlying disease.[41] In the neonate, group B streptococci, gram negative organisms, and *Candida* in addition to *S. aureus* are all possible causes of osteomyelitis. *Brucella melitensis* uncommonly causes osteomyelitis, but when it does, it has a predilection for the vertebral bodies.[24]

Radiographic evaluation may show soft tissue changes very early, but osteopenia does not occur until day 10 to 14. Radionuclide scanning (technetium-99m phosphate) provides a sensitive, if nonspecific method for the early detection of increased blood flow and bone uptake in the infected region (Fig. 12-4). It is particularly useful in localizing the lesion in osteomyelitis of the neonate or in infection of the axial skeleton. It is also of use in searching for subclinical areas of infection in multifocal osteomyelitis. A positive scan is not diagnostic of osteomyelitis, but a negative scan is unlikely in a child with bacterial osteomyelitis, except in the very early stages of the illness.

Other diagnostic tests should include a WBC count and differential as well as an ESR. Although these tests provide little help with diagnosis, they are useful measures in assessing effectiveness of therapy.

Treatment

In the absence of a specific indication to the contrary, the initial antibiotic treatment of osteomyelitis should be effective against *Staphylococcus aureus*. When culture results are available, appropriate intravenous antibiotic coverage for 4 to 6 weeks is recommended. Surgical treatment includes draining the subperiosteal and soft tissue abscesses and debriding

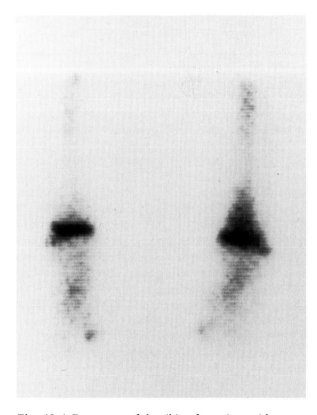

Fig. 12-4 Bone scan of the tibia of a patient with osteomyelitis showing increased uptake in the distal tibia on the left.

associated soft tissue lesions. Immobilization for relief of pain is useful, but weight bearing may be permitted as tolerated by the patient.

The most dreaded complication of acute osteomyelitis is chronic osteomyelitis. This should be suspected in a patient whose systemic symptoms respond slowly or incompletely to antibiotics or in whom there is a recurrence of pain at the affected site. Radiographic studies show a radiolucent involucrum (granulation tissue) surrounding dead (sclerotic) sequestered bone.

BRODIE'S ABSCESS

Subacute osteomyelitis, usually of staphylococcal origin, may develop after penetrating injury or by hematogenous spread in the metaphysis. It is characterized clinically by localized soft tissue swelling and tenderness with marked pain that may awaken the child at night. Radiographs show only soft tissue

swelling in the first week, but metaphyseal osteolytic lesions are visible by the second week. They are most common in the proximal or distal ends of the tibia[42,43] (Fig. 12-5). Cultures of the abscess contents may be negative. Treatment includes antibiotics, aspirin, and immobilization.

CHRONIC RECURRENT MULTIFOCAL OSTEOMYELITIS

The syndrome known as chronic recurrent multifocal osteomyelitis (CRMO), first described by Giedion in 1972,[44] mimics septic osteomyelitis. The etiology is unknown; cultures for bacteria always have negative results, although it has been speculated that either a virus or a fastidious slow-growing organism could be responsible for this syndrome.[45]

Clinically, patients with CRMO have the acute or insidious onset of multifocal bone pain, accompanied by fever. In a review of the anatomic distribution of 181 lesions in 35 patients, Gamble and Rinsky found the tibia to be most frequently affected[46] (Table 12-7). The disease is characterized by relapses and remissions. Radiographic changes are similar to those of septic osteomyelitis with osteolytic lesions surrounded by sclerosis (Fig. 12-6). Biopsy does not reveal an infectious organism, and histologic examination shows necrosis and new bone formation together with acute and chronic inflammatory cells with fibrosis.[46] These lesions heal without specific treatment but may recur months or years later. Antibiotics are unnecessary and ineffective; nonsteroidal anti-inflammatory drugs (NSAIDs) and occasionally corticosteriods may produce symptomatic relief. In a large series from Japan, Sonozaki et al. noted the presence of inflammatory oligoarthritis in one-quarter of the patients, and of sacroiliitis resembling ankylosing spondylitis in a small proportion.[47]

Bjorksten described a cutaneous complication, palmoplantar pustulosis, in six of nine patients,[48] and two of the seven patients reported by Laxer et al. had psoriasis.[49] The relationship of these skin changes to the bone lesions is not known.

Caffey's disease (infantile cortical hyperostosis), a rare disorder of infancy, may be confused with osteomyelitis. This disorder is characterized by fever, irritability, and swelling associated with hyperostosis of the mandible, clavicles, and long bones. The course is self-limited and the etiology is unknown. At one time this disease was quite

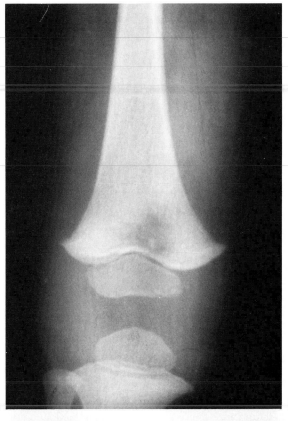

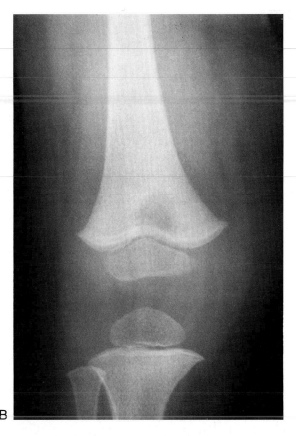

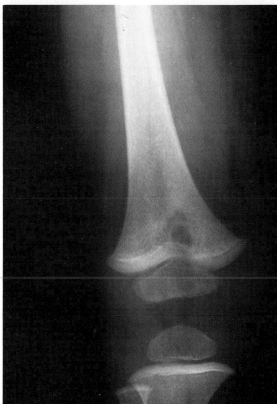

Fig. 12-5 Brodie's abscess. Radiographs of knee of 16-month-old boy with inadequately treated acute hematogenous osteomyelitis 1 month previously. (**A**) Shows central sequestration with surrounding ill-defined lytic margin. Patient appropriately treated with antibiotics at this stage. (**B**) One month later, sequestration has been removed by osteoclasts. (**C**) One month later, shows well-defined lesion with sclerotic borders. (Courtesy of Dr. B. Wood.)

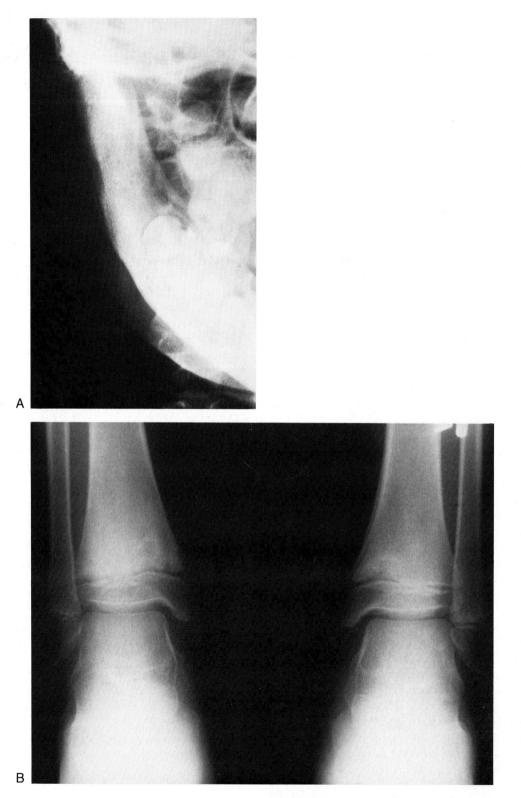

Fig. 12-6 Radiographs of a patient with chronic recurrent multifocal osteomyelitis affecting both distal tibiae. (**A**) There is subperiosteal new bone in the mandible, and (**B**) lytic lesions of both distal tibiae.

common but it has virtually disappeared, although a recent report documents a case[50] (see Ch. 14).

ARTHRITIS ASSOCIATED WITH ACNE

The association between arthritis and acne has been reviewed by Davis et al.[51] Most patients are male and have onset of musculoskeletal complications during adolescence. The syndrome includes severe truncal acne followed in several months by fever and arthralgia or arthritis, most often involving the hips, knees, and shoulders. We have observed one boy with pain and swelling in the sternoclavicular, knee and ankle joints and sacroiliac tenderness. Synovial histology was characterized by a nonspecific proliferative synovitis. Sacroiliac joint radiographs revealed early bilateral inflammatory changes. The patient was HLA-B27 positive. The possibility exists that this syndrome represents another example of reactive arthritis. Although in some patients arthritis lasts for only a few months, recurrences over many years have been documented.[51-53] Treatment with NSAIDs and antibiotics for control of the acne is indicated.

WHIPPLE'S DISEASE

Whipple's disease, first described in 1907,[54] is extremely rare in childhood. It is characterized by abdominal pain, weight loss, diarrhea, and, in 65 to 90 percent, by arthralgias or arthritis.[55,56] Whipple's disease occurs 10 times as often in men as in women and is most frequent in the fourth and fifth decades of life, although it has been identified in a 3-month-old boy[57] and a 7-year-old boy.[58] Migratory peripheral joint pain and inflammation, lasting hours to months, occur over a period of many years, often in association with fatigue, weight loss, and anemia. Joint swelling with increased synovial fluid and restriction of range of motion may occur,[59] although residual deformity does not.[56] The joints most frequently affected are ankles, knees, shoulders, and wrists,[59] and spondylitis has been reported in 20 percent.[60] Periodic acid–Schiff- (PAS-) positive material and bacteria are seen in macrophages infiltrating the upper small intestine and abdominal lymph nodes. Although the role of the bacteria, if any, is unknown, antimicrobial therapy (tetracycline, penicillin, streptomycin) has greatly improved the outcome in this disease.

SEPTIC ARTHRITIS CAUSED BY VIRUS, FUNGI, AND SPIROCHETES

Viral Arthritis

In general, viral arthritides are much more common in adults than in children. Arthralgia is more common than objective arthritis, and both are usually migratory and of short duration (1 to 2 weeks), disappearing without residual joint disease as a general rule. Small joints are most often affected by rubella, hepatitis B, and members of the arbovirus group (Ross River, chikugunya, etc.), whereas one or two large joints (usually the knee) are most often affected by mumps, varicella, and other viruses. In some viral arthritides, virus can be isolated from the joint space (rubella, varicella, herpes simplex, cytomegalovirus); in others only virus-containing immune complexes are found (hepatitis B, adenovirus 7); and in others the virus cannot be recovered from the joint. Whether this represents limitations of the recovery and culture techniques or whether culture-negative viral arthritis is "reactive" rather than "septic" is not known. A classification of viruses known to be associated with arthritis in humans is shown in Table 12-8. The togaviruses account for most of the identified viral arthritides.

ARTHRITIS ASSOCIATED WITH RUBELLA VIRUS

Now the most common virus-associated arthritis in North America, rubella-associated arthropathy was recognized by Osler.[61] Since that time it has been shown that musculoskeletal symptoms following natural rubella infection or immunization with rubella vaccine are relatively common occurrences in young women. They are very unusual, however, in preadolescent children and in males and are less frequent after rubella immunization than after the natural infection. Arthralgia usually begins within 7 days of the appearance of the rash or from 10 to 28 days after immunization. The joints of the fingers, followed by the knees, are most frequently affected. The arthralgia may be accompanied by warmth, erythema, and effusions, and tenosynovitis is not uncommon. Symptoms usually disappear within 3 to 4 weeks but occasionally persist for months or even

Table 12-8 Viruses That Can Cause Arthritis in Humans

Virus	Comment
Togaviruses	
Rubivirus	
Rubella	Global; most reports from North America and Europe
Alphaviruses	
Ross River	Australasia
Chikugunya	Africa, Asia
O'nyong-nyong	Africa
Mayaro	South America
Sindbis	Africa, Asia, Australia
Ockelbo	Sweden
Pogosta	Finland
Hepadnaviruses	
Hepatitis B	Global
Adenoviruses	
Adenovirus 7	Rare
Herpes viruses	
Epstein-Barr	Rare; suggested role in RA
Cytomegalovirus	Rare
Varicella zoster	Rare
Herpes simplex	Rare
Parvoviruses	Associated with fifth disease
Paramyxoviruses	
Mumps	Rare
Enteroviruses	
Echo	Rare
Coxsackie B	Rare
Orthopoxvirus	
Variola virus (smallpox)	Nonexistent today
Vaccinia virus	Rare

years. Rubella virus can be recovered from the synovial fluid of patients with rubella arthritis in many,[62,63] but not all,[64] instances. In a study of rubella in 37 teenage school students, 52 percent of the females and 8 percent of the males developed objective arthritis,[65] and an additional 13 percent of the females and 48 percent of the males developed arthralgia. In a group of young women who received RA 27/3 rubella vaccine, 14 percent developed acute polyarthritis. Not only was arthritis more common after natural infection; it was more severe and lasted longer.[65]

ARTHRITIS CAUSED BY ALPHAVIRUSES

In Australia, the islands of the South Pacific, Africa, and Asia, epidemic polyarthritis caused by infection with one of the alphaviruses is the most common viral-associated arthritis.[66] These viruses, which are closely related, are transmitted by arthropods, probably the mosquito, and cause an illness characterized by arthritis and a rash that may be macular, papular, vesicular, or purpuric. Although there are some virus-specific differences in these illnesses, in general they are uncommon and mild in children and occur with equal frequency in males and females. In Ross River virus disease, the wrist is most commonly affected, often accompanied by tenosynovitis and enthesitis at the plantar fascia insertion to the calcaneus.[66] The synovial fluid in Ross River virus disease is said to be highly characteristic with a predominance of vacuolated macrophages and very few polymophonuclear leukocytes.[66] In chikugunya, the knee is the most commonly affected joint, and back pain and myalgia are prominent. The arthritis lasts 1 to 2 weeks and is followed by complete recovery. The agent has not been recovered from synovial fluid, and diagnosis rests on the clinical presentation and elevated antibodies to the specific virus.

HEPATITIS B ARTHRITIS-DERMATITIS SYNDROME

In adults, up to 20 percent of infections with hepatitis B are characterized by a period of rash and arthritis, resembling serum sickness.[67] In a review of reported cases of arthritis associated with hepatitis B infection,[68] the age of the patients ranged from 14 to 56 years, and the sex ratio was 1.5 males to 1 female. The dermatitis, characterized by a macular papular rash, sometimes with petechiae, was most prominent on the lower extremities. The arthritis usually began abruptly and symmetrically and affected the interphalangeal joints in 82 percent, the knees in 30 percent, and the ankles in 24 percent. Although erythema and warmth were present, synovial effusions were uncommon. Joint symptoms lasted for 4 weeks on the average, responded well to NSAIDs, and disappeared without sequelae. The erythrocyte sedimentation rate is usually normal, although serum and synovial fluid complement levels are low in the early stages of the illness[69] and synovial fluid analysis has been reported to show a mononuclear cell predominance.[70] Electron microscopic evidence of hepatitis antigen in the synovial membrane has been reported.[71]

ADENOVIRUSES AND ARTHRITIS

There have been rare reports of arthritis associated with adenovirus type 7 infections, although virus was not isolated from the synovial fluid and diagnosis was made on clinical and serological grounds.[72,73]

HERPES VIRUSES AND ARTHRITIS

Four members of the herpes viruses have been associated with arthritis. Epstein-Barr virus has long been believed by some investigators to have a primary role in the etiology of rheumatoid arthritis, although direct evidence is lacking.[74] Arthritis is a rare complication of the infectious mononucleosis syndrome.[75,76]

Cytomegalovirus is occasionally associated with arthritis and has been isolated from synovial fluid in one instance.[77]

Varicella zoster infection is rarely complicated by arthritis.[78–81] There have, however, been instances of bacterial septic arthritis complicating chickenpox,[82,83] and in one instance varicella zoster virus has been grown from synovial fluid of an 8-year-old girl with acute painless monarthritis occurring 3 days after the onset of chickenpox.[84] The synovial fluid cells were predominantly lymphocytes.[80,81,84] Occasionally chickenpox is associated with the emergence of psoriatic arthritis.[85] Acute monarthritis has been reported in association with herpes zoster in two adults.[86,87]

Herpes simplex I virus has been isolated from the synovial fluid of one patient with arthritis and disseminated herpes simplex infection.[77]

PARVOVIRUS

Parvoviruses are the latest candidates in the list of viruses putatively involved in the etiology of rheumatoid arthritis in the adult, since parvovirus RA-1 has been isolated from synovial membrane of one patient with classical rheumatoid arthritis.[88] A second parvovirus (B19) is now known to be the agent responsible for erythema infectiosum (fifth disease or slapped cheek syndrome),[89] which is also sometimes accompanied by arthritis, not unlike that of rubella infection.[90–93] Parvovirus will undoubtedly be a subject of considerable interest in the next few years.

MUMPS

The paramyxovirus mumps rarely causes arthritis, and in a 1984 review, only 32 well-documented cases could be found.[94] Since then, 2 additional cases have been briefly reported.[95,96] The sex ratio is 3.6 males to 1 female, and the peak age of occurrence is in the 21- to 30-year group; 4 patients under 11 years of age and 7 between the ages of 11 and 20 years were noted. Arthritis occasionally preceded, but in general followed, parotitis by 1 to 3 weeks. In children, the arthritis was mild, affected few joints, and lasted 1 to 2 weeks. In postadolescent males, arthritis was often accompanied by orchitis and pancreatitis.[94] It is reported that the arthritis responds to ibuprofen or prednisone but not to aspirin.[94] The pathogenesis is unknown and no attempts at recovery of mumps virus from synovium or synovial fluid have been reported. Arthritis is not known to have occurred after mumps immunization.

ENTEROVIRUSES

Echoviruses[97–99] and Coxsackie B viruses[72,100] have been implicated on rare occasions as the cause of arthritis.

ORTHOPOXVIRUS

Smallpox (variola virus infection), now found only in the laboratory, was often accompanied by arthritis, especially in children under the age of 10 years, and may also follow smallpox vaccination.[101]

SYNDROMES PRESUMABLY RELATED TO VIRAL INFECTION: TRANSIENT SYNOVITIS

Transient or toxic synovitis of the hip is an idiopathic disorder often preceded by an upper respiratory tract infection. It occurs most commonly in boys

(70 percent) in the 3- to 10-year age group.[102] Pain in the hip, thigh, or knee may be of sudden or gradual onset and lasts for an average of 6 days.[103] Recurrences, often accompanied by low-grade fever, are quite common. Transient synovitis is bilateral in approximately 4 percent.[102] Examination of the hip reveals a loss of internal rotation and abduction, and the hip may be held in the flexed position. The ESR and WBC count are usually normal.[102,103] Radiographic examination may yield normal findings or may show widening of the joint space with lateral displacement of the femoral head that can be confirmed by computed tomography.[102] Radionuclide scanning may show transient decrease in uptake of technetium-99m phosphate. The investigation of transient synovitis may require aspiration of the hip joint to rule out bacterial sepsis. The synovial fluid has a normal or minimally increased cell count but may be under high pressure.[102] After aspiration, the pain and range of motion are dramatically improved, at least temporarily. Treatment includes the use of analgesic or NSAIDs, bed rest, and skin traction with the hip in 45 degrees of flexion to minimize intracapsular pressure.[102] Long-term sequelae include Legg-Calvé-Perthes disease in about 1.5 percent[104] and coxa magna and osteoarthritis.[105]

Fungal Arthritis

Arthritis caused by fungal infection is rare and in the pediatric population beyond the neonatal period is almost unknown. Candidal septic arthritis, often with osteomyelitis, is a recognized entity in the newborn[106,107] and occurs occasionally in the immunocompromised individual[26,27] and in infected prosthetic joints.[108]

Sporotrichosis (infection with *Sporothrix schenkii*) is a rare but significant occupational hazard of gardeners and field workers.[109,110] Monarthritis, or, less commonly, polyarthritis resembling rheumatoid arthritis, has been reported. Synovial biopsy is usually necessary in order to make the diagnosis. Other fungal infections are even less common causes of bone or joint infection, especially in children. The interested reader is referred to the review by Goldenberg and Cohen[110] and to the references listed in Table 12-9.[25,107,108,110,112-116]

Table 12-9 Fungal Organisms Causing Septic Arthritis or Osteomyelitis

Organism	Reference
Candida albicans	107, 108
Sporothrix schenkii	110
Actinomyces israelii	25
Aspergillus fumigatus	113
Histoplasma capsulatum	112
Cryptococcus neoformans	112
Blastomyces dermatitidis	114
Coccidioides immitis	115
Paracoccidioides brasiliensis	115
Pseudoallescheria boydii	116

PLANT-THORN SYNOVITIS

Synovitis caused by the penetration of plant thorns into the joint or surrounding structures is probably a reaction to the foreign material rather than an infection, although the circumstances of the injury may suggest the latter, and in the case of rose thorn penetration, *Sporothrix schenkii* may be the cause. Most commonly the thorn of the palm tree or blackthorn is implicated.[117] There are local signs of inflammation, and radiographs demonstrate periosteal new bone formation, a radiolucent defect in bone, or presence of the foreign material. Because this disorder may develop months after the initial injury the possibility of foreign body synovitis may be ignored. The synovial effusion is inflammatory, and culture may yield a relatively nonvirulent organism. Treatment should be directed at appropriate surgical exploration and removal of the foreign material.[117]

Arthritis Caused by Spirochetes

LYME DISEASE

The geographic and temporal clustering of cases of what was thought to be "juvenile rheumatoid arthritis" in Old Lyme, Connecticut, led Steere, Malawista, and their colleagues to the discovery and description of etiology, pathogenesis, and cure of what is now called Lyme disease. This work is one of the most important recent developments in rheumatology and provides a model for approaching the question of infectious etiology of other chronic arthritides of childhood.

Epidemiology

Although the disease was initially described in children,[118] all ages are affected, with approximately one-third of cases occurring in childhood and adolescence. In the original study by Steere et al., the prevalence of Lyme arthritis was 12.2 per 1,000, more than two orders of magnitude greater than that of juvenile rheumatoid arthritis.[118] The sex ratio is equal.[119-121] The disease most often has its onset in the summer months, the time of greatest exposure to the vector, the nymph stage of the tick *Ixodes dammini* or *Ixodes pacificum*.[22] There is pronounced geographical clustering, although as knowledge of the disorder expands, so does the number of areas in which it is found. It is now reported from many areas of the United States and Australia. The cutaneous component of Lyme disease, erythema chronicum migrans (ECM), has been described in the European literature since 1909,[123] and although it is associated with the bite of the tick *Ixodes ricinis*, it was rarely associated with arthritis in the European cases.[124]

Clinical Manifestations

Lyme disease occurs in three phases.[125] In phase 1 ECM is the characteristic finding. It begins as a red macule and expands peripherally with partial central clearing. The lesion is most common in the groin, axilla, and thigh (Fig. 12-7). It is warm, but not painful. approximately one-third of patients recall a tick bite at the site of the initial lesion up to a month previously. ECM may be accompanied by fever, chills, headache, malaise, fatigue, and regional lymphadenopathy. Approximately half of the patients develop multiple lesions like the first one but smaller, within days of the appearance of the initial lesion. These are not associated with a tick bite. A malar rash, urticaria, and conjunctivitis may develop along with these secondary lesions. These early signs and symptoms are typically intermittent and variable but disappear within 3 to 4 weeks.

Phase two is characterized by neurologic and cardiac manifestations. Although headache and meningismus may occur in phase one, neurologic lesions consisting of aseptic meningitis, chorea, cranial nerve palsy, radiculopathy, mononeuritis multiplex, or myelitis may occur several weeks to months after the

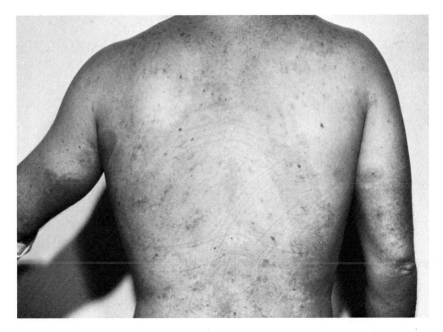

Fig. 12-7 Erythema chronicum migrans. Multiple lesions on the back of a teenage boy with Lyme disease. (Courtesy of Dr. J. Leyden.)

initial skin lesion. Although these lesions may last for months, they completely resolve. Cardiac abnormalities include various degrees of conduction disturbance from first-degree heart block, to Wenckebach phenomenon or complete heart block. These changes last 3 to 4 weeks but may recur.

Phase 3 is characterized by the development of recurrent and episodic arthritis in approximately two-thirds of patients. Although migratory polyarthralgia and myalgia may occur in phase 1, objective arthritis, affecting the knee most commonly, does not occur until 1 to 2 months after onset. Occasionally polyarthritis may mimic rheumatoid arthritis.[126] About 10 percent of patients with arthritis develop chronic disease with erosions.

Although the three-phase approach to understanding the clinical manifestations of Lyme disease is a useful one, it must be noted that there may be marked variation in the duration and sequence of events, and that "incomplete" Lyme disease may also occur. It may be that Lyme disease in children is most often restricted to arthritis alone.[127]

Borrelia infection of the pregnant woman may have serious consequences for the fetus. The offspring of 5 of 19 pregnant women who had Lyme disease during pregnancy had one of the following abnormal outcomes: prematurity, syndactyly, rash, cortical blindness and developmental delay, or intrauterine fetal death.[128]

Etiology and Pathogenesis

The organism *Borrelia burgdorferi* has been identified as the causative spirochete. It is transmitted to the susceptible host by the saliva of the tick *Ixodes dammini* or *Ixodes pacificum*. Its natural reservoir is the white-footed deer, although other animals (i.e., the field mouse) may also serve this function. *Borrelia burgdorferi* has occasionally been demonstrated in cerebrospinal fluid and blood,[129] and recently, by the use of silver stains, in synovial membrane.[130–132]

Laboratory Investigations

The erythrocyte sedimentation rate is usually elevated, especially in the early phase.[119] Serum immunoglobulin M (IgM) levels are also high,[132] and an elevation of hepatic enzymes may occur in some patients.[119] Microhematuria has been reported. Specific IgM titers to *Borrelia burgdorferi* peak between the third and sixth weeks of the illness. Synovial fluid may be quite large in volume, containing 4,000 to over 100,000 cells/mm^3, predominantly polymorphonuclear leukocytes.[133]

Treatment

Tetracycline, erythromycin, and penicillin have been shown to be effective in the treatment of Lyme arthritis. Of these, tetracycline is the most effective, and for adults this is the drug of choice. Because of the side effects of tetracycline in young children (<8 years of age), however, it is recommended that phenoxymethyl penicillin 50 mg/kg/day (minimum 1 g, maximum 2 g per day) be used for at least 10 days.[125] Even in late disease, neurologic manifestations or cardiac involvement should be treated with intravenous penicillin (20 million units) for at least 10 days. Prednisone and anti-inflammatory doses of aspirin may also be useful in treatment of patients with complete heart block.[134]

OTHER SPIROCHETES AND ARTHRITIS

Arthritis rarely complicates leptospirosis[135] and syphilis.[136] Congenital syphilis causes juxtaepiphyseal osteochondritis and periarthritis in infancy and syphilitic dactylitis in early childhood. Clutton's joints, relatively painless, recurrent, nonprogressive, symmetric synovitis of the knees, develop later.[137]

POSTINFECTIOUS ARTHRITIS

Arthritis-Dermatitis Syndrome Associated with Bowel Bypass

A syndrome characterized by recurrent episodes of polyarthritis, often with an associated pustular cutaneous vasculitis, occurs in 5 to 10 percent of adult patients undergoing surgical bypass of the distal jejunum and proximal ileum for the treatment of morbid obesity.[138] This syndrome includes arthritis or arthralgia in all patients, the cutaneous lesions in 75 percent, paresthesias (35 percent), Raynaud's phenomenon (29 percent), fever (14 percent), and pericarditis (3 percent).[139] Morning stiffness and severe periarthritis with warmth and swelling most commonly affected knees, ankles, fingers, wrists, shoulders, and elbows. The ESR is usually elevated, and cryoglobulins are present in one-third of patients. Rheumatoid factors and antinuclear antibodies are seldom detected and complement levels are usually normal.[139] The pathogenesis of this syndrome is not certain, although circulating immune complexes have been implicated and shown to contain antibody to *E. coli* and *B. fragilis*.[140,141] Treatment that has been found to be effective includes phenylbutazone, prednisone, and, if a blind-loop syndrome is suspected, tetracycline. To our knowledge, this syndrome has not been reported in children.

Musculoskeletal Manifestations of Systemic Bacterial Infections

Infective endocarditis frequently causes arthralgia or arthritis[142,143] and signs suggesting vasculitis (Osler nodes, Janeway lesions, Roth spots). The musculoskeletal signs and symptoms (arthralgia, arthritis, myalgia, low back pain) may precede other manifestations of infective endocarditis by weeks.[143] The arthritis is characteristically polyarticular and symmetrical, affecting large and small joints. An immune complex mediated pathogenesis is believed to be responsible, and the presence of hypocomplementemia,[144] circulating immune complexes,[145] and sometimes rheumatoid factors[144] supports this theory.

Bacterial infection of ventriculocaval shunts implanted for the management of hydrocephalus may also result in arthritis and nephritis.[146] Rheumatoid factors may be demonstrable in the serum of such patients.[146] Meningococcemia is complicated by arthritis in up to 10 percent of cases.[147] It is usually oligoarticular and occurs most frequently during the recovery phase when immune complexes can be demonstrated in the synovium.[148] It can also be complicated by acute septic arthritis in the early stage of the disease.

REACTIVE ARTHRITIS

Acute Rheumatic Fever and Related Disorders

The first complete description of the illness we now call acute rheumatic fever is ascribed to Thomas Sy-

denham in 1848.[149] In the last several decades, physicians in the United States, Canada, and Europe had come to believe that acute rheumatic fever was a disease of the past, although it remained a significant health problem elsewhere in the world, where the cardiac sequelae are the most important cause of heart disease.[150] A study of schoolchildren in Soweto, a black residential area in the Republic of South Africa, indicated a prevalence of 6.9 per 1,000 in 1975.[151] Since 1985 the disease has occurred in small epidemics in the United States.

EPIDEMIOLOGY

Acute rheumatic fever occurs with equal frequency in girls and boys, with a peak age of onset from 5 to 15 years. It is very uncommon under the age of 4 years. It is associated with poverty and crowding and is more common in urban than rural environments. It occurs in all races in all parts of the world. In the United States, the disease had, until very recently, almost disappeared.[152] An incidence rate of 0.5 to 1.88 per 100,000 population between the ages of 5 and 17 years was estimated in 1981.[153] Since the mid-1980s, however, there have been reports of three significant epidemics of the disease from widely scattered areas of the United States.[153–155] Initial mortality from rheumatic fever is approximately 1 percent; after 10 years, the cumulative mortality is 4 to 5 percent.

DEFINITIONS AND DIAGNOSTIC CRITERIA

Since no single manifestation of acute rheumatic fever is pathognomonic, a set of diagnostic criteria (the revised Jones criteria) form the basis for establishing a diagnosis[156] (Table 12-10). The Jones criteria were established at a time when acute rheumatic fever was the major cause of childhood arthritis. Today, when juvenile rheumatoid arthritis and other chronic arthritides of childhood are numerically much greater than acute rheumatic fever, the strict application of the Jones criteria can be misleading. Careful attention to the characteristics of the arthritis and the requirement for persistent arthritis in making the diagnosis of JRA by the American Rheumatism Association criteria will help prevent misdiagnosing patients with JRA or acute rheumatic fever (ARF).

Table 12-10 The Revised Modified Jones Criteria for the Diagnosis of Acute Rheumatic Fever[a]

Major Manifestations	Minor Manifestations
1. Carditis	1. Fever
2. Polyarthritis	2. Arthralgia
3. Chorea	3. Previous rheumatic carditis
4. Subcutaneous nodules	4. Prolonged PR interval
5. Erythema marginatum	5. Increased ESR or CRP

[a] Diagnosis requires the presence of two major criteria, or one major and two minor criteria, supported by evidence of a preceding streptococcal infection (increased ASO titer, positive pharyngeal culture, recent scarlet fever).[156]

CLINICAL MANIFESTATIONS

Streptococcal Pharyngitis

Classic streptococcal pharyngitis, characterized by fever, cervical lymphadenopathy, headache, erythema, and exudate on the oral pharynx, is readily recognizable during epidemics of streptococcal disease. Symptoms may be mild, however, and since other causes of pharyngitis may be exudative, a throat culture is necessary to make the diagnosis (Table 12-11).

The onset of clinical rheumatic fever may be either abrupt or insidious and follows the pharyngitis by 2 weeks. The onset is usually acute if articular symptoms predominate, insidious in patients who develop carditis alone (Fig. 12-8). Fever is frequent at the onset of the illness and is usually of a sustained type without wide swings. In most cases, the child's temperature returns to normal within 3 weeks of onset. Additional

Table 12-11 Clinical Characteristics of Acute Pharyngitis Due to Group A Beta-Hemolytic Streptococci ("Strep Throat")

Sudden onset of acute pharyngeal pain and malaise
Headache
Fever of 39°–40°C
Pharyngeal erythema and exudate; soft palate petechiae
Enlarged tender cervical lymph nodes
Sometimes, especially in younger children
    Abdominal pain
    Nausea and vomiting
    Acute otitis media
    Suppurative sinusitis
    Scarlatiniform rash

clinical findings include periumbilical pain and, rarely, erythema nodosum. Chronic rheumatic fever, the persistence of symptoms for longer than 6 months, occurs in less than 3 percent of cases and must be distinguished from recurrent attacks. The manifestations of second attacks usually mimic those of the initial episode, although the frequency of rheumatic heart disease increases with the number of acute attacks.

Arthritis

Arthritis is the most frequent major manifestation of rheumatic fever, occurring in approximately three-quarters of patients. Pain in the joints is frequently severe, whereas objective signs of joint inflammation may be minimal. The arthritis is typically polyarthric and migratory, affecting large joints in the lower extremities most commonly. The frequency of the arthritis increases with the patient's age and is higher in boys than in girls. Arthritis in any single joint persists for days to 1 or 2 weeks and is characteristically dramatically responsive to salicylate, leaving no residual joint disease.

Carditis

The most serious problem encountered in this disease, carditis, occurs most often in younger patients. In the United States and Canada the frequency of carditis is approximately 40 percent, although in other areas of the world[157] and in recent epidemics in the United States,[153] it appears to be considerably higher. In children, disappearance of the normal sinus arrhythmia may be the first sign of developing carditis. Persistent resting tachycardia without signs of heart failure may indicate myocarditis but must be cautiously interpreted in the presence of fever. The presence of a gallop rhythm, reduced intensity of the mitral first heart sound, and electrocardiographic abnormalities help to document the presence of carditis. As pointed out by many authors, prolongation of the PR interval correlates poorly with other signs of carditis. The detection of a new murmur is an important sign of cardiac involvement. An apical systolic murmur of mitral regurgitation is most common. Typically, it persists throughout systole and radiates toward the axilla. The second most common murmur is an apical middiastolic murmur, the Carey-Coombs murmur, which ends before the first heart sound and

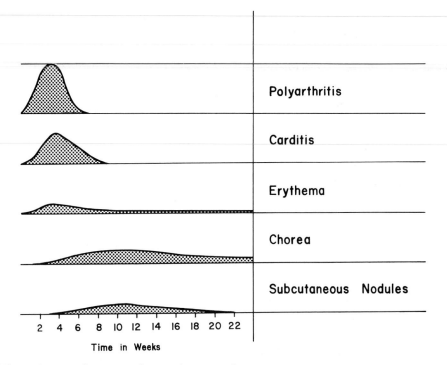

Fig. 12-8 The major manifestations of acute rheumatic fever. This diagram shows the expected occurrence of each of the major manifestations of acute rheumatic fever. The relative duration in weeks is indicated on the abscissa. In addition, the maximum clinical activity of each finding is represented by the peak of the shaded area. The expected frequency of each manifestation in any large number of cases is represented by the relative heights of each of the shaded areas. Arthritis and carditis in general are manifestations of acute early disease. Chorea, although it may be an early manifestation, is usually seen later (3 months) after the inciting episode of pharyngitis. It may be unaccompanied by the other manifestations of rheumatic fever. Erythema marginatum and subcutaneous nodules may occur for a longer period during and after the initial acute attack. In addition, these manifestations, although associated with severe disease, have become relatively infrequent in children in recent years.

results from relative mitral stenosis in relation to the left ventricular volume. It must be distinguished from the murmur of mitral stenosis that would indicate prior damage to the valve. The diastolic murmur of aortic regurgitation, often difficult to identify, is best heard at the left sternal border, starts with the second sound, and has a high-pitched decrescendo quality. Congestive heart failure is the most serious indication of cardiac disease and suggests a poor prognosis (Table 12-12). As late sequelae, mitral stenosis is more common in women, aortic valve disease in men (Fig. 12-9).

Pericarditis, characterized by precordial pain, a friction rub, or clinical, radiographic, and echocardiographic signs of effusion, almost always occurs in association with myocarditis and endocarditis.

Table 12-12 Estimated Occurrence of Rheumatic Heart Disease 5 years after Acute Rheumatic Fever

Initial Clinical Status	Subsequent Cardiac Disease (%)
No carditis	4
Soft apical systolic murmur	18
Loud apical systolic murmur	32
Diastolic murmur	47
Congestive heart failure or pericarditis	100

(Adapted from United Kingdom and United States Joint Report on Rheumatic Heart Disease,[172] with permission.)

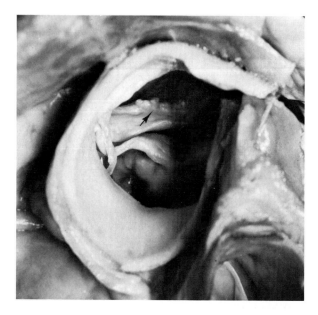

Fig. 12-9 Chronic rheumatic valvular heart disease. Verrucal endocardial thickening was present along the line of closure of the valve leaflets (arrow).

Many physicians believe that the presence of carditis dictates more aggressive therapy than that in children who have other manifestations of rheumatic fever and use corticosteroid drugs instead of acetylsalicylic acid.

Chorea

Sydenham's chorea (St. Vitus dance), the involuntary, purposeless movements associated with emotional lability that were formerly a common manifestation of acute rheumatic fever, is now seen in only 10 to 15 percent of patients. Chorea most commonly involves the muscles of the hands and face, including the tongue, resulting in dysarthria. It cannot be completely suppressed voluntarily but disappears during sleep and is not accompanied by pyramidal tract or sensory abnormalities. Emotional lability may be severe and must be distinguished from a psychological reaction to the chorea. Chorea is more common in girls than boys and, except in pregnancy, is uncommon after adolescence. When chorea is the only major manifestation of acute rheumatic fever, ESR, and C-reactive protein (CRP) findings may be normal and the interval between streptococcal infection and appearance of chorea is frequently far longer (up to 3

months) than that observed for the other manifestations. Rheumatic heart disease may occur in patients who have had only chorea as the initial clinical manifestation of their disease. The chorea of acute rheumatic fever may be difficult to distinguish from that which occurs in systemic lupus erythematosus (SLE). The presence of autoantibodies to nuclear antigens is diagnostically important in SLE. Sydenham's chorea usually lasts weeks to months.

Subcutaneous Nodules

Subcutaneous nodules are small (usually less than 1 cm in diameter) and painless. They occur over bony prominences, most often lasting for 1 or 2 weeks. They occur in less than 10 percent of patients, generally only in those with severe illness and carditis. They are currently seen almost exclusively in children with recurrent attacks. Clinically they are indistinguishable from the nodules of seropositive rheumatoid arthritis, which they also resemble histologically.[158]

Erythema Marginatum

Erythema marginatum, an uncommon (less than 10 percent) manifestation of acute rheumatic fever, is transient and occurs primarily on the trunk. The basic lesion is an erythematous macule that spreads with central clearing. Coalescence of several adjacent lesions results in the characteristic irregularly curved appearance (Fig. 12-10). Erythema marginatum is associated with carditis.

Analysis of the characteristics of the recent outbreaks of acute rheumatic fever shows that carditis is the most common manifestation (68 percent), followed by arthritis (57 percent), chorea (32 percent) erythema marginatum (7 percent), and nodules (5 percent).[153–155] The ages ranged from 3 to 17 years and there were 81 boys and 56 girls. Among the reasons for the resurgence are the presence of a susceptible population, or possibly, a change in the rheumatogenicity of the streptococcus.[159]

ETIOLOGY AND PATHOGENESIS

The clinical and pathologic manifestations of rheumatic fever occur as a direct consequence of prior infection with the group A beta-hemolytic streptococcus. Persistence of this infection for a minimum

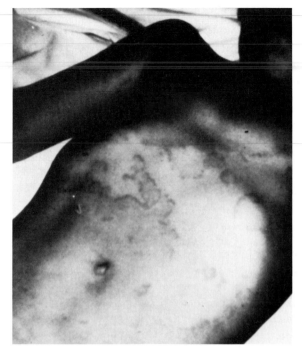

Fig 12-10 Acute rheumatic fever. This young boy developed the typical transient rash of erythema marginatum. The smaller lesions were closed, whereas larger areas showed marginated and serpiginous borders.

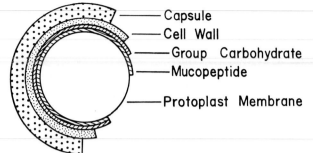

Fig. 12-11 Theoretic diagram of β-hemolytic *Streptococcus*. The successive layers of the *Streptococcus* are shown. The capsule is composed primarily of hyaluronic acid. The M protein is a component of the cell wall, along with the T and R antigens. The group carbohydrate sheath (Lancefield) is composed of *N*-acetyl glucosamine and rhamnose. The mucopeptide layer contains *N*-acetyl glucosamine, *N*-acetyl muramic acid, glutamic acid, alanine, lysine, and glycine. The protoplast membrane is composed of protein, lipid, and glucose.

period of 2 to 3 weeks appears to be necessary. The precise mechanisms by which antecedent infection leads to the multiple pathologic lesions of rheumatic fever have not been completely delineated. Studies during the past decade support the concept that hypersensitivity is central to the pathogenesis of this disease. Host factors are of importance since rheumatic fever occurs as a sequela of streptococcal pharyngitis in only 3 percent of the patients at risk.[160] Association with a high level of expression of a B cell antigen has been described.[161] Children who develop rheumatic fever demonstrate an exaggerated antibody response to toxins produced by the streptococcus (e.g., antistreptolysin O) compared to other patients who have recovered from streptococcal pharyngitis.[162,163] In addition, children who have had rheumatic fever are far more susceptible to recurrent attacks of the illness after a new streptococcal infection and again demonstrate exaggerated antibody responses.[164] Over 20 products of the streptococcus have been shown to be immunogenic in humans. The detection in serum of antibodies to these antigens es-

tablishes the relationship between such infections and the subsequent development of rheumatic fever. Antibody to M protein of the streptococcal cell wall is the only one to provide serotype-specific protection against subsequent streptococcal infection (Fig. 12-11).

Several studies have demonstrated that antistreptococcal antibodies cross-react with antigens found in cardiac muscle and valves[165–169] (Table 12-13, Fig. 12-12). It has also been demonstrated that antiheart antibodies are more readily detected in patients who have developed rheumatic carditis than in persons suffering from other manifestations of rheumatic fever. Antiheart antibodies bind to cardiac antigens in vivo, and their presence has been demonstrated in

Table 12-13 Cross-reactions between Streptococcal and Cardiac Antigens

Streptococcal Antigen	Cardiac Antigen
Cell wall M-associated protein	Myocardium
Cell membrane of all strains	Sarcolemma
Type I streptococcal cells	Intercalated disc
Acid extract of cell walls	Myocardium
Group A polysaccharide	Valve glycoprotein
Hyaluronic acid	Hyaluronic acid
Type I M protein	HLA antigens

(From DiSciascio and Taranta,[168] with permission.)

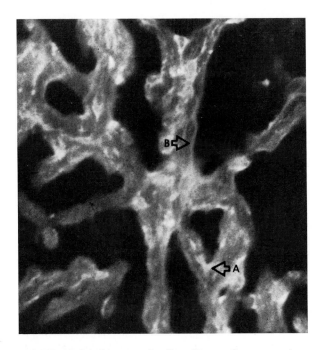

Fig. 12-12 Antiheart antibodies. Serum from a patient with acute rheumatic fever was incubated with a cryostat section of fetal heart tissue, and the pattern was developed with fluorescein-conjugated antihuman gamma globulins. The intense staining represents both the subsarcolemmal (**A**) and sarcolemmal (**B**) patterns of deposition of antibodies.

atrial tissue removed at the time of mitral valve surgery.[170] It has also been suggested that immune cross-reactivity between the streptococcal hyaluronate capsule and a hyaluronate-globulin complex in synovial fluid may be related to the pathogenesis of the acute arthritis of rheumatic fever. Toxic products generated by the organism may also cause tissue damage that, in turn, may lead to antibody formation to altered host antigens. Such antibody interactions are envisioned as activating or precipitating antigen-antibody mediated immunoinflammatory responses.

LABORATORY MANIFESTATIONS

Documentation of a preexistent streptococcal infection is essential to the diagnosis of rheumatic fever. This can be accomplished by the detection of streptococci by culture of pharyngeal secretions on sheep blood agar or by documentation of previous streptococcal infection by determination of ASO titers, which are elevated in 80 percent of patients. Addition of other antistreptococcal antibody assays such as antihyaluronidase, antistreptokinase, or antidesoxyribonuclease increases the sensitivity to 95 percent. Of most importance is the determination of a fourfold increase in titer. With the exception of patients with chorea, the ESR and CRP are elevated during an acute attack, and although these tests are nonspecific, if they are normal, the diagnosis of acute rheumatic fever is in doubt. Immunoglobulins are elevated, and antiheart antibodies can be demonstrated in two-thirds of patients with rheumatic carditis, although these antibodies are not specific for rheumatic fever.[171]

TREATMENT

Penicillin should be administered even in the absence of a positive throat culture after adequate differentiation between the signs of acute rheumatic fever and those of infective endocarditis has been made. This is particularly critical in children with a prior history of acute rheumatic fever. Bed rest is indicated during the acute attack, with resumption of full activity by 3 weeks. If carditis is present, however, a more prolonged period of bed rest may be indicated, depending upon the clinical situation. Acetylsalicylic acid controls fever and articular symptoms dramatically. Physicians should guard against salicylate intoxication in the young child since certain signs of toxicity may be confused with those associated with disease activity. A study of the treatment of rheumatic fever in the United Kingdom and the United States failed to establish an advantage of corticosteroids over acetylsalicylic acid.[172–174] Nonetheless in children with severe carditis, prednisone in an initial dose of 40 to 50 mg/day for 2 weeks may be indicated. Prophylaxis in the form of benzathine penicillin, 1.2 million units intramuscularly, should be given once a month until adulthood, and possibly throughout life if the patient is at high risk for exposure to streptococci. Oral penicillin G (200,000 units/day) or sulfisoxizole (1 g/day) is an effective alternative if compliance is assured. For surgical or dental procedures in children with known rheumatic heart disease, supplemental doses of penicillin should also be prescribed, and streptococcal pharyngitis should always be vigorously treated with a 10-day course of oral penicillin (1 million units/day) or the administration of intramuscular benzathine penicillin (1.2 million units as a single injection).

PROGNOSIS

The prognosis of acute rheumatic fever depends exclusively on the extent of cardiac involvement (Table 12-12). Residual articular disease probably never occurs, although there have been case reports of the development of Jaccoud periarthritis following acute rheumatic fever.[175–177]

POSTSTREPTOCOCCAL ARTHRITIS

There has been recent interest in a second post-streptococcal inflammatory joint syndrome. It differs significantly from acute rheumatic fever in the characteristics of the arthropathy, which tends to be polyarticular, to affect small joints as well as large, and to last for months. Emery et al.[178] described seven children with documented streptococcal pharyngitis who had arthritis in small joints of the hands, cervical spine, hips, and feet, as well as knees and ankles. In four there was a prompt response to salicylates, but in the remainder arthritis persisted. Carditis was present in six patients and persistent valve abnormalities occurred in four patients. This syndrome is arguably a variant of acute rheumatic fever.

Arthritis Following Infection with Enteric Bacteria

The reactive arthritides other than Reiter's syndrome and acute rheumatic fever are poorly documents in children. Four enteric pathogens, *Shigella flexneri*, *Yersinia enterocolitica*, *Salmonella* species and *Campylobacter jejuni*, give rise to infections that in some persons are followed by sterile arthritis. These same organisms are associated with Reiter's syndrome and the reactive arthritides following such infection may actually be incomplete forms of Reiter's syndrome; that is, they lack urethritis and conjunctivitis. On epidemiologic, genetic, and microbiologic grounds, this conclusion seems likely. It has been suggested that complete Reiter's syndrome is more common after *Shigella* infections than *Salmonella* or *Yersinia* (see Ch. 6).

REACTIVE ARTHRITIS AFTER *SHIGELLA INFECTION*

A period of high fever, with or without watery diarrhea and cramping abdominal pain lasting 48 to 72 h; may be followed in 7 to 21 days by the sudden onset of pauciarticular arthritis, most commonly affecting the knees and ankles. The arthritis is non-migratory and lasts from several weeks to 3 or 4 months.

Diagnosis requires a careful history, the demonstration of a sterile synovial fluid culture, the presence of agglutinins to *S. flexneri* serotype 2 or 2a,[179,180] and an attempt to isolate the organisms from the stool. Because of the interval between the diarrhea and the joint complaints, blood culture findings may be negative at the onset of the arthritis. Acute phase reactants are usually elevated, and rheumatoid factors and antinuclear antibodies are absent.

REACTIVE ARTHRITIS AFTER *SALMONELLA* INFECTION

The acute onset of pauciarticular arthritis, most frequently affecting the knees and ankles, may follow by 1 to 2 weeks an enteric infection with *S. typhimurium* or *S. enteritidis*. The enteric infection may be very mild, but the arthritis is usually accompanied by low-grade fever. Since *Salmonella* can cause osteomyelitis and septic arthritic as well as reactive arthritis, it is important to make certain that the joint fluid is sterile. The ESR is usually elevated, and the leukopenia that may accompany the acute infection is usually followed by a leukocytosis. Stool cultures are usually positive, even late in the disease course, but seroconversion to salmonella H and O antigens occurs in only 50 percent of patients. Response to aspirin or other nonsteroidal anti-inflammatory drugs is usually prompt and the prognosis is excellent.

POST-*YERSINIA* ARTHRITIS

A reactive arthritis of peripheral joints or spine follows infection with *Yersinia* in susceptible children. Although rarely reported from North America, the disease has been extensively studied in the Scandinavian countries.[181,182] Contact with the organism is through infected drinking water or milk. *Y. enterocolitica* produces gastroenteritis in young children and a syndrome of abdominal pain similar to that of appendicitis in older children and adolescents. The overall incidence of arthralgia or arthritis after *Yersinia* infection in childhood appears to be less than 5 percent,[183] but in a study of children who were hospitalized because of *Yersinia* infection, 35 percent had arthritis lasting 3 to 22 months (average 6.5 months). Of those with arthritis, 85 percent had HLA-B27.[184] Other uncommon systemic manifestations of infection with *Yersinia* include erythema nodosum, uveitis, episcleritis, conjunctivitis, and a myocarditis that must be distinguished from that of acute rheumatic fever. Laboratory investigations reveal evidence of acute inflammation, and synovial fluid cultures are sterile. Diagnosis rests on the demonstration of high, rising serum antibody titers to the bacterium. *Yersinia* can occasionally cause septic arthritis. It is of interest that antibodies to *Y. enterocolitica* serotypes 3 and 9, often associated with reactive arthritis, show a marked immunologic similarity to the agglutinins of *Brucella melitensis*.[185] *Brucella* infection is also associated with polyarthralgia, including pain in the lumbosacral spine and SI joints.[186,187] Treatment with nonsteroidal anti-inflammatory drugs results in complete disappearance of the signs of disease in days to weeks.

ARTHRITIS ASSOCIATED WITH *CAMPYLOBACTER JEJUNI* INFECTION

In an epidemic of *Campylobacter jejuni* enteritis in Finland, 2.3 percent of patients, all adults, developed pauci- or polyarthritis 4 days to 4 weeks after infection. The synovial fluid cultures were negative and 70 percent of arthritic patients had HLA-B27.[188]

Mycoplasma and Arthritis

Myalgia and arthralgia are frequent during pulmonary infection with *Mycoplasma pneumoniae*, and objective pauciarticular, polyarticular, or migratory arthritis has also been described.[189]

REFERENCES

1. Kunnamo I, Kallio P, Pelkonen P et al: Clinical signs and laboratory tests in the differential diagnosis of arthritis in children. Am J Dis Child 141:34, 1987
2. Welkon CJ, Long SS, Fisher MC et al: Pyogenic arthritis in infants and children: a review of 95 cases. Pediatr Infect Dis 5:669, 1986
3. Nelson JD, Koontz WC: Septic arthritis in infants and children: a review of 95 cases. Pediatrics 38:966, 1966
4. Wilson NIL, DiPaola M: Acute septic arthritis in infancy and childhood. 100 years' experience. J Bone Joint Surg 68B:584, 1986
5. Speiser JC, Moore TL, Osborn TG et al: Changing trends in pediatric septic arthritis. Semin Arthritis Rheum 15:132, 1985
6. Roca RP, Yoshikawa TT: Primary skeletal infections in heroin users. Clin Orthop 144:238, 1979
7. Morrey BF, Bianco AJ, Jr., Rhodes KH: Septic arthritis in children. Orthop Clin North Am 6:923, 1975
8. Fink CW, Nelson JD: Septic arthritis and osteomyelitis in children. Clin Rheum Dis 12:423, 1986
9. Dan M: Septic arthritis in young infants. Rev Infect Dis 6:147, 1984
10. Poznanski AK, Conway JJ, Shkolnik A et al: Radiological approaches in the evaluation of joint disease in children. Rheum Dis Clin North Am 13:57, 1987
11. Syriopoulou VP, Smith AL: Osteomyelitis and septic arthritis. In Feigin RD, Cherry JD (eds): Textbook of Pediatric Infectious Diseases. 2nd Ed. WB Saunders, Philadelphia, 1987
12. Tetzlaff TR, McCracken GH, Jr., Nelson JD: Oral antibiotic therapy for skeletal infections of children. II: Therapy of osteomyelitis and suppurative arthritis. J Pediatr 92:485, 1978
13. Ward JR, Atcheson SG: Infectious arthritis. Med Clin North Am 61:313, 1977
14. Nelson JD: Antibiotic concentrations in septic joint effusions. N Engl J Med 284:349, 1971
15. Griffin PP, Green WT: Hip joint infections in infants and children. Orthop Clin North Am 9:123, 1978
16. Fabry G, Meire E: Septic arthritis of the hip in children: poor results after late and inadequate treatment. J Pediatr Orthop 3:461, 1983
17. Chacha PB: Suppurative arthritis of the hip joint in infancy. J Bone Joint Surg 53A:538, 1971
18. Fink CW: Gonococcal arthritis in children. JAMA 194:237, 1965
19. Brogadir SP, Schimmer BM, Myers AR: Spectrum of the gonococcal arthritis-dermatitis syndrome. Semin Arthritis Rheum 8:177, 1979
20. Southwood TR, Hancock EJ, Petty RE et al: Tuberculous rheumatism (Poncet's disease) in a child. Arthritis Rheum 31:1311, 1988
21. Gomez-Reino FJ, Mateo I, Fuertes A et al: Brucellar arthritis in children and its successful treatment with trimethoprim-sulfamethoxazole (co-trimoxazole). Ann Rheum Dis 45:256, 1986
22. Gotuzzo E, Alarcon GS, Bocanegra TS et al: Articular involvement in human brucellosis: a retrospective analysis of 304 cases. Semin Arthritis Rheum 12:245, 1982
23. Thapar MK, Young EJ: Urban outbreak of goat cheese brucellosis. Pediatr Infect Dis 5:640, 1986
24. Young EJ: Human brucellosis. Rev Infect Dis 5:821, 1983

25. Hart PD, Russell E, Jr., Remington JS: The compromised host and infection. II: Deep fungal infection. J Infect Dis 120:169, 1969

26. Lipstein-Kresch E, Isenberg HD, Singer C et al: Disseminated *Sporothrix schenkii* infection with arthritis in a patient with acquired immunodeficiency syndrome. J Rheumatol 12:805, 1985

27. Ricciardi DD, Sepkowitz DV, Berkowitz LB et al: Cryptococcal arthritis in a patient with acquired immune deficiency syndrome. Case report and review of the literature. J Rheumatol 13:455, 1986

28. Sapico FL, Montgomerie JZ: Pyogenic vertebral osteomyelitis: report of nine cases and review of the literature. Rev Infect Dis 1:754, 1979

29. Hensey OJ, Coad N, Carty HM et al: Juvenile discitis. Arch Dis Child 58:983, 1983

30. Fischer GW, Popich GA, Sullivan DE et al: Diskitis: a prospective diagnostic analysis. Pediatrics 62:543, 1978

31. Spiegel PG, Kengla KW, Isaacson AS et al: Intervertebral disc-space inflammation in children. J Bone Joint Surg 54A:284, 1972

32. Rocco HD, Eyring EJ: Intervertebral disk infections in children. Am J Dis Child 123:448, 1972

33. Alexander CJ: The aetiology of juvenile spondylarthritis (discitis). Clin Radiol 21:178, 1970

34. Nade S: Acute haematogenous osteomyelitis in infancy and childhood. J Bone Joint Surg 65B:109, 1983

35. Cole WG, Dalziel RE, Leitl S: Treatment of acute osteomyelitis in childhood. J Bone Joint Surg 64B: 218, 1982

36. Morrissy RT, Shore SL: Bone and joint sepsis. Pediatr Clin North Am 33:1551, 1986

37. Elliott SJ, Aronoff SC: Clinical presentation and management of Pseudomonas osteomyelitis. Clin Pediatr 24:556, 1985

38. Seeler RA, Metzger W, Mufson MA: Diplococcus pneumoniae infections in children with sickle cell anemia. Am J Dis Child 123:8, 1972

39. Mallouh A, Talab Y: Bone and joint infection in patients with sickle cell disease. J Pediatr Orthop 5:158, 1985

40. Kauffman CA, Watanakunakorn C, Phair JR: Pneumococcal arthritis. J Rheumatol 3:409, 1976

41. Hadari I, Dagan R, Gedalia A et al: Pneumococcal osteomyelitis. An unusual cluster of cases. Clin Pediatr 24:143, 1985

42. Green NE, Beauchamp RD, Griffin PP: Primary subacute epiphyseal osteomyelitis. J Bone Joint Surg 63A:107, 1981

43. Gledhill RB: Subacute osteomyelitis in children. Clin Orthop 96:57, 1973

44. Giedion A, Holthusen W, Masel LF et al: Subacute and chronic "symmetrical" osteomyelitis. Ann Radiol 15:329, 1971

45. Speer DP: Chronic multifocal symmetrical osteomyelitis (editorial). Am J Dis Child 138:340, 1984

46. Gamble JG, Rinsky LA: Chronic recurrent multifocal osteomyelitis: a distinct clinical entity. J Pediatr Orthop 6:579, 1986

47. Sonozaki H, Mitsui H, Miyanaga Y et al: Clinical features of 53 cases with pustulotic arthro-osteitis. Ann Rheum Dis 40:547, 1981

48. Bjorksten B, Gustavson K-H, Eriksson B et al: Chronic recurrent multifocal osteomyelitis and pustulosis palmoplantaris. J Pediatr 93:227, 1978

49. Laxer RM, King S, Manson D et al: Chronic recurrent multifocal osteomyelitis (CRMO)—a review of seven cases. Arthritis Rheum 30:s80, 1987

50. Marshall GS, Edwards KM, Wadlington WB: Sporadic congenital Caffey's disease. Clin Pediatr 26:177, 1987

51. David DE, Viozzi FJ, Miller OF et al: The musculoskeletal manifestations of acne fulminans. J Rheumatol 8:317, 1981

52. Hunter LY, Hensinger RN: Destructive arthritis associated with acne fulminans: a case report. Ann Rheum Dis 39:403, 1980

53. Cros D, Gamby T, Serratrice G: Acne rheumatism. Report of a case. J Rheumatol 8:336, 1981

54. Whipple GH: A hitherto undescribed disease characterized anatomically by deposits of fat and fatty acids in the intestinal and mesenteric lymphatic tissues (intestinal lipodystrophy). Bull Johns Hopkins Hosp 18:382, 1907

55. LeVine ME, Dobbins WO, III: Joint changes in Whipple's disease. Semin Arthritis Rheum 3:79, 1973

56. Maizel H, Ruffin JM, Dobbins WO, III: Whipple's disease. A review of 19 patients from one hospital and a review of the literature since 1950. Medicine 49:175, 1970

57. Aust CH, Smith EB: Whipple's disease in a three month old infant. Am J Clin Pathol 37:66, 1962

58. Barahat AY, Bitar J, Nassar VH: Whipple's disease in a seven year old child. Am J Proctol 24:312, 1973

59. Caughey OE, Bywaters EGL: The arthritis of Whipple's syndrome. Ann Rheum Dis 22:327, 1963

60. Kelly JJ, III, Weisiger BB: The arthritis of Whipple's disease. Arthritis Rheum 6:615, 1963

61. Osler W: Principles and Practice of Medicine. 6th Ed. Appleton, East Norwalk, CT, 1906

62. Ogra PL, Herd JK: Arthritis associated with induced rubella infection. J Immunol 107:810, 1971

63. Chantler JK, Ford DK, Tingle AJ: Persistent rubella infection and rubella-associated arthritis. Lancet 1:1323, 1982

64. Spruance SL, Metcalf R, Smith CB et al: Chronic

arthropathy associated with rubella vaccination. Arthritis Rheum 20:741, 1977

65. Tingle AJ, Allen M, Petty RE et al: Rubella-associated arthritis. Comparative study of joint manifestations associated with natural rubella infection and RA 27/3 rubella immunization. Ann Rheum Dis 45:110, 1986

66. Fraser JRE: Epidemic polyarthritis and Ross River virus disease. Clin Rheum Dis 12:369, 1986

67. Alarcon GS, Townes AS: Arthritis in viral hepatitis. Report of two cases and review of the literature. J Hopkins Med J 132:1, 1973

68. Inman RD: Rheumatic manifestations of Hepatitis B virus infection. Semin Arthritis Rheum 11:406, 1982

69. Alpert E, Isselbacher KJ, Schur PH: The pathogenesis of arthritis associated with viral hepatitis. Complement component studies. N Engl J Med 285:185, 1971

70. Duffy J, Lidsky MD, Sharp JT et al: Polyarthritis, polyarteritis and hepatitis B. Medicine 55:19, 1976

71. Schumacher HR, Gall EP: Arthritis in acute hepatitis and chronic active hepatitis. Pathology of the synovial membrane with evidence for the presence of Australia antigen in synovial membranes. Am J Med 75:655, 1974

72. Rahal JJ, Millian SJ, Noriega ER: Coxsackievirus and adenovirus infection. Association with acute febrile and juvenile rheumatoid arthritis. JAMA 235:2496, 1976

73. Panush RS: Adenovirus arthritis. Arthritis Rheum 17:534, 1974

74. Bluestein HG, Hasler F: Epstein-Barr virus and rheumatoid arthritis. Surv Immunol Res 3:70, 1984

75. Pollack S, Enat R, Barzilai D: Monarthritis with heterophil-negative infectious mononucleosis. Arch Intern Med 140:1109, 1980

76. Adebonojo FO: Monarticular arthritis. An unusual manifestation of infectious mononucleosis. Clin Pediatr 11:549, 1972

77. Friedman HM, Pincus T, Gibilisco P et al: Acute monarticular arthritis caused by herpes simplex virus and cytomegalovirus. Am J Med 68:241, 1980

78. Friedman A, Naveh Y: Polyarthritis associated with chicken pox. Am J Dis Child 122:179, 1971

79. Brook I: Varicella arthritis in childhood. Clin Pediatr 16:1156, 1977

80. Mulhern LM, Friday GA, Perri JA: Arthritis complicating varicella infection. Pediatrics 48:827, 1971

81. Ward JR, Bishop B: Varicella arthritis. JAMA 212:1954, 1970

82. Buck RE: Pyarthrosis of the hip complicating chicken pox. JAMA 206:135, 1968

83. Sethi AS, Schloff I: Purulent arthritis complicating chickenpox. Clin Pediatr 13:280, 1974

84. Priest JR, Urick JJ, Groth KE et al: Varicella arthritis documented by isolation of virus from joint fluid. J Pediatr 93:990, 1978

85. Shore A, Ansell BM: Juvenile psoriatic arthritis—an analysis of 60 cases. J Pediatr 100:529, 1982

86. Cunningham AL, Fraser JRE, Clarris BJ et al: A study of synovial fluid and cytology in arthritis associated with herpes zoster. Aust NZ J Med 9:440, 1979

87. Devereaux MD, Hazleton RA: Acute monarticular arthritis in association with herpes zoster. Arthritis Rheum 26:236, 1983

88. Simpson RW, Smith CA, Godzeski CW et al: Association of parvoviruses with rheumatoid arthritis in humans. Science 224:1425, 1984

89. Anderson MJ, Jones SE, Fisher-Hoch SP et al: Human parvovirus, the cause of erythema infectiosum (fifth disease)? Lancet 1:1378, 1983

90. Semble EL, Agudelo CA, Pegram PS: Human parvovirus B19 arthropathy in two adults after contact with childhood erythema infectiosum. Am J Med 83:560, 1987

91. Reid DM, Reid TMS, Brown T et al: Human parvovirus-associated arthritis: a clinical and laboratory description. Lancet 1:422, 1985

92. White DG, Woolf AD, Mortimer PP et al: Human parvovirus arthropathy. Lancet 1:419, 1985

93. Smith CA, Woolf AD, Lenci M: Parvoviruses: infections and arthropathies. Rheum Dis Clin North Am 13:249, 1987

94. Gordon SC, Lauter CB: Mumps arthritis: a review of the literature. Rev Infect Dis 6:338, 1984

95. Fontebasso M: Mumps polyarthritis. J R Coll Gen Pract 35:152, 1985

96. Moffatt CD: Mumps arthropathy. J R Coll Gen Pract 36:230, 1986

97. Blotzer JW, Myers AR: Echovirus-associated polyarthritis. Arthritis Rheum 21:978, 1978

98. Kujak G, Newman JH: Isolation of echovirus type 11 from synovial fluid in acute monocytic arthritis. Arthritis Rheum 28:98, 1985

99. Ackerson BK, Raghurathan R, Kreller MA et al: Echovirus 11 arthritis in a patient with x-linked agammaglobulinemia. Pediatr Infect Dis J 6:485, 1987

100. Roberts-Thomson P, Southwood TR, Moore BW et al: Adult onset Still's disease or coxsackie polyarthritis? Aust NZ J Med 16:509, 1986

101. Holtzman CB: Postvaccination arthritis. N Engl J Med 280:111, 1969

102. Wingstrand H: Transient synovitis of the hip in the child. Acta Orthop Scand, Suppl., 57:219, 1986

103. Hardinge K: The etiology of transient synovitis of the hip in childhood. J Bone Joint Surg 52B:100, 1970

104. Spock A: Transient synovitis of the hip joint in children. Pediatrics 24:1042, 1959

105. Wynne-Davis R, Gormley J: The aetiology of Perthes disease. Genetic, epidemiological and growth factors in 310 Edinburgh and Glasgow patients. J Bone Joint Surg 60B:6, 1978

106. Klein JD, Yamauchi T, Horlick SP: Neonatal candidiasis, meningitis and arthritis. Observations and a review of the literature. J Pediatr 81:31, 1972

107. Poplack DG, Jacobs SA: Candida arthritis treated with Amphotericin B. J Pediatr 87:989, 1975

108. MacGregor RR, Schimmer BM, Steinberg ME: Results of combined amphotericin B-5-fluorocytosine therapy for prosthetic knee joint infected with *Candida parapsilosis*. J Rheumatol 6:451, 1979

109. Crout JP, Brewer NS, Tompkins RB: Sporotrichosis arthritis: clinical features in seven patients. Ann Intern Med 86:294, 1977

110. Goldenberg DL, Cohen AS: Arthritis due to tuberculous and fungal microorganisms. Clin Rheum Dis 4:211, 1978

111. Bayer AS, Choi C, Tillman DB et al: Fungal arthritis. V: Cryptococcal and histoplasmal arthritis. Semin Arthritis Rheum 9:218, 1980

112. Tack KJ, Rhame FS, Brown B et al: Aspergillus osteomyelitis. Report of four cases and review of the literature. Am J Med 73:295, 1982

113. Sanders LL: Blastomycosis arthritis. Arthritis Rheum 10:91, 1969

114. Bayer AS, Yoshikawa TT, Galpin JE et al: Unusual syndromes of coccidioidomycosis: diagnostic and therapeutic considerations. Medicine 55:131, 1976

115. Castaneda OJ, Alarcon GS, Garcia MT et al: *Paracoccidioides brasiliensis* arthritis. Report of a case and review of the literature. J Rheumatol 12:356, 1985

116. Ansari RA, Hindson DA, Stevens DL et al: *Pseudoallescheria boydii* arthritis and osteomyelitis in a patient with Cushing's disease. South Med J 80:90, 1987

117. Sugarman M, Stobie DG, Quismorio FP et al: Plant thorn synovitis. Arthritis Rheum 20:1125, 1977

118. Steere AC, Malawista SE, Snydman DR et al: Lyme arthritis: an epidemic of oligoarticular arthritis in children and adults in three Connecticut communities. Arthritis Rheum 20:7, 1977

119. Steere AC, Bartenhagen NH, Craft JE et al: The early clinical manifestations of Lyme disease. Ann Int Med 99:76, 1983

120. Bowen GS, Schulze TL, Parkin WL: Lyme disease in New Jersey, 1978–1982. In Steere AC, Malawista SE, Craft JE et al (eds); Lyme Disease. First International Symposium. Yale Journal of Biology and Medicine, New Haven, 1984, p. 211

121. Osterholm MT, Forfang JC, White KE et al: Lyme disease in Minnesota: epidemiologic and serologic findings. In Steere AC, Malawista SE, Craft JE et al (eds): Lyme Disease. First International Symposium. Yale Journal of Biology and Medicine, New Haven, 1984, p. 227.

122. Burgdorfer W: Discovery of the Lyme disease spirochete and its relation to tick vectors. In Steere AC, Malawista SE, Craft JE et al (eds): Lyme Disease. First International Symposium. Yale Journal of Biology and Medicine, New Haven, 1984, p. 65

123. Afzelius A: Verhandlungen der dermatologischen Gesellschaft zu Stockholm, December 1909. Arch Dermatol Syphil (Berlin) 101:405, 1910

124. Schmid GP: The global distribution of Lyme disease. In Steere AC, Malawista SE, Craft JE et al (eds): Lyme Disease. First International Symposium. Yale Journal of Biology and Medicine, New Haven, 1984, p. 167

125. Steere AC, Malawista SE, Bartenhagen NH et al: The clinical spectrum and treatment of Lyme disease. In Steere AC, Malawista SE, Craft JE et al (eds): Lyme Disease. International Symposium. Yale Journal of Biology and Medicine, New Haven, 1984, p. 3

126. Steere AC, Gibofsky A, Patarroyo ME et al: Chronic Lyme arthritis: clinical and immunogenetic differentiation from rheumatoid arthritis. Ann Intern Med 90:286, 1979

127. Steere AC, Taylor E, Wilson ML et al: Longitudinal assessment of the clinical and epidemiological features of Lyme disease in a defined population. J Infect Dis 154:295, 1986

128. Markowitz LE, Steere AC, Benach JL et al: Lyme disease during pregnancy. JAMA 255:3394, 1986

129. Steere AC, Grodzicki RL, Kornblatt AN et al: The spirochetal etiology of Lyme disease. N Engl J Med 308:733, 1983

130. Johnston YE, Duray PH, Steere AC et al: Lyme arthritis: spirochetes found in synovial microangiopathic lesions. Am J Pathol 118:26, 1985

131. Snydman DR, Schenkein DP, Berardi VP et al: *Borrelia burgdorferi* in joint fluid in chronic Lyme arthritis. Ann Intern Med 104:798, 1986

132. De Koning J, Bosma RB, Hoogkamp-Korstanje JAA: Demonstration of spirochaetes in patients with Lyme disease with a modified silver stain. J Med Microbiol 23:261, 1987

133. Culp RW, Eichenfield AH, Davidson RS et al: Lyme arthritis in children. J Bone Joint Surg 69A:96, 1987

134. Steere AC, Malawista SE, Newman JH et al: Antibiotic therapy in Lyme disease. Ann Intern Med 93:1, 1980

135. Sutliff WD, Shepard R, Dunham WB: Acute leptospira pomona arthritis and myocarditis. Ann Intern Med 39:134, 1953

136. Reginato AJ, Schumacher HR, Jiminez S et al: Syn-

ovitis in secondary syphilis. Arthritis Rheum 22:170, 1979

137. Argen RJ, Dixon ASJ: Clutton's joints with keratitis and periostitis: a case report with histology of synovium. Arthritis Rheum 6:341, 1963

138. Shagrin JW, Frame B, Duncan H: Polyarthritis in obese patients with intestinal bypass. Ann Intern Med 75:377, 1971

139. Stein HB, Schlappner OLA, Boyko W et al: The intestinal bypass arthritis-dermatitis syndrome. Arthritis Rheum 24:684, 1981

140. Ginsberg J, Quismorio FP, De Wind LT et al: Musculoskeletal symptoms after jejunoileal shunt surgery for intractable obesity; clinical and immunologic studies. Am J Med 67:443, 1979

141. Wands JR, LaMont JT, Mann E et al: Arthritis associated with intestinal-bypass procedure for morbid obesity. N Engl J Med 294:121, 1976

142. Churchill MA, Geraci JE, Hunder GG: Musculoskeletal manifestations of bacterial endocarditis. Ann Intern Med 87:754, 1977

143. Levo Y, Nashif M: Musculoskeletal manifestations of bacterial endocarditis. Clin Exp Rheumatol 1:49, 1983

144. Williams RC, Jr., Kunkel HG: Rheumatoid factor, complement and conglutinin aberrations in patients with subacute bacterial endocarditis. J Clin Invest 41:666, 1962

145. Bayer AS, Theophilopoulos AN, Eisenberg R et al: Circulating immune complexes in infective endocarditis. New Engl J Med 295:1500, 1977

146. Pinals RS, Tunnessen WW: Shunt arthritis. J Pediatr 91:681, 1977

147. Schaad UB: Arthritis in disease due to *Neisseria meningitidis*. Rev Infect Dis 2:880, 1980

148. Greenwood BM, Whittle HC, Bryceson ADM: Allergic complications of meningococcal disease. II: Immunological investigations. Br Med J 2:737, 1973

149. Sydenham T: The works of Thomas Sydenham. Vol. 1. RG Latham: Trans London Sydenham Society, London, 1848, p. 254

150. El Kholy A, Rotta J, Wannamaker LW et al: Recent advances in rheumatic fever control and future prospects. A WHO memorandum. WHO Bull 56:887, 1978

151. McLaren MJ, Hawkins DM, Koorhop HJ et al: Epidemiology of rheumatic heart disease in black schoolchildren of Soweto, Johannesburg. Br Med J 3:474, 1975

152. Gordis L: The virtual disappearance of rheumatic fever in the United States: lessons in the rise and fall of disease. Circulation 72:1155, 1985

153. Veasey LG, Wiedmeier SE, Orsmond GS et al: Resurgence of acute rheumatic fever in the intermountain area of the United States. N Engl J Med 316:421, 1987

154. Hosier DM, Craenen JM, Teske DW et al: Resurgence of acute rheumatic fever. Am J Dis Child 141:730, 1987

155. Congeni B, Rizzo C, Congeni J et al: Outbreak of acute rheumatic fever in northeast Ohio. J Pediatr 111:176, 1987

156. Stollerman GH, Markowitz M, Taranta A et al: Jones criteria (revised) for guidance in the diagnosis of rheumatic fever. Circulation 32:664, 1965

157. Markowitz M, Gordis L: Rheumatic Fever. 2nd Ed. WB Saunders, Philadelphia, 1972, p. 62

158. Bywaters EGL, Glynn LE, Zeldis A: Subcutaneous nodules of Still's disease. Ann Rheum Dis 27:278, 1958

159. Ferrieri P: Acute rheumatic fever. The come-back of a disappearing disease. Am J Dis Child 141:725, 1987

160. Sigel AC, Johnson EE, Stollerman GH: Controlled studies of streptococcal pharyngitis in a pediatric population. I: Factors related to the attack rate of rheumatic fever. N Engl J Med 265:559, 1961

161. Khanna AK, Buskirk DR, Williams RC, Jr. et al: Presence of a non-HLA B cell antigen in rheumatic fever patients and their families as defined by a monoclonal antibody. J Clin Invest 83:1710, 1989

162. Taranta A, Wood HF, Feinstein AR et al: Rheumatic fever in children and adolescents. IV: Relation of the rheumatic fever recurrence rate per streptococcal infection to the titers of streptococcal antibodies. Ann Intern Med 60:47, 1964

163. Schulman ST, Ayoub EM, Victorica BE et al: Differences in antibody response to streptococcal antigens in children with rheumatic and non-rheumatic mitral valve disease. Circulation 50:1244, 1974

164. Taranta A, Kleinberg RE, Feinstein AR et al: Rheumatic fever in children and adolescents. V: Relation of the rheumatic fever recurrence rate per streptococcal infection to pre-existing clinical features of the patients. Ann Intern Med 60:suppl. 5, 58, 1964

165. Kaplan MH: Immunologic relation of streptococcal and tissue antigens. I: Properties of an antigen in certain strains of group A streptococci exhibiting an immunologic cross reaction with human heart tissue. J Immunol 90:595, 1963

166. Kaplan MH, Suchy ML: Immunologic relation of streptococcal and tissue antigens. II: Cross reactions of antisera to mammalian heart tissue with a cell wall constituent of certain strains of group A streptococci. J Exp Med 119:643, 1964

167. Kaplan MH, Meyereserian M, Kushner I: Immunologic studies of heart tissue. IV: Serologic reactions with human heart tissue as revealed by immunoflu-

orescent methods: Isoimmune, Wassermann, and auto-immune reactions. J Exp Med 113:17, 1961

168. Di Sciascio G, Taranta A: Rheumatic fever in children. Am Heart J 99:635, 1980

169. Van de Rijn I, Zabriskie JB, McCarty M: Group A streptococcal antigens cross-reactive with myocardium. Purification of heart-reactive antibody and isolation and characterization of the streptococcal antigen. J Exp Med 146:579, 1977

170. Goldstein I, Halpern B, Robert L: Immunological relationship between streptococcus A polysaccharide and the structural glycoproteins of heart valve. Nature 213:44, 1976

171. Das S, Cassidy JT, Petty RE: Antibodies against heart muscle and nuclear constituents in cardiomyopathy. Am Heart J 83:159, 1972

172. United Kingdom and United States Joint Report on Rheumatic Heart Disease: The evolution of rheumatic heart disease in children. Five-year report of a cooperative clinical trial of ACTH, cortisone and aspirin. Circulation 22:503, 1960

173. United Kingdom and United States Joint Report of Rheumatic Heart Disease: The natural history of rheumatic fever and rheumatic heart disease. Ten-year report of a cooperative clinical trial of ACTH, cortisone and aspirin. Circulation 32:457, 1965

174. Wannamaker LW, Rammelkamp CH, Jr., Denny FW et al: Prophylaxis of acute rheumatic fever by treatment of the preceding streptococcal infection with various amounts of depot penicillin. Am J Med 10:673, 1951

175. Bywaters EGL: The relation between heart and joint disease including "rheumatoid heart disease" and chronic post-rheumatic arthritis (type Jaccoud). Br Heart J 12:101, 1950

176. Grahame R, Mitchell ABS, Scott JT: Chronic post-rheumatic fever (Jaccoud's) arthropathy. Ann Rheum Dis 29:622, 1970

177. Levin EB: Jaccoud's arthritis. Post-rheumatic fever complication—not rheumatoid arthritis. Calif Med 112:19, 1970

178. Emery H, Wagner-Weiner L, Magilavy D: Resurgence of childhood post-streptococcal rheumatic syndromes. Arthritis Rheum 30:s80, 1987

179. Davies NE, Haverty JR, Boatwright M: Reiter's disease associated with shigellosis. South Med J 62:1011, 1969

180. Singsen BH, Bernstein BH, Koster-King KG et al: Reiter's syndrome in childhood. Arthritis Rheum, suppl. 20:402, 1977

181. Arvastson B, Damgaard K, Winblad S: Clinical symptoms of infections with *Yersinia enterocolitica*. Scand J Infect Dis 3:37, 1971

182. Ahvonen P: Human yersiniosis in Finland. II. Clinical features. Ann Clin Res 4:39, 1972

183. Maki M, Vesikari T, Rantala I et al: Yersiniosis in children. Arch Dis Child 55:861, 1980

184. Leino R, Makela A-L, Tiilikainen A et al: Yersinia arthritis in children. Scand J Rheum 9:245, 1980

185. Ahvonen P, Sievers K, Aho K: Arthritis associated with *Yersinia enterocolitica* infection. Acta Rheum Scand 15:232, 1969

186. Rotes-Querol J: Osteo-articular sites of brucellosis. Ann Rheum Dis 16:63, 1957

187. Hodinka L, Gomer B, Meretey K et al: HL-A27 associated spondyloarthritis in chronic brucellosis. Lancet 1:499, 1978

188. Kosunen TU, Ponka A, Kauranen O et al: Arthritis associated with *Campylobacter jejuni* enteritis. Scand J Rheumatol 10:77, 1981

189. Broughton RA: Infections due to *Mycoplasma pneumoniae* in childhood. Pediatr Infect Dis 5:71, 1986

Table 14-7 Classification of Pseudoxanthoma Elasticum

Type	Inheritance[a]	Clinical Characteristics			
		Skin	Skeleton	Eye	Vascular Disease
I	AD	Flexural rash	None	Angioid streaks	+ + +
II	AD	Macular rash	Hyperextensible joints; arched palate	Angioid streaks; blue sclerae	+
III	AR	Flexural rash	Hyperextensible joints; arched palate	Angioid streaks	+ +
IV	AR	Generalized cutis laxa	None	None	–

[a] AD = autosomal dominant; AR = autosomal recessive.
(Data from Pope.[81])

pain and effusion, and arachnodactyly become increasingly obvious by the second decade.[1,4] Many patients are only mildly affected. Children with Marfan's syndrome are tall, their arm span exceeds their height, and the pubis-to-heel measurement is greater than the crown-to-pubis distance. The palate is high and arched, and there may be other skeletal abnormalities such as moderate to severe kyphoscoliosis, pectus carinatum, slipped capital femoral epiphysis, and talipes equinovarus. Muscular hypotonia is common. Skin lesions include striae distensae and elastosis perforans serpiginosa. Ectopia lentis with iridodonesis and cardiovascular abnormalities occur in about one-third of patients. The latter include aortic root dilation, aneurysm formation, mitral valve prolapse, and conduction defects. Affected patients often die suddenly from cardiac complications. Collagen turnover is increased and a cross-linking defect has been proposed. The disease is inherited in an autosomal dominant pattern.

A number of other disorders may be confused with Marfan's syndrome. Children with the *Stickler syndrome* have a marfanoid body habitus, congenital hyperextensibility of the joints, and a positive family history (autosomal dominant).[1,4] Enlargement of the knees, ankles, and wrists, often congenital, can be misdiagnosed as JRA or NOMID. Associated but variable clinical features include deafness, myopia, cataracts, and retinal degeneration and detachment. Midfacial hypoplasia, cleft palate, and micrognathia are often observed. Intelligence is normal. Radiographs in the newborn show characteristic "dumbbell-shaped" long bones with enlarged epiphyses and metaphyses. With increasing age, the epiphyses become fragmented. There may be mild platyspondyly and steeply sloping ribs. No specific biochemical defect has been identified.

Homocystinuria is easily confused with Marfan's syndrome because of the excessive height and other abnormalities that begin to appear just after the neonatal period.[1,5] However, affected children lack normal pigmentation and are light-skinned and blond. Cutaneous ulcerations and livedo reticularis are common. Hypotonia is present, but the joints may be stiff rather than hyperextensible. Progressive osteoporosis, mental retardation, and ocular anomalies (ectopia lentis, myopia, and peripheral retinal degeneration) are characteristic. Arterial or venous thromboses may lead to death. The basic biochemical defect is a deficiency of cystathionine synthetase that is inherited as an autosomal recessive trait. There is an accumulation in tissues of the sulfur-containing amino acids homocystine, homocysteine, serine, and methionine. There may also be a defect in collagen cross-linking.

Congenital contractural arachnodactyly may be confused with arthrogryposis or with Marfan's syndrome.[82] As in arthrogryposis, there are congenital contractures of the knees, elbows, and PIP joints, but the hands and feet are long and the head is elongated. Linear growth is accelerated. Early and progressive kyphoscoliosis may develop. The helix of the ear is abnormal. This disorder is inherited as an autosomal dominant trait. The contractures tend to improve as the child grows older.

The *cerebro-oculofacioskeletal syndrome* resembles contractural arachnodactyly except that microcephaly, microphthalmia, and blepharophimosis are present in addition to the features described previously.[83] Inheritance is autosomal recessive.

Children with the *Weill-Marchesani syndrome* are short and have short hands and feet and stiff joints. Thickening of the skin contributes to the limitation of joint mobility and contractures of the fingers, knees, and elbows. Ectopia lentis and microspherophakia occur. Inheritance is autosomal recessive.[1,4]

MISCELLANEOUS DISORDERS

Osteochondritis Dissecans

Osteochondritis dissecans affecting specific bones in children must be differentiated from other rheumatic conditions. For example, *Kohler's disease* develops predominantly in young school-age boys with the insidious onset of foot pain and a limp; the affected child characteristically walks with weight bearing on the lateral foot.[84] On physical examination, tenderness of the dorsal foot directly over the tarsal navicular is present, and films of both feet reveal that on the painful side that bone is narrowed, of increased density, and sometimes fragmented. *Freiburg's disease* occurs in adolescents, usually girls, who develop foot pain with weight bearing.[85] Tenderness and often swelling are found in the region of the second metatarsal head. Radiographs reveal increased density or flattening of the affected metatarsal head.

Thiemann's Disease

Thiemann's disease (osteonecrosis of the phalangeal epiphyses) is characterized by progressive, painless enlargement during adolescence of the epiphyses of the PIP joints of the hands and the interphalangeal joints of the first toes.[86-88] Flexion contractures of the large joints also occur. Radiologically, there is irregularity of the epiphyses of the digits. Results of tests for the acute phase reactants are normal. Disability is only minimal. The condition may be familial in some cases.[89-91]

Osteo-Onychodysostosis

In the *nail-patella syndrome*, inherited as an autosomal dominant trait, dysplasia of the nails, hypoplasia of the patella, bony horns and hypoplasia of the iliac bones, and scapular hypoplasia are found.[1-4] Elbow joint movement may be restricted because of dislocation of the radial head and malformation of the radiohumeral joint.[92]

Brachydactyly

Shortness of the phalanges may occur in some children with JRA in relation to premature epiphyseal closure. It may also develop as a result of trauma or infarction of the epiphyseal plate (sickle cell anemia) or as a congenital anomaly (Moore–Federman syndrome).[93]

The term *clinodactyly* refers to the presence of a short middle phalanx of the fifth finger (brachymesophalangy). It may occur as an isolated finding, be inherited as an autosomal dominant trait, or constitute part of Down's syndrome or the oral-facial-digital syndrome. It is asymptomatic and requires no treatment.

Congenital Soft Tissue Contractures

Soft tissue contractures in the absence of primary joint disease are characteristic of several syndromes. In *arthrogryposis multiplex congenita,* congenital contractures affect all four extremities in about half of the children and the lower limbs in most of the others; 10 percent of cases have only the arms involved. The axial skeleton is frequently spared, but scoliosis may be present. Characteristically, the elbows are fixed in extension, the wrists are flexed, the arms are held in internal rotation, the knees are contracted in flexion, and the feet are held in a position of talipes equinovarus. Extremity muscles are underdeveloped. The joints are rigid and fibrosed and their normal contours are lost. Other congenital anomalies, especially those associated with oligohydramnios, may be present as well. Although the classic syndrome is not a diagnostic problem, incomplete forms may be confused with rheumatic diseases because of decreased range of movement. This disorder may result from immobility of the fetus in utero. Although most cases are sporadic, a few may have an hereditary basis.[1,4,94] The results of surgical attempts to correct the multiple deformities are often unsatisfactory.

In *Léri's pleonosteosis,* a rare disorder that develops after the neonatal period, the toes and thumbs become broad and stiff, and the hands and feet are short and broad.[95,96]

The child tends to be short, with limited range of motion at the wrists, elbows, hips, and knees. The upper limbs may be held in a semiflexed position of internal rotation and the lower limbs in external rotation. The face has a mongoloid appearance. Pleonosteosis may not be as rare as reported and is inherited as an autosomal dominant trait. The basic defect may reside in thickening of the capsular connective tissues.

The term *camptodactyly* refers to the presence of congenital or acquired flexion contractures of the PIP joints resulting from soft tissue tightening without limitation of flexion.[97,98] It is most common in the fifth finger but may occur in all digits of the hand except the thumb. The etiology is not certain but appears to be related to fibrotic changes in the subcutaneous tissue of the palmar aspect of the joint. Radiographs reveal neither bony nor articular abnormalities per se.

Camptodactyly may be seen with diseases such as Marfan's syndrome and has been reported in association with familial arthritis by Malleson et al.[99] Three children in one family had iridocyclitis, and one boy died suddenly at the age of 4 years. Postmortem examination revealed chronic synovitis and granulomatous arteritis affecting the aorta, coronary arteries, myocardium, and pericardium. A family in which five children had camptodactyly and arthritis, together with pericarditis in three of the children, has also been noted.[100]

Children with the *fetal alcohol syndrome* have a characteristic facial appearance (flattening of the midface, hypertelorism, and smooth, elongated upper lip) but may also have flexion contractures of the elbows, restricted motion at the metacarpophalangeal (MCP) joints, camptodactyly, and clinodactyly. Developmental delay, impaired linear growth, and cardiac septal defects are associated problems.[101]

REFERENCES

1. McKusick VA: Heritable Disorders of Connective Tissue. 4th Ed. CV Mosby, St. Louis, 1972, p. 521
2. Wynn-Davies R: Heritable Disorders in Orthopaedic Practice. Blackwell Scientific Publications, Oxford, England, 1973, p. 231
3. Horan F, Beighton P: Orthopaedic Problems in Inherited Skeletal Disorders. Springer-Verlag, New York, 1982
4. Smith DW, Jones KJ: Recognizable Patterns of Human Malformation. Genetic, Embryologic and Clinical Aspects. 4th Ed. WB Saunders, New York, 1988
5. Stanbury JB, Wyngaarden JB, Fredrickson DS et al: The Metabolic Basis of Inherited Disease. 6th Ed. McGraw-Hill, New York, 1989
6. Poznanski AK: The Hand in Radiologic Diagnosis. WB Saunders, Philadelphia, 1974, p. 588
7. Wynn-Davies R, Fairbank TJ: Fairbank's Atlas of General Afflictions of the Skeleton. 2nd Ed. Churchill Livingstone, Edinburgh, 1976, p. 262
8. Gordon IRS, Ross FGM: Diagnostic Radiology in Paediatrics. Butterworths, London, 1977, p. 384
9. Kozlowski K, Lewis IC, Kennedy J et al: Progressive pseudorheumatoid arthritis. Paediatr Indones 25:237, 1985
10. Wynne-Davies R, Hau C, Ansell BM: Spondylo-epiphyseal dysplasia tarda with progressive arthropathy. J Bone Joint Surg 64B:442, 1982
11. Bradley JD: Pseudoseptic pseudogout in progressive pseudorheumatoid arthritis of childhood. Ann Rheum Dis 46:709, 1987
12. McKusick VA: Metaphyseal dyostosis and thin hair: a new recessively inherited syndrome? Lancet 1:832, 1964
13. Maudsley RH: Dysplasia epiphysialis multiplex: a report of fourteen cases in three families. J Bone Joint Surg 37B:22, 1955
14. Patrone NA, Kredich DW: Arthritis in children with multiple epiphyseal dysplasia. J Rheumatol 12:145, 1985
15. Shapiro: Epiphyseal disorders. N Engl J Med 317:1702, 1987
16. Brenton DP, Dent CF: Idiopathic juvenile osteoporosis. In Bickel H, Stern J (eds): Inborn Errors of Calcium and Bone Metabolism. University Press, Baltimore, 1976, p. 222
17. Gluck J, Miller JJ, III: Familial osteolysis of the carpal and tarsal bones. J Pediatr 81:506, 1972
18. Erickson CM, Hirschbever M, Stickler GB: Carpal-tarsal osteolysis. J Pediatr 93:779, 1978
19. Brown DN, Bradford DS, Gorlin RJ et al: The acro-osteolysis syndrome: morphologic and biochemical studies. J Pediatr 88:573, 1976
20. Beals RK, Bird CB: Carpal and tarsal osteolysis: a case report and review of the literature. J Bone Joint Surg 57A:681, 1975
21. Gorham LW, Stout AP: Massive osteolysis (acute spontaneous absorption of bone, phantom bone, disappearing bone): its relationship to hemangiomatosis. J Bone Joint Surg 37A:985, 1955
22. Shurtleff DB, Sparkes RS, Clawson DK: Hereditary

osteolysis with hypertension and nephropathy. JAMA 188:363, 1964

23. Elias AN, Pinals RS, Anderson HC et al: Hereditary osteodysplasia with acro-osteolysis (the Hajdu-Cheney syndrome). Am J Med 65:627, 1978

24. Pease CN: Focal retardation and arrestment of growth of bones due to vitamin A intoxication. JAMA 182:980, 1962

25. Christensen WR, Liebman C, Sosman MC: Skeletal and periarticular manifestations of hypervitaminosis. Am J Roentgenol 65:27, 1951

26. Shapiro JR, Fallat RW, Tsang RC: Achilles tendinitis and tenosynovitis: a diagnostic manifestation of familial type II hyperlipoproteinemia in children. Am J Dis Child 128:486, 1974

27. Buckingham RB, Bole GG, Bassett DR: Polyarthritis associated with type IV hyperlipoproteinemia. Arch Intern Med 135:286, 1975

28. Rosenbloom AL, Frias JL: Diabetes, short stature and joint stiffness—a new syndrome. Clin Res 22:92A, 1974

29. Rosenbloom AL, Silverstein JH, Lezotte DC et al: Limited joint mobility in childhood diabetes mellitus indicates increased risk for microvascular disease. N Engl J Med 305:191, 1981

30. Grgic A, Rosenbloom AL, Weber FT et al: Joint contracture–common manifestation of childhood diabetes mellitus. J Pediatr 88:584, 1976

31. Ansell BM: Rheumatic Disorders in Childhood. Butterworths, London, 1980, p. 194

32. Vijanto JA: Duputren's contracture: a review. Semin Arthritis Rheum 3:155, 1973

33. Buckingham BA, Uitto J, Sandborg C et al: Scleroderma-like syndrome and the non-enzymatic glucosylation of collagen in children with poorly controlled insulin dependent diabetes. Pediatr Res 15:626, 1981

34. De Seye S, Solnica J, Mitrovic D et al: Joint and bone disorders and hypoparathyroidism in hemochromatosis. Semin Arthritis Rheum 2:71, 1972

35. Clouse ME, Gramin HF, Legg M et al: Diabetic osteoarthropathy. Clinical and roentgenographic observations in 90 cases. Am J Roentgenol 121:22, 1974

36. Rusolf MJC, Genel M, Tamborlane WV et al: Juvenile rheumatoid arthritis in children with diabetes mellitus. J Pediatr 99:519, 1981

37. Howell RR: Juvenile gouty arthritis. Am J Dis Child 139:547, 1985

38. Treadwell BLJ: Juvenile gout. Ann Rheum Dis 30:279, 1971

39. Lesch M, Nyhan WL: A familial disorder of uric acid metabolism and central nervous system function. Am J Med 26:561, 1964

40. Seegmiller JE, Rosenbloom RM, Kelly WN: An enzyme defect associated with a sex-linked neurological disorder and excessive purine synthesis. Science 1555:1682, 1967

41. Kelly WN, Greene NL, Rosenbloom JM et al: Hypoxanthine-guanine phosphoribosyltransferase deficiency in gout. Ann Intern Med 70:155, 1969

42. O'Brien WM, LaDu BN, Bunim JJ: Biochemical, pathologic and clinical aspects of alcaptonuria, ochronosis and ochronotic arthropathy. Review of world literature (1584–1962). Am J Med 34:813, 1963

43. Weinberg AG, Curranino G: Sickle cell dactylitis: histopathologic observations. Am J Clin Pathol 58:518, 1972

44. Ramgren O: Haemophilia in Sweden. III: Symptomatology with special reference to differences between haemophilia A and B. Acta Med Scand 171:237, 1962

45. Arnold WD, Hilgartner MW: Hemophilic arthropathy: current concepts of pathogenesis and management. J Bone Joint Surg 59A:287, 1977

46. Ahlberg A, Silwer JP: Arthropathy in von Willebrand's disease. Acta Orthop Scand 41:539, 1970

47. Handelsman JE: The knee joint in hemophilia. Orthop Clin North Am 10:139, 1979

48. Kisker CT, Burke C: Double-blind studies on the use of steroids in the treatment of acute hemarthrosis in patients with hemophilia. N Engl J Med 282:639, 1970

49. Sokoloff L: Endemic forms of osteoarthritis. Clin Rheumat Dis 11:187, 1985

50. Lee YW, Mirocha CJ, Shroeder DJ et al: TDP-1, a toxic component causing tibial dyschondroplasia in broiler chickens, and trichothecenes from *Fusarium roseum* 'graminearum'. Appl Env Microbiol 50:102, 1985

51. Nesterov AI: The clinical course of Kashin-Beck disease. Arthritis Rheum 7:29, 1964

52. Takamori T: Kashin-Beck's Disease. The Professor Tokio Takamori Foundation, University School of Medicine, Japan, 1968

53. Sokoloff L: Kashin-Beck disease. Rheum Dis Clin North Am 13:101, 1987

54. Lockitch G, Fellingham SA, Wittman W et al: Mseleni joint disease: the pilot study. S Afr Med J 1:2283, 1973

55. Lockitch G, Fellingham SA, Elphinstone CD: Mseleni joint disease: a radiological study of two affected families. S Afr Med J 1:2366, 1973

56. Hers HG: Inborn lysosomal diseases. Gastroenterology 48:625, 1965

57. Kelly TE: Hurler-like disorders in infancy. Clin Perinatol 3:115, 1976

58. Fisher RC, Horner RL, Wood VE: The hand in

mucopolysaccharide disorders. Clin Orthop 104:191, 1974

59. Morquio L: Sur une forme de dystrophie osseuse familiale. Bull Soc Pédiatr Paris 27:145, 1929

60. Scheie HG, Hambrick GW, Jr, Barness LA: A newly recognized forme fruste of Hurler's disease (gargoylism). Am J Ophthalmol 53:753, 1962

61. Maroteaux P, Lamy M: La pseudo-polydystrophie de Hurler. Presse Méd 74:2889, 1966

62. Farber S, Cohen J, Uzman JL: Lipogranulomatosis. A new lipoglycoprotein "storage" disease. J Mt Sinai Hosp 24:816, 1957

63. Toppet M, Vamos-Hurwitz E, Jonniaux G et al: Farber's disease as a ceramidosis: clinical, radiological and biochemical aspects. Acta Paediatr Scand 67:113, 1978

64. Zayid I, Farraj J: Familial histiocytic dermatoarthritis. Am J Med 54:793, 1973

65. Winchester PH, Grossman H, Wan NL et al: A new acid mucopolysaccharidosis with skeletal deformities simulating rheumatoid arthritis. Am J Roentgenol 106:121, 1969

66. Hollister DW, Rimoin DL, Lachman RS et al: The Winchester syndrome: a nonlysosomal connective tissue disease. J Pediatr 84:701, 1974

67. Kniest W: Zur Abgrenzung der Dysostosis enchondralis von der Chondrodystrophie. Z Kinderheilk 70: 663, 1952

68. Sconyers SM, Rimoin DL, Lachman RS et al: A distinct chondrodysplasia resembling Kniest dysplasia: clinical, roentgenographic, histologic, and ultrastructural findings. J Pediatr 12:898, 1985

69. Dyggve HV, Melchoir JC, Clausen J: Morquio-Ullrich's disease. Arch Dis Child 37:525, 1962

70. Jimenez SA, Lally EV: Disorders of collagen structure and metabolism. Bull Rheum Dis 30:1016, 1979–1980

71. Uitto J, Murray LW, Blumberg B, et al: Biochemistry of collagens in diseases. Ann Intern Med 105:740, 1986

72. Pope FM, Nicholls AC, McPheat J et al: Collagen genes and proteins in osteogenesis imperfecta. J Med Genet 22:466, 1985

73. Sykes B: Molecular diagnostics: genetics cracks bone disease. Nature 330:607, 1987

74. Sillence DO, Senn A, Banks DM: Genetic heterogeneity in osteogenesis imperfecta. J Med Genet 16: 101, 1979

75. Castells S, Yasumura S, Fusi MA et al: Plasma osteocalcin levels in patients with osteogenesis imperfecta. J Pediatr 109:88, 1986

76. Castells S, Colbert C, Chakrabarti C et al: Therapy of osteogenesis imperfecta with synthetic salmon calcitonin. J Pediatr 95:807, 1979

77. Beighton P: The Ehlers-Danlos Syndrome. William Heinemann Medical Books, London, 1970

78. Osborn TG, Lichtenstein JR, Moore TL et al: Ehlers-Danlos syndrome presenting as rheumatic manifestations in the child. J Rheumatol 8:79, 1981

79. Lewkonia RM, Pope FM: Joint contractures and acroosteolysis in Ehlers-Danlos syndrome type IV. J Rheumatol 12:140, 1985

80. Byers PH, Siegel RC, Holbrook KA: X-linked cutis laxa. Defective cross-link formation in collagen due to decreased lysyl oxidase activity. N Engl J Med 303:61, 1980

81. Pope FM: Two types of autosomal recessive pseudoxanthoma elasticum. Arch Dermatol 110:209, 1974

82. Mirise RT, Shear S: Congenital contractural arachnodactyly: description of a new kindred. Arthritis Rheum 22:542, 1979

83. Pena SDJ, Shokeir MHK: Autosomal recessive cerebro-oculo-facio-skeletal (COFS) syndrome. Clin Genet 5:285, 1974

84. Giannestras NJ: Problems of the tarsal portion of the foot in the adolescent and the adult. In Giannestras NJ (ed): Foot Disorders. Lea & Febiger, Philadelphia, 1973, p. 565

85. Giannestras NJ: Other problems of the forepart of the foot. In Giannestras NJ (ed): Foot Disorders. Lea & Febiger, Philadelphia, 1973, p. 410

86. White J: Osteochondritis dissecans in association with dwarfism. J Bone Joint Surg 39B:261, 1957

87. Gewanter H, Baum J: Thiemann's disease. J Rheumatol 12:150, 1985

88. Molloy MG, Hamilton EBD: Thiemann's disease. Rheumatol Rehabil 17:179, 1978

89. Allison AC, Blumberg BS: Familial osteoarthropathy of the fingers. J Bone Joint Surg 40B:538, 1958

90. Stougaard J: Familial occurrence of osteochondritis dissecans. J Bone Joint Surg 46B:542, 1964

91. Robinson RP, Franck WA, Carey EJ, Jr. et al: Familial polyarticular osteochondritis dissecans masquerading as juvenile rheumatoid arthritis. J Rheumatol 5:190, 1978

92. Valduveza AF: The nail-patella syndrome. A report of three families. J Bone Joint Surg 55B:145, 1973

93. Moore WT, Federman DD: Familial dwarfism and "stiff joints." Arch Intern Med 115:398, 1965

94. Lloyd-Roberts GC, Lettin AWF: Arthrogryposis multiplex congenita. J Bone Joint Surg 52B:494, 1970

95. Léri A, Joanny J: Une affection non décrite des os: hyperostose "en coulée" sur toute la longueur d'un membre ou "mélorhéostose." Bull Med Soc Hop Paris 46:1141, 1922

96. Beauvais P, Faure C, Montagne JP et al: Léri's me-

lorheostosis: three pediatric cases and a review of the literature. Pediatr Radiol 6:153, 1977

97. Welch JP, Temtamy SA: Hereditary contractures of the fingers (camptodactyly). J Med Genet 3:104, 1966

98. Laxer RM, Cameron BJ, Chaisson D et al: The camptodactyly arthropathy-pericarditis syndrome: case report and literature review. Arthritis Rheum 29:439, 1986

99. Malleson P, Schaller JG, Dega F et al: Familial arthritis and camptodactyly. Arthritis Rheum 24:1199, 1981

100. Martínez-Lavín M, Buendía A, Delgado E et al: A familial syndrome of pericarditis, arthritis, and camptodactyly. N Engl J Med 309:224, 1983

101. Jones KL: The fetal alcohol syndrome. Addict Dis 2:79, 1975

Appendix

Table A-1 Clinical Manifestations of the Connective-Tissue Diseases

	Juvenile Rheumatoid Arthritis	Systemic Lupus Erythematosus	Polyarteritis	Dermatomyositis	Scleroderma	Rheumatic Fever
Female/male ratio	2:1	5:1	1:3	2:1	2:1	1:1
Constitutional symptoms	+++	+++	+++	+++	+	+++
Arthritis	+++	++	+	+	+	+++
Skin						
Rash	+	+++	+	+++	-	+
Photosensitivity	-	++	-	+	-	-
Purpura	-	+++	++	-	-	-
Telangiectasia	-	+	-	+	+++	-
Pigmentation	-	+	-	++	++	-
Calcinosis	-	-	-	++	++	-
Subcutaneous nodules	+	+	+	-	+	+
Alopecia	-	++	-	+++	+	-
Mucous membranes	-	++	-	+	-	-
Raynaud's phenomenon	-	+++	+++	++	+++	-
Vasculitis	+	+++	+++	+++	+	+
Myositis	+	+	+	+++	++	-

	C1	C2	C3	C4	C5	C6
Serositis	++	+++	+	+	−	+
Cardiac						
Pericardial	++	+++	+	−	−	+
Myocardial	+	+	++	−	++	++
Endocardial	−	++	−	−	−	+++
Pulmonary disease	+	++	++	+	+++	+
Gastrointestinal						
Dysphagia	−	−	−	++	+++	−
Abdominal pain	+	++	+++	++	+	++
Malabsorption	−	−	−	−	+++	−
Hepatomegaly	+	+	−	−	−	+
Splenomegaly	+	++	−	−	−	−
Lymphadenopathy	+	+++	+	++	−	−
Nephritis	+	+++	+++	+	+	−
Hypertension	−	++	+++	−	+	−
Ocular disease	++	++	++	+	−	−
Nervous system						
Peripheral	−	+	+++	−	−	−
Central	−	+++	+	−	−	−
Chorea	−	+	−	−	−	++

−, absent; +, minimal; ++, moderate; +++, severe.

Table A-2 Laboratory Abnormalities in the Rheumatic Diseases of Childhood

Abnormality	Juvenile Rheumatoid Arthritis			Systemic Lupus Erythematosus	Dermatomyositis	Scleroderma	Vasculitis	Rheumatic Fever
	Polyarthritis	Oligoarthritis	Systemic Onset					
Anemia	+	−	++	++	+	+	++	+
Leukopenia	−	−	−	+++	−	−	−	−
Thrombocytopenia	−	−	−	++	−	−	−	−
Leukocytosis	+	−	+++	−	+	−	+++	+
Thrombocytosis	+	−	++	−	+	−	+	+
Antinuclear antibodies	+	++	−	+++	+	++	−	−
Anti-DNA antibodies	−	−	−	+++	−	+	−	−
Rheumatoid factors	+	−	+	++	−	+	+	−
Anti-streptococcal antibodies	+	−	−	−	−	−	−	+++
Hypocomplementemia	−	−	−	+++	−	−	++	−
Elevated hepatic enzyme levels	+	−	++	+	+	+	+	−
Elevated muscle enzyme levels	−	−	−	+	+++	++	+	−
Abnormal urinalysis	+	−	+	+++	+	+	++	−

−, absent; +, minimal; ++, moderate; +++, severe.

Table A-3 Clinical Manifestations of the Common Forms of Spondyloarthropathy Compared to Juvenile Rheumatoid Arthritis

	Juvenile Ankylosing Spondylitis	Psoriatic Arthropathy	Reiter's Syndrome	Juvenile Rheumatoid Arthritis
Clinical course of disease				
Arthritis				
Peripheral	+ +	+ + +	+ +	+ + +
Axial				
Sacroiliac	+ + +	+	+ +	±
Lumbar	+ +	+	+	−
Thoracic	+ +	−	−	+
Cervical	+	+	−	+ + +
Skin and mucous membranes	−	+ + +	+ + +	+
Genital tract	−	+	+ +	−
Ocular disease	+ +	+	+ +	+ +
Heart	+	−	+	+
Vasculitis	−	−	−	+
Pulmonary disease	+	−	−	+
Rheumatoid nodules	−	−	−	+
Pathologic findings				
Acute synovitis	+	+	+ + +	+ +
Mononuclear cell infiltrate	+ +	+	+	+ +
Pannus	+	+	+	+ +
Bursitis and tendinitis	+ +	−	+ +	+ +
Ankylosis	+ +	−	+	+ +
Laboratory abnormalities				
Acute phase response	+	+ +	+ +	+ + +
Anemia	+	+	+	+ + +
Leukocytosis	−	+	+ +	+ +
Rheumatoid factors	−	−	−	+
Antinuclear antibodies	−	+	−	+ + +

Absent −, variable, rare ±, minimal +, moderate + +, severe + + +.

Table A-4 Characteristics of Synovial Fluid in the Rheumatic Diseases

Group	Condition	Synovial Complement	Color/Clarity	Viscosity	Mucin Clot	WBC Count	PMN (%)	Miscellaneous Findings
Noninflammatory	Normal	N[a]	Yellow Clear	N	N	<200	<25	
	Traumatic arthritis	N	Xanthochromic Turbid	N	N	<2,000	<25	Debris
	Osteoarthritis	N	Yellow Clear	N	N	1,000	<25	
Inflammatory	SLE	→	Yellow Clear	N	N	5,000	10	LE cells
	Rheumatic fever	N – ↑	Yellow Cloudy	→	Fair	5,000	10–50	
	Juvenile rheumatoid arthritis	N – →	Yellow Cloudy	→	Poor	15,000–20,000	75	
	Reiter's syndrome	↑	Opaque	→	Poor	20,000	80	Reiter's cells
Pyogenic	Tuberculous arthritis	N – ↑	Yellow Cloudy	→	Poor	25,000	50–60	Acid-fast bacteria
	Septic arthritis	↑	Serosanguinous Turbid	→	Poor	80,000–200,000	75	Low glucose, bacteria

[a] N = normal.

572

Table A-5 The Major Neuromuscular Diseases in Children

	Inheritance	Onset	Symptoms	Course	Treatment
Muscular dystrophy					
Pseudohypertrophic (Duchenne)	Sex-linked recessive	Early childhood	Swayback, waddling gait, difficulty in rising from the floor and climbing stairs; fat deposits replace wasting muscle in the calves	Rapid, involving all the voluntary muscles; death usually occurs in 10–15 years	None
Fascioscapulohumeral (Landouzy-Déjerine)	Autosomal dominant	Early adolescence	Lack of facial mobility, difficulty in raising arms over head, forward slope of shoulders	Very slow; average life span rarely shortened	None
Limb-girdle (juvenile dystrophy of Erb)	Autosomal recessive	First to third decade	Weakness of proximal muscles of pelvic and shoulder girdles	Variable	None
Congenital dystrophy	Familial	Congenital	Small, weak muscles, multiple contractures	Rapid, leading to early death	None
Myotonias					
Myotonia congenita (Thomsen)	Autosomal dominant	Early childhood	Difficulty in relaxing muscles, hypertrophy	Mild, lifelong disability	Drug therapy and repetitive exercises
Myotonic dystrophy (Steinert)	Autosomal dominant	Youth	Weakening of hand and forearm muscles, myotonic stiffness and inability to relax; handgrip, eye, and tongue muscles often affected; cataracts, temporal baldness, testicular atrophy	Variable, but reaches severe disability 15–20 years after onset	Myotonic symptoms relieved by drugs; no treatment for dystrophic process
Myopathies					
Central core disease	Familial	Congenital	Hypotonic muscles and slowness in learning to walk; later, diffuse proximal weakness	Very slow except in central core disease, which is nonprogressive	None
Nemaline myopathy					
Mitochondrial disease					
Myotubular myopathy					
Idiopathic myopathy					

(continued)